T0237110

Health Informatics

This series is directed to healthcare professionals leading the transformation of healthcare by using information and knowledge. For over 20 years, Health Informatics has offered a broad range of titles: some address specific professions such as nursing, medicine, and health administration; others cover special areas of practice such as trauma and radiology; still other books in the series focus on interdisciplinary issues, such as the computer based patient record, electronic health records, and networked healthcare systems. Editors and authors, eminent experts in their fields, offer their accounts of innovations in health informatics. Increasingly, these accounts go beyond hardware and software to address the role of information in influencing the transformation of healthcare delivery systems around the world. The series also increasingly focuses on the users of the information and systems: the organizational, behavioral, and societal changes that accompany the diffusion of information technology in health services environments.

Developments in healthcare delivery are constant; in recent years, bioinformatics has emerged as a new field in health informatics to support emerging and ongoing developments in molecular biology. At the same time, further evolution of the field of health informatics is reflected in the introduction of concepts at the macro or health systems delivery level with major national initiatives related to electronic health records (EHR), data standards, and public health informatics.

These changes will continue to shape health services in the twenty-first century. By making full and creative use of the technology to tame data and to transform information, Health Informatics will foster the development and use of new knowledge in healthcare.

More information about this series at http://www.springer.com/series/1114

Jessica D. Tenenbaum • Piper A. Ranallo
Editors

Mental Health Informatics

Enabling a Learning Mental Healthcare System

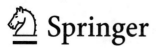 Springer

Editors
Jessica D. Tenenbaum
Duke University
Durham, NC
USA

Piper A. Ranallo
Six Aims for Behavioral Health
Minneapolis, MN
USA

ISSN 1431-1917   ISSN 2197-3741   (electronic)
Health Informatics
ISBN 978-3-030-70560-2   ISBN 978-3-030-70558-9   (eBook)
https://doi.org/10.1007/978-3-030-70558-9

© Springer Nature Switzerland AG 2021
This work is subject to copyright. All rights are reserved by the Publisher, whether the whole or part of the material is concerned, specifically the rights of translation, reprinting, reuse of illustrations, recitation, broadcasting, reproduction on microfilms or in any other physical way, and transmission or information storage and retrieval, electronic adaptation, computer software, or by similar or dissimilar methodology now known or hereafter developed.
The use of general descriptive names, registered names, trademarks, service marks, etc. in this publication does not imply, even in the absence of a specific statement, that such names are exempt from the relevant protective laws and regulations and therefore free for general use.
The publisher, the authors and the editors are safe to assume that the advice and information in this book are believed to be true and accurate at the date of publication. Neither the publisher nor the authors or the editors give a warranty, expressed or implied, with respect to the material contained herein or for any errors or omissions that may have been made. The publisher remains neutral with regard to jurisdictional claims in published maps and institutional affiliations.

This Springer imprint is published by the registered company Springer Nature Switzerland AG
The registered company address is: Gewerbestrasse 11, 6330 Cham, Switzerland

Preface

There is a paradoxical tension in healthcare between the desire to differentiate the field of mental health from physical health — "But mental health is different!"— and the recognition that mental and physical health are inextricably and causally linked. In many ways, physical and mental health *are* different. Most of the technologies used to detect, diagnose, and treat mental health conditions are fundamentally different from those used to detect, diagnose, and treat medical conditions. Scientists and practitioners in the field of mental health come from a wider variety of scientific disciplines, train through a wider variety of educational programs, and embrace a wider variety of theoretical models about the mechanisms underlying mental health and illness.

Mental healthcare systems around the world are also more likely to exist in a different structural, sociocultural, or financial environment than the country's medical health systems. Even in countries where physical and mental healthcare systems are structurally integrated (e.g., in national health systems), resources allocated to mental healthcare are rarely proporionate to the relative burden of illness of mental health conditions.

And yet, despite the differences between the fields of mental and physical healthcare, there are significant commonalities as well. Both fields are significantly impacted by technological developments, from the adoption of electronic health records to smartphone-enabled mHealth to genomic-era high-throughput biological assays. Both fields are increasingly focused on the use of evidence-based treatments. Both fields are moving increasingly toward "precision" healthcare—focusing on understanding which interventions are most effective for which people in which contexts. Both fields are increasingly emphasizing the need to accelerate the rate at which new discoveries in basic science are applied at the bedside. Both fields are increasingly collecting granular patient level data to leverage the advances made in the era of big data. And finally, both fields are increasingly recognizing the need to expand the scope of phenomena factored into their models to phenomena they have not traditionally included.

Biomedical and health informatics as a field has existed for several decades. Yet, there are very few mental health informaticians in the world. We think that needs to change. In the past decade, a rich variety of books with titles that include the terms "mental health," "psychiatry," or "behavioral health" along with the term "informatics" have appeared. These books signify the start of a trend. They represent the recognition of both the importance of this interdisciplinary combination and of its potential. Many of these books provide a welcome survey of advanced topics in mental health informatics along with a deep dive into promising new methods and technologies. Some frame the specialty areas they address in the context of the need for a more coherent, integrated subdiscipline of what is variously referred to as *psychiatry informatics*, *behavioral health informatics*, or *mental health informatics*. As we reviewed the existing texts available to burgeoning mental health informaticians, we found a gap in texts that systematically introduce fundamental informatics methods and technologies of the field, covering the spectrum of phenomena from molecules to populations. We thought it important to develop a textbook to do just that.

This book is intended to be used in an introductory course to this relatively nascent field, whether that course is aimed at undergraduates, graduate students, or postdoctoral scholars. We expect many (but not all) readers of this book to have had some formal training in either mental health or informatics, but likely not in both. We created this book in part to cross-train both informaticians and mental health professionals in these topics.

In the first section of the book, we cover foundational concepts. We set the stage for this interdisciplinary field, looking at what is meant by mental health and informatics and providing clinical context. We also set out a framework for the rest of the topics in the book involving translational research, precision medicine, and the learning health system.

The second section is a broad survey of topics around turning data into information and information into knowledge. This includes discussion of how data are collected, analyzed, visualized, and stored. It also spans different data types relevant to mental health, from biological to clinical, behavioral to imaging.

The third section covers informatics at the point of care—turning knowledge into action. Finally, we conclude with broader implications of the field, using an ethical, legal, and social lens, and looking ahead at the future of the field.

It is often said that "absence of evidence is not evidence of absence." And yet you will see statements in more than one chapter of this book regarding what is not (yet) known in mental health research, or not (yet) done in clinical practice. In some cases, we include reference to peer-reviewed articles that have made these assertions. In other cases, these unprovable assertions are made based on significant study of the literature as well as discussion with mental health experts and care practitioners. We welcome feedback from readers who may be, or become, aware of evidence to refute these assertions. And we certainly look forward to revising these statements in future versions of this book, as knowledge and practice in mental health continue to advance.

Durham, NC   Jessica D. Tenenbaum
Minneapolis, MN   Piper A. Ranallo

Acknowledgments

We are grateful to the esteemed collection of authors whose expertise and hard work, during a global pandemic no less, has made this book a reality. As mentioned above, there are not many mental health informaticians in the world. But of those that do exist, a significant portion have contributed to this book. Many others have contributed to this book in less direct ways. We are grateful to be part of this community.

This book would not have been written without the inspiration, insight, and encouragement of many people. We want to especially thank Christopher Chute who, despite the immense demands that come with being a renowned thinker and leader in the field of biomedical informatics, agreed to advise and mentor a new graduate student who became adamantly convinced that improving systems for concept and knowledge representation was the most important next step in improving outcomes for mental health. Without his mentorship and encouragement—and strong support for this text—this book may never have been written. We also thank (and blame) Rachel Richesson, who made editing a first edition textbook in a burgeoning field seem like, on balance, a good idea.

We are thankful the following people who have so generously shared their time, knowledge, and passion for informatics and mental health and inspired our thinking and commitment to this field over the years: Terry Adam and Genevieve Melton-Meaux for their long-standing, friendship, support and guidance. Jim Case for generously sharing his time and passion for terminology. Ed Hammond for his mentorship, friendship, and collegiality. Thanks to Stan Huff, Jim Cimino, Swapna Abhyankar, Dan Vreeman, Philip RO Payne, Peter Embi, Neil Sarkar, Ted Shortliffe, Robert Krueger, Katharine Nelson, and Moira Rynn. The AMIA Mental Health Workgroup. Members of the SNOMED Mental and Behavioral Health Clinical Reference Group, especially the dedicated core team of Laura Fochtmann, Uma Vaidyanathan, and Michael First. The folks at SNOMED International who provided a forum for work and patiently guided and mentored members of our CRG, especially Ian Green, Jane Millar, and Elaine Wooler. Finally, we thank our families – our children and our spouses – for putting up with us during the writing and editing of this book, and for going above and beyond the call of duty to make family life work during the process.

We hope this book proves useful for inspiring the next generation to train in this exciting field, and contributing to the expansion of this much-needed workforce in years to come.

Contents

1 Precision Medicine and a Learning Health System for Mental Health 1
Piper A. Ranallo and Jessica D. Tenenbaum

2 What Is Informatics? 31
Elizabeth S. Chen

3 The Mental Health System: Definitions and Diagnoses 55
John L. Beyer and Mina Boazak

4 The Mental Healthcare System: Organization and Structure 81
John L. Beyer and Mina Boazak

5 The Mental Health System: Access, Diagnosis, Treatment, and Monitoring 97
Mina Boazak and John L. Beyer

6 Mental Health Informatics 121
Piper A. Ranallo and Jessica D. Tenenbaum

7 Technologies for the Computable Representation and Sharing of Data and Knowledge in Mental Health 155
Piper A. Ranallo and Jessica D. Tenenbaum

8 Use of Medical Imaging to Advance Mental Health Care: Contributions from Neuroimaging Informatics 191
Randy L. Gollub and Nicole Benson

9 Informatics Technologies for the Acquisition of Psychological, Behavioral, Interpersonal, Social and Environmental Data 217
Elena Tenenbaum, Piper A. Ranallo, and Janna Hastings

10 Data to Information: Computational Models and Analytic Methods 235
Shyam Visweswaran and Mohammadamin Tajgardoon

11 Bioinformatics in Mental Health: Deriving Knowledge
    from Molecular and Cellular Data 265
    Krithika Bhuvaneshwar and Yuriy Gusev

12 Integrative Paradigms for Knowledge Discovery in Mental
    Health: Overcoming the Fragmentation of Knowledge
    Inherent in Disparate Theoretical Paradigms 295
    Janna Hastings and Rasmus Rosenberg Larsen

13 Natural Language Processing in Mental Health Research and
    Practice.. 317
    Sam Henry, Meliha Yetisgen, and Ozlem Uzuner

14 Information Visualization in Mental Health Research and
    Practice 355
    Harry Hochheiser and Anurag Verma

15 Big Data: Knowledge Discovery and Data Repositories 393
    Sumithra Velupillai, Katrina A. S. Davis, and Leon Rozenblit

16 Electronic Health Records (EHRS) and Other
    Clinical Information Systems in Mental Health................. 427
    Tyler Anne Hassenfeldt and Ross D. Martin

17 Informatics Technologies in the Diagnosis and
    Treatment of Mental Health Conditions....................... 453
    Wendy Marie Ingram, Rahul Khanna, and Cody Weston

18 Ethical, Legal, and Social Issues (ELSI) in Mental Health
    Informatics.. 479
    Vignesh Subbian, Hannah K. Galvin, Carolyn Petersen,
    and Anthony Solomonides

19 The Future of Mental Health Informatics 505
    Gregory K. Farber, Joshua A. Gordon,
    and Robert K. Heinssen

Index 521

Chapter 1
Precision Medicine and a Learning Health System for Mental Health

Piper A. Ranallo and Jessica D. Tenenbaum

Abstract More than any other field of healthcare, mental health is in dire need of efficient models for integrating the people, paradigms, and technologies required to acquire and apply new knowledge. In this chapter, we introduce the need for precision mental healthcare. We address the critical role of health information technology (HIT) and the application of informatics technologies on the journey towards precision mental healthcare. We describe the Learning Health System (LHS)—a health system in which data generated during the routine delivery of care is used to generate the evidence upon which new knowledge can be built and fed seamlessly back into the system. We describe how the LHS model aligns with, and integrates, the core informatics cycle of knowledge acquisition within and among basic research, clinical research, and real-world clinical practice. Finally, we introduce the idea of a precision healthcare agenda for mental health—what it is, how it relates to the LHS, and how it is made possible by the science of informatics.

Keywords Learning health system · Precision medicine · Precision healthcare · Mental health · Behavioral health

P. A. Ranallo (✉)
Six Aims for Behavioral Health, Minneapolis, USA
e-mail: pranallo@sixaims.org; sven0018@umn.edu

J. D. Tenenbaum
Duke University, Durham, NC, USA
e-mail: jessie.tenenbaum@duke.edu

© Springer Nature Switzerland AG 2021
J. D. Tenenbaum, P. A. Ranallo (eds.), *Mental Health Informatics*, Health Informatics, https://doi.org/10.1007/978-3-030-70558-9_1

1.1   Introduction

Mental Health Informatics, as you will see throughout this book, is the science fundamentally concerned with capturing data relevant to mental health, turning these data into actionable knowledge, and applying this newly acquired knowledge to optimize the mental health of individuals and communities. Mental Health Informatics is an essential science in the journey to safe, high quality, precision mental healthcare. In this text, we introduce you to the people, the paradigms, the methods, and the technologies that make this journey possible. As in any journey, there are many paths, and many steps along each path, to get us to our ultimate destination. In this chapter, we introduce a map for our journey. The map we present is a well-known model for aligning and integrating the people, paradigms, tools, and technologies needed to acquire and apply new knowledge to optimize mental health. This model, called the *Learning Health System* (LHS), is one in which knowledge is continuously generated as a by-product of healthcare. In this chapter, we describe the LHS — a healthsytem in which data generated during the routine delivery of care is used to generate the evidence upon which new knowledge can be built and fed seamlessly back into the system. We describe how the LHS model aligns with and integrates the core informatics cycle of knowledge acquisition within and among basic research, clinical research, and real-world clinical practice. Finally, we introduce the idea of precision healthcare for mental health—what it is, how it relates to the LHS, and how it is made possible by the science of informatics.

1.2   The Need for Precision Mental Healthcare

It is widely acknowledged that the practice of mental healthcare is less precise than that of physical healthcare[1] [1–3]. Mental health conditions enumerated in current diagnostic classification systems are commonly described as representing broad heterogeneous syndromes rather than discrete disorders with a common underlying etiology [4–9]. There are few definitive tests for clearly identifying the underlying etiology of many mental health conditions. Even when such tests exist, they tend to be used primarily for establishing diagnoses for research and are infrequently used in routine practice. Consequently, diagnosis for many mental health conditions consists of identifying the broad, heterogeneous category into which a person's presenting signs and symptoms fall, rather than identifying a specific disorder defined in terms of a presumed underlying pathological dysfunction. Treatment generally

---

[1] A few words on terminology: "Biomedical healthcare" is a mouthful, "general medicine" usually refers to general health problems, as opposed to those addressed by a specialist, and "physical medicine" is generally associated with rehabilitation and physiatry. For purposes of this textbook, we use the term "physical healthcare" to refer to care provided in the context of physical health and illness, in contrast with care provided in the mental health context.

focuses on mitigating symptoms by targeting one or more of the presumed etiologies of the disorder for the entire diagnostic category as a whole, rather than targeting the known etiology of the condition in the individual person being treated. Depressive disorders are a good example. While there are multiple theories about the underlying etiology of depressive disorders, and a handful of diagnostic tests used in research, there is no comprehensive diagnostic protocol used in routine practice for identifying the specific etiology in any given person presenting with one of these syndromes. Treatment often draws on techniques from multiple theories, or from the theory to which the clinician providing care most subscribes. For example, cognitive behavioral theorists argue that depression is the result of maladaptive (depressive) thought processes [10]. Consequently, cognitive behavioral therapies target patterns of thought as a means to reducing depression. Biological theories of depression posit disruption in neurochemicals and/or neural circuitry as the source of depression [11–13], and biological therapies focus on mitigating symptoms by either altering the level of various neurotransmitters [14–19] or disrupting electrophysiological patterns [20–22] in the brain. Attachment theories of depression theorize that disrupted attachment relationships in childhood result in maladaptive working models of self and other [23, 24] and focus on repairing these models by providing a secure base in the therapeutic relationship from which the person can develop more adaptive working models of self and other [25, 26].

This is in contrast to physical healthcare, where, over the past several decades, there have been significant gains in the ability to precisely diagnose and treat many previously intractable medical conditions. Heterogeneous diagnostic categories for many medical conditions have been increasingly refined over time, and these refinements used as the basis for updates to both diagnostic classification systems and treatment guidelines. A commonly cited example is the leukemias. Acute Myeloid Leukemia (AML), a cancer involving the blood cells, was previously classified using the French-American-British (FAB) classification system [27]. This system classified leukemia into 9 subtypes based on the physical appearance of person's blood cells when viewed under a microscope. Researchers learned over time that the FAB classification system did not include many factors later found to be important in effectively predicting response to treatment and both short- and long-term prognosis. The World Health Organization (WHO) developed a new classification to take these factors into account [28]. This classification system is based on both the specific genetic mutations seen in people with AML, as well as information about specific genes and proteins expressed by the cancer cells. In the case of most of the leukemias, disease classification has been refined to the point that the precise diagnosis is rarely made, and treatment plans rarely finalized, until genomic and proteomic testing has confirmed the specific etiology of the person's leukemia. The sophistication of tools used to detect pathology, the specificity with which diseases are being diagnosed, and the targeted nature of interventions has increased significantly in this domain.

Unfortunately, this has not been true for mental health. To a greater degree than in physical healthcare, mental healthcare around the world is currently practiced without clear insight into which interventions are most likely to work for whom [1, 29, 30]. It is increasingly recognized that despite significant increases in knowledge about the human brain and mind, researchers have struggled to translate this knowledge into meaningful advances to improve mental health [3]. Unlike in physical healthcare, where newly identified phenotypes have made their way into clinical nosologies and clear linkages have been made in both research and practice between refined phenotypes and interventions, insight into refined phenotypes in mental health have not been clearly linked to interventions. Consequently, evidence from clinical effectiveness trials often represents what we know about the average patient and the average presentation of the syndrome with which they are diagnosed.

It is important to consider that the root cause of this lack of actionable knowledge is not necessarily a shortage of data from which to generate knowledge. In the past decade, numerous data repositories have been created, many with some coverage of mental health conditions (Chap. 15). Thousands of empirical studies have been published about the etiology and/or treatment of mental health conditions. There are scores of approved drugs, evidence-based psychosocial treatments, and brain stimulation devices [31–33] in use around the world. However, it is increasingly recognized that despite the increasing number and variety of pharmacological, neuromodulatory, and psychosocial interventions available, knowledge about *which* interventions are most appropriate for *which* people has not accompanied the increase in available treatments [1–3]. Despite the exponential growth in *information* about the mind, brain, and mental health, the mental healthcare system has not yet produced the *actionable knowledge* required to produce the outcomes one would expect from such an investment [3, 34]. Moreover, while personalized treatment is becoming a reality in physical healthcare, it is increasingly acknowledged that in mental healthcare selecting the right treatment remains largely a process of trial and error [1, 29, 30].

A primary premise of this text, a premise that has been articulated by many others in the field [1, 3], is that we have reached a tipping point in mental health research and healthcare, a tipping point that promises near-term, exponential increases in our ability to precisely diagnose and more precisely treat mental health conditions. We have arrived at this tipping point as the result of the confluence of several factors. One factor is the evolution of increasingly sophisticated technologies for capturing and analyzing both genomic and neurocircuitry data (Chap. 11), as well as methods for linking these biological processes to mental processes (Chaps. 9, 12). Another factor is the widespread adoption of health information technologies, such as electronic health records (Chap. 16), clinical research databases (Chap. 15), and smart devices (Chap. 17). These technologies have made possible the real-time capture of all kinds of data relevant to mental health and illness. Related to health information technologies for capturing and storing data is the growth and increasing sophistication of foundational informatics technologies, such as standards for representing and transmitting these data (Chap. 7), as well as those for aggregating, analyzing, and visualizing these data (Chaps. 10, 14, and 19). As discussed in more detail in Chap. 15, these technologies are essential for being able to pool and aggregate data so they can be analyzed to acquire meaningful knowledge.

Another key factor in the arrival at this important tipping point is a conceptual shift within the behavioral sciences and psychology in particular. This conceptual shift is an emphasis on the dimensional nature of mental health and illness, in which signs and symptoms of mental health conditions—as well as most aspects of normative human development—are conceived as occurring along a nuanced continuum, rather than in distinct categories with well-defined boundaries [35–37]. The dimensional approach emphasizes the existence of fundamental dimensions of functioning underlying both normative and pathological processes. Not only has there been an emphasis on the dimensional nature of mental, emotional, behavioral, and social functions, there has also been an increasing emphasis on identifying the complex interactions between multiple correlates of human psychological functions, ranging from molecular and cellular phenomena, to more complex physiological and behavioral observations [3]. The final factor bringing us to this tipping point in mental health is the growing recognition that precision medicine is an aspirational ideal of healthcare research and practice [38].

We believe that mental health is an area of both dire need and tremendous opportunity for impactful change not only through increased adoption of health information technology (HIT) but, more importantly, through the more systematic application of informatics technologies. However, if the field of mental health is to benefit from these powerful technologies and paradigm shifts, it will require a new workforce that is equipped to integrate fundamental knowledge and technologies from informatics on the one hand, and the behavioral and social sciences on the other. That is, the promise of an LHS in mental health will only be achieved through the widespread, intentional, and systematic development, enhancement, and application of informatics technologies and paradigms in this domain.

1.2.1 Informatics: A Brief Preview

To understand the significance of the LHS model, we must first understand a bit about informatics. The science and practice of informatics will be described in detail in Chap. 2, and mental health informatics in Chap. 6. In this section, however, we present a brief preview of informatics to frame our discussion of the LHS.

Informatics is the science concerned with how humans acquire data and transform it into knowledge to solve real world problems. As you will see in Chap. 2,

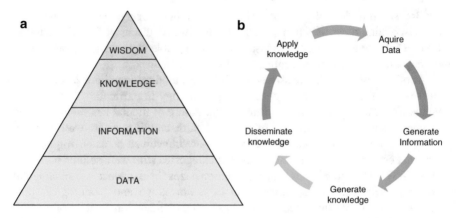

Fig. 1.1 Data-Information-Knowledge-Wisdom or Action (often abbreviated as DIKW or DIKA)

health informatics is the science concerned with developing and using technologies to capture health-related data and transform these data into actionable knowledge to improve health outcomes. This core process is depicted in Fig. 1.1. Figure 1.1a depicts the way that information, knowledge, and wisdom are sequentially derived from a foundation of data. Figure 1.1b depicts the cyclical nature of the process, in which applied knowledge serves as the basis for new data.

As you will see in Chap. 6, mental health informatics is the science of informatics applied specifically in the domain of mental health. The ultimate goal of mental health informatics is to increase our capacity to both identify and capture the data most relevant to mental health, transform these data into actionable knowledge, and apply this newly acquired knowledge to optimize the mental health of individuals and communities. As you will see in subsequent chapters, the science of informatics is grounded in theories of human knowledge acquisition and strives to develop paradigms, tools, and technologies to optimize the entire knowledge acquisition process.

1.3   The Path to the Learning Health System

A Learning Health System (LHS) is one that acquires knowledge as a by-product of the regular process of clinical care (Box 1.1). The concept of the LHS was first introduced by the Institute of Medicine (IOM, now the National Academy of Medicine, or NAM) in 2007 [39]. Compared to traditional models of knowledge discovery, the LHS model is intended to be more efficient and cost effective, and to generate more immediately and broadly actionable knowledge. This, in part, is because an LHS relies heavily on clinical data produced in the routine delivery of care as an essential data source for generating high quality, actionable knowledge.

Box 1.1 Definitions of Learning Health System and Related Paradigms
Learning Health System

In the initial report on LHSs, the IOM defined an LHS as a "healthcare system that 'learns'—one in which knowledge generation is so embedded into the core of the practice of medicine that it is a natural outgrowth and product of the healthcare delivery process and leads to continual improvement in care." ([39], p. 6) In a subsequent report, the IOM defined an LHS as a system "in which science, informatics, incentives, and culture are aligned for continuous improvement and innovation, with best practices seamlessly embedded in the care process, patients and families active participants in all elements, and new knowledge captured as an integral by-product of the care experience." [40].

Evidence Based Medicine

Introduced in JAMA in 1992 by the "Evidence-Based Medicine Working Group," evidence-based medicine was intended to "de-emphasize… intuition, unsystematic clinical experience, and pathophysiologic rationale as sufficient grounds for clinical decision making and stress… the examination of evidence from clinical research." [41] Admirable goals, certainly. It is important to note, however, that it has not always been viewed in a positive light. Critics have offered objections since just after the term was introduced that it was not actually novel, or that it was meant to promote "cookie cutter" medicine, purely to save costs, and to take away physician autonomy and judgement in decision making [42].

Evidence Generating Medicine

Embi and Payne defined Evidence Generating Medicine (EGM) in 2013 as "The systematic consideration and incorporation of research and improvement activities into the organization and practice of healthcare to accelerate biomedical discovery and improve the health of individuals and populations." [43] In EGM, clinical practice is not only informed by the results of research findings, but is also practiced in such a way as to facilitate generation of data for secondary use, shape research questions, and inform the ability to answer those questions.

Several key distinguishing features of an LHS are described in Box 1.2 below.

Box 1.2 Key Features of a Learning Health System

- Emphasis on effectiveness research over efficacy research. *Efficacy* research measures how an intervention performs under ideal and controlled conditions. *Effectiveness* research, on the other hand, measures how, an intervention performs under "real world" conditions.
- Evidence focuses on the needs of decision makers in the healthcare system itself. This may be contrasted with the needs and interests of, for example, a drug company.
- Focus on narrowing the research-practice divide. This convergence has important ethical implications as these different tasks have different primary concerns, namely the needs of the patient vs. the acquisition of new, generalizable knowledge [44].
- Research is conducted in typical clinical practice environments with unselected populations, again to emphasize effectiveness and increase generalizability.

It is helpful to understand how the LHS model differs from, builds upon, and ultimately integrates with, more traditional methods for knowledge discovery in order to appreciate the full value of the LHS model. Figure 1.2 below shows some of the primary paradigms used for knowledge discovery over the past several decades and highlights some key events in the evolution of the LHS paradigm.

In the sections that follow we describe this evolution from a system in which research and clinical care occurred in relative isolation from each other, and health professionals learned of new discoveries often years after they were made, to one in which research and clinical care are designed to be highly synchronized with minimal lapses of time between new discoveries and their direct application in clinical care.

1.3.1 The Traditional Model for the Discovery and Application of Knowledge in Healthcare

In both physical and mental healthcare, acquiring knowledge about how to prevent, detect, diagnose and treat illness involves many of the same core activities (Table 1.1). Through basic research, scientists in the physical, biological, behavioral, and social sciences discover new phenomena and obtain new insights into the complex interactions among them. They disseminate this new knowledge through multiple venues ranging from publications to professional conferences. Clinical researchers use this knowledge to formulate and test hypotheses about how it might

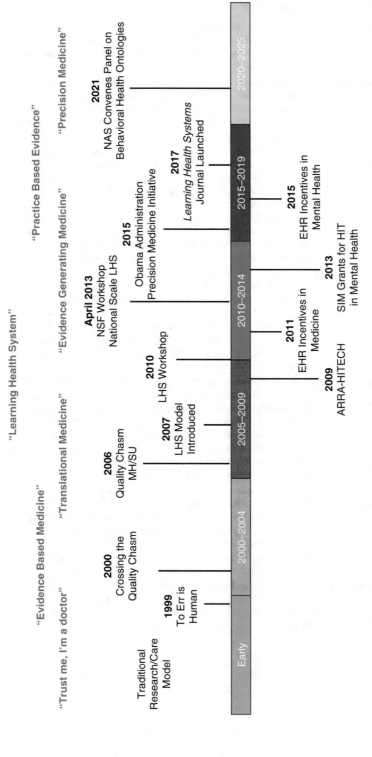

Fig. 1.2 Timeline of precision medicine and learning health system milestones and phases

Table 1.1 Knowledge discovery in healthcare

Basic research	Basic research is research performed to obtain knowledge about phenomena relevant to human health. The goal of basic research is to gain greater insight into these phenomena, not to develop specific applications or products [45].
Clinical research	Clinical research is research performed to produce knowledge about how discoveries made in basic research can be applied to improve human health. The goal of clinical research is to acquire knowledge about how basic science discoveries can be applied to prevent, detect, diagnose, and treat human disease [46].
Randomized controlled trial (RCT)	Randomized controlled trials are studies in which the primary variable of interest (the independent variable) is controlled by the researcher, and study participants are randomly assigned to different groups (or "arms") of the study. In RCTs there is always a group (the "control" group) that is not exposed to the independent variable. Typically, both the researcher and study participant are "blind" as to which arm they are in. This type of design increases the likelihood that differences between groups are causally related to the independent variable, rather than systemic differences between the groups. RCTs are the historical gold standard in biomedical research.
Observational research	Observational research is research in which the primary variable of interest (the independent variable) is not controlled by the researcher. In observational research, observations about differences between the groups (the dependent variables) are recorded and analyzed. However, the causal relationship between the independent variable and the dependent variables cannot be assumed, as they may be attributed to natural differences between the observed groups.
Pragmatic clinical trial (PCT)	Pragmatic clinical trials (PCTs) combine the scientific rigor of RCTs with the real-world nature of observational studies. PCTs are clinical trials that draw samples from real-world practice often in groups rather than patient by patient. For example, one arm may include one set of clinical practices, and the other arm another set of practices. They do not have the strict, and often unrealistic, inclusion and exclusion criteria of RCTs, making them more likely to reflect reality. PCTs often focus on identifying correlations between treatments and outcomes rather than causal mechanisms [47].
Comparative effectiveness research (CER)	Comparative effectiveness research is research that compares two or more interventions to identify relative risks and benefits of each intervention. CER relies on head-to-head comparisons of active treatments and focuses both on study populations typical of day-to day clinical practice, and evidence about the effects of the intervention relative to specific characteristics of individual people. CER can be performed using observational research paradigms or randomized controlled trials [48].
Implementation science	The US National Institutes of Health (NIH) defines implementation science as "the study of methods to promote the adoption and integration of evidence-based practices, interventions and policies into routine health care and public health settings" [49]

be applied to prevent, detect, diagnose, or treat illness. The clinical applications uncovered by these researchers may take the form of new clinical methods (such rooming a mother with her newborn to facilitate attachment) or new products (such as medical devices and equipment, pharmaceutical agents, and clinical treatment regimens). Clinical researchers, in turn, disseminate newly acquired clinical knowledge through publications, professional conferences, and product marketing channels. Healthcare professionals implement this knowledge, and both clinical researchers and health services researchers study the outcomes obtained from broad implementation of this new clinical knowledge.

For discoveries in basic research to benefit people, they must move through this entire process, with effective hand-offs between each phase. Clinical implications of basic knowledge must be recognized and the findings "picked up" and carried forward by clinical researchers. Similarly, the knowledge acquired by clinical researchers must be picked up not only by health professionals, but also by payers who ultimately approve reimbursement for use of these products and services. Most importantly, to minimize the time it takes for new knowledge to make its way to the people who will benefit from its clinical application, new knowledge must be acted upon quickly and seamlessly at each step in the process.

While the traditional model of knowledge discovery has generated a vast body of healthcare knowledge, it has been increasingly recognized that the hand-offs between disciplines are not well synchronized. Instead, they are inefficient and too often serendipitous instead of systematic. The dissemination of new knowledge through venues ranging from publications to professional conferences is inefficient and unsystematic. In fact, one frequently cited study demonstrated that, on average, 17 years elapsed between the time new knowledge was discovered and this knowledge was routinely implemented in practice [50]. In 2000, the IOM (now NAM) released the landmark report, "Crossing the Quality Chasm: A New Health System for the twenty-first Century", highlighting this substantial gap between known best healthcare practices, and healthcare that is routinely delivered [51] (Table 1.2A).

1.3.2 Translational Science

The mid-2000's saw increasing recognition that despite significant research funding, and subsequent knowledge discovery, scientific discoveries were not resulting in sufficient tangible improvement in health for the general population [54]. Elias Zerhouni, Director of NIH at the time, framed efforts to address gaps in clinically actionable knowledge in terms of the need to accelerate the *translation* of scientific discoveries from the laboratory to the patient, or "from bench to bedside". The focus of the translational model was on identifying ways to decrease the time it took for research to move through the many stages required to get new discoveries safely

Table 1.2 Problems with the traditional model of knowledge discovery

Problem	Solution
Gaps in application of existing knowledge: There is a significant delay in moving new knowledge into action, with one study suggesting that on average, it takes 17 years for new knowledge to make its way to the bedside [50].	**Translational science ("Bench to bedside"):** Create a standard process for quickly moving discoveries from the "bench" (basic science) to the "bedside".
Gaps in availability of knowledge: Providers frequently discover gaps in knowledge needed to make a clinical decision.	**"Bedside to bench":** Create a venue for quickly feeding important information back to the research enterprise based on gaps in knowledge discovered at the point of care. This venue becomes the mechanism for better synchronizing (and prioritizing) activities occurring in research settings with the immediate, real-time needs of patients and clinicians.
	Practice based evidence: Generate information and support therapeutic decision making by using data in EHR-based clinical repositories [52, 53].

from the laboratory to the people who stand to benefit from the new knowledge. These stages are traditionally defined in terms of increasingly applied levels (Table 1.3).

The translational model emphasizes the need to better synchronize and systematize the hand-offs of activities performed within one enterprise, by one type of scientist or health professional, with those performed within another enterprise, by another type of scientist or health professional (Fig. 1.3).

1.3.2.1 Limitations of Translational Research

Translational research is a valuable paradigm, responsible for countless discoveries and advances in clinical care, but it also has certain drawbacks. The first is that it is expensive and resource intensive. It requires significant money, time, and labor to set up experiments, recruit participants, obtain informed consent, and enroll participants, as well as follow up over time for longitudinal studies [58]. Studies are often designed to try to minimize variance in factors other than the one[s] being evaluated, with extensive exclusion criteria, resulting in a very special cohort that is not representative of the general population. For example, studies often exclude patients with various comorbidities or who take or have taken a specific drug. Unfortunately, this precludes the acquisition of knowledge about effectiveness of the intervention in people with comorbidities.

A number of large-scale, "moon-shot" type initiatives have been launched in the past decade or so to facilitate translational research. Notable examples include the NIH's "All of Us" project (formerly the Precision Medicine Initiate) [60], Google's

Table 1.3 Definitions of key terms used in translational medicine

Key terms	
Translational science	The process of moving scientific knowledge from basic scientific discovery to applications in human populations.
Translational research	Research that "fosters the multidirectional and multidisciplinary integration of basic research, patient-oriented research, and population-based research, with the long-term aim of improving the health of the public." [55]
T0 research	T0 research is "basic" research. It includes preclinical trials and animal studies, but not studies involving humans [56].
T1 research	T1 research takes basic research and applies it to humans. T1 research is performed in a highly controlled setting. T1 research includes phase 1 clinical trials [56].
T2 research	T2 research takes research that has been demonstrated to be safe in humans and applies it to samples of people for whom the discovery is designed, using controlled studies to generate empirical evidence supporting broad clinical application. T2 research includes phase 2 and 3 clinical trials. The goal of T2 research is to demonstrate the suitability of the new knowledge for incorporation into evidence-based guidelines [56].
T3 research	T3 research takes research that has been demonstrated to be effective in patients and applies it more broadly in practice. Comparative effectiveness research, post-marketing studies, clinical outcomes research, as well as health services, and dissemination and implementation research are all examples of T3 research [56].
T4 research	T4 research takes research that has been demonstrated to be both safe and effective and applies it broadly to communities. Population level outcomes research is an example of T4 research, which includes monitoring of morbidity, mortality, benefits, and risks, and impacts of policy and change [56].

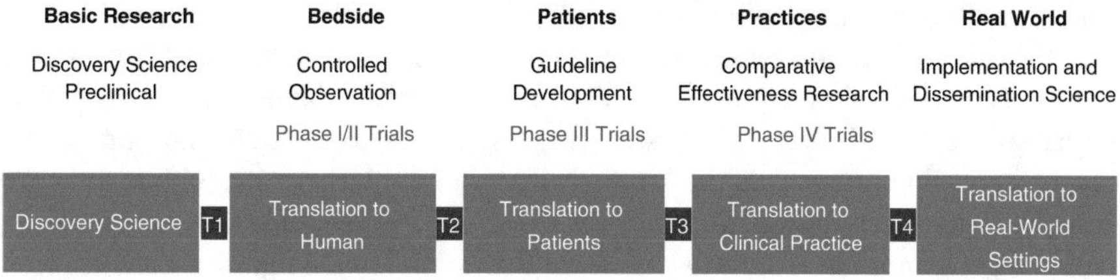

Fig. 1.3 Translational flow (adapted from [57])

Project Baseline [61], Leroy Hood's "Scientific Wellness" study [62], and the Department of Veteran Affairs' Million Veteran's Program [63], to name just a few in the United States alone. These are all exciting initiatives and will no doubt generate considerable new scientific knowledge. However, in addition to the significant costs associated, engagement over time can be a big challenge. The Scientific Wellness study cited above was preceded by a pilot study in 108 participants [64]. Those participants were given Fitbit trackers to monitor their sleep, but only 64% of participants were still using those devices after 40 days, a drop-off seen in other studies as well [62].

Another problem not solved by the translational model is the need for better flow of information from the "bedside to the bench" [65]. Neither the traditional nor the translational model address the need to better prioritize research based on known gaps in knowledge faced by front-line health professionals. Currently, there is no systematic process for prioritizing basic and clinical research agendas based on the here-and-now needs of patients and healthcare professionals (Table 1.2B). Rather, prioritizing and synchronizing work being performed by basic and clinical research-ers with the needs for new knowledge to support clinical practice occurs indirectly and is largely driven by advocacy groups, the goals and values of funding agencies, and, sadly, opportunities for profits.

1.3.3   The Learning Health System Paradigm

The traditional and translational models for knowledge discovery are linear, going "from bench to bedside." The learning health system, on the other hand, is cyclical [66]. In its purest (aspirational) form, the core activities in an LHS occur as tightly integrated cycles explicitly designed for knowledge discovery (Fig. 1.4). Two of the essential features of this model are the continuity of both the specific people, i.e., the "learning community" (Fig. 1.4) and the specific activities involved (Fig. 1.5).

We can also think of the LHS as activities that are not (yet) explicitly linked via a single learning community and continuous cycle. This way of thinking about an LHS (Fig. 1.6) acknowledges a looser integration between research and prac-tice, and views the (interim) system as a more bi-directional with research and clinical care occurring in distinct cycles, but research explicitly informing clinical care, and clinical care explicitly informing research. This way of thinking about an LHS acknowledges the reality of the way in which knowledge discovery occurs in most healthcare delivery systems. That is, few health systems have formal rela-tionships with institutes for research (especially basic research), and similarly, few research institutes have the kinds of integrated relationships with healthcare delivery systems required to enable a true LHS. It represents what could be thought of as an interim state as organizations work towards implementing a true LHS model [69].

A robust LHS depends on an infrastructure of informatics technologies [70–72]. One especially important type of technologies is those for concept and knowledge representation (described in detail in Chap. 7). These technologies make it possible to represent and manipulate clinical data, information, and knowledge computation-ally . Many other informatics technologies have been developed, and continue to evolve, to transform this new rich, and high-volume, source of clinical data into information and actionable knowledge (Table 1.4). Some of these technologies are focused on data capture and enable both more complete and accurate capture of health-related data, as well as the capture of new sources of data. These technolo-gies include imaging (Chap. 8) and genomics technologies (Chap. 11), mobile and "smart" device technologies (Chap. 17), and technologies for improved

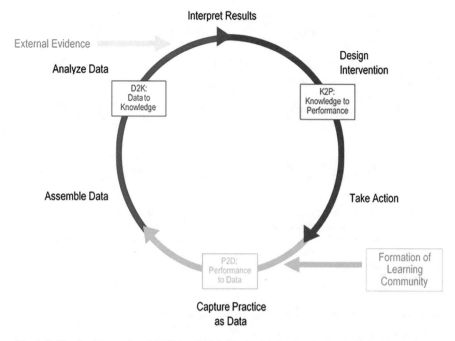

Fig. 1.4 The fundamental activity in an LHS is a complete cycle of study and change carried out by a single learning community. That community comprises all stakeholders affected by and needed to ensure the successful implementation of knowledge, including consumers of care. According to Friedman, the cycle begins not at the top with K2P, but at the bottom right with P2D. That is, the first step is to form the learning community, then to begin collecting baseline data about what the system is currently doing. Reproduced with permission from [67]

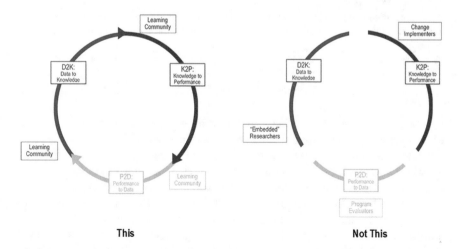

Fig. 1.5 In an LHS, each of the core knowledge discovery components is highly synchronized with the next. Moreover, the "community that discovers is also the community that implements." Reproduced with permission from [67]

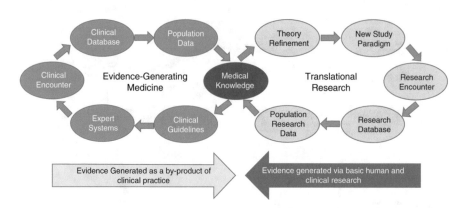

Fig. 1.6 The bidirectional cycle of the Learning Health System. Basic and translational research informs clinical care, translating knowledge from "bench to bedside" (lower path of cycle from research encounter to clinical encounter). Conversely, data captured through clinical practice may be used to inform research, effectively generating evidence through clinical care (upper path of dual cycle from clinical encounter to research encounter). Evidence generating medicine cycle adapted from [68]

Table 1.4 Informatics aspects of the different components of an LHS

LHS component	Role of informatics
Clinical encounter	Electronic health record to enable data capture, information retrieval, and real-time clinical decision support (see "Expert Systems" below)
Clinical data repositories and data integration	Data standards, mappings, and storage technologies
Data analysis and knowledge extraction	Analytic methods to transform data to information to knowledge
New medical knowledge informs new clinical guidelines	Standards for knowledge representation to facilitate computable guidelines, enabling automated clinical decision support (CDS)
Expert systems	Standards for knowledge representation, such CDS "hooks", to enable development of real-time clinical decision support technologies based on empirical, real-world evidence.

psychometric measurement (Chap. 9). Other informatics technologies making an LHS possible are technologies for transforming the new rich source of data into actionable knowledge. This includes National Language Processing (NLP), described in Chap. 13, and new computational models and analytics methods (Chap. 10), particularly those used in "Big-Data" paradigms (Chap. 15). Collectively, these technologies have allowed researchers to fully leverage EHR—and other sources of data generated outside the health system—for knowledge discovery. These technologies also expand our repertoire of knowledge discovery methods to support "evidence-based medicine" by introducing paradigms for "evidence-generating medicine" and "medicine-based evidence" [43] (see Box 1.1).

One of the earliest examples in the scientific literature of the LHS approach was work by Frankovich et al. at Stanford University [59]. They introduce the article by highlighting the fact that many doctors pride themselves on their practice of evidence-based medicine. They note, however, that doctors, and pediatricians in particular, often find themselves in a situation in which they must make a therapeutic decision for which no evidence base exists. They encountered such a situation with a 13-year-old patient with lupus who was admitted to the hospital with a number of factors that increased her risk for thrombosis. In deciding whether to treat this patient with anti-coagulants, which come with their own risk of bleeding, the care team was able to draw on an "electronic cohort" of pediatric lupus patients and calculate a significantly increased chance of thrombosis among patients with similar risk factors. They were thus able to use a data-driven approach to make the decision to treat the patient with anti-coagulants. This approach has been generalized at Stanford through a so-called "Green Button" (Table 1.2B) or "Informatics Consult" approach [52, 53] which enables clinicians to use aggregate patient data to inform therapeutic decisions. In addition to informing decisions in the absence of gold-standard evidence, this approach can also serve to help prioritize which questions to study using a more traditional randomized prospective approach. The authors do note that the "privacy rule in [HIPAA] may require revision to support this novel use of patient data." [52] (See Chap. 18.)

1.3.3.1   Limitations of the Learning Health System Paradigm

It is important to note that the LHS paradigm has its limitations as well. While formal LHS paradigms use data explicitly modeled and generated as part of the knowledge discovery cycle, less formal LHS paradigms consume whatever data is available in EHRs. These EHR data are notoriously noisy data that have been demonstrated time and again to have various weaknesses, including inaccuracy, incompleteness, and bias [73–76]. Indeed, the acquisition of robust, actionable, high quality knowledge will depend largely on the quality of the data captured during the routine delivery of care.

Just as the ability to acquire actionable knowledge from a tissue sample or radiographic image depends on the care taken, and instruments used, in obtaining and storing the specimen or image, the ability to acquire actionable knowledge from clinical documentation depends on the care taken in obtaining the data. A clinical finding of "mood swings" for example, based on clinical interview may be a useful data point for some purposes. An additional clinical finding of "increased emotional stability" two months into a regimen of a mood stabilizing drug might also be useful information. A series of metrics based on the results of one or more validated instruments for assessing emotional lability (mood swings) and affect (emotion) regulation, however, is more likely to yield actionable knowledge about the magnitude of improvement and the specific dimensions of affect regulation affected by the drug. If data from many different people, seeing many different types of providers were pooled and aggregated, the knowledge obtained from data of the second type will be far more actionable than that obtained from data of the first type.

This brings us to another potential limitation of the LHS paradigm: the benefits of collection of such data, especially in a structured manner, are balanced by significant literature showing the increase in time spent on clinical documentation when such systems are implemented, and in some cases an accompanying decrease in time spent on patient care and interaction [68, 77, 78] Still, mental health must struggle with this tension right along with the rest of the various specializations within physical health.

The LHS paradigm also raises important privacy concerns, as well as issues around autonomy and the right (or lack thereof?) to opt out of having one's data used for research, even in a "de-identified" manner. (We use that term in quotes because some believe that in this day and age, de-identification is a "reassuring myth." [79]). Finally, engagement with the health system tends to occur primarily when people are ill, which may provide a skewed picture of their overall health. Even during routine preventive care encounters, healthcare providers may be less likely to document findings indicative of excellent health or health promoting variables than there are to document findings indicative of poor health or risk factors for disease. The LHS does not replace traditional gold and silver standard clinical trials, rather it alters their role within the overarching health system.

1.3.4   Foundational Requirements of a Learning Health System in Mental Health

Building a robust LHS in mental health depends on a number of things. First, clinicians must be able to acquire and capture relevant clinical information during the routine delivery of care. To do this, a consensus set of core functional systems relevant to mental health and a common set of clinical findings, assessments, and interventions related to each of these systems must be defined (see Chap. 7). Relevant functional systems must be evaluated according to some consensus level of empirical rigor dictated by the purpose of the encounter, the presumed or rule-out condition, or the treatment regimen being undertaken. As in physical healthcare, some minimal set of clinical observations must be acquired using validated instruments, and must be captured with as much empirical specificity as possible. While clinical interviews may be sufficient for screening, clinical assertions about signs or symptoms leading a clinician to diagnose or rule-out a mental health conditions must be assessed with the same empirical rigor used when diagnosing or ruling out physical conditions (see Chaps. 5, 6, and 9). The instrument(s) and method(s) used to determine the existence, severity, and other dimensions of clinical findings must be documented along with the finding itself. Ideally, the instruments used to empirically assess signs and symptoms would be relatively consistent across clinicians and health systems, but empirical measurement of any type is an important first step in mental health (see Chaps. 6, 9).

Clinicians must also be able to capture detailed information about interventions performed during the routine delivery of care. In order to do this, the essential elements of each treatment regimen, protocol, or program must be identified, and a consensus set of core data elements sufficient to describe the treatment performed must be developed [80]. Data elements necessary for capturing the intensity, frequency, timing, and "dose" of each intervention must also be defined [80]. For example, Dialectical Behavior Therapy (DBT) [81], a psychosocial treatment commonly recommended for people suffering from chronic suicidal ideation includes several specific behavioral interventions designed to decrease the frequency of suicidal behavior. These interventions include—among *many* others—simple behavioral techniques such as reinforcement, shaping, punishment, and extinction [81]. If we hope to use data captured during the routine delivery of DBT to identify which people are most likely to benefit from DBT, which people may not benefit from DBT, or how we might tailor the intervention based on specific characteristics of a person and his or her underlying problems, we need more information than just that the treatment regimen was DBT and that sessions occurred weekly. We may want, for example, information about each time reinforcement or punishment was used, what the reinforcing or punishing stimulus was, and what behavior was being targeted.

Second, clinicians must have access to a robust health information technology (HIT) infrastructure on par with what is currently available in physical healthcare. EHRs must be available—and used—in all settings where mental health related information is generated, and these systems must be configured to allow for the capture and exchange of the entire gamut of mental health information described above. Moreover, EHRs must also be able to capture this information in a structured—or at least "structure-able" [82]— way (e.g., through use of NLP). Meeting the latter requirement will be a much greater challenge than the former, as it will require us to fill immense gaps that exist in technologies for the computable representation of both concepts (clinical observations) and knowledge (theoretical models and known best practices) (see Chap. 7) in mental health [83, 84].

Finally, clinical data captured in EHRs must be amenable to pooling and aggregation, and once aggregated, amenable to analysis . The former will be driven by the quality of standards for the representation and exchange of data (see Chap. 7) as well as the ability and willingness of clinicians to document the clinical encounter. The latter will require routine use of technologies ranging from simple query, report, and visualization tools (for internal analyses such as monitoring how a person is responding to treatment [85] or how frequently a provider deviates from evidence based guidelines) to complex analytic paradigms that can effectively integrate and analyze multi-site data sets comprised of observations of phenomena as diverse as genes, neural circuits, phenomenological experiences, behavior, and complex physical and social environments. Analytic methods must be designed not only to answer specific questions, but also to stimulate new ones. For example, through the use of visualization tools (see Chap. 14) patterns and relationships detected through data analysis can generate knowledge in the form of new hypotheses that can then be tested (i.e., hypothesis generation). These hypotheses must then be validated through clinical trials, whether randomized or pragmatic, as described above.

Collectively, the structures and activities described above create an LHS. The LHS has become an aspirational goal for improving the value of healthcare through rapid learning and translation of new knowledge into practice. In the context of the Triple Aim in healthcare—lowering cost, improving the health of populations, and improving satisfaction both for those providing and receiving care [86]—the LHS represents a cost-effective way to obtain data from which actionable knowledge can be acquired.

1.3.5 Learning Health System Models: The Role of Informatics

Both Translational Science and Learning Health Systems models depend on informatics technologies [70–72]. As described in Chap. 2, informatics comprises methods and technologies for the capture, storage, analysis, and retrieval of data, and for turning that data into information and information into knowledge. As such, each step in the LHS has important informatics components (Table 1.4).

1.4 Precision Medicine in Mental Health

Precision medicine is not a new concept. "Precision medicine" is only the latest aspirational moniker for a concept that has existing for almost 30 years and is being increasingly recognized as an ideal in healthcare [38]. Though different sources give different formal definitions, precision medicine essentially boils down to using more data (both higher quantities of data and more diverse types and sources of data) to deliver the right *intervention* to the right *person* at the right *time*. That is, rather than treating all people diagnosed with, for example, bipolar disorder the same way, we look at the unique features of the condition in each person, along with those things that make each person unique—demographics, lifestyle, living environment, genotype, presumed underlying etiology of the condition, personal goals and preferences—and use that rich and varied information to select the optimal therapeutic intervention. Other terms used for the same, or at least similar, concepts include *personalized medicine*, *"P4" medicine* (predictive, preventative, personalized, participatory), *stratified medicine*, *genomic medicine*, and *individualized medicine*, to name a few (Table 1.5). Each term may reflect a specific, nuanced focus, but all terms refer to a similar goal: use more data to prevent and treat illness in people, and do it in ways that align with their personal goals and preferences, using interventions designed to effectively target their unique health condition.

While the concept of precision medicine was used heavily following the release of the human genome, with an emphasis on the use of genetic data to inform clinical decision making, precision medicine is much broader than the use of genetic data to

Table 1.5 Precision medicine and related terms

Term	Description	PubMed Hits 10/04/2020
Precision Medicine	Use of clinical, demographic, molecular (including genomic), environmental, and lifestyle, and personal preferences and goals data to inform treatment [87, 88].	34,688
Personalized Medicine	Used interchangeably with Precision Medicine, though sometimes (mis)interpreted to refer to therapies developed specifically for an individual as opposed to a group with certain characteristics [89–91].	18,731
Genomic Medicine	Focus on genetic data in particular [92, 93].	14,787
Individualized Medicine	No meaningful difference from Personalized or Precision Medicine [94].	2000
Precision Health	Use of clinical, demographic, molecular (including genomic), environmental, lifestyle, and personal preferences and goals data to inform health maintenance and disease prevention [95].	988
Stratified Medicine	Focus on breaking down heterogeneous phenotypes into biologically meaningful subtypes, e.g., likely responders to a given therapy [96, 97].	660
Precision Psychiatry	Psychiatry founded in precise, empirical measurement and based on a "highly sophisticated and intricate classification system, where infinitesimal categories will, ideally, attain perfection in a detailed multidimensional classification" [2].	113
P4 Medicine	Coined by Leroy Hood; predictive, preventative, personalized, participatory [98].	111
Personalized Psychiatry / Personalized Mental Health / Personalized Mental Healthcare	Treatment of patients based on individual characteristics including genomic information [99].	68
Genomic Psychiatry	A term primarily associated with research performed using genetic and clinical data from a cohort of more than 30,000 people who have been diagnosed with mental health conditions and have seen at academic health centers in the US. [100].	22
Precision Mental Health	An approach to prevention and treatment of mental health conditions that focuses on the unique needs and preferences of the individual, tailors interventions to the individual, is aligned with the current scientific evidence, and uses a data-driven approach to clinical decision-making [101].	17
Stratified Psychiatry	An approach that conceives of mental health conditions as unique combinations of dysfunction occurring along multiple dimensions of human functioning (rather than discrete disorders as defined by current nosologies), and outcomes as "multidimensional constructs that can expose within- and between-patient differences in response" [102].	5

https://ghr.nlm.nih.gov/primer/precisionmedicine/precisionvspersonalized

Table 1.6 Intuitive versus precision medicine [104]

Intuitive Medicine	The provision of care for conditions diagnosed on the basis of symptoms, rather than known etiology, and treated using therapies for which the efficacy is unknown.
Precision Medicine	The provision of care for conditions with known etiology that can be precisely diagnosed and treated using therapies of known, and predictable effectiveness.

inform healthcare. Precision medicine is also broader than the idea of providing targeted interventions to treat illness and disease—it focuses on identifying people at risk for disease, and facilitating early intervention to prevent illness. This point is acknowledged specifically in the term "precision *health*" and in the "preventive" P of P4 medicine, but is implied in many of these paradigms. Williams [95] highlights the distinction made by Christensen et al. [104] between *intuitive medicine and precision medicine* (Table 1.6).

While personalized treatment is becoming a reality in the medical domain, selecting the right treatment in mental health remains largely a process of trial and error [103]. For example, when a person seeks care for depression, a psychiatrist may prescribe an anti-depressant. Which anti-depressant to prescribe is often based more on the doctor's personal preference and typical side effect profiles than on actual knowledge of which medication the patient is most likely to respond to. In a discussion of precision medicine.

Though there are companies that offer genetic testing for response to psychiatric drugs, their value is controversial. The FDA issued a Safety Communication in 2019 warning against reliance on these tests with insufficient clinical evidence to support claims that they can predict patient response to different drugs [105]. Drugs to treat depression were called out specifically as an example in that statement. Some insurance companies reimburse for these tests, while others do not.

Genetic and genomic biomarkers have seen the most press and hype in recent years, but other molecular biomarkers have shown promise as well [106, 107], and imaging biomarkers are commonly used in a number of different medical specialties, including neurology. Authorities differ on whether biomarkers are yet clinically actionable in mental health. In the imaging space, the American Psychiatry Association took the position in 2018 that neuroimaging had not yet had a significant impact on diagnosis or treatment in clinical settings [108]. Another group disagreed, pointing out that putting aside the very high bar of a pathognomonic signature of disease (i.e. a marker that specifically indicates a particular disease or condition), neuroimaging can in fact be useful to visualize certain biological contributors to conditions that might masquerade as psychiatric disorders. They also describe how certain imaging modalities, namely single photon emission computed tomography (SPECT) and positron emission tomography (PET), may be used for differential diagnosis Alzheimer's disease and other dementias, and ADHD [109].

In an ideal world, with realization of precision medicine, there would be reliable clinical evidence to enable a clinician to take into account not only the person's genetics but also use their demographics, lifestyle, co-morbidities, and other medications taken to inform the best choice for therapeutic intervention, whether pharmaceutical, therapy-based, or some combination of these and other treatments.

1.4.1 The Role of Informatics in Precision Medicine

Research involving human beings is already far more complex than for other systems like single cells or even animal models where most variables can be held constant. Testing a drug or diet change in genetically identical mice who live in the same cage under the same conditions allows a researcher to determine if that variable made a difference or not using only tens of animals. Testing a single hypothesis in human beings is more difficult, since people's genetics, diet, environment, and even adherence to the protocol may differ. With that increased variation, much larger numbers of people must be included to extract signal from noise. With the additional variables being considered in the precision medicine approach – genetics, environment, and lifestyle, this multiple hypothesis testing challenge is even greater. To address this issue, both experimental design and statistical approaches must be used. Experimentally, far more data points are needed. That is, instead of tens of animals we need tens of thousands of people, or more. In addition, statistical analysis approaches have been developed to correct for multiple hypothesis testing.

Precision medicine researchers require more data than they will ever be able to generate, and also, paradoxically, generate more data than they can possibly use [70]. Informatics plays a key role throughout the research process: electronic consent and specimen management, data standards for data integration, computational methods for reproducible biomarker discovery, knowledge representation for computable guidelines, and EHR enhancement both to enable decision support, and to capture clinical data in the course of practice. These components are shown in Fig. 1.7, adapted from an article on an "informatics research agenda to support precision medicine." Commonalities between the cycle depicted in this figure and the cyclic nature of the LHS as shown in Fig. 1.4 are not a coincidence. In both cases, informatics facilitates the transformation of data to information to knowledge, enabling knowledge to inform action, and then capturing data from that guided action to inform additional knowledge acquisition.

As described above, it is extremely expensive, with high costs in both time and labor, to conduct research with tens of thousands of participants using traditional methods of recruiting, informed consent, etc. A number of initiatives are doing just that. However, the LHS offers a complementary approach in which we are able to extract new knowledge from the data points collected every time a patient sees his or her doctor. This approach raises significant ethical, legal and social questions that must be addressed and answered in such a way as to maintain the trust of patients, their advocates, and society at large. These issues are discussed in detail in Chap. 18. The LHS approach also requires attention to data quality, fit for use, and many possible sources of bias.

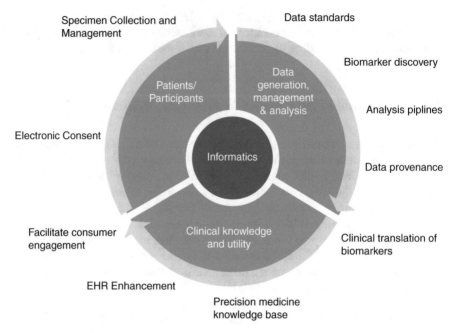

Fig. 1.7 The many roles of informatics throughout the research and translational cycle in precision medicine. Adapted from [70]

1.4.2 A Learning Heath System for Precision Mental Health

Mental health lags other fields in medicine not only in the use of high-quality translational science workflows, but also in developing a robust LHS. A significantly lower proportion of mental health practitioners have adopted electronic health records. Even when they have embraced EHRs, much of the data that is captured is recorded as free text. Though this does not preclude the use of this data for secondary analysis, it does require extra steps and expertise to extract information that is computable, and there are significant opportunities for inaccurate interpretation. A number of tools exist, both proprietary and open source, to facilitate such work, and natural language processing is a promising area for recent deep learning approaches. However, factors such as misspellings, homonyms, negation, lack of complete sentences or proper grammar, use of overloaded acronyms, and many others introduce complexity and noise in the data (Chap. 13).

That said, there is a body of work around secondary analysis of data from psychiatric EHRs. For example, researchers have successfully used EHR data to stratify patients based on symptoms [110], to extract Research Domain Criteria concepts [3] from notes and correlate those concepts with outcomes [111, 112], and to identify adolescents at risk for suicide [113]. However, few of the findings to date reach the bar for actionability. In addition, clinical decision support functionality is not common in psychiatric EHR systems.

In some cases, quantitative assessments may be stored as structured data. Initiatives such as the National Network of Depression Centers (NNDC)'s Mood Outcome Program (MOP) promotes the use and aggregation of such measures, with an explicit aim of creating "a nationwide 'learning health system' for mood disorders" [114].

1.5 Summary and Conclusions

If we can harness the LHS model to inform precision healthcare in mental health, we can significantly improve health outcomes. In order to do that, we need researchers and practitioners with expertise in both mental health *and* informatics – researchers and practitioners who can effectively communicate with, and translate between experts in each. Even with such resources, differences in knowledge acquisition between the behavioral and biological sciences are expected to introduce unique challenges for informaticians working in translational research— from "bench to bedside"—in mental health. Arguably the most significant challenge facing mental health informaticians is the complexity and fragmented nature of the landscape of theoretical models of psychopathology, exacerbated by a lack of computable representations (such as ontologies) of existing theoretical models through which to integrate them. In addition, the volume of instruments used within a given corpus of research, the variation in instruments used across studies, and the classification of research participants using coarse, heterogeneous diagnostic categories make it difficult to aggregate data for knowledge discovery.

For informaticians working to apply informatics best practices to enable a learning health system through "evidence generating medicine", the greatest challenges are introduced by the complexity of the landscape of treatment models in mental health and a ubiquitous reliance on clinical impression rather than use of objective laboratory, imaging or psychometric assessment techniques. In addition, lack of standards for clinical documentation, predominance of narrative notes, limited use of structured documentation, lack of standards for encoding clinical data, as well as the inconsistent and idiosyncratic approaches to diagnosis, means that data generated during routine clinical care is inaccessible or of limited usability. These issues will need to be addressed in order to make a robust LHS in mental health a reality.

Equipped with the knowledge and concepts presented in this book, trainees will be able to advance the field and to take on the numerous challenges that lie between where we are today and where we aspire to be.

References

1. Redish AD, Gordon JA. Computational psychiatry: new perspectives on mental illness. Strüngmann forum reports. Cambridge, MA: The MIT Press; 2016. xii, 408 pages
2. Fernandes BS, et al. The new field of 'precision psychiatry'. BMC Med. 2017;15(1):80.
3. Insel TR. The NIMH research domain criteria (RDoC) project: precision medicine for psychiatry. Am J Psychiatry. 2014;171(4):395–7.
4. Goldberg D. The heterogeneity of "major depression". World Psychiatry. 2011;10(3):226–8.
5. Gillan CM, Fineberg NA, Robbins TW. A trans-diagnostic perspective on obsessive-compulsive disorder. Psychol Med. 2017;47(9):1528–48.
6. Hyett MP, McEvoy PM. Social anxiety disorder: looking back and moving forward. Psychol Med. 2018;48(12):1937–44.
7. Kelly JR, et al. Dimensional thinking in psychiatry in the era of the research domain criteria (RDoC). Ir J Psychol Med. 2018;35(2):89–94.
8. Brazil IA, et al. Classification and treatment of antisocial individuals: from behavior to bio-cognition. Neurosci Biobehav Rev. 2018;91:259–77.
9. Allsopp K, et al. Heterogeneity in psychiatric diagnostic classification. Psychiatry Res. 2019;279:15–22.
10. BECK AT. Thinking and depression: I. Idiosyncratic content and cognitive distortions. Arch Gen Psychiatry. 1963;9(4):324–33.
11. Dean J, Keshavan M. The neurobiology of depression: an integrated view. Asian J Psychiatr. 2017;27:101–11.
12. Felger JC, Lotrich FE. Inflammatory cytokines in depression: neurobiological mechanisms and therapeutic implications. Neuroscience. 2013;246:199–229.
13. Drevets WC, Price JL, Furey ML. Brain structural and functional abnormalities in mood disorders: implications for neurocircuitry models of depression. Brain Struct Funct. 2008;213(1–2):93–118.
14. Kraus C, et al. Serotonin and neuroplasticity–links between molecular, functional and structural pathophysiology in depression. Neurosci Biobehav Rev. 2017;77:317–26.
15. Kryst J, Kawalec P, Pilc A. Efficacy and safety of intranasal esketamine for the treatment of major depressive disorder. Expert Opin Pharmacother. 2020;21(1):9–20.
16. Pitsillou E, et al. The cellular and molecular basis of major depressive disorder: towards a unified model for understanding clinical depression. Mol Biol Rep. 2020;47(1):753–70.
17. Fornaro M, et al. Brexpiprazole for treatment-resistant major depressive disorder. Expert Opin Pharmacother. 2019;20(16):1925–33.
18. Chong PS, et al. Therapeutic potential of Hericium erinaceus for depressive disorder. Int J Mol Sci. 2019;21(1):163.
19. Pochwat B, Nowak G, Szewczyk B. An update on NMDA antagonists in depression. Expert Rev Neurother. 2019;19(11):1055–67.
20. Iseger TA, et al. A frontal-vagal network theory for major depressive disorder: implications for optimizing neuromodulation techniques. Brain Stimul. 2020;13(1):1–9.
21. George MS. Whither TMS: a one-trick pony or the beginning of a neuroscientific revolution? Am J Psychiatry. 2019;176(11):904–10.
22. Li M, et al. Effects of electroconvulsive therapy on depression and its potential mechanism. Front Psychol. 2020;11:80.
23. Cawnthorpe D, West M, Wilkes T. Attachment and depression: the relationship between the felt security of attachment and clinical depression among hospitalized female adolescents. Can Child Adolesc Psychiatry Rev. 2004;13(2):31–5.
24. Klohnen EC, John OP. Working models of attachment: a theory-based prototype approach. In: Attachment theory and close relationships. New York, NY, US: The Guilford Press; 1998. p. 115–40.
25. Zilcha-Mano S, et al. Identifying the most suitable treatment for depression based on patients' attachment: study protocol for a randomized controlled trial of supportive-expressive vs. supportive treatments. BMC Psychiatry. 2018;18(1):362.

26. Gunlicks-Stoessel M, et al. The role of attachment style in interpersonal psychotherapy for depressed adolescents. Psychother Res. 2019;29(1):78–85.
27. Bennett JM, et al. Proposals for the classification of the acute leukaemias. French-American-British (FAB) co-operative group. Br J Haematol. 1976;33(4):451–8.
28. Vardiman JW, Harris NL, Brunning RD. The World Health Organization (WHO) classification of the myeloid neoplasms. Blood. 2002;100(7):2292–302.
29. Arango C, Kapur S, Kahn RS. Going beyond "trial-and-error" in psychiatric treatments: OPTiMiSE-ing the treatment of first episode of schizophrenia. Schizophr Bull. 2015;41(3):546–8.
30. McMahon FJ. Prediction of treatment outcomes in psychiatry–where do we stand ? Dialogues Clin Neurosci. 2014;16(4):455–64.
31. Trapp NT, et al. A new device to improve target localization for transcranial magnetic stimulation therapy. Brain Stimul. 2019;12(6):1600–2.
32. Oliveira-Maia AJ, et al. Comparative efficacy of repetitive transcranial magnetic stimulation for treatment of depression using 2 different stimulation devices: a retrospective open-label study. J Clin Psychiatry. 2016;77(6):743–4.
33. Souza VH, et al. Development and characterization of the InVesalius navigator software for navigated transcranial magnetic stimulation. J Neurosci Methods. 2018;309:109–20.
34. Institute of Medicine Committee on Crossing the Quality Chasm. Adaptation to Mental, H. and D. Addictive, The national academies collection: reports funded by national institutes of health, in improving the quality of health care for mental and substance-use conditions: quality chasm series. Washington (DC): National Academy of Sciences; 2006. National Academies Press (US) Copyright © 2006.
35. Kotov R, et al. The hierarchical taxonomy of psychopathology (HiTOP): a dimensional alternative to traditional nosologies. J Abnorm Psychol. 2017;126(4):454–77.
36. Waszczuk MA, et al. Redefining phenotypes to advance psychiatric genetics: implications from hierarchical taxonomy of psychopathology. J Abnorm Psychol. 2020;129(2):143–61.
37. Strickland CM, et al. Categorical and dimensional conceptions of personality pathology in DSM-5: toward a model-based synthesis. J Personal Disord. 2019;33(2):185–213.
38. Dzau VJ, Ginsburg GS. Realizing the full potential of precision medicine in health and health care. JAMA. 2016;316(16):1659–60.
39. Medicine Io. In: Olsen L, Aisner D, McGinnis JM, editors. The learning healthcare system: workshop summary, vol. 374. Washington, DC: The National Academies Press; 2007.
40. Medicine, I.o., Roundtable on value & science-driven health care. 2012.
41. Evidence-Based Medicine Working, G. Evidence-based medicine. A new approach to teaching the practice of medicine. JAMA. 1992;268(17):2420–5.
42. Sackett DL, et al. Evidence based medicine: what it is and what it isn't. British Med J. 1996;312:71–2.
43. Embi PJ, Payne PR. Evidence generating medicine: redefining the research-practice relationship to complete the evidence cycle. Med Care. 2013;51(8 Suppl 3):S87–91.
44. Piasecki J, Dranseika V. Research versus practice: the dilemmas of research ethics in the era of learning health-care systems. Bioethics. 2019;33(5):617–24.
45. NIH. Notice of intent to publish parent funding opportunity announcements for basic experimental studies with humans. 2018 10/26/18 [cited 2020 5/2/20]; Available from: https://grants.nih.gov/grants/guide/notice-files/NOT-OD-19-024.html.
46. Ommaya A, Korn A, Tunis S. The role of purchasers and payers in the clinical research enterprise: workshop summary. National Academies Press; 2002.
47. Tunis SR, Stryer DB, Clancy CM. Practical clinical trials: increasing the value of clinical research for decision making in clinical and health policy. JAMA. 2003;290(12):1624–32.
48. Sox HC, Goodman SN. The methods of comparative effectiveness research. Annu Rev Public Health. 2012;33(1):425–45.
49. Health, U.N.I.o. Implementation science news, resources and funding for global health researchers. 2020 [cited 2020 October 5, 2020]; Available from: https://www.fic.nih.gov/ResearchTopics/Pages/ImplementationScience.aspx.

50. Green LW, et al. Diffusion theory and knowledge dissemination, utilization, and integration in public health. Annu Rev Public Health. 2009;30:151–74.
51. Institute of Medicine Committee on Quality of Health Care in, A in crossing the quality chasm: a new health system for the 21st Century. 2001, National Academies Press (US) Copyright 2001 by the National Academy of Sciences. All rights reserved.: Washington (DC).
52. Longhurst CA, Harrington RA, Shah NH. A 'green button' for using aggregate patient data at the point of care. Health Aff (Millwood). 2014;33(7):1229–35.
53. Schuler A, et al. Performing an informatics consult: methods and challenges. J Am Coll Radiol. 2018;15(3 Pt B):563–8.
54. Zerhouni EA. Translational and clinical science–stime for a new vision. N Engl J Med. 2005;353(15):1621–3.
55. Rubio DM, et al. Defining translational research: implications for training. Acad Med. 2010;85(3):470.
56. University of Wiscon-Madison, U.I.f.C.a.T.R. What are the T0 to T4 research classifications? 2020 [cited 2020 Ocotber 4, 2020]; Available from: https://ictr.wisc.edu/what-are-the-t0-to-t4-research-classifications/
57. National Academies of Sciences, E., et al. in Exploring strategies to improve cardiac arrest survival: proceedings of a workshop. 2016, National Academies Press (US) Copyright 2017 by the National Academy of Sciences. All rights reserved.: Washington (DC).
58. Tenenbaum JD. Translational bioinformatics: past, present, and future. Genomics, Proteomics & Bioinformatics. 2016;14(1):31–41. ISSN 1672-0229. https://doi.org/10.1016/j.gpb.2016.01.003.
59. Frankovich J, Longhurst CA, Sutherland SM. Evidence-based medicine in the EMR era. N Engl J Med. 2011;365(19):1758–9.
60. Denny JC, et al. The "all of us" research program. N Engl J Med. 2019;381(7):668–76.
61. Manos D. Rocking the baseline: verily, Duke, and Stanford aim to make medicine more predictive with a new baseline study. New Rochelle, NY: Mary Ann Liebert, Inc.; 2017.
62. Cross R. 'Scientific wellness' study divides researchers. Science. 2017;357(6349):345.
63. Gaziano JM, et al. Million veteran program: a mega-biobank to study genetic influences on health and disease. J Clin Epidemiol. 2016;70:214–23.
64. Price ND, et al. A wellness study of 108 individuals using personal, dense, dynamic data clouds. Nat Biotechnol. 2017;35(8):747.
65. Ledford H. Translational research: the full cycle. Nature. 2008;453(7197):843–5.
66. Friedman C. Envisioning the learning health system. Lecture conducted as part of the Institute for Health Informatics Invited Speaker Series at the University of Minnesota, United States.
67. Guise J-M, Savitz LA, Friedman CP. Mind the gap: putting evidence into practice in the era of learning health systems. J Gen Intern Med. 2018;33(12):2237–9.
68. Carayon P, Wetterneck TB, Alyousef B, et al. Impact of electronic health record technology on the work and workflow of physicians in the intensive care unit. Int J Med Inform. 2015;84(8):578–94. https://doi.org/10.1016/j.ijmedinf.2015.04.002. [published Online First: Epub Date]
69. Chute C. Lecture conducted as part of the Institute for Health Informatics Invited Speaker Series at the University of Minnesota, United States.
70. Tenenbaum JD, et al. An informatics research agenda to support precision medicine: seven key areas. J Am Med Inform Assoc. 2016;23:791–5.
71. Skiba DJ. Informatics and the learning healthcare system. Nurs Educ Perspect. 2011;32(5):334–6.
72. McLachlan S. Innovation in health informatics. J Innov Health Inform. 2018;25(1):11.
73. Pivovarov R, et al. Identifying and mitigating biases in EHR laboratory tests. J Biomed Inform. 2014;51:24–34.
74. Weiner SJ, et al. How accurate is the medical record? A comparison of the physician's note with a concealed audio recording in unannounced standardized patient encounters. J Am Med Inform Assoc. 2020;27:770–5.
75. Botsis T, et al. Secondary use of EHR: data quality issues and informatics opportunities. Summit Transl Bioinform. 2010;2010:1–5.

76. Hersh WR, et al. Caveats for the use of operational electronic health record data in comparative effectiveness research. Med Care. 2013;51(8 Suppl 3):S30–7.

77. Baumann LA, Baker J, Elshaug AG. The impact of electronic health record systems on clinical documentation times: A systematic review. Health Policy. 2018;122(8):827–36. https://doi.org/10.1016/j.healthpol.2018.05.014. [published Online First: Epub Date]

78. Joukes E, Abu-Hanna A, Cornet R, de Keizer NF. Time spent on dedicated patient care and documentation tasks before and after the introduction of a structured and standardized electronic health record. Appl Clin Inform. 2018;9(1):46–53. https://doi.org/10.1055/s-0037-1615747. [published Online First: Epub Date]

79. Kulynych, J. and H. Greely Every patient a subject: when personalized medicine, genomic research, and privacy collide. Slate.com, 2014.

80. Gonzalez ML, Butler AS, England MJ. Psychosocial interventions for mental and substance use disorders: A framework for establishing evidence-based standards. Washington, DC: National Academies Press; 2015.

81. Linehan MM, Cochran BN, Kehrer CA. Dialectical behavior therapy for borderline personality disorder. In: Barlow DH, editor. Clinical handbook of psychological disorders: a step-by-step treatment manual, vol. 3. New York: The Guilford Press; 2001. p. 470–522.

82. Chute CG. Clinical classification and terminology: some history and current observations. J Am Med Inform Assoc. 2000;7(3):298–303.

83. Ranallo PA, et al. Behavioral health information technology: from chaos to clarity. Health Aff (Millwood). 2016;35(6):1106–13.

84. Ranallo PA, et al. Psychological assessment instruments: a coverage analysis using SNOMED CT, LOINC and QS terminology. AMIA Annu Symp Proc. 2013;2013:1333–40.

85. Lambert MJ. Prevention of treatment failure: The use of measuring, monitoring, and feedback in clinical practice. Washington, DC: American Psychological Association; 2010.

86. Berwick DM, Nolan TW, Whittington J. The triple aim: care, health, and cost. Health Aff (Millwood). 2008;27(3):759–69.

87. Collins FS, Varmus H. A new initiative on precision medicine. N Engl J Med. 2015;372(9):793–5.

88. Jameson JL, Longo DL. Precision medicine–personalized, problematic, and promising. N Engl J Med. 2015;372(23):2229–34.

89. Hamburg MA, Collins FS. The path to personalized medicine. N Engl J Med. 2010;363(4):301–4.

90. Ginsburg GS, McCarthy JJ. Personalized medicine: revolutionizing drug discovery and patient care. Trends Biotechnol. 2001;19(12):491–6.

91. Pauker SG, Kassirer JP. Decision analysis. N Engl J Med. 1987;316(5):250–8.

92. Guttmacher AE, Collins FS. Genomic medicine–a primer. N Engl J Med. 2002;347(19):1512–20.

93. Feero WG, Guttmacher AE, Collins FS. Genomic medicine–an updated primer. N Engl J Med. 2010;362(21):2001–11.

94. Evans WE, Relling MV. Moving towards individualized medicine with pharmacogenomics. Nature. 2004;429(6990):464–8.

95. Williams MS. Informatics for a precision learning healthcare system, in personalized and precision medicine informatics, Adam T. and A. C.,. Cham: Springer; 2020.

96. Trusheim MR, Berndt ER, Douglas FL. Stratified medicine: strategic and economic implications of combining drugs and clinical biomarkers. Nat Rev Drug Discov. 2007;6(4):287–93.

97. Schumann G, et al. Stratified medicine for mental disorders. Eur Neuropsychopharmacol. 2014;24(1):5–50.

98. Hood L, Friend SH. Predictive, personalized, preventive, participatory (P4) cancer medicine. Nat Rev Clin Oncol. 2011;8(3):184–7.

99. Amare AT, Schubert KO, Baune BT. Pharmacogenomics in the treatment of mood disorders: strategies and opportunities for personalized psychiatry. EPMA J. 2017;8(3):211–27.

100. Pato MT, et al. The genomic psychiatry cohort: partners in discovery. Am J Med Genet B Neuropsychiatr Genet. 2013;162b(4):306–12.

101. Bickman L, Lyon AR, Wolpert M. Achieving precision mental health through effective assessment, monitoring, and feedback processes: introduction to the special issue. Adm Policy Ment Health. 2016;43(3):271–6.
102. Joyce DW, et al. Realising stratified psychiatry using multidimensional signatures and trajectories. J Transl Med. 2017;15(1):15.
103. Zanardi R, et al. Precision psychiatry in clinical practice. Int J Psychiatry Clin Pract. 2020;25:1–9.
104. Christensen, C.M., J.H. Grossman, and J. Hwang, The innovator's prescription.. A disruptive Solution for, 2010.
105. FDA. The FDA warns against the use of many genetic tests with unapproved claims to predict patient response to specific medications. 2019.; Available from: https://www.fda.gov/medical-devices/safety-communications/fda-warns-against-use-many-genetic-tests-unapproved-claims-predict-patient-response-specific.
106. Bi J, et al. Altered cellular metabolism in gliomas–an emerging landscape of actionable co-dependency targets. Nat Rev Cancer. 2020;20(1):57–70.
107. Doll S, Gnad F, Mann M. The case for proteomics and Phospho-proteomics in personalized cancer Medicine. Proteomics Clin Appl. 2019;13(2):e1800113.
108. First MB, et al. Clinical applications of neuroimaging in psychiatric disorders. Am J Psychiatry. 2018;175(9):915–6.
109. Henderson TA, et al. Functional neuroimaging in psychiatry—aiding in diagnosis and guiding treatment. What the American Psychiatric Association does not know. Front Psych. 2020;11(276):0415.
110. Liu Q, et al. Symptom-based patient stratification in mental illness using clinical notes. J Biomed Inform. 2019;98:103274.
111. McCoy TH Jr, et al. High throughput phenotyping for dimensional psychopathology in electronic health records. Biol Psychiatry. 2018;83:997–1004.
112. McCoy TH, et al. A clinical perspective on the relevance of research domain criteria in electronic health records. Am J Psychiatry. 2015;172(4):316–20.
113. Velupillai S, et al. Identifying suicidal adolescents from mental health records using natural language processing. Stud Health Technol Inform. 2019;264:413–7.
114. Zandi PP, et al. Development of the National Network of depression centers mood outcomes program: a multisite platform for measurement-based care. Psychiatr Serv. 2020;71(5):456–64.

Chapter 2
What Is Informatics?

Elizabeth S. Chen

Abstract Biomedical informatics is a discipline dating back to the 1950s that continues to evolve with the growth of data and advances in technology in biomedicine and health care. This field brings together foundational approaches from many scientific and technological disciplines that can be applied across the spectrum from molecules to individuals to populations. In the context of the learning healthcare system, this chapter highlights frameworks and methods for transforming data to knowledge, putting knowledge into practice through evidence-based technology innovations, and evaluating the impact of those innovations.

Keywords (MeSH): Informatics · Natural language processing · Data mining Machine learning · Health information interoperability · Decision support systems Clinical · Information technology · Evaluation studies as topic

2.1 History and Role in Biomedicine and Health

Since its origins in the 1950s, the field of biomedical informatics has continued to evolve with rapid advances in technology and exponential growth of data in biomedicine and health care. While the terms *informatika* (Russian), *informatik* (German), and *informatique* (French) were being used in the 1950s and 1960s (and now refer to the field of computer science), the English term *informatics* was formally defined in the 1970s with applications in biology and medicine referred to as *bioinformatics* and *medical informatics* respectively (Table 2.1a-c) [1–6]. As these sub-disciplines advanced in parallel, *biomedical informatics* emerged as an umbrella term in the 1990s to encompass the breadth and depth of methods applied across the

E. S. Chen (✉)
Brown University, Providence, RI, USA
e-mail: liz_chen@brown.edu

© Springer Nature Switzerland AG 2021
J. D. Tenenbaum, P. A. Ranallo (eds.), *Mental Health Informatics*, Health Informatics, https://doi.org/10.1007/978-3-030-70558-9_2

31

Table 2.1 Formal terms and definitions

Term	Definition
(a) Informatics	Discipline of science which investigates the structure and properties (not specific context) of scientific information, as well as the regularities of scientific information activity, its theory, history, methodology, and organization [2]. Branch of study that deals with the structure, properties, and communication of information and with means of storing or processing information [8].
(b) Bioinformatics	Branch of science concerned with information and information flow in biological systems, esp. the use of computational methods in genetics and genomics [9]. Conceptualizing biology in terms of macromolecules (in the sense of physical-chemistry) and then applying "informatics" techniques (derived from disciplines such as applied maths, computer science, and statistics) to understand and organize the information associated with these molecules, on a large-scale [10].
(c) Medical Informatics	Field that concerns itself with the cognitive, information processing, and communication tasks of medical practice, education, and research, including the information science and the technology to support these tasks [3]. Comprises the theoretical and practical aspects of information processing and communication, based on knowledge and experience derived from processes in medicine and health care [11]. Develop and assess methods and systems for the acquisition, processing, and interpretation of patient data with help of knowledge that is obtained in scientific research [12].
(d) Biomedical Informatics	Scientific field that deals with the storage, retrieval, sharing, and optimal use of biomedical information, data, and knowledge for problem solving and decision making. It touches on all basic and applied fields in biomedical science and is closely tied to modern information technologies, notably in the areas of computing and communication [13]. Interdisciplinary field that studies and pursues the effective uses of biomedical data, information, and knowledge for scientific inquiry, problem solving and decision making, motivated by efforts to improve human health [7]. Science of information applied to, or studied in the context of biomedicine [14].

spectrum from molecules to individuals to populations (Table 2.1d) [7]. More about the origins of informatics and biomedical informatics can be found in *A History of Medical Informatics in the United States* [1, 2].

Biomedical informatics brings together foundational approaches that can be applied in a range of contexts, thus representing a continuum from basic research to applied research and practice [13]. Methods, techniques, and theories from many scientific and technological disciplines (e.g., cognitive science, computer science, decision science, engineering, epidemiology, implementation science, management science, social and behavioral sciences, and statistics) are leveraged and advanced to support applications in domain disciplines (e.g., basic biomedical science, clinical science, and public and population health science) [13]. From an education and training perspective, core competencies are being defined that reflect the needs for knowledge, skills, and attitudes in the domains of health, information science and technology, and social and behavioral science as well as the intersection of these domains [7, 15–17].

There are hundreds of informatics subdisciplines both outside the biomedical and healthcare domains (e.g., biodiversity informatics, business informatics, and museum informatics) and within [18]. While there may be variability in terms (particularly the modifier or adjective preceding "informatics" [19]), definitions, and organization of the many subdisciplines of biomedical informatics (sometimes referred to as *biomedical and health informatics*), they share the same foundation and diverge in how the theories, paradigms, and technologies are applied. The spectra along which informatics may be delineated can be thought of as dimensional axes that refer to the: (1) *scale* of the object of study (from molecules to populations) [20], (2) *translational spectrum* (from bench to bedside to community) [21], and (3) *continuum* from data to information to knowledge to wisdom or action [22]. Additional qualifiers may refer to disease area, modality of data acquisition, or functional system of interest. Location along these three axes, along with one or more qualifiers, circumscribe the specific informatics approaches commonly used within a particular informatics subdiscipline.

The axes of scale and translational spectrum are illustrated in Fig. 2.1 with examples: (A) Genomic research that identifies a single nucleotide variant (SNV) with a small hazards ratio of 1.1 is molecular in scale, but not actionable and at the research end of the translational spectrum; (B) Use of RNA-based biomarkers for drug repositioning is at the molecular scale, but done for the purpose of impacting health outcomes and therefore translational; (C) A clinically actionable genotype is molecular in scale, but impacts actual clinical and community care; (D) Retrospective

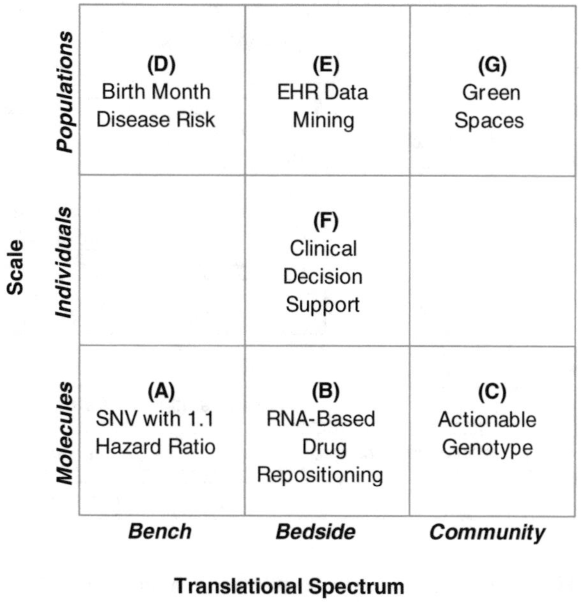

Fig. 2.1 Axes and translational spectrum of biomedical informatics

Scale	Bench	Bedside	Community
Populations	(D) Birth Month Disease Risk	(E) EHR Data Mining	(G) Green Spaces
Individuals		(F) Clinical Decision Support	
Molecules	(A) SNV with 1.1 Hazard Ratio	(B) RNA-Based Drug Repositioning	(C) Actionable Genotype

Translational Spectrum

data mining of electronic health record (EHR) data that identifies a correlation between month of birth and subsequent diagnoses is at the population level, but not yet actionable [23]; (E & F) Depending on the objective or application, mining EHR data may be translational in nature, and fall anywhere between individuals and populations on the scale axis, for informing clinical decision support; and (G) Installation of recreational facilities or green spaces in order to improve physical and mental well-being is an actionable intervention at the population scale.

Four major informatics subdisciplines are: (1) *bioinformatics* (molecular and cellular processes), (2) *imaging informatics* (tissues and organs), (3) *clinical informatics* (patients), and (4) *public health informatics* (populations and society) [13, 24]. Together, the latter two are referred to as *health informatics* with *medical informatics*, *nursing informatics* [25, 26], and *dental informatics* [27] considered subdisciplines of clinical informatics. Other subdisciplines span these areas such as *consumer health informatics* (people) [28, 29] and *translational informatics* (bench-to-bedside research) [30] that is further subdivided into *translational bioinformatics* [31–33] and *clinical research informatics* [34]. Global health informatics studies not just a single population but populations across the world, particularly in low and middle income countries [35]. Informatics specializations focused on specific clinical specialties, disease states, functional systems, and populations are also becoming more prevalent (e.g., *cancer informatics* [36], *immunoinformatics* [37], *mental health informatics* [38, 39], *pediatric informatics* [40], *pathology informatics* [41, 42], and *veterinary informatics* [43]). Chap. 4 further describes how mental health informatics relates to biomedical informatics and its major subdisciplines (Fig. 2.2).

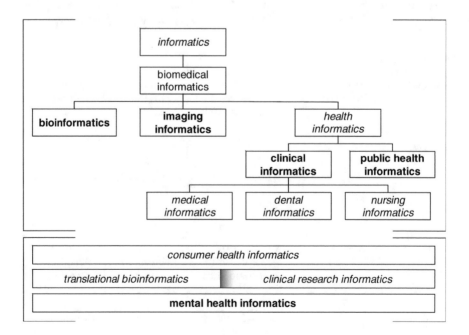

Fig. 2.2 Organization and specialization of informatics subdisciplines

Chap. 11 and Chap. 12 provide in depth looks at bioinformatics and neuroinformatics respectively.

Biomedical informatics is core to supporting a continuously learning healthcare system (LHS) where "progress in science, informatics, and care culture align to generate new knowledge as an ongoing, natural by-product of the care experience, and seamlessly refine and deliver best practices for continuous improvement in health and health care" [44, 45] (Chap. 6). Through a cyclical process, data are transformed into knowledge (Data to Knowledge [D2K]), knowledge is applied to implement change (Knowledge to Performance [K2P]), and changed performance generates new data (Performance to Data [P2D]) that feeds into the next learning cycle [46, 47]. Each of these flows is associated with a series of steps for: collecting, assembling, and analyzing data; interpreting results; representing, managing, and applying knowledge; and taking action to change practice [47].

This chapter covers core frameworks and methodologies for supporting the D2K, K2P, and P2D flows and corresponding steps of the LHS where some may be applicable to multiple flows and steps (e.g., all flows involve standards and evaluation) (Fig. 2.3). A case study in the context of mental health is transforming electronic health record (EHR) data for suicidal thoughts and behaviors (STB) into knowledge, developing an evidence-based clinical decision support (CDS) tool in the EHR for STB, and evaluating the impact of this tool. A comprehensive review of methods and applications in biomedical informatics can be found in *Methods in Biomedical Informatics: A Pragmatic Approach* [48] and *Biomedical Informatics: Computer Applications in Health Care and Biomedicine* [13].

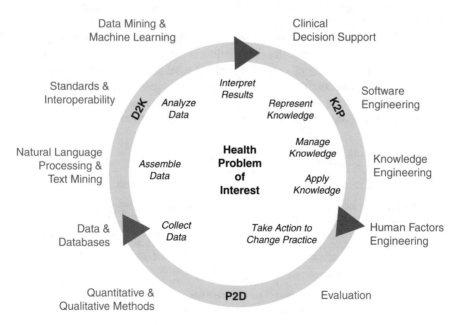

Fig. 2.3 Biomedical informatics in support of a learning healthcare system (cycle diagram adapted from [47] and enhanced with addition of chapter topics)

2.2   From Data to Knowledge (D2K)

The discovery of knowledge in data requires a range of processes and techniques that are summarized in this chapter and further described in Section 2 of this book (Fig. 2.4). This section provides an overview of knowledge discovery frameworks, data and databases, techniques such as natural language processing and machine learning, and foundational concepts in standards and interoperability. Visualization and visual analytic techniques that can be used to facilitate exploration and interpretation of data, information, and knowledge are described in Chap. 16. Ethical, legal, and social implications that underlie the overall process are described in Chap. 22.

2.2.1   Knowledge Discovery Process

The Data, Information, Knowledge, and Wisdom (DIKW) hierarchy, formalized by Ackoff in 1989 [49], provides a representation of relationships and transformations between these levels [50, 51]. *Data* are defined as facts or observations with no meaning that are transformed to *information* to provide meaning and value. *Knowledge* builds upon data and information by incorporating understanding, experience, learning, and expertise. Finally, *wisdom* (or *action*) involves determining how best to apply knowledge in a given context. The DIKW or DIKA model, including definitions and relationships, continues to evolve and be refined for use in biomedical informatics [14] and its subdisciplines (e.g., nursing informatics [52, 53] and public health informatics [54]).

As a clinical example, lab values for a person are *data*, those representing a person's absolute neutrophil count levels over time is *information*, levels that are trending lower and have fallen below the threshold of what is considered a normal range is *knowledge*, and discontinuation of clozapine in adherence to a guideline for people with schizophrenia is turning knowledge into *wisdom* or *action*. From a basic research perspective, expression levels from an RNA sequencing assay are *data*.

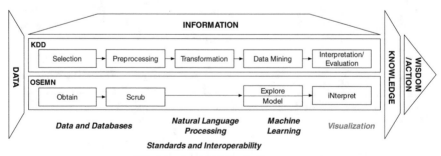

Fig. 2.4 Knowledge discovery framework

Associating those expression levels with specific genes is *information*. Observing that the set of genes with increased expression in blood samples from people with schizophrenia are enriched for a specific biological pathway turns that information into the *knowledge* of what may be a promising molecular target for therapeutic intervention. The knowledge in this sense is not a certainty, but rather is a hypothesis about how the biology works. The researcher can then use *wisdom* or take *action* by designing follow-up experiments meant to test the newly formed hypothesis.

Knowledge Discovery in Databases (KDD) as a formal process for discovering knowledge from data was also defined in 1989 [55]. KDD is the "nontrivial process of identifying valid, novel, potentially useful, and ultimately understandable patterns in data" that uses techniques from fields such as statistics, databases, artificial intelligence, and visualization [56]. The KDD process consists of a series of interactive and iterative steps for data selection, preprocessing, transformation, data mining, and interpretation/evaluation [57]. More recently, analogous data science processes such as OSEMN (Obtain, Scrub, Explore, Model, and iNterpret) have been introduced and are being widely adopted [58, 59].

2.2.2 Data and Databases

The exponential growth and digitization of data in all domains has resulted in the era of data including big data [60–62]. At a fundamental level, big data are characterized by 3Vs: (1) *Volume* reflecting the size or scale of data, (2) *Variety* representing different forms of data, and (3) *Velocity* referring to the speed at which these data are generated [63]. The 3Vs model has been enhanced with additional Vs such as *Veracity* to consider data quality issues and *Value* to highlight the worth of data [60]. Data are collected or generated in many contexts using different technologies in biomedicine and health care (e.g., biomedical researchers conducting and publishing experiments, clinicians documenting in the EHR, public health practitioners monitoring health behaviors, and individuals recording symptoms and activity). As a result, there are a wealth of data sources including biological (Chap. 7); psychological, behavioral, social, and environmental (Chap. 8); clinical (Chap. 19); and public health [64]. While these collectively reflect heterogeneous data, a core set of techniques and technologies can be used for acquisition, representation, storage, sharing, and analysis [65–70].

Data are categorized as structured, semi-structured, or unstructured [68]. *Structured* data are discrete elements that adhere to a data model and typically organized in a database. *Unstructured* data are not organized according to a data model and can be in a variety of forms such as free-text narrative, images, audio, and video. *Semi-structured* data have some organization and can be formatted as delimited files (e.g., comma-separated value [CSV] or tab-separated value [TSV]) or using a data interchange format such as eXtensible Markup Language (XML) or

Table 2.2 Categories of data

Structured				Semi-Structured	Unstructured
Id	**Attribute**	**Value**	**Units**	\<patient id = 123\>	The patient's height is
123	Height	140	Cm	\<height \> 140\</	140 centimeters and
123	Weight	63.5	Kg	height \> \<weight \> 63.5\</weight\>	weight is 63.5 kilograms.
				\</patient\>	

Javascript Object Notation (JSON). Semi-structured and unstructured data can be converted into structured data through additional processing and techniques such as natural language processing (Sect. 2.2.3 and Chap. 15). Table 2.2 provides examples of structured, semi-structured, and unstructured data. Various types of *metadata* (data about data) are needed to support discovery, identification, and use of data [71]. For example, *descriptive metadata* for articles in PubMed include title, authors, and MeSH keywords while *structural metadata* describe tables and columns for the PubMed database [72]. Metadata are critical to achieving the Findable, Accessible, Interoperable, and Reusable (FAIR) guiding principles for scientific data management and stewardship [73].

Database management systems (DBMS) are used to define, create, query, update, and administer databases [74]. With a Relational DBMS (RDBMS), data are stored in tables consisting of columns (fields) and rows (records) where keys are used to indicate relationships between tables [75]. The Structured Query Language (SQL, pronounced "sequel") is used to define and query these tables. Other database models such as NoSQL (Not Only SQL; originally non SQL or non relational) and specific types such as graph databases are growing in popularity as alternatives to the relational model [76]. Data may initially be stored in a database that is referred to as the *data repository* for real-time or transactional use, which go through an extraction, transformation, and load (ETL) process to populate a *data warehouse* for reporting and analytic purposes or *data mart* for subject-specific purposes [77]. An alternative approach is populating a *data lake* with structured, semi-structured, and unstructured data in their raw formats for subsequent use [77–79].

Regardless of the format (e.g., delimited files or database), there is often a need to first select or obtain a subset of data from one or more data sources. Algorithms for *case detection* define how to identify cases of interest based on inclusion and exclusion criteria [80]. *Computable phenotyping* [81–86] is focused on developing algorithms to identify patient cohorts using clinical data in the EHR and ancillary data sources such as Research Electronic Data Capture (REDCap [87]), health information exchanges [88, 89], or claims databases [90]. Development of standardized EHR phenotyping algorithms is critical to supporting a wide range of applications (e.g., precision medicine, clinical trials, quality improvement, and health services research) [91]. Open questions and challenges include addressing data quality and standardization issues, using natural language processing to enable use of unstructured or narrative data, and exploring machine learning compared with manual expert-generated rules [91].

2.2.3 Natural Language Processing and Text Mining

Unstructured data are abundant and reported to make up 80–90% of data in some domains. Natural language processing (NLP) combines aspects of artificial intelligence and linguistics. Natural language understanding (NLU) is a subset of NLP that involves transforming narrative into structured data while natural language generation (NLG) is focused on turning structured data into narrative form [92, 93]. A more comprehensive discussion of NLP methods and applications, evaluation, and challenges can be found in Chap. 15 and [13, 48].

Within biomedicine and health care, narrative or free-text data are generated by clinicians (e.g., clinical notes and reports in EHR systems), biomedical researchers (e.g., abstracts, titles, and full-text for biomedical literature in PubMed/MEDLINE and PubMed Central, study criteria and results in ClinicalTrials.gov, and molecular sequence metadata in GenBank), public health specialists (e.g., global reporting by the Program for Monitoring Emerging Diseases [ProMED]), and consumers (e.g., social media and text messaging). The sublanguages in these different sources of text resulted in development of specialized areas of NLP such as clinical NLP, biomedical NLP, and social media NLP, which can be collectively referred to as health NLP [94–98]. *Text mining* leverages NLP for the discovery of patterns in textual data (analogous to data mining) with similar specializations (e.g., clinical text mining and biomedical text or biomedical literature mining) [99–102].

A major application area of NLP, particularly NLU, is *information extraction* (IE) that involves extracting, encoding, and structuring named entities (e.g., genes, diseases, and medications) as well as relationships between these entities (e.g., gene-disease, disease-disease, or disease-medication) in narrative text [13, 48] (Table 2.3). Earlier systems for named entity recognition (NER) were knowledge-based involving creation and maintenance of dictionaries or rules that could be time consuming and manually intensive [103]. Over time, more automated statistical or machine learning based NLP emerged as an alternative approach. However, given the advantages and disadvantages of both approaches, a hybrid approach is commonly used. For clinical NLP, numerous systems have been developed for extraction of entities from clinical text, many of which leverage open-source frameworks (e.g., General Architecture for Text Engineering [GATE] or Unstructured Information Management Architecture [UIMA]) and normalize these entities to established knowledge source (e.g., Unified Medical Language System [UMLS] concepts) [104].

Other related application areas include *information retrieval* (IR) for indexing or categorizing documents in large collections (e.g., articles in PubMed/MEDLINE or clinical notes in the EHR), *question answering* that essentially combines IE and IR

Table 2.3 Examples of text and entity recognition

Clinical Text [105]	Biomedical Text [106]	Social Media Text [107]
The patient denied any suicidal ideation or homicidal ideation.	Risk and protective factors underlying depression and suicidal ideation in autism Spectrum disorder.	It didn't make any sense to me, the suicide thing. I refuse to believe that that is actua...

approaches for understanding and addressing natural language questions (e.g., responses to clinical questions using biomedical literature), and *text summarization* that synthesizes information from multiple sources of narrative text (e.g., patient summaries from the EHR). Consumer-oriented applications include *text simplification* to facilitate health literacy as well as *sentiment analysis* and *emotion detection* using social media and other consumer-generated text.

2.2.4   Data Mining and Machine Learning

In the context of the knowledge discovery process, *data mining* is the analysis step for discovering patterns using database, statistical, and machine learning methods that typically requires human intervention [56]. As a subfield of artificial intelligence, *machine learning* incorporates algorithms and models for automatically learning and improving at a given objective without explicit programming [108–111]. While there is significant overlap between data mining and machine learning, a distinguishing factor is the more exploratory nature and goal of discovering previously unknown knowledge of the former (e.g., trajectory of a mental health condition) compared with the more predictive nature and goal of reproducing known knowledge of the latter (e.g., prediction of a mental health condition) [112]. A more comprehensive discussion of methods and their applications, evaluation, and challenges can be found in Chap. 10 and [48].

Methods used for data mining and machine learning are categorized as supervised, unsupervised, and reinforcement [113, 114]. *Supervised learning* techniques are focused on learning a function (model) for mapping input variables (features) to an output variable (label) using a training dataset (Fig. 2.5a). The model is then optimized using a validation dataset and evaluated with a test dataset. Regression models such as linear regression are used for prediction of continuous values (e.g., age, weight, or healthcare cost) while classification models such as logistic

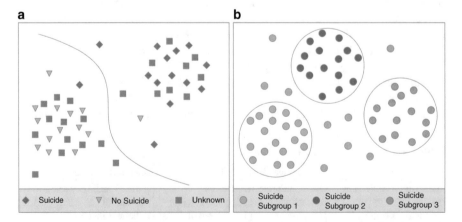

Fig. 2.5   Supervised learning (Classification) (**a**) and unsupervised learning (Clustering) (**b**)

regression, support vector machines, and decision trees focus on categorical values (e.g., presence/absence of disease, mortality, or re-admission). *Unsupervised learning* techniques aim to identify patterns from an input dataset without an output variable or label (Fig. 2.5b). For example, clustering techniques such as hierarchical and k-means can be used to identify groupings based on similarity (e.g., disease subgroups). With *reinforcement learning*, an agent learns from positive and negative feedback to arrive at an output based on provided input. *Semi-supervised learning* combines supervised and unsupervised learning by training on labeled and unlabeled data. *Deep learning* is a subset of machine learning where the methods are based on artificial neural networks that use multiple layers [115, 116].

2.2.5   Standards and Interoperability

With the range of data sources in a domain comes the challenge of too many ways to say the same thing. Standards are thus essential for supporting exchange, interpretation, integration, and use of data within and across disparate systems [13, 117]. *Syntactic interoperability* is concerned with the structure of data while *semantic interoperability* focuses on the meaning of data through common coding systems [118]. Such standards underlie common data models adopted by national and international informatics initiatives (e.g., Observational Medical Outcomes Partnership [OMOP] and Informatics for Integrating Biology & the Bedside [i2b2] [119–121]). This section provides an overview of syntactic and semantic standards that are further described in Chap. 6 and [13, 122].

There are many standards development organizations (SDO) that are responsible for developing standards in biomedicine and health care [123]. Health Level 7 International (HL7) is an SDO established in 1987 to provide "a comprehensive framework and related standards for the exchange, integration, sharing, and retrieval of electronic health information" [124]. Primary standards for integration and interoperability include HL7 Version 2.x, Version 3.x, and Fast Healthcare Interoperability Resources (FHIR, pronounced "fire") for messaging or transfer of data to support all healthcare workflows (e.g., administrative, financial, and clinical) [125]. There are many implementation guides describing how these standards can be applied in a range of contexts such as clinical genomics, clinical trials, quality reporting, and public health reporting [126]. Other standards include those focused on clinical decision support (Sect. 2.3.1 and Chap. 18). The Interoperability Standards Advisory provides guidance in the use of interoperability standards and implementation specifications for clinical, quality, public health, and research purposes [127].

Coding systems are standard sets of codes and terms that are needed to promote semantic interoperability [128]. There are coding systems for different aspects of biomedicine and health care that are distinguished as being a terminology, vocabulary, controlled vocabulary, taxonomy, thesaurus, or ontology [129]. Table 2.4 depicts some examples including those defined in the United States Core Data for

Table 2.4 Example coding systems

Abbreviation	Name	Example Code: Term
CPT	Current procedural terminology	96127: Administering, scoring, and documenting a brief behavioral or emotional screening, including measures for suicide risk
GO	Gene ontology	0003677: DNA binding
HGNC	HUGO gene nomenclature committee	5401: SP110 nuclear body protein
ICD-9/10-CM	International classification of diseases, clinical modifications	V62.94: Suicidal ideation R45.851: Suicidal ideation
ICNP	International classification for nursing practice	1002295: Suicidal ideation
LOINC	Logical observation identifiers names and codes	93245–9: Columbia–Suicide severity rating scale–Lifespan recent [C-SSRS]
MeSH	Medical subject headings	D059020: Suicidal ideation
SNOMED CT	Systematized nomenclature of medicine–Clinical terms	6471006: Suicidal thoughts (finding)
UMLS	Unified medical language system	C0424000: Feeling suicidal (finding)

Interoperability (USCDI) [130, 131]. Resources such as the Unified Medical Language System (UMLS) Knowledge Sources [132, 133] and BioPortal [134, 135] aim to facilitate mapping of data to standardized concepts as well as support integration and linkage of disparate data sources. Grouping of related terms or concepts is often needed and can be facilitated by categorization schemes such as the UMLS Semantic Network [136], Clinical Classifications Software (CCS) [137], and phecode groupings [138, 139].

2.3 From Knowledge to Performance (K2P)

The development of evidence-based innovations based on results from the D2K flow involves processes and techniques that are summarized in this chapter and further described in Chaps. 18, 19, and 20. Rapid advances in information and communications technology have resulted in increased use of digital health solutions involving health information technology (e.g., EHR, HIE, and personal health record [PHR]), mobile and wireless devices (e.g., cell phone and tablet), wearables (e.g., activity tracker and smartwatch), and telehealth and telemedicine technologies (e.g., videoconferencing and remote monitoring) [140–142]. This section highlights the role of software, knowledge, and human factors engineering in the development of technology-based innovations such as CDS tools in the EHR. In-depth discussions of related methods and applications for CDS can be found in *Improving*

Outcomes with Clinical Decision Support: An Implementer's Guide [143], *Clinical Decision Support: The Road to Broad Adoption* [144], and *Optimizing Strategies for Clinical Decision Support* [145].

2.3.1 Clinical Decision Support

The overall goal of clinical decision support (CDS) is to provide "clinicians, staff, patients, or other individuals with knowledge and person-specific information, intelligently filtered or presented at appropriate times, to enhance health and health care" [143, 145]. The CDS Five Rights framework provides guidance for creating a CDS program or implementing a CDS intervention to consider: (1) what information to provide (*the right information*), (2) who should receive the information to take action (*the right person*), (3) how to format the information (*in the right intervention form*), (4) where to deliver the information (*through the right channel*), and (5) when to present the information (*at the right time in workflow*) [146].

CDS can be broadly categorized as passive (e.g., tools for information management) and active (e.g., tools for focusing attention such as alerts and reminders) [147]. Categories of CDS include interventions to facilitate: (1) *data entry* such as order sets and documentation templates in EHR systems, (2) *data review* such as real-time reports and dashboards, (3) *assessment and understanding* such as "infobuttons" [148] that aim to address information needs by providing context-specific links to medical knowledge sources, and (4) *triggered by user task* such as alerts about abnormal results or medications as well as reminders about vaccinations and preventative care [144]. This latter category typically involves an event that initiates the execution of logic on provided data to present notifications or possible actions to an end-user.

2.3.2 Software and Knowledge Engineering

The software or systems development life cycle (SDLC) is a formal process describing phases in the life cycle of a software application or information system [48, 149]. The basic phases are: (1) requirements analysis, (2) feasibility study, (3) design, (4) implementation, (5) testing, (6) installation/deployment, and (7) maintenance [150]. There are several different SDLC methods or models that incorporate the same or similar phases but differ in how they are executed [151]. The *waterfall model* is the oldest model where there is interdependence between the phases that are performed sequentially while the *agile model* has gained in popularity due to its flexible and adaptable approach of iterative and incremental development. To promote usability, usefulness, and satisfaction with a system, user-centered design (UCD) frameworks focus on understanding users, tasks, and environment by engaging end-users (e.g., providers and patients) through a cooperative or participatory design process [152, 153].

Knowledge engineering focuses on the development of knowledge-based or expert systems and involves formal methods for acquisition, representation, management, and validation of knowledge [154]. Early CDS efforts such as MYCIN [155] involved the development of stand-alone systems such as rule-based expert systems that include several core components: *knowledge base* including facts and rules for a domain; *inference engine* for performing reasoning using the knowledge base and user-provided data; and, *user interface* for interacting with users [144]. To facilitate the sharing and exchange of CDS, knowledge representation standards were developed such as the Arden Syntax, introduced in 1989 and later adopted by HL7 in 1999, to encode rules needed to make a decision as Medical Logic Modules (MLMs) [156, 157] (Chap. 6). This resulted in the emergence of standards-based systems as well as facilitated the integration of CDS into EHR and other systems [158, 159].

The latest generation of CDS explores use of service-oriented architecture that leverages web application programming interfaces (API) [160]. In 2009, Substitutable Medical Applications, Reusable Technologies (SMART) emerged as an open platform for third-party applications that are immediately "tangible, interoperability supporting, and vendor-independent" [161]. Leveraging HL7 standards, SMART on FHIR apps can interface with or be integrated into systems (e.g., EHR, PHR, or HIE) [162] and SMART CDS Hooks can be used for additional decision support services (e.g., executing rules on patient data and providing a response) [163, 164]. More recently, SMART Markers was created as a framework for patient-generated health data [165].

2.3.3 Human Factors Engineering

Considering human factors and ergonomics is essential in the process of developing a technology-based solution [166–169]. Human factors engineering (HFE) is a "scientific discipline that provides insights into design (or redesign) of healthcare systems and processes impacting patient safety and quality of care" and focuses on "improving human performance by accounting for their cognitive and physical limitations" [170]. At the macro-level, models such as the Systems Engineering Initiative for Patient Safety (SEIPS) can be used to study the interactions between the work system (e.g., clinicians interacting with a CDS tool in the EHR), effects on healthcare processes, and outcomes such as patient safety and healthcare quality [171].

Micro-level efforts focus on specific problems in a given context and involve use of HFE approaches that can be used to study complex environments in biomedicine and health care [168]. For example, Task, User, Presentation, and Function (TURF) is a unified framework developed for understanding EHR usability that is defined as "how useful, usable, and satisfying a system is for the intended users to accomplish goals in the work domain by performing certain sequences of tasks" [172]. Cognitive and usability engineering methods such as cognitive task analysis, cognitive walk-throughs, and heuristic evaluation can be used to identify or inspect usability issues based on conducting specific tasks in laboratory or naturalistic settings during the design phase [173, 174]. In contrast, usability testing methods include direct observations and think aloud protocols of users interacting with a system and performing tasks for characterizing usability problems.

2.4   From Performance to Data (P2D)

The adoption and sustainability of evidence-based innovations developed as part of the K2P flow involve processes and techniques that are summarized in this chapter and further in *Evaluation Methods in Biomedical Informatics* [175], *Evidence-Based Health Informatics* [176], and *Cognitive Informatics in Health and Biomedicine* [177]. Many of these are used in implementation science that is focused on "the scientific study of methods to promote the systematic uptake of research findings and other evidence-based practices into routine practice, and, hence, improve the quality and effectiveness of health services" [178]. There is overlap with approaches in quality improvement (e.g., Lean and Six Sigma) that also has a goal of improving the quality of healthcare, but is typically driven by a particular problem in a specific healthcare system [179, 180]. Dissemination is also a related activity that is focused on the spread of information about an evidence-based innovation through education and training [179, 180]. This section highlights some frameworks, methods, and metrics used in biomedical informatics and implementation science for the evaluation of technology-based innovations such as CDS tools in the EHR.

2.4.1   Evaluation Models

There are numerous theories, models, and frameworks for promoting the translation of knowledge into practice as well as testing the efficacy and effectiveness of interventions in optimal and real-world settings respectively [179, 181, 182]. A range of methods can be used to evaluate the implementation process, impact, and uptake of a technology-based solution by identifying and addressing barriers and facilitators [176, 183, 184]. Technology assessment is "any process of examining and reporting properties of a medical technology used in health care, such as safety, efficacy, feasibility, and indication for use, costs, and cost effectiveness, as well as social, economic, and ethical consequences, whether intended or unintended" [185].

Evaluation studies can involve characterization of use before, during, and after implementation (*process evaluation*), assessment of user needs and requirements prior to or during implementation (*formative evaluation*), and measurement of outcomes and impact after implementation (*summative evaluation*) [175, 179]. Process models such as Reach, Efficacy, Adoption, Implementation, Maintenance (RE-AIM) study the impact of an intervention at the individual, organizational, and community levels [186, 187]. The Practical, Robust Implementation and Sustainability Model (PRISM) model extends RE-AIM to facilitate the integration of research findings into practice by considering a range of factors (e.g., organizational, patient, environment, and infrastructure) [188]. The Consolidated Framework for Implementation Research (CFIR) brings together implementation theories, including those for process, formative, and summative evaluation, into a comprehensive framework for facilitating the translation of research findings into practice [189]. CFIR incorporates constructs in five domains: (1) intervention characteristics, (2) outer setting, (3) inner setting, (4) characteristics of the individuals involved, and (5) and process of implementation.

2.4.2   Quantitative and Qualitative Methods

Quantitative, qualitative, and mixed methods can be used for evaluation throughout the learning healthcare system process (D2K, K2P, and P2D). Objectivist studies typically involve comparisons of variables (independent and dependent) with and without an innovation using quantitative statistical methods [175]. A contingency table, particularly a 2x2 table, can be used to characterize accuracy (true positives [TP] and true negatives [TN]) and errors (false positives [FP] and false negatives [FN]) associated with an innovation compared with a gold or reference standard. These can be used to calculate sensitivity (TP/TP + FN), specificity (TN/FP + FN), and area under the receiver operating characteristic curve based on plotting sensitivity and 1-sensitivity at different thresholds. In cases where true negatives cannot be determined, recall (TP/TP + FN), precision (TP/TP + FP), and area under the precision-recall curve can be calculated [190]. These represent some metrics that are commonly used for assessing the performance of techniques such as NLP and machine learning as part of the D2K flow as well as technology-based innovations such as CDS tools developed as part of the K2P flow.

Engagement of stakeholders as part of the software development process in the K2P flow or implementation and dissemination process in the P2D flow involves the use of surveys and qualitative methods for data collection and analysis [174, 191]. A content or thematic analysis involves identifying patterns in data collected from subjectivist methods such as surveys, interviews, focus groups, and observations [192]. Other approaches such as grounded theory provide more formal frameworks that are guided by specific theories, research questions, and data collection and analysis procedures [193].

2.5   Summary

Biomedical informatics is a transdisciplinary field that is concerned with the effective use of data, information, and knowledge, often leveraging information and communications technology, to improve human health. This chapter highlights some of the frameworks and methods in the context of a learning healthcare system. The foundations and applications of biomedical informatics will continue to advance and play a critical role in supporting health and health care, including mental health care.

References

1. Collen MF. A history of medical informatics in the United States, 1950 to 1990, vol. xv. Indianapolis, IN: American Medical Informatics Association; 1995. p. 489.
2. J Ball M. The history of medical informatics in the United States. New York, NY: Springer Berlin Heidelberg; 2015.
3. Greenes RA, Shortliffe EH. Medical informatics. An emerging academic discipline and institutional priority. JAMA. 1990;263(8):1114–20.
4. Hagen JB. The origins of bioinformatics. Nat Rev Genet. 2000;1(3):231–6.
5. Martin-Sanchez F, et al. Synergy between medical informatics and bioinformatics: facilitating genomic medicine for future health care. J Biomed Inform. 2004;37(1):30–42.
6. Maojo V, et al. Medical informatics and bioinformatics: European efforts to facilitate synergy. J Biomed Inform. 2001;34(6):423–7.
7. Kulikowski CA, et al. AMIA board white paper: definition of biomedical informatics and specification of core competencies for graduate education in the discipline. J Am Med Inform Assoc. 2012;19(6):931–8.
8. Oxford English Dictionary, O.E., "*informatics, n.*". Oxford University Press.
9. Oxford English Dictionary, O.E., "*bioinformatics, n.*". Oxford University Press.
10. Luscombe NM, Greenbaum D, Gerstein M. What is bioinformatics? A proposed definition and overview of the field. Methods Inf Med. 2001;40(4):346–58.
11. van Bemmel JH. The structure of medical informatics. Med Inform (Lond). 1984;9(3–4):175–80.
12. Bemmel JHv, Musen MA, Helder JC. Handbook of medical informatics, vol. xl. AW Houten, Netherlands, Heidelberg, Germany: Bohn Stafleu Van Loghum: Springer Verlag; 1997. 621 p.
13. Shortliffe E, Cimino J. Biomedical informatics, vol. 12. London: Springer London; 2014. https://doi.org/10.1007/978-1-4471-4474-8.
14. Bernstam EV, Smith JW, Johnson TR. What is biomedical informatics? J Biomed Inform. 2010;43(1):104–10.
15. Valenta AL, et al. AMIA board white paper: AMIA 2017 core competencies for applied health informatics education at the master's degree level. J Am Med Inform Assoc. 2018;25(12):1657–68.
16. Mantas J, et al. Recommendations of the international medical informatics association (IMIA) on education in biomedical and health informatics. First revision. Methods Inf Med. 2010;49(2):105–20.
17. Jaspers MW, et al. IMIA accreditation of biomedical and health informatics education: current state and future directions. Yearb Med Inform. 2017;26(1):252–6.

18. Chen ES, Sarkar IN. Informatics: identifying and tracking informatics sub-discipline terms in the literature. Methods Inf Med. 2015;54(6):530–9.
19. Hersh W. A stimulus to define informatics and health information technology. BMC Med Inform Decis Mak. 2009;9:24.
20. Kuhn KA, et al. Informatics and medicine–from molecules to populations. Methods Inf Med. 2008;47(4):283–95.
21. Payne PR, Embi PJ, Sen CK. Translational informatics: enabling high-throughput research paradigms. Physiol Genomics. 2009;39(3):131–40.
22. Payne PRO, Bernstam EV, Starren JB. Biomedical informatics meets data science: current state and future directions for interaction. JAMIA Open. 2018;1(2):136–141.
23. Boland MR, et al. Birth month affects lifetime disease risk: a phenome-wide method. J Am Med Inform Assoc. 2015;22(5):1042–53.
24. Sarkar IN. Biomedical informatics and translational medicine. J Transl Med. 2010;8:22.
25. Ball MJ, Hannah KJ. Nursing informatics: where technology and caring meet, Health informatics, vol. xxxi. 4th ed. London; New York: Springer; 2011. p. 482.
26. Saba VK, McCormick KA. Essentials of nursing informatics, vol. xxiii. 6th ed. New York: McGraw-Hill Education; 2015. p. 886.
27. Abbey LM, Zimmerman JL. Dental informatics: integrating technology into the dental environment. Computers in health care, vol. xiii. New York: Springer; 1992. p. 348.
28. Lewis D. Consumer health informatics: informing consumers and improving health care. Health informatics. New York: Springer; 2005. p. xxi, 258 p.
29. Consumer informatics and digital health: solutions for health and health care. 2018, New York, NY: Springer Science+Business Media, LLC. pages cm.
30. Payne PR, Embi PJ. Translational informatics: realizing the promise of knowledge-driven healthcare: Springer; 2014.
31. Butte AJ. Translational bioinformatics: coming of age. J Am Med Inform Assoc. 2008;15(6):709–14.
32. Sarkar IN, et al. Translational bioinformatics: linking knowledge across biological and clinical realms. J Am Med Inform Assoc. 2011;18(4):354–7.
33. Tenenbaum JD. Translational bioinformatics: past, present, and future. Genomics Proteomics Bioinformatics. 2016;14(1):31–41.
34. Richesson RL, Andrews JE. Clinical research informatics. Health informatics, vol. ix. London; New York: Springer; 2012. 419 pages.
35. Dixon BE, et al. What's past is prologue: a scoping review of recent public health and Global Health informatics literature. Online J Public Health Inform. 2015;7(2):e216.
36. Silva JS. Cancer informatics: essential technologies for clinical trials. Health informatics, vol. xxvi. New York: Springer; 2002. p. 377.
37. Oli AN, et al. Immunoinformatics and vaccine development: an overview. Immunotargets Ther. 2020;9:13–30.
38. Hanson A, Levin BL. Mental health informatics, vol. x. New York: Oxford University Press; 2013. p. 274.
39. Diederich J, Song I. Mental health informatics: current approaches, in Mental Health Informatics: Springer; 2014. p. 1–16.
40. Lehmann CU, Kim GR, Johnson KB. Pediatric informatics: computer applications in child health. Health informatics series, vol. xxiv. Dordrecht; New York: Springer; 2009. 483 p.
41. Pantanowitz L, et al. Pathology informatics: theory & practice, vol. xvi. Chicago, Ill: American Society for Clinical Pathology Press; 2012. 352 p.
42. Sinard JH. Practical pathology informatics: demystifying informatics for the practicing anatomic pathologist, vol. xix. New York: Springer Science+Business Media; 2006. p. 393.
43. Lustgarten J. et al. Veterinary informatics: forging the future between veterinary medicine, human medicine, and One Health initiatives—a joint paper by the Association of Veterinary Informatics (AVI) and the CTSA One Health Alliance (COHA). JAMIA Open, 2020.
44. Institute of Medicine (U.S.). Roundtable on Value & Science-Driven Health Care, et al. Digital infrastructure for the learning health system: the foundation for continuous improvement in health and health care: workshop series summary. Learning health system series, vol. xxvi. Washington, D.C: National Academies Press; 2011. 308 p.

45. Friedman C, et al. Toward a science of learning systems: a research agenda for the high-functioning learning health system. J Am Med Inform Assoc. 2015;22(1):43–50.
46. Friedman CP, Rubin JC, Sullivan KJ. Toward an information infrastructure for Global Health improvement. Yearb Med Inform. 2017;26(1):16–23.
47. Flynn AJ, et al. The knowledge object reference ontology (KORO): a formalism to support management and sharing of computable biomedical knowledge for learning health systems. Learn Health Syst. 2018;2(2):e10054.
48. Sarkar IN. Methods in biomedical informatics: a pragmatic approach. Amsterdam: Elsevier/AP, Academic Press is an imprint of Elsevier; 2014. p. xvi, 571 pages.
49. Ackoff RL. From data to wisdom. J Appl Syst Anal. 1989;16(1):3–9.
50. Zins C. Conceptual approaches for defining data, information, and knowledge. J Am Soc Info Sci Tech. 2007;58(4):479–93.
51. Rowley J. The wisdom hierarchy: representations of the DIKW hierarchy. J Inf Sci. 2007;33(2):163–80.
52. Matney S, et al. Philosophical approaches to the nursing informatics data-information-knowledge-wisdom framework. ANS Adv Nurs Sci. 2011;34(1):6–18.
53. Ronquillo C, Currie LM, Rodney P. The evolution of data-information-knowledge-wisdom in nursing informatics. ANS Adv Nurs Sci. 2016;39(1):E1–18.
54. Dammann O. Data, information, evidence, and knowledge:: a proposal for health informatics and data science. Online J Public Health Inform. 2018;10(3):e224.
55. Piateski G, Frawley W. Knowledge discovery in databases. 1991: MIT press.
56. Fayyad U, Piatetsky-Shapiro G, Smyth P. From data mining to knowledge discovery in databases. AI Mag. 1996;17(3):37.
57. Kurgan LA, Musilek P. A survey of knowledge discovery and data mining process models. Knowl Eng Rev. 2006;21(1):1–24.
58. Mason H, Wiigins C. A taxonomy of data science. Available from: http://www.dataists.com/2010/09/a-taxonomy-of-data-science/.
59. Janssens J, editor. Data science at the command line, vol. xvii. 1st ed. Sebastopol, CA: O'Reilly; 2014. 191 pages.
60. Yin S, Kaynak O. Big data for modern industry: challenges and trends [point of view]. Proc IEEE. 2015;103(2):143–6.
61. Jagadish H. Big data and science: myths and reality. Big Data Res. 2015;2(2):49–52.
62. Berman JJ. Principles of big data: preparing, sharing, and analyzing complex information, vol. xxvi. Amsterdam: Elsevier, Morgan Kaufmann; 2013. 261 pages.
63. Zikopoulos P. Understanding big data: analytics for enterprise class Hadoop and streaming data, vol. xxxi. New York: McGraw-Hill; 2012. 141 pages
64. Weber GM, Mandl KD, Kohane IS. Finding the missing link for big biomedical data. JAMA. 2014;311(24):2479–80.
65. Tan SS, Gao G, Koch S. Big data and analytics in healthcare. Methods Inf Med. 2015;54(6):546–7.
66. Ross MK, Wei W, Ohno-Machado L. "Big data" and the electronic health record. Yearb Med Inform. 2014;9:97–104.
67. Chen ES, Sarkar IN. Mining the electronic health record for disease knowledge. Methods Mol Biol. 2014;1159:269–86.
68. Gandomi A, Haider M. Beyond the hype: big data concepts, methods, and analytics. Int J Inf Manag. 2015;35(2):137–44.
69. Collen MF. Computer medical databases: the first six decades (1950–2010). Health informatics, vol. xix. London; New York: Springer; 2012. 288 p.
70. Beam AL, Kohane IS. Big data and machine learning in healthcare. JAMA. 2018;319(13):1317–8.
71. Riley J. Understanding metadata. National Information Standards Organization, 2017.
72. Zhang AB, Gourley D. Creating digital collections: a practical guide. Chandos information professional series. 2009, Oxford: Chandos Pub xiv, 234 p.
73. Wilkinson MD, et al. The FAIR guiding principles for scientific data management and stewardship. Sci Data. 2016;3:160018.
74. Ramakrishnan R, Gehrke J. Database management systems, vol. xxxii. 3rd ed. Boston: McGraw-Hill; 2003. p. 1065.

75. Codd EF. The relational model for database management: version 2, vol. xxii. Reading, Mass: Addison-Wesley; 1990. 538 p
76. Jatana N, et al. A survey and comparison of relational and non-relational database. Int J Eng Res Tech. 2012;1(6):1–5.
77. Sholle ET, et al. Secondary use of Patients' electronic records (SUPER): an approach for meeting specific data needs of clinical and translational researchers. AMIA Annu Symp Proc. 2017;2017:1581–8.
78. Stein B, Morrison A. The enterprise data lake: Better integration and deeper analytics.
79. Gorelik A. The enterprise big data lake: delivering the promise of big data and data science, vol. xiii. 1st ed. Sebastopol, California: iO'Reilly Media, Inc; 2019. 205 pages.
80. Ford E, et al. Extracting information from the text of electronic medical records to improve case detection: a systematic review. J Am Med Inform Assoc. 2016;23(5):1007–15.
81. Richesson RL, et al. Electronic health records based phenotyping in next-generation clinical trials: a perspective from the NIH health care systems Collaboratory. J Am Med Inform Assoc. 2013;20(e2):e226–31.
82. Hripcsak G, Albers DJ. Next-generation phenotyping of electronic health records. J Am Med Inform Assoc. 2013;20(1):117–21.
83. Shivade C, et al. A review of approaches to identifying patient phenotype cohorts using electronic health records. J Am Med Inform Assoc. 2014;21(2):221–30.
84. Wei WQ, Denny JC. Extracting research-quality phenotypes from electronic health records to support precision medicine. Genome Med. 2015;7(1):41.
85. Richesson RL, et al. Clinical phenotyping in selected national networks: demonstrating the need for high-throughput, portable, and computational methods. Artif Intell Med. 2016;71:57–61.
86. Pendergrass SA, Crawford DC. Using electronic health records to generate phenotypes for research. Curr Protoc Hum Genet. 2019;100(1):e80.
87. Harris PA, et al. Research electronic data capture (REDCap)–a metadata-driven methodology and workflow process for providing translational research informatics support. J Biomed Inform. 2009;42(2):377–81.
88. Devine EB, et al. Health information exchange use (1990-2015): a systematic review. EGEMS (Wash DC). 2017;5(1):27.
89. Menachemi N, et al. The benefits of health information exchange: an updated systematic review. J Am Med Inform Assoc. 2018;25(9):1259–65.
90. Peters A, et al. The value of all-payer claims databases to states. N C Med J. 2014;75(3):211–3.
91. Electronic Health Records-Based Phenotyping. Available from: https://rethinkingclinicaltrials.org/resources/ehr-phenotyping/.
92. Jurafsky D, Martin JH. Speech and language processing: an introduction to natural language processing, computational linguistics, and speech recognition, Prentice Hall series in artificial intelligence, vol. xxxi. 2nd ed. Upper Saddle River, N.J: Pearson Prentice Hall; 2009. 988 p.
93. Allen JF. Natural language processing. 2003.
94. Filannino M, Uzuner O. Advancing the state of the art in clinical natural language processing through shared tasks. Yearb Med Inform. 2018;27(1):184–92.
95. Velupillai S, et al. Using clinical natural language processing for health outcomes research: overview and actionable suggestions for future advances. J Biomed Inform. 2018;88:11–9.
96. Cohen KB, Demner-Fushman D. *Biomedical natural language processing*. Natural language processing (NLP), vol. x. Amsterdam; Philadelphia: John Benjamins Publishing Company; 2014. 160 pages.
97. Doan S, et al. Natural language processing in biomedicine: a unified system architecture overview. Methods Mol Biol. 2014;1168:275–94.
98. Conway M, Hu M, Chapman WW. Recent advances in using natural language processing to address public Health Research questions using social media and ConsumerGenerated data. Yearb Med Inform. 2019;28(1):208–17.

99. Hearst MA. Untangling text data mining. In Proceedings of the 37th annual meeting of the Association for Computational Linguistics on Computational Linguistics. 1999. Association for Computational Linguistics.

100. Zweigenbaum P, et al. Frontiers of biomedical text mining: current progress. Brief Bioinform. 2007;8(5):358–75.

101. Shatkay H, Feldman R. Mining the biomedical literature in the genomic era: an overview. J Comput Biol. 2003;10(6):821–55.

102. Kumar VD, Tipney HJ. Biomedical literature mining. Methods in molecular biology, vol. xii. New York: Humana Press; 2014. 288 p.

103. Nadkarni PM, Ohno-Machado L, Chapman WW. Natural language processing: an introduction. J Am Med Inform Assoc. 2011;18(5):544–51.

104. Wang Y, et al. Clinical information extraction applications: a literature review. J Biomed Inform. 2018;77:34–49.

105. Available from: http://medicaltranscriptionwordhelp.synthasite.com/mental-status-exam-common-words-and-phrases.php.

106. Hedley D, et al. Risk and protective factors underlying depression and suicidal ideation in autism Spectrum disorder. Depress Anxiety. 2018;35(7):648–57.

107. Sentiment140 dataset with 1.6 million tweets. Available from: https://www.kaggle.com/kazanova/sentiment140.

108. Russell SJ, Norvig P. Artificial intelligence: a modern approach. Fourth edition. Ed. Pearson series in artificial intelligence. Hoboken: Pearson. pages cm; 2021.

109. Shalev-Shwartz S, Ben-David S. Understanding machine learning: from theory to algorithms, vol. xvi. New York, NY, USA: Cambridge University Press; 2014. 397 pages.

110. Bishop CM. Pattern recognition and machine learning. Information science and statistics. New York: Springer; 2006. p. xx, 738 p.

111. Yu KH, Beam AL, Kohane IS. Artificial intelligence in healthcare. Nat Biomed Eng. 2018;2(10):719–31.

112. Witten IH, Witten IH. Data mining: practical machine learning tools and techniques, vol. xxxii. 4th ed. Amsterdam: Elsevier; 2017. p. 621.

113. Maini V, Sabri S, Machine learning for humans. Online: https://medium.com/machine-learning-for-humans, 2017.

114. Rajkomar A, Dean J, Kohane I. Machine learning in medicine. N Engl J Med. 2019;380(14):1347–58.

115. Wang F, Casalino LP, Khullar D. Deep learning in medicine-promise, Progress, and challenges. JAMA Intern Med. 2019;179(3):293–4.

116. Esteva A, et al. A guide to deep learning in healthcare. Nat Med. 2019;25(1):24–9.

117. Chen ES, Melton GB, Sarkar IN. Translating standards into practice: experiences and lessons learned in biomedicine and health care. J Biomed Inform. 2012;45(4):609–12.

118. Dolin RH, Alschuler L. Approaching semantic interoperability in health level seven. J Am Med Inform Assoc. 2011;18(1):99–103.

119. Overhage JM, et al. Validation of a common data model for active safety surveillance research. J Am Med Inform Assoc. 2012;19(1):54–60.

120. Murphy SN, et al. Serving the enterprise and beyond with informatics for integrating biology and the bedside (i2b2). J Am Med Inform Assoc. 2010;17(2):124–30.

121. Klann JG, et al. Data model harmonization for the all of us research program: transforming i2b2 data into the OMOP common data model. PLoS One. 2019;14(2):e0212463.

122. Schulz S, Stegwee R, Chronaki C. Standards in healthcare data, in fundamentals of clinical data science, P. Kubben, M. Dumontier, and A. Dekker, Editors. 2019: Cham (CH). p. 19–36.

123. Hammond WE. The making and adoption of health data standards. Health Aff (Millwood). 2005;24(5):1205–13.

124. About HL7. Available from: https://www.hl7.org/about/index.cfm?ref=nav.

125. Benson T. Principles of health interoperability: snomed ct, hl7 and fhir. New York, NY: Springer Berlin Heidelberg. pages cm; 2016.

126. HL7 Implementation Guides. Available from: https://www.hl7.org/implement/standards/product_section.cfm?section=22&ref=nav.
127. Interoperability Standards Advisory. Available from: https://www.healthit.gov/isa/.
128. Cimino JJ. Review paper: coding systems in health care. Methods Inf Med. 1996;35(4–5):273–84.
129. Cimino JJ, Zhu X. The practical impact of ontologies on biomedical informatics. Yearb Med Inform. 2006:124–35.
130. U.S. Core Data for Interoperability (USCDI). Available from: https://www.healthit.gov/isa/us-core-data-interoperability-uscdi.
131. Bodenreider O, Cornet R, Vreeman DJ. Recent developments in clinical terminologies - SNOMED CT, LOINC, and RxNorm. Yearb Med Inform. 2018;27(1):129–39.
132. Lindberg C. The unified medical language system (UMLS) of the National Library of medicine. J Am Med Rec Assoc. 1990;61(5):40–2.
133. McCray AT, Nelson SJ. The representation of meaning in the UMLS. Methods Inf Med. 1995;34(1–2):193–201.
134. Noy NF, et al. BioPortal: ontologies and integrated data resources at the click of a mouse. Nucleic Acids Res. 2009;37(Web Server issue):W170–3.
135. Musen MA, et al. The National Center for biomedical ontology. J Am Med Inform Assoc. 2012;19(2):190–5.
136. McCray AT, Burgun A, Bodenreider O. Aggregating UMLS semantic types for reducing conceptual complexity. Stud Health Technol Inform. 2001;84(Pt 1):216–20.
137. Salsabili M, Kiogou S, Adam TJ. The evaluation of clinical classifications software using the National Inpatient Sample Database. AMIA Jt Summits Transl Sci Proc. 2020;2020:542–51.
138. Wu P, et al. Mapping ICD-10 and ICD-10-CM codes to Phecodes: workflow development and initial evaluation. JMIR Med Inform. 2019;7(4):e14325.
139. Wei WQ, et al. Evaluating phecodes, clinical classification software, and ICD-9-CM codes for phenome-wide association studies in the electronic health record. PLoS One. 2017;12(7):e0175508.
140. Digital health. Scaling healthcare to the world. New York, NY: Springer Berlin Heidelberg. pages cm; 2017.
141. Digital Health. Available from: https://www.fda.gov/medical-devices/digital-health.
142. World Health Organization, W.H., Recommendations on Digital Interventions for Health System Strengthening. 2019.
143. Osheroff JA, et al. A roadmap for national action on clinical decision support. J Am Med Inform Assoc. 2007;14(2):141–5.
144. Greenes RA. Clinical decision support: the road to broad adoption, vol. xxxix. 2nd ed. Amsterdam Boston: Academic; 2014. p. 887.
145. Tcheng JE, National Academy of Medicine (U.S.). Optimizing strategies for clinical decision support: summary of a meeting series, in The learning health system series. Washington, DC: National Academy of Medicine; 2017. p. 1 online resource
146. Osheroff JA, Healthcare Information and Management Systems Society. Improving outcomes with clinical decision support: an implementer's guide, vol. xxiii. 2nd ed. Chicago, IL: HIMSS; 2012. p. 323.
147. Bell GC, et al. Development and use of active clinical decision support for preemptive pharmacogenomics. J Am Med Inform Assoc. 2014;21(e1):e93–9.
148. Cook DA, et al. Context-sensitive decision support (infobuttons) in electronic health records: a systematic review. J Am Med Inform Assoc. 2017;24(2):460–8.
149. Introduction to Software Engineering/Process/Life Cycle. Available from: https://en.wikibooks.org/wiki/Introduction_to_Software_Engineering/Process/Life_Cycle.
150. Kushniruk A. Evaluation in the design of health information systems: application of approaches emerging from usability engineering. Comput Biol Med. 2002;32(3):141–9.
151. Sommerville I. Software engineering, vol. xv. 9th ed. Boston: Pearson; 2011. p. 773.
152. Luna D, et al. User-centered design to develop clinical applications. Literature review. Stud Health Technol Inform. 2015;216:967.

153. Kushniruk A, Nohr C. Participatory design, user involvement and health IT evaluation. Stud Health Technol Inform. 2016;222:139–51.
154. Payne PR. Chapter 1: Biomedical knowledge integration. PLoS Comput Biol. 2012;8(12):e1002826.
155. Shortliffe EH, et al. Computer-based consultations in clinical therapeutics: explanation and rule acquisition capabilities of the MYCIN system. Comput Biomed Res. 1975;8(4): 303–20.
156. Pryor TA, Hripcsak G. The Arden syntax for medical logic modules. Int J Clin Monit Comput. 1993;10(4):215–24.
157. Hripcsak G. Writing Arden syntax medical logic modules. Comput Biol Med. 1994;24(5):331–63.
158. Wright A, Sittig DF. A four-phase model of the evolution of clinical decision support architectures. Int J Med Inform. 2008;77(10):641–9.
159. Wright A, Sittig DF. A framework and model for evaluating clinical decision support architectures. J Biomed Inform. 2008;41(6):982–90.
160. Loya SR, et al. Service oriented architecture for clinical decision support: a systematic review and future directions. J Med Syst. 2014;38(12):140.
161. Mandl KD, et al. The SMART platform: early experience enabling substitutable applications for electronic health records. J Am Med Inform Assoc. 2012;19(4):597–603.
162. Mandel JC, et al. SMART on FHIR: a standards-based, interoperable apps platform for electronic health records. J Am Med Inform Assoc. 2016;23(5):899–908.
163. Spineth M, Rappelsberger A, Adlassnig KP. Implementing CDS hooks communication in an Arden-syntax-based clinical decision support platform. Stud Health Technol Inform. 2018;255:165–9.
164. Dolin RH, Boxwala A, Shalaby J. A pharmacogenomics clinical decision support service based on FHIR and CDS hooks. Methods Inf Med. 2018;57(S 02):e115–23.
165. Sayeed R, Gottlieb D, Mandl KD. SMART markers: collecting patient-generated health data as a standardized property of health information technology. NPJ Digit Med. 2020;3:9.
166. Pelayo S, et al. Human factors and sociotechnical issues. Yearb Med Inform. 2019;28(1):78–80.
167. Patel VL, Kannampallil TG. Human factors and health information technology: current challenges and future directions. Yearb Med Inform. 2014;9:58–66.
168. Kushniruk A, Nohr C, Borycki E. Human factors for more usable and safer health information technology: where are we now and where do we go from here? Yearb Med Inform. 2016;1:120–5.
169. Turner P, Kushniruk A, Nohr C. Are we there yet? Human factors knowledge and health information technology - the challenges of implementation and impact. Yearb Med Inform. 2017;26(1):84–91.
170. Carayon P, et al. Human factors systems approach to healthcare quality and patient safety. Appl Ergon. 2014;45(1):14–25.
171. Carayon P, et al. Work system design for patient safety: the SEIPS model. Qual Saf Health Care. 2006;15(Suppl 1):i50–8.
172. Zhang J, Walji MF. TURF: toward a unified framework of EHR usability. J Biomed Inform. 2011;44(6):1056–67.
173. Kushniruk AW, Patel VL. Cognitive and usability engineering methods for the evaluation of clinical information systems. J Biomed Inform. 2004;37(1):56–76.
174. Borycki EM, et al. Use of qualitative methods across the software development lifecycle in health informatics. Stud Health Technol Inform. 2011;164:293–7.
175. Friedman CP, Wyatt J. Evaluation methods in biomedical informatics, Health informatics, vol. xvii. 2nd ed. New York: Springer; 2006. p. 386.
176. Ammenwerth E, Rigby M. Evidence-based health informatics: promoting safety and efficiency through scientific methods and ethical policy. Studies in health technology and informatics, vol. xv. Amsterdam; Washington, DC: IOS Press; 2016. 369 pages.
177. Cognitive informatics in health and biomedicine. Understanding and modeling health behaviors. New York, NY: Springer Berlin Heidelberg. pages cm; 2017.

178. Eccles M, Mittman B. Welcome to implementation science. Implement Sci. 2006:**1**(1).
179. Bauer MS, et al. An introduction to implementation science for the non-specialist. BMC Psychol. 2015;3:32.
180. Bauer MS, Kirchner J. Implementation science: what is it and why should I care? Psychiatry Res. 2020;283:112376.
181. Nilsen P. Making sense of implementation theories, models and frameworks. Implement Sci. 2015;10:53.
182. Tabak RG, et al. Bridging research and practice: models for dissemination and implementation research. Am J Prev Med. 2012;43(3):337–50.
183. World Health Organization, Monitoring and evaluating digital health interventions: a practical guide to conducting research and assessment. 2016.
184. Murray E, et al. Evaluating digital health interventions: key questions and approaches. Am J Prev Med. 2016;51(5):843–51.
185. Institute of Medicine (U.S.). Committee for Evaluating Medical Technologies in Clinical Use., Institute of Medicine (U.S.). Division of health sciences policy., and Institute of Medicine (U.S.). division of health promotion and disease prevention., Assessing medical technologies, vol. xvii. Washington, D.C.: National Academy Press; 1985. p. 573.
186. Gaglio B, Shoup JA, Glasgow RE. The RE-AIM framework: a systematic review of use over time. Am J Public Health. 2013;103(6):e38–46.
187. Glasgow RE, et al. RE-AIM planning and evaluation framework: adapting to new science and practice with a 20-year review. Front Public Health. 2019;7:64.
188. Feldstein AC, Glasgow RE. A practical, robust implementation and sustainability model (PRISM) for integrating research findings into practice. Jt Comm J Qual Patient Saf. 2008;34(4):228–43.
189. Damschroder LJ, et al. Fostering implementation of health services research findings into practice: a consolidated framework for advancing implementation science. Implement Sci. 2009;4:50.
190. Tharwat A. Classification assessment methods. Applied Computing and Informatics, 2018.
191. Hamilton AB, Finley EP. Qualitative methods in implementation research: an introduction. Psychiatry Res. 2019;280:112516.
192. Anderson JG, Aydin CE. Evaluating the organizational impact of healthcare information systems. 2nd ed. health informatics series. New York, NY: Springer. xv; 2005. p. 344.
193. Cummings E, Borycki EM. Grounded theory evolution and its application in health informatics. Stud Health Technol Inform. 2011;164:286–92.

Chapter 3
The Mental Health System: Definitions and Diagnoses

John L. Beyer and Mina Boazak

Abstract The way we define health and well-being has shifted throughout human history. This chapter reviews three primary views of health and illness (pathogenic, salutogenic, and halogenic models) and how each view influences our understanding of mental health and illness. We discuss the idea that health and illness may be viewed both as a continuum of wellness, and as distinct, but related, concepts. Next, we review various theories of psychopathology (biological, psychological, and social theories) and introduce the current biopsychosocial theory of illness. Finally, we review the two primary nosologies used for diagnosing mental health conditions, and estimating their prevalence, in the United States.

Keywords Mental health · Mental wellbeing · Diagnostic standards · DSM-5 ICD-10 · Theories of psychopathology

3.1 Introduction

It has been a widely reported and replicated finding that diagnosable mental health conditions affect approximately 23% of the adult population at any given time [1], and that up to half of all adults in developed countries meet the criteria for an anxiety, mood, or substance use disorder at some point in their lives [2]. Further, it is frequently observed that these problems are universal. They affect people of all countries, cultures, ages, gender, socioeconomic status, and geographical environments. Globally, over 500 million people suffer from a mental disorder [3].

The impact of poor mental health on individuals' lives, social relationships, and the global economy is profound. According to the World Health Organization

J. L. Beyer · M. Boazak (✉)
Duke University School of Medicine, Department of Psychiatry
and Behavioral Sciences, Durham, NC, USA
e-mail: john.beyer@duke.edu; mina.boazak@duke.edu

© Springer Nature Switzerland AG 2021
J. D. Tenenbaum, P. A. Ranallo (eds.), *Mental Health Informatics*, Health
Informatics, https://doi.org/10.1007/978-3-030-70558-9_3

(WHO), mental health conditions contribute 14% to the global burden of disease, though it is estimated that the real contribution is even higher due to the complex interaction of physical and mental illness. In the US, the suicide rate is 13.5 per 100,000 people and rising. It is the 10th leading cause of death for all ages (and the second-leading cause of death among people between the age of 10–34) [4]. Even when suicide is excluded from mortality statistics, those living with mental health conditions have been shown to have a lower average life expectancy than the general population and a higher rate of co-occuring health conditions.

Unfortunately, access to high quality mental healthcare is a major public health issue. Even in the twenty-first century, there is significant stigma and discrimination attached to mental helath conditions, particularly compared with physical health conditions. The WHO estimates that between 35–50% of people experiencing severe mental health problems in developed countries and 76–85% in developing countries receive no treatment [5].

Given the complex issues and multiple challenges facing clinicians, researchers, and policy makers working in the mental health field, an essential starting point for dicussion is how we define and identify mental health conditions. How do we measure whether a person is suffering from a "mental health condition", much less measure whether a person is "mentally healthy"? Are mental health and mental "illness" just opposite points on the same continuum, or is there a discrete boundary between health and illness? For those interested in mental health informatics, we must begin by asking the questions: What is mental health and what is mental "illness"?

3.2   Defining Mental Health and Mental Illness

3.2.1   The Concept of Mental Health

In general, when we talk about mental health, most of us use a rather vague working definition that identifies mental health as an individual's sense of psychological well-being. Unfortunately, while this may work in general conversations, it does not meet the needs of healthcare professionals attempting to determine what constitutes successful treatment, nor public health experts attempting to formulate policies for effective social interventions, nor researchers attempting to discover the sources of mental illnesses. Because treatment, research, and policy all require specific, replicable, and measurable definitions, a subjective "sense of psychological well-being" is not an adequate working model for mental health. Unfortunately, creating an exact definition of mental health has varied widely over time and among different groups, often due to cultural differences, subjective assessments, patient expectations, or competing professional theories [6, 7].

Box 3.1 Quick Facts about Mental Health and Illness
- As many as 500 million people suffer from a mental or behavioral disorder [3]
- Nearly 800,000 people worldwide commit suicide every year
- Four of the six leading causes of years lived with disability are due to neuropsychiatric disorders (depression, alcohol-use disorders, schizophrenia, bipolar disorder).
- In the United States, in any given year, one in five people have a mental disorder.
- Family members are often the primary caregivers of people with mental disorders. This has a significant impact on the family's quality of life.
- In addition to the health and social costs, those suffering from mental illnesses are also victims of human rights violations, stigma, and discrimination, both inside and outside of psychiatric institutions.
- The cost of mental health problems in developed countries is estimated to be between 3% and 4% of the GNP. Yet, in developed countries with well-organized health care systems, between 44% and 70% of people with mental disorders do not receive treatment. In developing countries, the treatment gap is closer to 90%. However, the average annual costs, including medical, pharmaceutical and disability costs for employees with depression may be 4.2 times higher than those incurred by a typical beneficiary.

3.2.2 Health and Disease

The concept of mental health is intrinsically interwoven with our understanding of the broader concepts of health and disease. The basic theory of health is embodied in the myth of Asclepius, the Greek god of medicine [8]. According to Greek mythology, Asclepius was the son of Apollo trained by the centaur Chiron in the healing arts. People from across the world would come to his temple to be treated for their illnesses. During his rounds, Asclepius was accompanied by his two daughters Panacea (the goddess/personification of universal remedies) and Hygieia (the goddess/personification of good health, cleanliness, and hygiene). The daughters symbolize complimentary models of healthcare [8, 9]. The first, represented by Panacea, is the **pathogenic** approach. This concept, derived from the Greek word *pathos* (meaning suffering or an emotion evoking sympathy), views health as the absence of suffering, the absence of disability, or the absence of disease. Health is restored when a disease is treated by a "panacea". Thus, a pathogenic understanding of mental health would be the absence of a mental illness or disorder.

Alternatively, a second understanding of health, represented by Hygieia, is the **salutogenic** approach. This concept, derived from the Latin word *salus* (meaning health), views health not as the absence of disease, but rather as the presence of

Fig. 3.1 Hygieia, daughter
of Asclepius,
personification of good
health and hygiene.
Courtyard of the Hamburg
city hall,
Hamburg, Germany

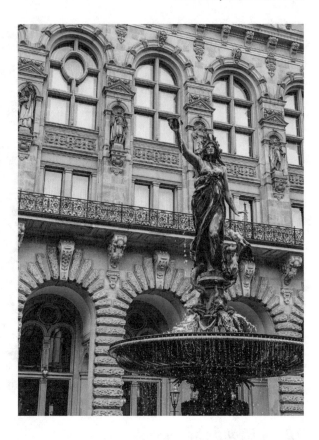

positive states of human capacities and functioning (emotions, cognitive abilities,
behaviors) that derive from "hygienic" or health promotion [10]. Thus, a salutogenic understanding of mental health includes ideas about subjective well-being,
perceived self-efficacy, autonomy, competence, intergenerational dependence and
recognition of the ability to realize one's intellectual and emotional potential [11]
(Fig. 3.1).

3.2.3 Definitions of Mental Health

Until recently in our history, mental health was primarily defined by the pathogenic
view. To be mentally healthy, was to have an absence of psychopathology. However,
this idea has evolved over the past several decades. In 1999, Dr. David Satcher
published the first ever US Surgeon General's Report on Mental Health [1]. In it,
mental health was defined as:

"A state of successful performance of mental function, resulting in productive activities, fulfilling relationships with other people, and the ability to adapt to change and to cope with adversity."

In 2004, the WHO [12] echoed this concept in its published report on mental health promotion. In it, they defined mental health not merely as the absence of mental illness, but as:

"A state of well-being in which the individual realizes his or her own abilities, can cope with the normal stresses of life, can work productively and fruitfully, and is able to make a contribution to his or her community."

These definitions affirm a more positive view of mental health than just the pathogenic view; that mental health is not the same thing as the absence of mental illness or the absence of a disability. It also involves the salutogenic concept of subjective well-being.

Researchers note that the hybridizing of both pathogenic and salutogenic concepts create a third and complementary conception of health. Derived from word "hale" (meaning "to be whole") the **halogenic** approach to mental healthcare involves treatments (panaceas) and mental health promotion (hygiene). However, it is not limited just to "positive feelings" about oneself nor the absence of disease. Rather, the new definition of mental health includes an outward meaningful expression of social interaction. The World Health Organization [7] emphasizes that the process of promoting mental health is also the process of enhancing competencies of individual and communities, enabling them to achieve their self-determined goals. Thus, mental health is a concern not just for those who suffer from a mental disorder, but for the whole community.

3.2.4   Mental Health and Somatic Health

One key point in defining mental health is our understanding of the mind/body connection. Our everyday language tends to encourage the misperception that "mental health" is separate (if not unrelated) to "physical health". This partitioning has been further codified by a health insurance system that often "carves out" the management (and payment) for mental healthcare to separate systems from those that manage (and pay for) physical healthcare. This concept of splitting the mind from the body can be traced to the seventeenth century philosopher Rene Descartes, who conceptualized the "mind" as the concern of organized religion, whereas the body was seen as the concern of physicians [13].

However, the mind and the body are intimately interrelated [14, 15]. The US Surgeon General's Report on Mental Health (1999), in an effort to de-emphasize this tendency toward dichotomizing the mind and body, advocated for the use of more neutral terms "somatic health" and "mental health" (soma being the medical term for "body"). For example, when discussing the brain, one would note that it performs both somatic functions (such as movement, balance, regulation of body functions) as well as mental functions (such as thoughts, mood, and behaviors). A stroke may cause a lesion in the brain that disrupts the ability to talk or move. When these symptoms are considered, the stroke is perceived as a somatic condition. However, when a stroke causes a lesion that produces alterations of thoughts, mood, or behavior, it is considered a mental condition (e.g. dementia).

In summary, a working definition of mental health focuses not on just an absence of illness, but it encompasses one's internal assessment of themselves, one's internal mental abilities (such as cognition, emotions, perceptions), and one's applications of the internal structures to daily life problems. Mental health is the foundation then for effective and meaningful functioning for individuals and communities.

3.3 The Concept of Mental Illness

In addition to their increased emphasis on recognizing a more holistic view of mental health, both the US Surgeon General and the WHO also identify well-characterized, specific types of mental disorders. Yet agreement about what constitutes mental "illness" has proved elusive. Similar to the challenge of defining mental health, the definition of a mental illness may vary extensively based on cultural differences, subjective assessments, and professional theories.

As noted previously, the pathogenic model of medicine attempts to define mental health in contrast to mental illness. In this view mental illness is a discrete entity not present in the mentally healthy. However the salutogenic model attempts to define mental health in terms of mental functioning. In this view, mental illness could potentially be any less-than-optimal mental performance. Considered together, these models demonstrate the challenge of defining a "mental disorders". One model emphasizes the presence of concrete pathological disorders, while the other takes a much more fluid approach. Before we look at how scientists have defined specific mental disorders, we must first consider how mental health and mental illness may be on a continuum. This can be summarized by discussing the differences in our understanding of mental distress, mental health challenges, and mental disorders.

3.3.1 The Continuums of Mental Health and Illness

Mental distress can be defined as the inner signal of anxiety or "stress" that occurs when a person is presented with a challenge. Stressors are normal daily events experienced by everyone, such as being in a new situation, socially interacting with others, or participating in some novel event that takes a person out of his or her comfort zone and requires them to develop or expand a life skill. When confronted with a stressor, a "stress response" is evoked. The individual will experience this on several levels. These include emotional responses (such as worry, excitement, unhappiness, irritability), cognitive reactions (thoughts such as "I can do this" or "I don't want to do this"), physical symptoms (such as arousal, increased heart rate, shallower breathing, or "butterflies in one's stomach"), and/or behavior actions (such as avoidance or engagement). Once a person has successfully overcome the challenge, the distress goes away.

Mental health challenges refer to more severe stressors in which "distress" signs and symptoms are present, though of insufficient intensity or duration to meet the criteria for a mental disorder (Surgeon General 1999). Almost everyone has experienced mental health problems as part of normal life events, such as the death of a loved one, a serious physical illness, or a move to a new geographic location. The response may cause significant difficulties in emotions (sadness, grief, anger), negative cognitions (such as "I am not good enough" or "it is too much for me to bear"), physical symptoms (sleep problems, low energy, non-specific aches/pains), and/or behaviors (social withdrawal, decreased activities, anger outbursts). These mental health challenges do not usually require treatment (such as medications or psychotherapy) but often respond to the presence of support or guidance from significant others.

Mental disorders, on the other hand, are health conditions characterized by significant dysfunction in emotions (depression, panic disorder, mania), cognition (delusions, psychosis, hopelessness, suicidal thoughts), physical states (fatigue, weight changes, excessive movements), and/or behaviors (withdrawal from others, poor self-care, suicidal behaviors, etc.). When these dysfunctions co-occur in specific constellations, persist for an extended period of time, or exceed some threshhold level of intensity and frequency, they can impair a person's overall functioning, and may require treatment by trained professionals.

As can be seen in the above examples, mental stress, challenges, and disorders all involve changes in emotions, cognitions, physical states, and/or behaviors. For the most part, the differences are ones of intensity of symptoms, duration, or the effect on overall functioning. One could thus consider them as different positions along a continuum of experience. However, some researchers suggest that mental health and illness are better understood, not as residing on a single continuum, but rather in a dual continuum model [16]. This theory suggests that mental health and mental illness belong to two separate but correlated dimensions, one continuum indicating the presence and absence of positive mental health, the other indicating the presence and absence of symptoms of mental illness [17, 18].

There are three important implications of this model:

1. The absence of a mental health condition does not imply the presence of mental health. This was supported by the finding that while just over 75% of people were free of the most common forms of mental disorders (major depressive episodes, panic attacks, and generalized anxiety disorder) during the previous year, only 20% were described as "flourishing".

2. The presence of a mental health condition does not imply the absence of mental health. In studies of the roughly 23% of adults who experienced a mental illness, 14.5% were identified as having "moderate mental health", while 1.5% were identified as "flourishing" [16, 19, 20]. In this model, an individual with optimal mental health can also have a mental health condition, and an individual who has no mental health condition can also have poor mental health.
3. If mental health and mental illnesses are separate entities, then there should be a differentiation of functioning for those with different levels of mental health who are free of mental illness. This indeed is seen in studies that show adults and adolescents who are classified as anything less than "flourishing", have worse physical health outcomes, health utilization, missed days of work, and poorer psychosocial functioning.

3.4 Theories of Psychopathology

Over the centuries, there have been many different theories about the causes of mental illness. Most of these are reflected by the contemporary social philosophies of their times. Ancient cultures often attributed mental illnesses to supernatural or mystical forces. They were most often, but not always, viewed as the result of spiritual disfavor, a curse, or moral failing. Treatment was often focused on spiritual intervention.

Between the 5th and 3rd centuries BCE, the Greek physician Hippocrates and the Latin physician Galen suggested that mental illnesses were due to somatic pathologies. They emphasized that mental illness was a disease state of the body, not the "spirit". Specifically, they believed that mental illness was the result of an imbalance of one or more of four essential fluids or "humors" of the body —blood, yellow bile, phlegm and black bile. As a result of this theory, treatment was changed from spiritual practices to physical interventions, such as bleeding or purging in an effort to rebalance the humors (Table 3.1).

3.4.1 Biological Theories of Psychopathology

This emphasis on a physical cause of mental illness was important because it brought the study and treatment of mental health and illness into the domain of science rather than religion, eventually leading to the development of the **biological theory** of mental illness in the late twentieth century. From a biological perspective, mental health conditions are illnesses like any other physical disease, except they are diseases of the brain. Therefore, the biological theory demanded that scientists

Table 3.1 Major theoretical models of psychopathology

Theory	Common assertions
Biological theories	
Major assumptions	Mental health conditions are primarily disorders of the brain. They are caused by any number of malfunctions in the nervous system, including disrupted neural connections, chemical imbalances, protein regulation problems, and abnormal genetic regulation.
Psychological theories	
Major assumptions	Mental health conditions are primarily dysfunctions in mental, cognitive, emotional, or behavioral processes.
Psychoanalytic (Psychodynamic)	Mental health conditions are primarily dysfunctions in internal mental ("intrapsychic") processes, particularly drives and motivation. They are caused by distressing early childhood events, unresolved internal conflicts, unconscious processes that drive behavior, and an over-reliance on defense mechanisms that undermine mental health.
Behavioral theories	Mental health conditions are primarily dysfunctions in behavior and the mental processes leading to behavior. They are the result of interactions with the environment that establish and maintain dysfunctional behavior (e.g., modeling, conditioning, and external "contingencies" such as reinforcement and punishment).
Cognitive theories	Mental health conditions are primarily dysfunctions in cognitive processes that lead to inaccurate or distorted perceptions of external events or internal experiences. They are the result of both specific interactions with the environment and the ways a person cognitive "constructs", or interprets, these experiences.
Humanistic (Positive psychology) theories	Mental health conditions are the result of internal processes or external influences that undermine a person's natural tendency to grow and develop. The humanist approach is less of a theoretical model of "mental illness" and more of a philosophical approach to working with people to achieve optimal mental health.
Social and social psychological theories	
Major assumptions	Mental health conditions are primarily dysfunctions in the relationship between an *individual person* and some *social entity*—whether that entity be a close interpersonal relationship, a peer group, an organization, or an entire society. Mental health conditions may be caused by distressing or maladaptive psychological states and processes that arise from an incompatibility between the needs of the individual and the needs of social entities. They may also be caused by psychological injuries inflicted by social entities.
Stress theories	Mental health conditions are caused by the stress created by incompatibilities between the needs of the individual and the needs of social entities, particularly larger social entities such as organizations, communities and the broader society.
Structural strain theories	Mental health conditions are caused by a person's efforts to either adapt or accommodate to the needs of social entities.
Labeling/Social reaction theories	Mental health conditions are either things that exist only in the minds of those who label others as "mentally ill"; or they are real conditions causes by the distress and real-world consequences of being labeled and discriminated against.
Biopsychosocial theories	
Major assumptions	Mental health conditions result from a complex interaction between biological, environmental, psychological, and behavioral factors.

and clinicians unravel the mysteries of the brain to determine how disruptions in brain functioning might lead to the development of mental health conditions [21].

The biological theory of mental illness stimulated development of a new field of study, the neurosciences. The neurosciences are an amalgamation of various disciplines focused on understanding how neurons communicate, form connections, and give rise to thoughts and behaviors [6]. Neuroscience encompasses several areas of study, such as brain structure and function (neuroanatomy and neurotransmitter systems), brain activity (neurocircuitry), gene effects (genetics) and other biological factors (such as prenatal development, infections, toxins, or injuries).

The most common metaphor neuroscientists use to describe the brain and how it functions is "the neural network". In this conceptualization, the brain is an integrated system of command centers composed of nerve cells communicating with each other through electrical impulses and chemical exchanges. The organization of the system is regulated by genetic determinism, developmental modulations, and environmental exposures. When activated and coordinated, it is these chemical exchanges that provided the biological substrate of thought, emotions, memory, judgement, and feeling. The biological theory suggests that mental disorders arise when there are malfunctions at any point in the system, such as disrupted neural connections, chemical imbalances, protein regulation problems, abnormal genetic regulation, or some disruption in the myriad of other brain processes that occur. Treatment therefore is focused on physical interventions to correct the malfuction, usually using medications or some type of neuromodulation.

The strength of the biological model is that it is based on a maturing field of neuroscience, which has provided a rich understanding of the workings of the human brain. It empirically investigates how specific brain abnormalities are associated with signs and symptoms of specific mental disorders. Further, biological treatments that have been developed are often relatively rapid in effect, comparatively inexpensive, easy to administer, and moderately effective in managing serious mental health conditions. The biological model has also contributed significantly to the destigmatization of mental disorders by identifying and treating them as somatic, or physical, diseases.

However, critics of a pure biological theory of mental illness have also pointed out significant weaknesses in the model. First, they note that despite extensive research, few true biological markers identifying specific mental health conditions have been discovered. Though we understand much of the biology of the brain, we have not successfully been able to pair specific biological abnormalities consistently with specific mental health conditons. Secondly, they argue that current medication treatments, though often effective in managing symptoms, do not appear to "cure" the underlying dysfunction for which they are prescribed. Critics suggest that while the biological theory has been the most influential model for determining the way people with mental health conditions are treated, at best it can provide only a partial explanation of mental illness.

3.4.2   Psychological Theories of Psychopathology

As the biological model was developing, the 19th and 20th centuries also saw the rise of several **psychological theories** of mental illness. Numerous theories have been proposed, but four of the most widely used models are the psychoanalytic model, the behavioral model, the cognitive model, and the humanistic/existential models. Each theory contains its own, unique set of assumptions about human nature and about what drives human behavior, how behaviors become abnormal, and how dysfunction can be prevented or corrected [22]. In contrast to the biological model which focuses on the physical functioning of the neural network, psychological models focus on the meta-network grounded in this neural substrate [23]. This network, commonly referred to as the "mind", perform many functions, such as learning, perception, and reasoning as well as formation of beliefs, attitudes, and internal mental models of the world, people, and relationships. Using these functions, psychological models attempted to explain how phenomena as diverse as identity, emotion, cognition, and behaviors develop.

The **psychoanalytic model** was developed by Sigmund Freud in the early twentieth century. As a neurologist by training, he viewed people as closed energy systems. He believed there were two primary psychological energies: libido and aggression. As energy, these drives were always present and could never be eliminated; however, they could be transformed and redirected. He theorized that people had three parts to their personality: the id, the superego, and the ego which modulated the energies. The id is the impulsive part that expresses our sexual and aggressive instincts. The superego is the internal representation of our values, expectations, moral standards. It represents our conscience. The ego attempts to mediate the desires of the id against the demands of reality and the moral limitations of the superego. According to Freud, while the three parts of the personality generally work well together, if conflict is not resolved, intrapsychic conflicts arise and lead to mental disorders. Treatment is aimed at helping persons develop insight, thus bringing conflicts and motives into conscious awareness. Psychoanalysis (or the "talking cure") developed several strategies for revealing unconscious conflicts such as free association, dream interpretation, and transference relationship. Since Freud's original work, many others have proposed their own versions of psychoanalysis.

The **learning or behavioral model** is quite different from the psychoanalytic model in that it developed from scientists' observations about patterns of physical and behavioral responses to external events. Researchers observed that people constantly interact with the world and that our responses are influenced and shaped by prevailing patterns of rewards and punishments. Behavioral theorists emphasize several psychological processes that lead to learning. These include classical conditioning in which people come to associate particular emotional reactions with neutral stimuli (remember Pavlov's dogs). Operant conditioning is the process by which people associate responses with consequences. If the consequences are positive or reinforcing, then the behavior is more likely to be repeated. If the consequence is negative or painful, then the behaviors are less likely to be repeated. Finally, there is vicarious conditioning, or modeling, in which people learn behaviors by watching others. If the modeled behavior is rewarded, then people are more likely to behave similarly. In the behavioral model's perspective, mental disorders develop due to inappropriate responses to conditioning. Treatment therefore is aimed at changing the behaviors.

Closely associated with the behavioral model is the **cognitive model**. Cognitive theories of psychopathology evolved out of the observation that people think conceptually about the world, and it is in the context of our thoughts (or cognitions) that learning occurs, emotions are evoked, and behaviors are generated [3, 24]. Cognitive theorists posit that cognitions are organized into schemas [24, 25], or complex interrelated sets of beliefs – beliefs about ourselves, other people, and the world in general [26]. According to the cognitive model, each person develops a unique set of schemas based on his or her life experiences, but the processes involved in schema formation and maintenance appear to be driven by common set of principles across people. There are many different ideas about what these principles are, and how commonly or idiosyncratically, these principles operate. According the cognitive model, mental health conditions arise as the result of inflexible or maladaptive schemas, with specific disorders being linked to specific kinds of maladaptive schema [27]. Treatments based on cognitive models of psychopathology focuses primarily on changing these maladaptive schemata and patterns of thought [27–30].

In the 1980s and 1990s, researchers began to integrate behavioral and cognitive theories of human behavior into a single, integrated model [31–33]. This combined model, the **cognitive-behavioral model**, and its corresponding approach to psychotherapy, Cognitive Behavioral Therapy (CBT) [34, 35], is one of the most widely accepted models in clinical practice today [35]. Cognitive behavioral theory conceptualizes human behavior as arising from complex interpersonal, cognitive and behavioral processes through which a person interacting with the world develops internal schemata of the world, then uses these schemata not only as the basis for future behavior, but also as the filter through which the world is subsequently perceived and experienced [31–36]. The principles of learning articulated by the behavioral model (imitation, conditioning, reinforcement, punishment, etc.) are included in this theory as cognitive representations within schemata. Cognitive behavioral theorists argue that mental health problems develop as the result of the complex ways in which life experiences, patterns of thought, and learned behavior interact to produce maladaptive thoughts, ineffectual behaviors, or distressing emotional states.

Another major psychological model is the **humanistic or existential perspective** [35, 37]. This model emerged in the 1960s and 1970s as an alternative to the largely deterministic view of personality espoused by psychoanalysis and emphasized by behaviorism. Key features of this model include a belief in human perfectibility, personal fulfillment, valuing self-disclosure, placing feelings over intellect, and an emphasis on the present [38]. Key figures in developing this model are Abraham Maslow and Carl Rogers, who taught that people strive to make the most of their potential in a process called self-actualization [39]. This emphasis on self-actualization is very different from other psychological perspectives in that it emphasizes understanding the goals people have, their conscious choices in setting them, and the choices they make to achieve them.

3.4.3 Social Theories of Psychopathology

In the mid-twentieth century, theories about the relationships between social and psychological phenomena and their implications for mental health and illness began to appear in the scientific literature. These theories arose at the interface of the fields of sociology and psychology and gave rise to the field of social psychology—a field concerned with the empirical study of how a person's thoughts, emotions, and behavior are influenced by the presence of other people as well as mental representations of others [40]. Social and social psychological theories of mental health and "illness" emphasize the ways that social structures and social interactions—ranging from interactions in close interpersonal relationships to informal social interactions and passive exposure to images and messaging—influence thoughts, emotions, and behavior. There are many theories in this space, differing primarily in terms of the specific social and psychological phenomena emphasized, assumptions about the ways in which these phenomena influence each other, and assertions about the mechanism that either bolster or undermine mental health.

Social psychological theories place internal psychological (mental, cognitive, emotional) processes at the center of their theoretical models, and focus on the way that social situations and experiences influence and are influenced by psychological processes [41]. Interpersonal schema [42], working models of self and other [43, 44], learned helplessness [45], and locus of control [46] are key constructs in social psychological theories of mental health.

Stress theories focuses on the accumulations of stress and its role in precipitating mental health problems. Social stress theories focus specifically on stress arising from social structures, social experiences, and social status. Evidence cited for the critical role of stress in mental health and illness is the high correlation between social disadvantage and social discrimination on the one hand and measures of mental health and distress on the other [47–52].

Strain theories, including general strain theories [53] and role strain theories [54], emphasize the ways in which social institutions and broad societal norms influence behavior through pressure to conform with role expectations [55]. Role strain theory and its variants emphasize the stress inherent in social pressure to conform to either multiple, conflicting roles; to roles that conflict with internal values; or to desired roles with many barriers for attainment [56–59]. Clinical applications of role strain theories emphasize interventions aimed at identifying and mitigating sources of social strain [60–62].

Labeling, or social reaction, theories emphasize the way that labels others apply to people influence the way a person perceives, thinks, and feels about him or herself, and the way these self-perceptions and feelings in turn influence the person's behavior and mental health [63]. *Identity, stigma, stereotyping, self-fulfilling prophesy*, and *social norms* are key constructs commonly referenced in labeling theories. One particularly relevant labeling theory argues that "mental illness" is a label applied to people whose behavior deviates from the values and norms embraced by those applying the label. The internalization of the label, along with the real-world consequences of the ways others interact with people labeled "mental ill", can have effect of inducing the very thoughts, emotions, and behaviors that undermine a person's mental health [64].

3.4.4 The Biopsychosocial Theory of Psychopathology

More recently, the primary model of contemporary mainstream Western psychiatry has been the **biopsychosocial model** (Fig. 3.2) [65]. This view suggests that it is the dynamic interplay between biological, psychological, and social factors that contribute to mental illness (and mental health) [66]. Thus there are many different factors that can contribute to good mental health, such as a family history of illness (genetics factors), lifestyle/health behaviors (e.g., smoking, exercise, substance use), environmental stressors or traumas, exposure to toxins, personal life experience and history, access to supports (e.g. timely healthcare, social supports), or coping skills [67]. It is the complex interplay of these factors that determine one's individual mental health state.

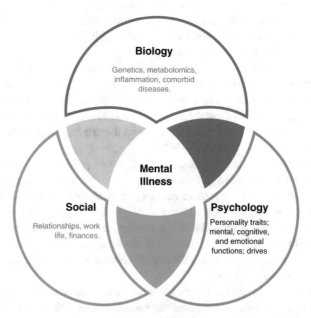

Fig. 3.2 George Engel's conceptualization of health and well-being posits that illness develops due to a mixture of biological, psychological, and social predisposing factors

3.5 Defining Mental Disorders

Thus far, we have noted that mental health and illness can be conceived as lying on a continuum of emotional, physical, cognitive, and behavioral functioning, with mental health at one end of the continuum and mental "illness" at the other. We have noted that mental health and illness can also be concieved as non-mutually exclusive concepts existing on two different dimensions. That is, overall strong mental health can co-exist with even serious mental health conditions, and poor mental health can occur even in the absence of any diagnosable mental health condition. Finally, we have reviewed several major theories of mental health and illness. In this section, we provide an overview of two major nosologies that conceive of mental health and illness in terms of a finite set of discrete, pathological disorders.

As the biopsychosocial model of illness asserts, we cannot separate life experience, perceptions, thoughts, and emotions from our physical body. The brain is the physical substrate from which the mind emerges [68] and the substrate upon which the enviroment acts. Somehow the genetic programming underlying brain development unfolds in a two-way interaction with our environment, with the external environment influencing the brain's cellular structure and function, and the brain's cellular function and structure in turn influencing the environment through our behavior. Somehow, too, as the brain develops, the mind becomes capable of conceiving of itself and the world. When problems arise in the functioning of either the brain, the mind, or the environment – and the larger system comprising the three is not able to effectively compensate – the potential for a mental "disorder" develops.

Given the limitations in our understanding of the brain, the mind, and and complex ways in which they interact, the precise causes of most mental health conditions remain largely unknown. Few lesions or physiologic abnormalities (biomarkers) have been identified that positively identify a mental disorder. Thus, the "gold-standard" method by which diagnose physical conditions cannot be used for diagnosing mental health conditions [69]. Consequently, diagnosis of mental health conditions is based primarily on the use of diagnostic nosologies that define mental disorders based primarily in terms of signs, symptoms, and functional impairment.

3.5.1 Diagnostic Classification Systems Used in Mental Healthcare: DSM-5 and ICD-11

Beginning in the late 19th and early twentieth century, in an effort to collect health statistics in mental health institutions the American Medico-Psychological Association, now the American Psychiatric Association (APA), started to codify mental disorders. This resulted in publication of a narrow manual used primarily for diagnosing serious mental health conditions. In 1952, the APA published the first version of the Diagnostic and Statistical Manual of Mental Disorders was published.

This manual has continued to be refined over time, with the current version of the manual being the DSM-5 [70]. While the DSM-5 is the primary manual in use within the United States, most of the rest of the world uses the nosology developed by the World Health Organization (WHO), the ICD-11 [71], when diagnosing mental health conditions.

> **Box 3.2 A Note on ICD-10, ICD-11, and DSM-5**
> ICD-11 was released in 2019 by the World Health Organization and is expected to become the primary diagnostic code for much of the world. It should be noted that ICD-11 and DSM-5 were co-developed, so that codes for DSM-5 disorder map to ICD11 disorders. However, in the United States, ICD-10 is still used for billing purposes while DSM-5 is used for diagnostic coding.

The DSM-5 and the ICD-11 are more than listings of mental disorders. They are an attempt to codify major mental disorders based on their key symptoms. For example, anxiety disorders are identified by certain patterns of experiences and behaviors associated with a stress response; depressive disorders are identified by certain symptoms and behaviors indicating sadness and despair; substance disorders are identified by certain patterns of an individual unable to control cravings; psychotic disorders are identified by certain symptoms of altered perceptions. Further, the onset and time course of symptoms, the degree of functional impairment, and the presence (or absence) of specific causes of symptoms are also used to determine whether and how to classify clusters of symptoms as specific disorders. The goals of these manuals are to improve the reliability of psychiatric diagnoses, respond to the multiple of theoretic models of mental illness, and to distinguish "true mental disorders" from non-disorders. How well these goals have been achieved is a continuing source of debate and cause for the subsequent revisions [72].

Over the past four decades, the definition of mental disorders published in versions of the DSM has been fairly consistent (See Box 3.3). The definition used by the APA is based on work by Spitzer and colleagues [73] who focused on developing coherent and valid distinctions between "mental disorders" and "non-disorders". They make four key assertions in their definition of a mental disorder [69]. First, they assert that a mental disorder is not simply emotional distress following an environmental stressor, but rather an internal condition characterized by a significant disturbance in mental or behavioral functioning. Second, the internal condition (inferred from manifest symptoms) is due to some underlying physical or mental dysfunction. That is, the states and proceses that result in disturbances in mental and behavioral functioning are attributable to some underlying function that is not performing the way it does in people without a disorder. Third, the dysfunction is harmful – it causes distress or interferes with functioning. Finally, the harm is a direct result of the underlying dysfunction itself (it is not the result of others' responses to the person and his or her way of thinking or behaving). These operational definitions are used by the APA to distinguish a mental disorder from mental distress and mental health problems.

> **Box 3.3 DSM-5 Definition of Mental Disorder**
>
> - A mental disorder is a syndrome characterized by clinically significant disturbance in an individual's cognition, emotional regulation, or behavior that reflects a dysfunction in the psychological, biological, or developmental processes underlying mental functioning.
> - Mental disorders are usually associated with significant distress or disability in social, occupations, or other important activities.
> - An expectable or culturally approved response to a common stressor or loss, such as the death of a loved one, is not a mental disorder.
> - Socially deviant behavior (e.g., political, religious, or sexual) and conflicts that are primarily between the individual and society are not mental disorders unless the deviance or conflict results from a dysfunction in the individual, as described above.
>
> NOTE: The diagnosis of a mental disorder is not equivalent to a need for treatment [74].

In the past several decades, there have been extensive critiques of the DSM's and ICD's symptom-based approach to diagnosis. Many critics argue that symptom "cutoffs" within diagnostic categories are arbitrary, leading to missed diagnosis in some instances and over diagnosis in others. Others note that for many diagnoses, presenting symptoms may broadly vary, resulting in marked diversity between individuals with the same diagnosis and pointing to the reality that heterogenous groups of disorders are erroneously treated as if they are one and the same.

Finally, and most importantly, critics argue that the symptom-based approach to diagnosis carves up the universe of mental health conditions based on symptoms, rather than precise, underlying etiological mechanisms that can serve as targets for treatment. Both the DSM and the ICD define mental disorders using this symptom based approach. Thus, a diagnosis made using either of these systems cannot be viewed as a specific mental health condition, but rather a label representing a heterogenous group of conditions with a similar phenotypic expressions. For example, recent evidence suggests that there is not just one "major depressive disorder", but rather multiple underlying conditions that produce the cluster of symptoms currently defined as "major depressive disorder" [75]. This would also suggest, of course, that not all of the conditions we currently diagnose as major depressive disorder can be effectively be treated using the same intervention.

A vigorous debate continues about whether to continue to use this categorical approach to diagnosis or to embrace new systems (see further discussion in Chap. 5). One framework that has been proposed is the Hierarchical Taxonomy of Psychopathology

(HiToP), an alternate framework for conceptualizing, describing, and measuring psychopathology [76, 77]. The HiToP emphasizes the dimensional nature of mental health and illness and addresses the difficulties inherent in the diagnostic categorization model [78]. It overcomes the limitations of current nosologies by empirically deriving homogenous groups from clusters of signs and symptoms, then empirical deriving syndromes from traits, and finally deriving two high level classes (called "spectra") – internalizing and externalizing disorders – from syndromes [76, 77].

The National Institute of Mental Health (NIMH) has addressed the need for a knowledge base to support the development of more refined diagnostic systems by developing a framework for research capable of generating insights into the biological underpinnings of specific mental, emotional, behavioral, and social processes [79, 80]. This framework, the Research Domain Criteria (RDoC), represents the new standard for NIH funded research. RDoC does not represent a set of diagnostic categories, nor does it replace the DSM-5 or ICD-10 categorizations of mental illness in the clinical setting. Instead RDoC is a *research* framework that attempts to stimulate reasearch into the many dimensions of mental health and illlness by shifting the focus of mental health research away from heterogeneous diagnostic categories to specific mental, emotional, behavioral, and social constructs.

Despite the critiques, most agree that the DSM and ICD systems, though flawed, are a valuable source of information and guidance. In the United States, the DSM-5 continues to be the predominant diagnostic standard used in clinical practice. However, the informatician should be aware that though diagnoses are most often derived from the DSM-5, the ICD-10-CM is the *coding* standard set by the United States Department of Health and Human Services. Thus, datasets that list diagnoses may be drawn from the DSM diagnostic category or from the coded ICD-10. While these two systems are very similar, they are not directly interchangeable. To address this challenge, DSM-5 to ICD-10 "crosswalks" have been developed, representing a key value dataset of the DSM-5 diagnosis and their ICD-10 coded counterparts (Table 3.2).

Regardless of the systems currently used to define and classify mental disorders, it is likley that the definition of mental "disorder", the universe of known mental health conditions, and our approach to classifying these conditions will continue to be refined over time.

3.5.2 Mental Health Conditions

As noted above, mental health conditions are conditions characterized by disturbances in thinking, emotion, or behavior in which there is also significant distress and/or impaired functioning. The current version of the DSM, the DSM-5, defines 18 broad categories of mental disorder and 157 specific disorders [82] (Table 3.3).

The most comprehensive epidemiologic surveys assessing the prevalence and treatment of mental heatlh conditions performed in the United States to date are the National Comorbidity Study (NCS) in 1994, and the National Comorbidity Study – Replication Survey (NCS-R) in 2004 [83]. It should be noted that the NCS-R

Table 3.2 Categorization of Major Depressive Episode by the DSM-5 (American Psychiatric Association and [74]) and ICD-10 (World Health Organization [81])

DSM-5	ICD-10
Five (or more) of the following symptoms have been present during the same two-week period and represent a change from previous functioning; at least one of the symptoms is either (1) depressed mood or (2) loss of interest or pleasure. • Depressed mood most of the day, nearly every day, as indicated by either subjective report (eg, feels sad, empty, hopeless) or observations made by others (eg, appears tearful). (NOTE: In children and adolescents, can be irritable mood.) • Markedly diminished interest or pleasure in all, or almost all, activities most of the day, nearly every day (as indicated by either subjective account or observation) • Significant weight loss when not dieting, or weight gain (e.g., a change of more than 5% of body weight in a month), or decrease or increase in appetite nearly every day. (NOTE: In children, consider failure to make expected weight gain.) • Insomnia or hypersomnia nearly every day • Psychomotor agitation or retardation nearly every day (observable by others, not merely subjective feelings of restlessness or being slowed down) • Fatigue or loss of energy nearly every day • Feelings of worthlessness or excessive or inappropriate guilt (which may be delusional) nearly every day (not merely self-reproach or guilt about being sick) • Diminished ability to think or concentrate, or indecisiveness, nearly every day (either by their subjective account or as observed by others) • Recurrent thoughts of death (not just fear of dying), recurrent suicidal ideation without a specific plan, or a suicide attempt or a specific plan for committing suicide. The symptoms cause clinically significant distress or impairment in social, occupational, or other important areas of functioning. The episode is not attributable to the direct physiological effects of a substance or to another medical condition. The occurrence of the major depressive episode is not better explained by schizoaffective disorder, schizophrenia, schizophreniform disorder, delusional disorder, or other specified and unspecified schizophrenia spectrum and other psychotic disorders. There has never been a manic or hypomanic episode.	In typical depressive episodes[…]the individual usually suffers from depressed mood, loss of interest and enjoyment, and reduced energy leading to increased fatiguability and diminished activity. Marked tiredness after only slight effort is common. Other common symptoms are: (a)reduced concentration and attention; (b)reduced self-esteem and self-confidence; (c)ideas of guilt and unworthiness (even in a mild type of episode); (d) bleak and pessimistic views of the future; (e)ideas or acts of self-harm or suicide; (f) disturbed sleep (g)diminished appetite. The lowered mood varies little from day to day, and is often unresponsive to circumstances, yet may show a characteristic diurnal variation as the day goes on. As with manic episodes, the clinical presentation shows marked individual variations, and atypical presentations are particularly common in adolescence. In some cases, anxiety, distress, and motor agitation may be more prominent at times than the depression, and the mood change may also be masked by added features such as irritability, excessive consumption of alcohol, histrionic behaviour, and exacerbation of pre-existing phobic or obsessional symptoms, or by hypochondriacal preoccupations. For depressive episodes of all three grades of severity, a duration of at least 2 weeks is usually required for diagnosis, but shorter periods may be reasonable if symptoms are unusually severe and of rapid onset. Some of the above symptoms may be marked and develop characteristic features that are widely regarded as having special clinical significance. The most typical examples of these "somatic" symptoms are: Loss of interest or pleasure in activities that are normally enjoyable; lack of emotional reactivity to normally pleasurable surroundings and events; waking in the morning 2 hours or more before the usual time; depression worse in the morning; objective evidence of definite psychomotor retardation or agitation (remarked on or reported by other people); marked loss of appetite; weight loss (often defined as 5% or more of body weight in the past month); marked loss of libido. Usually, this somatic syndrome is not regarded as present unless about four of these symptoms are definitely present. […] The presence of dementia (F00-F03) or mental retardation (F70-F79) does not rule out the diagnosis of a treatable depressive episode, but communication difficulties are likely to make it necessary to rely more than usual for the diagnosis upon objectively observed somatic symptoms, such as psychomotor retardation, loss of appetite and weight, and sleep disturbance.

Table 3.3 DSM major
categories of mental disorders

Neurodevelopmental disorders
Schizophrenia Spectrum and other psychotic disorders
Bipolar and related disorders
Depressive disorders
Anxiety disorders
Obsessive-compulsive and related disorders
Trauma- and stressor-related disorders
Dissociative disorders
Somatic symptom and related disorders
Feeding and eating disorders
Elimination disorders
Sleep-wake disorders
Sexual dysfunctions
Gender Dysphoria
Disruptive, impulse-control, and conduct disorders
Substance-related and addictive disorders
Neurocognitive disorders
Personality disorders
Paraphilic disorders
Other mental disorders
Medication-induced movement disorders and other adverse effects of medication
Other conditions that may be a focus of clinical attention

utilized the DSM-IV categorization of mental disorders for its interviews (not the more current DSM-5). Further, while the most comprehensive, it did not assess all mental disorders, but focused primarily on the prevalence of mood disorders (major depression, dysthymia, mania), anxiety disorders (generalized anxiety disorder, panic disorder, phobias, obsessive-compulsive disorder, posttraumatic stress disorder), addictive disorders (alcohol abuse, drug abuse and dependence) psychotic disorders (schizophrenia, schizophreniform disorder, schizoaffective disorder, delusional disorder, brief reactive psychotic reaction) and somataform disorders (disorders characterized by distressing physical symptoms having no clear biological etiology). More recent surveys, such as the 2017 Global Burden of Disease study, have evaluated the prevalence of mental health conditions around the world (including in the United States) [84].

Table 3.4 depicts the lifetime and 12-month prevalence of the mental health conditions evaluated as part of the NCS-R [83]. The most prevalent lifetime conditions were major depression, alcohol abuse, specific phobia, and social phobia. Anxiety disorders were the most prevalent class of disorders, followed by disruptive behavior disorders, mood disorders, and substance abuse disorders.

Table 3.4 Estimates of Lifetime and 12-month prevalence of DSM-IV* disorders in the NCS-R ([85]; Updated 2007)

Mental disorder	Lifetime %	12-Month %
Anxiety Disorders		
Panic disorder	4.7	2.7
Agoraphobia without panic	1.3	0.9
Specific phobia	12.5	9.1
Social phobia	12.1	7.1
Generalized anxiety disorder	5.7	2.7
Posttraumatic stress disorder	6.8	3.6
Obsessive-compulsive disorder	2.3	1.2
Adult/child separation anxiety disorder	9.2	1.9
Any anxiety disorder	31.2	19.1
Mood Disorders		
Major depressive disorder	16.9	6.8
Dysthymia	2.5	1.5
Bipolar I/II disorders	4.4	2.8
Any mood disorder	21.4	9.7
Disruptive Behavior Disorders		
Oppositional-defiant disorder	8.5	1.0
Conduct disorder	9.5	1.0
Attention-deficit/hyperactivity disorder	8.1	4.1
Intermittent explosive disorder	7.4	4.1
Any disruptive disorder	25.0	10.5
Substance Abuse Disorders		
Alcohol abuse with or without dependence	13.2	3.1
Drug abuse with or without dependence	8.0	1.4
Nicotine dependence	29.6	11.0
Any substance disorder	35.3	13.4
Any Disorder		
Any disorder	57.4	32.4
Two or more disorders	27.7	5.8
Three or more disorders	17.3	6.0

Results suggest that mental health conditions are highly prevalent in the general population with the lifetime prevalence of any condition being 47.4%. (Again, note that not all identified disorders were surveyed.) These estimates are broadly consistent with other community surveys in the US [86, 87] and elsewhere in the world ([5]; WHO International Consortium in Psychiatric Epidemiology, 2000). It should also be noted that comorbidity for mental health conditions was common. 27.7% of respondents had two or more lifetime disorders and 17.3% had three or more.

Upon first view, the prevalence of mental disorders (47.4%) might initially seem remarkable, but it should be understood that the DSM and ICD classification systems are very broad and include a number of disorders that are usually self-limiting and not severely impairing (such as specific phobias). Further, the study's author also suggested that one should be no more surprised to find that half the population have met criteria for a mental health condition in their lifetime than to find that the vast majority of the population have experienced the flu or some other common physical illness at some time in their life [88].

What is surprising is that although many people have experienced mental health conditions at some time in their life, the major burden of illness is concentrated in the relatively small proportion of people who have more than one condition (comorbidity). These observations suggest that the prevalence rates of individual disorders may be less important than the prevalence of functional impairment, comorbidity, and chronicity. To focus on this subgroup, the National Advisory Mental Health Council [89] created a category defining those who struggle with "severe and persistent mental illness" (SPMI). Similarly, the Substance Abuse and Mental Health Service Administration (1993) created a working definition for "serious mental illness" (SMI). SPMI commonly refers to a collection of mental health conditions that usually affect people in early adulthood and may have profound effects on family relationships, educational attainment, occupational productivity, and social role functioning over the course of their lifetimes. Disorders typically subsumed under this rubric include schizophrenia, schizoaffective disorder, bipolar disorder, major depression, autism, and obsessive-compulsive disorder (National Advisory Mental Health Council [NAMHC], [89]). As opposed to the NCS-R 1-year prevalence of 32.4% for any mental disorder, the 1-year prevalence of SPMI and SMI are approximately 3% and 6% respectively [90].

One interesting pattern of the NCS-R findings is that most mental health conditions begin at an early age, peak in adulthood, and decrease in prevalence in the older population [91]. This pattern is opposite to that found for most chronic physical illnesses where conditional risk increases with age [92].

3.6   Conclusions

The way we define health and well-being has shifted throughout human history. This chapter reviewed three primary views of health and illness (pathogenic, salutogenic, and halogenic models) and how each view influences our understanding of mental health and illness. We discussed the idea that health and illness may be viewed both as a continuum of wellness, and as non-mutually exclusive concepts residing on two different continua. We review various theories of psychopathology and introduced the biopsychosocial theory of health and illness. Finally, we introduced the two primary nosologies used for diagnosing mental health conditions and estimating their prevalence, in the United States.

As we have seen, the definition of mental health continues to evolve and our approach to diagnosing and conceptualizing mental disorders is undergoing a revolutionary change. While the last 50 years we have focused on codifying heterogenic disorders based on similar symptoms presentations, recent approaches to classification have focused on identifying more homogenous groups based on dimensions of mental, emotional, social, and emotional functioning. Moreover, advances in our understanding of the brain have allowed us to add additional variables to empirical studies as we work to elucidate the underlying causes, rather than just the symptoms, of mental disorders.

Mental health informatics as a field is in its infancy, but has the potential to influence not only the development of treatment and policies for delivery of mental healthcare, but also the very definitions of mental health and illness.

References

1. Department of Health and Human Services, Office of the Surgeon General, Center for Mental Health Services, and National Institute of Mental Health (U.S.). Mental Health: A Report of the Surgeon General, 1999.
2. OECD. Sick on the Job? Myths and Realities about Mental Health and Work, Mental Health and Work. Paris: OECD Publishing; 2012. https://doi.org/10.1787/9789264124523-en.
3. Beck AT. Cognitive therapy and the emotional disorders. London: Penguin; 1979.
4. Hedegaard H, et al. Suicide rates in the United States continue to increase. NCHS data brief no. 309. National Center for Health Statistics; 2018. Available at www.cdc.gov/nchs/products/databriefs/db309.htm.
5. Demyttenaere K, Bruffaerts R, Posada-Villa J, Gasquet I, Kovess V, Lepine JP, Angermeyer MC, Bernert S, de Girolamo G, Morosini P, Polidori G, Kikkawa T, Kawakami N, Ono Y, Takeshima T, Uda H, Karam EG, Fayyad JA, Karam AN, Mneimneh ZN, Medina-Mora ME, Borges G, Lara C, de Graaf R, Ormel J, Gureje O, Shen Y, Huang Y, Zhang M, Alonso J, Haro JM, Vilagut G, Bromet EJ, Gluzman S, Webb C, Kessler RC, Merikangas KR, Anthony JC, Von Korff MR, Wang PS, Brugha TS, Aguilar-Gaxiola S, Lee S, Heeringa S, Pennell BE, Zaslavsky AM, Ustun TB, Chatterji S. WHO world mental health survey consortium. Prevalence, severity, and unmet need for treatment of mental disorders in the World Health Organization world mental health surveys. JAMA. 2004 Jun 2;291(21):2581–90.
6. Cowen EL. The enhancement of psychological wellness: challenges and opportunities. Am J Community Psychol. 1996;22:149–79.
7. World Health Organization. Mental health: strengthening our response;2014. Retrieved 4 May 2014.
8. Keyes CLM. Mental health as a complete state: how the salutogenic perspective completes the picture. In: Bauer GF, Hammig O, editors. Bridging occupational, organizational and public health: a Transdisciplinary approach. Springer Science & Business Media: Dordrecht; 2014.
9. Hart GD. Asclepius, god of medicine. Can Med Assoc J. 1965;92:232–6.
10. Antonovsky A. The salutogenic model as a theory to guide health promotion. Health Promot Int. 1996;11(1):11–8.
11. World Health Organization. Investing in mental health. Geneva: World Health Organization; 2003.
12. World Health Organization. Promoting mental health: concepts, emerging evidence, practice (summary report). Geneva: World Health Organization; 2004.
13. Eisendrath SJ, Feder A. The mind and somatic illness: psychological factors affecting physical illness. In: Godman HH, editor. Review of general psychiatry. 5th ed. Norwalk, CT: Appleton & Lange; 2000.
14. Baum A, Posluszny DM. Health psychology: mapping biobehavioral contributions to health and illness. Annu Rev Psychol. 1999;50:137–63.

15. Cohen S, Herbert TB. Health psychology: psychological factors and physical disease from the perspective of human psychoneuroimmunology. Annu Rev Psychol. 1996;47:113–42.
16. Keyes CLM. The mental health continuum: from languishing to flourishing in life. J Health Soc Behav. 2002;43:207–22.
17. Downie RS, Fyfe C, Tannahill A. Health promotion: models and values. Oxford, England: Oxford University Press; 1990.
18. Health and Welfare Canada. *Mental health for Canadians: Striking a balance.* Ottawa, Canada: Supply and Service Canada, 1988.
19. Keyes CLM. Mental illness and/or mental health? Investigating axioms of the complete state model of health. J Consult Clin Psychol. 2005;73:539–48.
20. Keyes CLM. Promoting and protecting mental health as flourishing: a complementary strategy for improving national mental health. Am Psychol. 2007;62:95–108.
21. Andreasen N. The broken brain: the biological revolution in psychiatry. New York: Harper & Row; 1984.
22. Peterson C. Psychological approaches to mental illness. In TL Scheid & TN Brown (Eds) *A* Handbook for the study of mental health: social contexts, theories, and systems (2nd Ed). Cambridge University Press: New York, NY, 2010.
23. Kinderman P. A psychological model of mental disorder. Harv Rev Psychiatry. 2005 Jul-Aug;13(4):206–17.
24. BECK AT. Thinking and depression: I. Idiosyncratic content and cognitive distortions. Arch Gen Psychiatry. 1963;9(4):324–33.
25. Piaget, J., Piaget's theory, in Piaget and his school. 1976, Springer: New York. p. 11-23.
26. Epstein S. Cognitive-experiential self-theory. In: Advanced personality. Boston, MA: Springer; 1998. p. 211–38.
27. Beck AT, Weishaar M. Cognitive therapy. In: Comprehensive handbook of cognitive therapy. Boston, MA: Springer; 1989. p. 21–36.
28. Beck AT. Cognitive therapy of depression. New York: Guilford Press; 1979.
29. Hawke LD, Provencher MD. Schema theory and schema therapy in mood and anxiety disorders: a review. J Cogn Psychother. 4:257–76.
30. Young JE, Klosko J, Weishaar M. Schema therapy. New York: Guilford; 2003. p. 254.
31. Rachman S. The evolution of cognitive behaviour therapy. In: Clark DM, Fairburn CG, editors. Science and practice of cognitive behaviour therapy. Oxford: Oxford University Press; 1997.
32. Kendall PC. Toward a cognitive-behavioral model of child psychopathology and a critique of related interventions. J Abnorm Child Psychol. 1985;13(3):357–72.
33. Carvalho S, et al. The evolution of cognitive behavioural therapy–The third generation and its effectiveness. Eur Psychiatry. 2017;41(S1):s773–4.
34. Kendall PC, Hollon SD. Cognitive-behavioral interventions: theory, research, and procedures, vol. 21. Saint Louis: Academic Press; 2013.
35. Cain DJ. Humanistic psychotherapies: handbook of research and practice. Washington, DC: American Psychological Association; 2002.
36. Craske MG. Cognitive–behavioral therapy. Washington, DC: American Psychological Association; 2010.
37. Rogers C. Client centered therapy (New Ed). London: Hachette UK; 2012.
38. Bugental JF. The third force in psychology. J Humanist Psychol. 1964;4(1):19–26.
39. Maslow AH. A theory of human motivation. Psychol Rev. 1943;50(4):370.
40. Allport GW, Clark K, Pettigrew T. The nature of prejudice. New York: Basic Books; 1954.
41. Fiske ST, Taylor SE. Social cognition. London: McGraw-Hill Book Company; 1991.
42. Fiske ST. Schema-triggered affect: applications to social perception. In: Affect and cognition: 17th Annual Carnegie Mellon symposium on cognition. Hillsdale: Lawrence Erlbaum; 1982.
43. Pietromonaco PR, Barrett LF. The internal working models concept: what do we really know about the self in relation to others? Rev Gen Psychol. 2000;4(2):155–75.
44. Klohnen EC, John OP. Working models of attachment: a theory-based prototype approach. In: Attachment theory and close relationships. New York: The Guilford Press; 1998. p. 115–40.

45. Maier SF, Seligman ME. Learned helplessness: theory and evidence. J Exp Psychol Gen. 1976;105(1):3.
46. Lefcourt HM. Locus of control. New York: Academic Press; 1991.
47. Brondolo E, et al. Racism and mental health: examining the link between racism and depression from a social cognitive perspective. In: Alvarez AN, Liang CTH, Neville HA, editors. The cost of racism for people of color: contextualizing experiences of discrimination. Washington, DC: American Psychological Association; 2016.
48. Carter RT. Racism and psychological and emotional injury: recognizing and assessing race-based traumatic stress. Couns Psychol. 2007;35(1):13–105.
49. Harrell SP. A multidimensional conceptualization of racism-related stress: implications for the well-being of people of color. Am J Orthopsychiatry. 2000;70(1):42–57.
50. Harrell CJP, et al. Multiple pathways linking racism to health outcomes. Du Bois Rev Soc Sci Res Race. 2011;8(1):143.
51. Cyrus K. Multiple minorities as multiply marginalized: applying the minority stress theory to LGBTQ people of color. J Gay Lesbian Ment Health. 2017;21(3):194–202.
52. McConnell EA, et al. Multiple minority stress and LGBT community resilience among sexual minority men. Psychol Sex Orientat Gend Divers. 2018;5(1):1.
53. Agnew R. Pressured into crime: an overview of general strain theory. Oxford: Oxford University Press; 2007.
54. Goode WJ. A theory of role strain. Am Sociol Rev. 1960;42:483–96.
55. Thoits PA. Sociological approaches to mental illness. In: A handbook for the study of mental health. New York: Cambridge University Press; 1999. p. 121–38.
56. Marks SR. Multiple roles and role strain: some notes on human energy, time and commitment. Am Sociol Rev. 1977;42:921–36.
57. Acosta LM, et al. Testing traditional machismo and the gender role strain theory with Mexican migrant farmworkers. Hisp J Behav Sci. 2020;42(2):215–34.
58. Levant RF, Powell WA The gender role strain paradigm. 2017.
59. McGee E, Griffith D, Houston S II. "I know I have to work twice as hard and hope that makes me good enough": exploring the stress and strain of Black doctoral students in engineering and computing. Teach Coll Rec. 2019;121(4):1–38.
60. Silverstein LB, Auerbach CF, Levant RF. Contemporary fathers reconstructing masculinity: clinical implications of gender role strain. Prof Psychol Res Pract. 2002;33(4):361.
61. O'Driscoll MP, et al. Family-responsive interventions, perceived organizational and supervisor support, work-family conflict, and psychological strain. Int J Stress Manag. 2003;10(4):326.
62. Piquero NL, et al. Gender, general strain theory, negative emotions, and disordered eating. J Youth Adolesc. 2010;39(4):380–92.
63. Goffman E. The presentation of self in everyday life. London: Harmondsworth; 1978.
64. Szasz T. The myth of mental illness. In: Biomedical ethics and the law. New York: Springer; 1976. p. 113–22.
65. Ghaemi SN. Paradigms of psychiatry: eclecticism and its discontents. Curr Opin Psychiatry. 2006;19(6):619–24.
66. Carey B. When will we solve mental illness? The New York Times. 2018;19
67. Canadian Centre for Occupational Health and Safety (CCOHS). Mental Health–Introduction. http://www.ccohs.ca/) What is mental health and mental illness? Workplace Mental Health Promotion; 2015. wmhp.cmhaontario.ca. Retrieved 2019-07-09.
68. Redish AD. The mind within the brain: how we make decisions and how those decisions go wrong. Oxford: Oxford University Press. xii; 2013. 377 pages.
69. Wakefield JC, Schmitz MF. The measurement of mental disorder. In: Scheid TL, Brown TN, editors. A handbook for the study of mental health: social contexts, theories, and systems. 2nd ed. New York, NY: Cambridge University Press; 2010.
70. Association AP. Diagnostic and statistical manual of mental disorders (DSM-5®). Arlington, VA: American Psychiatric Pub; 2013.
71. Organization WH International classification of diseases for mortality and morbidity statistics (11th Revision). 2019; Available from https://icd.who.int/en.

72. Kirk SA, Kutchins H. The selling of the DSM: the rhetoric of science in psychiatry. New York: Aldine de Gruyter; 1992.
73. Spitzer RL, Endicott I. Medical and mental disorder: proposed definition and criteria. In: Spitzer RL, Klein DF, editors. Critical Issues in Psychiatric Diagnosis. New York, NY: Raven Press; 1978. p. 15–40.
74. American Psychiatric Association. Diagnostic and statistical manual of mental disorders. 5th ed. DC: Washington; 2013.
75. Dinga R, et al. Evaluating the evidence for biotypes of depression: methodological replication and extension of. Neuroimage Clin. 2019;22:101796.
76. Kotov R, et al. The Hierarchical Taxonomy of Psychopathology (HiTOP): a dimensional alternative to traditional nosologies. J Abnorm Psychol. 2017;126(4):454–77.
77. Waszczuk MA, et al. Redefining phenotypes to advance psychiatric genetics: Implications from hierarchical taxonomy of psychopathology. J Abnorm Psychol. 2020;129(2):143–61.
78. Kotov R, Krueger RF, Watson D. A paradigm shift in psychiatric classification: The Hierarchical Taxonomy of Psychopathology (HiTOP). World Psychiatry. 2018;17(1):24–5. https://doi.org/10.1002/wps.20478
79. National Institute of Mental Health. Research Domain Criteria (RDoC). NIMH strategic research priorities 2012 November 9 [cited 2012 November 23]; Available from http://www.nimh.nih.gov/research-funding/rdoc/index.shtml.
80. Insel TR. The NIMH Research Domain Criteria (RDoC) Project: precision medicine for psychiatry. Am J Psychiatry. 2014;171(4):395–7.
81. World Health Organization. ICD-10: international statistical classification of diseases and related health problems: tenth revision, 2nd ed. World Health Organization; 2004. https://apps.who.int/iris/handle/10665/42980
82. McCarron RM. The DSM-5 and the art of medicine: certainly uncertain. Ann Intern Med. 2013;159(5):360–1.
83. Kessler RC, Merikangas KR. The National Comorbidity Survey Replication (NCS-R): Background and aims. International Journal of Methods in Psychiatric Research. 2004;13(2):60–8. https://doi.org/10.1002/mpr.166
84. Global Burden of Disease Collaborative Network. Global Burden of Disease Study 2017 (GBD 2017) Reference life table. Seattle, USA: Institute for Health Metrics and Evaluation (IHME); 2018.
85. Kessler RC, Berglund P, Demler O, Jin R, Merikangas KR, Walters EE. Lifetime prevalence and age-of-onset distributions of DSM-IV disorders in the National Comorbidity Survey Replication. Arch Gen Psychiatry. 2005;62:593–602.
86. Kessler RC. The National Comorbidity Survey of the United States. Int Rev Psychiatry. 1994;4:81–94.
87. Regier DA, Kaelber CT, Rae DS, Farmer ME, Knauper B, Kessler RC, et al. Limitations of diagnostic criteria and assessment instruments for mental disorders: implications for research and policy. Ach Gen Psychiatry. 1988;55:109–15.
88. Kessler RC. The presence of mental illness. In: Scheid TL, Brown TN, editors. A handbook for the study of mental health: social contexts, theories, and systems. 2nd ed. New York, NY: Cambridge University Press; 2010.
89. National Advisory Mental Health Council. Basic behavioral science research for mental health: a national investment (NIH Pub. No. 95–3682) Washington DC: US Government Printing Office; 1995.
90. Kessler RC, Berglund PA, Walters EE, Leaf PJ, Kouzis AC, Bruce ML, et al. Estimation of the 12-month prevalence of serious mental illness (SMI) (NCS Working Paper #8). Ann Arbor: University of Michigan, Institute for Social Research; 1995.
91. Kessler RC, Birnbaum H, Bromet E, Hwang I, Sampson N, Shahly V. Age differences in major depression: results from the National Comorbidity Survey Replication (NCS-R). Psychol Med. 2010 Feb;40(2):225–37.
92. Murray CJL, Lopez AD. Global health statistics. Cambridge, MA: Harvard University Press; 1996.

Chapter 4
The Mental Healthcare System: Organization and Structure

John L. Beyer and Mina Boazak

Abstract Mental healthcare is delivered in a wide variety of settings by a wide variety of mental healthcare professionals. This chapter outlines and defines the many faces of mental healthcare in the United States. We start by introducing the healthcare professionals who make up the field of mental health, emphasizing how they differ in their roles, training, and approaches to mental health. We review the settings in which mental healthcare is delivered, and discuss how decisions about appropriate care setting are made. Finally, we discuss how mental healthcare is funded in the United States, and describe public health disparities related to both funding and workforce shortages.

Keywords Mental health workforce · Mental health providers · Treatment settings Funding · Workforce disparity

4.1 Introduction

If we were to create an ideal mental health system, we would create it to have several specific qualities. First, it would be a culturally integrated organization. It would be viewed as a natural part of the larger healthcare system and appropriately adapted to the culture of the society which it serves. Secondly, the system would accurately identify those affected with a mental health condition, as discussed in the last chapter. Thirdly, the system would be empowered to intervene for those in distress, and it would do so by delivering high-quality, affordable care for all people across a wide range of treatment needs. Fourthly, the mental healthcare system would emphasize mental health promotion and preventive care. Finally, the system

J. L. Beyer · M. Boazak (✉)
Department of Psychiatry and Behavioral Sciences, Duke University School of Medicine, Durham, NC, USA
e-mail: john.beyer@duke.edu; mina.boazak@duke.edu

© Springer Nature Switzerland AG 2021
J. D. Tenenbaum, P. A. Ranallo (eds.), *Mental Health Informatics*, Health Informatics, https://doi.org/10.1007/978-3-030-70558-9_4

would seamlessly integrate world-class healthcare research while facilitating access to new technologies, medicines, and therapies as they are developed. Unfortunately, social and economic factors have created significant obstacles to fulfilling of vision of an ideal mental healthcare system. The mental healthcare system in the US has evolved over the past several hundred years into a patchwork system of providers and programs often divided by funding source, geographic location, political philosophies, and theoretical orientations of providers and administrators.

In 2011, the US spent $113 billion on mental healthcare, about 5.6% of the national healthcare spending [1]. Despite this level of expenditure, mental healthcare remains less accessible than physical healthcare services. For example, 89.3 million Americans live in federally-designated Mental Health Professional Shortage Areas (MHPSA), compared to 55.3 million Americans living in similarly designated primary-care shortage areas, and 44.6 million in dental health shortage areas (see Fig. 4.1). Further, mental healthcare is prohibitively expensive for many people, with 45% of those untreated citing cost as a barrier to care [2]. Finally, the cultural stigma of mental illness remains a significant barrier to the creation of an integrated system with physical healthcare, access to treatment, and acceptance as a priority for funding [3, 4].

The mental healthcare system is a formidable amalgam of healthcare providers offering many types of services, based on multiple and divergent theoretical models of mental health and illness, provided in a variety of settings, and financed by a complicated patchwork of insurers. For those interested in mental health informatics, an understanding of some basic building blocks of the mental healthcare system may be helpful. While an extensive review of these topics is beyond the scope of this chapter, here we provide a basic introduction to mental healthcare providers, settings, and payment models.

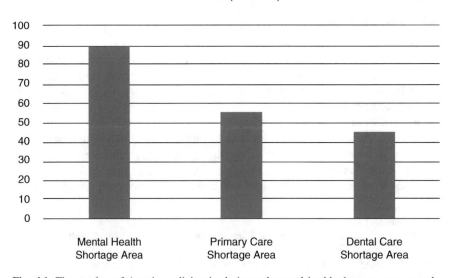

Fig. 4.1 The number of Americans living in designated mental health shortage areas grossly exceeds those in primary care and dental care shortage areas

4.2   Mental Healthcare Professionals

4.2.1   Types of Mental Healthcare Professionals

The mental healthcare workforce is comprised of many types of healthcare professionals with varying skills, training, licenses, and foci of care. As in physical healthcare, this variety ensures that healthcare professionals are sufficiently qualified to perform the activities required to meet the entire range of needs of people seeking mental healthcare services. The diversity in skills, training and foci of care in the mental healthcare workforce has an additional dimension less frequently seen in physical healthcare: a diversity rooted not in the variety of consensus diagnostic and treatment approaches to known health conditions, but a diversity rooted in fundamentally different beliefs about the etiology of mental health conditions, and how best to diagnose and treat them. In order to understand the mental healthcare system, it is important to understand not only the types of healthcare professionals, but also the variety of theoretical and philosophical approaches to conceptualizing and treating mental health conditions. In Chap. 3 we provided an overview of the major theoretical models embraced by mental healthcare professionals. In subsequent chapters (Chaps. 6, 9) we touch on the implications of the variety of theoretical approaches to mental healthcare for mental health research and care. In this section, we focus on types of providers. In the US, licensing for healthcare professionals, including mental healthcare professionals, is regulated at the state level. While there is variation in the specific educational, training, and competency evaluation requirements – as well as the titles used to describe each role – across states, the mental healthcare workforce across the US is generally comprised of a core set of healthcare professionals. The most common mental healthcare specialties along with corresponding training and licensure requirements and typical roles within the mental healthcare system are enumerated in Table 4.1.

Table 4.1   Mental health professionals

Discipline	Degree	Services
Medicine		
Psychiatrists	MD with applicable residency	Medical doctors who specialize in the diagnosis and treatment of mental illness. A psychiatrist can prescribe medications, provide therapy and counseling. They are licensed by their state medical boards. There are four subspecializations of psychiatrists: Addiction medicine specialists, child/adolescent psychiatrists, forensic psychiatrists, and Geropsychiatrists.
Advanced practice providers Nurse practitioner Physician assistant	MSN PA	Nurse practitioners or physician assistants who specialize in mental health. They usually work under the authority of, but relatively independent from, a psychiatrist. They also can prescribe medications, provide therapy and counseling. They are licensed by their state nursing or medical boards.
Psychiatric nurse	RN, BSN	A nurse who specializes in mental health, and cares for people of all ages experiencing mental illnesses or distress. They are licensed by their state nursing or medical boards

(continued)

Table 4.1 (continued)

Discipline	Degree	Services
Psychology		
Clinical psychologists	PhD or PsyD with applicable internship	Mental health specialists with a doctoral degree who diagnose and treat by various psychotherapeutic interventions. They are licensed by various psychology boards or committees of their state.
Mental health counselors Licensed mental health counselor (LMHC) Licensed professional counselor (LPC) Licensed professional clinical counselor (LPCC)	B.S., B.A.	Mental health specialists that use various psychotherapeutic interventions, usually with supervision by one of the specialists described above. Licensing varies by state
School psychologist School counselor	M.A., M.S., M.Ed., Ed.S., S.S.P., Ph.D., Psy.D., or Ed.D.	Mental health specialists that work primarily in school systems with students, parents and administrators. They do psychological testing, psychoeducational assessments, counseling, and consultations. Licensing varies by state
Certified alcohol and drug abuse counselor (addiction or substance abuse counselors)	Varies	Specialists that devise and implement treatment plans for drug and alcohol abuse problems. Various levels of certification are available from different certifying bodies. Some states require a license in addition to certification
Social work		
Social workers	MSW BSW	These represent a subsector of social work that also use various psychotherapeutic interventions. Licensing varies by state.
Paraprofessionals		
Psychiatric aides and technicians	HS diploma, GED	Psychiatric technicians and aides work in psychiatric hospitals, residential mental health facilities, and related healthcare settings caring for people who have mental illness and developmental disabilities.
Certified peer specialist	Varies	A certified peer specialist is a someone with personal experience in a mental health problem who supports others struggling with mental health, psychological trauma, or substance use. Various state certifications.
Psychiatric rehabilitation case manager Homeless outreach specialist Parent aides	Varies	These represent additional groups that support the mental healthcare process.

Medical Providers. In the United States *psychiatrists* have traditionally been afforded the lead professional role in mental healthcare among medical providers. They are medical doctors who have completed their medical training and four or more additional years of psychiatric residency. As medical doctors, their work may span a variety of activities including diagnostic consultation, therapy, administration, or medication prescribing. While traditionally the role of prescriber (the most restrictive of roles in mental healthcare due to the required specialized training and licensure) was delegated solely to physicians, the limited availability of physicians has promoted a gradual opening of this role to additional provider types, such as nurse practitioners and physician assistants, grouped together this group is referred to as Advanced Practice Providers (APPs) (Table 4.1).

In the 1960's advanced practice provider programs for *nurse practitioners* and *physician assistants* were developed to meet the resource demands of the public health system. Originally, Advanced Practice Providers (APPs) were intended to meet the growing disparity in healthcare providers, by functioning as prescribers under the supervision of a physician. More recently, however, an increasing number of states have been changing regulations to allow for the independent practice of APPs. Unfortunately, while there are 11,650 psychiatric APP's [5] practicing in the mental health field in the United States, there remains a disparity of prescribing providers in mental health. Due to the persistent challenges in relation to the aforementioned disparity, New Mexico enacted legislation in the early 2000s that gave appropriately trained psychologists privileges to prescribe medication for certain mental health conditions. Since then, Iowa, Idaho, Illinois, and Louisiana have also passed similar laws.

Psychiatrists and APPs work in a variety of settings including private practices, group practices with other professionals, inpatient wards at hospitals, or any clinic in which medical treatment of mental illnesses are required. As noted above, psychiatrists and APPs can perform many rolls within the mental health system, but they have increasingly been focused on providing medical consultation and medication management of mental disorders. In the United States, this represents an increasingly important role in the treatment of mental healthcare, with 12.2% of American adults receiving prescription medication for mental illness in 2018, a number that has steadily risen from 10.5% in 2002 [2].

Psychologists. While licensed *psychologists* (LPs) function in a plethora of roles, we focus here specifically on clinical psychologists working in a healthcare delivery role. Practicing clinical psychologists are mental health professionals who provide comprehensive mental healthcare to individuals and families [1]. They provide a number of services including diagnostic evaluations, formal psychological testing, and of course, treatment for mental health conditions and concerns. Psychologists assess and diagnose mental health conditions using a wide variety of both formal and informal assessment tools and methods. Formal psychological testing is typically performed by psychologists with specialized training in psychometric assessment. These psychologists use formal psychometric instruments and methods to aid in the diagnosis of mental health conditions, or to evaluate intellectual skills, vocational aptitude and preference, and neuropsychological functioning. Psychologists help people maintain or improve their mental health through the use of psychosocial (rather than physiological) interventions. These interventions are often referred to simply as "therapy". Some psychologists approach therapy using a combination of interventions they have acquired through training and practice, using what is called an "eclectic" or "integrative" [2] approach to treatment. Other psychologists use a more proscriptive set of interventions as part of a circumscribed treatment regimen. These regimens are often referred to as "manualized interventions" or "manual-based treatments" [3]. Regardless of the type of therapy provided, most psychotherapy in the United States takes the form of a seated, face-to-face verbal interaction between the therapist and the person (or people) seeking mental health services in a private office or room. The duration and frequency of therapy "sessions" vary according depending on a number of factors such as the condition for which a person is seeking care, the type of therapy he or she is receiving, the setting in which he or she is receiving care, and logistical considerations related to both personal and health system resources. The licensure requirements for psychologists vary by region, but in the United States, all psychologists complete a doctoral level training program (PhD, PsyD, or EdD) followed by an extended period of supervised practice (analogous to the residency programs required for new medical school graduates). Other practicing psychologists work in a variety of settings, including schools, colleges and universities, hospitals and medical clinics, prisons, veterans' medical centers, community health and mental health clinics nursing homes, and rehabilitation and long-term care centers.

Box 4.1 A Note on Psychotherapists

While the term "psychotherapy" is often primarily associated with psychologists, many different types of mental health professionals provide psychotherapy. In fact, the term "psychotherapist" has become a general term for any health professional licensed to provide therapy for mental health conditions. This includes not only psychologists, but also healthcare professionals such as social workers, marriage and family therapists, licensed professional counselors, certified prevention specialists, pastoral therapists, etc. Other terms commonly used to describe these mental healthcare professionals are "counselor", "clinician", and "therapist".

Social Workers. While psychiatrists, APPs, and psychologists often have the largest breadth in their license to provide care, they are not the most predominant members of the mental health workforce. In fact, while psychiatrists, APP's, and psychologists together comprise approximately 144,000 [5–7] of the mental health workforce, another 232,900 [8] is comprised of social workers. Social workers, due to their number and broad roles, represent a pivotal component of the mental health system. The role of social workers in the mental healthcare system varies significantly according to their training and area of expertise. Some, such as clinical social workers, receive training to provide therapy and counselling. Others, such as case managers, focus on helping people navigate the social system. Others may implement government health policies or become advocates for mental health services.

Clinical social workers typically complete a master's degree program and extensive supervised post graduate training (analogous to the residency programs new medical school graduates complete prior to independent practice), while case managers and people working in non-clinical social work positions may complete either a bacchelors or masters degree program [19].

Psychiatric aides technicians and aids. Psychiatric technicians and aides work with people experiencing mental health conditions or living with developmental disabilities. They work in psychiatric hospitals, residential mental health facilities, and related healthcare settings, providing physical care, monitoring, or support. Typically, these members of the mental healthcare team have obtained a postsecondary certificate and succesfully completed on-the-job training.

4.3   Mental Healthcare Settings

The A 2017 SAMSHA survey of mental healthcare noted that of the 46.6 million adults diagnosed with a mental health condition, 42.6% received some type of mental health services. Most of this was provided as counseling or some type of outpatient care. Only about one third of mentally ill adults received some type of psychiatric medications (prescribed primarily by psychiatrists or other physicians). 3.3% of adult mentally ill were treated at an inpatient hospital facility [2].

Because individuals with mental disorders may vary widely in severity of their illness or the capability of their social support system, treatments must be adapted to the level of need. While most disorders do not require constant high-intensive treatment in specialized centers, they may require different levels of care at different points in the illness. For example, individuals with severe substance abuse disorders may require acute inpatient treatment at detoxification facilities (usually located either in psychiatric or general hospitals) since withdrawal from alcohol can be life-threating and may require medical supervision. Afterward, they may be referred to **Acute Residential Treatment (ART) programs,** which are short-term, highly focused treatment programs that help individuals solidify their recovery and sobriety. Finally, some people may then transition to an Intensive Outpatient Programs (IOP), which allows them to work, go to school, and continue their regular activities while also providing services and supports, such as a 12-step program to remain sober. Similarly, people who are depressed and experiencing suicidal ideation or suicidal behaviors may require an acute inpatient hospitalization for both safety and treatment. Depending upon their response, they may then move to a different level of care, such as an outpatient practice or more intensive treatment through a partial hospital program.

The four primary types of mental health treatment settings are (1) hospital inpatient (including VA hospital, state or county mental hospitals, private psychiatric hospitals, or psychiatric units in general or community hospitals), (2) residential, (3) outpatient facilities (private clinics, partial hospital programs, intensive outpatient programs, and community mental health centers), and (4) telehealth (with present telehealth options of care spanning each of the aforementioned options). Table 4.2 lists the settings in which most mental healthcare is provided.

Table 4.2 Mental healthcare settings

Setting	Description
Adult Family Care Home (AFCH)	A residential home designed to provide personal care services to peopler requiring assistance. The provider lives in the home and offers personal care services for up to 5 residents.
Assisted Living Facility	A housing facility for people with disabilities or for adults who cannot or who choose not to live independently.
Community Mental Health Center	A community-sponsored (i.e., publicly funded) organization that provides services to people without health insurance.
Hospice	A type of healthcare that focuses on the palliation of a terminally ill person's pain and symptoms as well as attending to their emotional and spiritual needs at the end of life.
Hospital	A healthcare facility providing patient treatment with specialized medical and nursing staff and medical equipment.
Intensive Outpatient Program (IOP)	A program that provides intensive treatment to people experiencing mental health or substance use problems such as addiction, depression, or eating disorders that do not require detoxification or round-the-clock supervision.
Intermediate Care Faciltiy for the Developmentally Disabled (ICF/DD)	A facility with a capacity of 4 to 15 beds that provides 24-hour personal care, habilitation, developmental, and supportive health services to people with developmental disabilities who have intermittent recurring needs for nursing services, but have been certified by a physician as not requiring availability of continuous skilled nursing care.
Outpatient Clinic / Private Practice Office	A private office or clinic with one or more mental healthcare professionals who offer diagnostic or therapeutic services.
Partial Hospitalization Program (PHP)	A program that provides treatment for an extended part of the day, for most or all days of the week, to people experiencing mental health or substance abuse problems. The person resides at home and commutes to the treatment center.
Residential Treatment Facility (RTF)	A live-in healthcare facility providing therapy for people experiencing substance abuse, mental health, or behavioral problems.
Skilled Nursing Facility	An in-patient rehabilitation and medical treatment center staffed with trained medical professionals who provide the medically-necessary services of licensed nurses, physical and occupational therapists, speech pathologists, and audiologists.
State Mental Hospital	A public psychiatric hospital operated by a state government.

4.3.1 Inpatient Settings

Hospital Inpatient Setting Inpatient treatment facilities involve an overnight or longer treatment outside a person's home, usually because of safety concerns to the individual or others. There are two basic types of inpatient facilities: those that focus on acute stabilization and those that provide longer term care. Acute stabilization usually occurs in psychiatric hospitals or general medical and surgical hospitals that may have a psychiatric inpatient unit (and/or a substance abuse unit). Psychiatric hospitals are facilities that treat only mental health conditions. They may also have some more specialized care units, such as drug and alcohol detoxification units, or eating disorders, geriatric, child and adolescent services. Typically, stays in acute inpatient settings are shorter than 30 days. A person living with a chronic mental health condition or experiencing a severe mental health crisis may require inpatient care lasting longer than 30 days. In these instances, the person may transition to a long-term treatment facility. This may be at another facility or in a different setting within the psychiatric hospital. People living with chronic mental health conditions who cannot affort extended stays in private treatment facilities often end up in (see Box 4.2 on Deinstitutionalization).

Residential Settings. Residential mental health treatment facilities generally provide longer-term care hospitalizations or longer-term care. Unlike acute inpatient units, residential facilities are designed to accommodate long-term care in a medical setting. However, they are primarily designed to be more comfortable and less like a hospital ward. Examples include psychiatric residential centers (some of

---

Box 4.2 On Deinstitutionalization

In reading the history of mental health treatment over the centuries, you will often find reports of good faith attempts to treat the mentally ill that have resulted in more difficulties or unintended consequence with sometimes tragic results. This includes the deinstitutionalization effort of the 1960s and 70s. At their peak psychiatric state hospitals in the United States housed over 500,000, or 0.3% of the then population [9]. Many of these people were housed against their will, and the vast majority (roughly 75%) were hospitalized for at least 2 years [9]. Many of these facilities were grossly underfunded which created undignified conditions, allowed for abusive practices, and provided only limited clinical care. With advent of psychiatric medications, there was great hope that many individuals receiving these new treatments could live a relatively independent life outside of the state hospitals. In 1963 President Kennedy signed the Community Mental Health Care Act. This law significantly decreased funding for state mental health institutions and increased funding to alternative community care centers. It intended to provide treatment to people experiencing mental health conditions in a manner that maintains the civil freedoms of the person by making services available in the least restrictive environment. Since the passing of the law there has been a significant decrease in beds available in the state hospitals, and the majority of state mental health institutions closed. Unfortunately, an equivalent number of community care centers have not adequately developed programs capable of providing the outpatient services to meet the needs of the people released from these instiutions. The result for many people with severe and persistent mental illness (SPMI) has been a shift from housing in the state hospitals to jails and prisons. In fact, a report from the National Sheriff's Association and the Treatment Advocacy Center has found that jails now hold three times as many SPMI individuals as hospitals (Torrey et al. n.d.).

which may be specialized to treat certain disorders such as schizophrenia, eating disorders, obsessive compulsive disorder, mood disorders) or alcohol and drug rehabilitation centers. In addition, nursing homes may also accept people suffering from mental health conditions. They usually have psychiatric consultation available as needed.

4.3.2   Outpatient Settings

Outpatient Settings. Most of the mental healthcare provided in the United States is conducted in outpatient settings. While there is wide variety in the types of outpatient settings, they all focus on treatment at the provider's facility with no overnight stay. Depending on the particular clinic, individual therapy, group therapy and medication management may be available. These services may be based in private offices, community mental health centers, or psychiatric and/or general hospitals where individuals visit an outpatient clinic for an appointment. **Partial hospitalization programs (PHPs)**, also called "day programs," refer to outpatient programs that people attend for six or more hours a day, every day or most days of the week. These programs, which are less intensive than inpatient hospitalization, may focus on specific mental health conditions and/or substance abuse. They will commonly offer group therapy, educational sessions, and individual counseling. **Intensive outpatient programs (IOPs)** are similar to PHPs but are only attended for three to four hours and often meet during evening hours to accommodate persons who are working. Most IOPs focus on either substance abuse or mental health issues.

A **Community or County Mental Healthcare Center** provides mental healthcare services for people who cannot afford private mental healthcare services. These centers are operated by local governments to meet the needs of people whose mental health condition seriously impacts their daily functioning. Most of the people getting services from a community or county mental healthcare center receive Social Security disability benefits and rely on Medicaid to fund their treatment needs. Some of the services a person might receive from a community or county mental health center include outpatient services, medication management, case management services and intensive community treatment services. Often centers manage contracts with mental health service providers and refer clients for employment, day program services, residential treatment services, therapeutic residential services and supportive residential services.

Telepsychiatry or Telehealth Services refer to the remote delivery of mental health assessment and care, or psychological support and services, via telephone or the Internet using email, online chat, or videoconferencing. Most commonly, these services improve access to care for people living in remote locations or underserved areas, or who can't leave home due to illness, emergencies, or mobility problems. 2020 marked a turn in the utilization of telehealth services in the United States and around the world. Due to the COVID-19 pandemic many clinics turned to utilizing telehealth services to meet their communities' healthcare needs. According to a Civic Science survey of over 118,000 Americans, while the number that had used

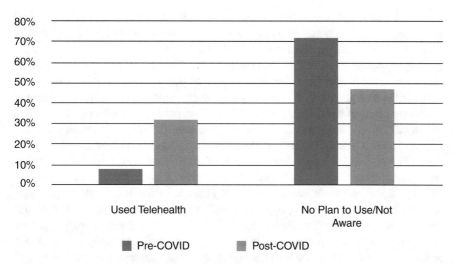

Fig. 4.2 Subsequent to the COVID-19 crisis the percentage of Americans utilizing telehealth services increased by 24% and those with no plans to utilize or were not aware of telehealth services decreased by 25% [10]

telehealth services prior to the COVID crisis was 8%, subsequent to the crisis 32% of Americans utilized telehealth services [10]. Furthermore, this was marked by a 25% drop in the number of Americans who either did not plan to or were unaware of telehealth services [10] (Fig. 4.2). While much of the increase in telehealth utilization will likely persist past the COVID-19 pandemic much needs to be done to improve service quality. This is most evident in a separate CivicScience assessment of American perceptions of service quality, in which 52% of people reported they found the quality of telehealth service to be lower than that of in-person care [10].

4.4   Disparities in the Mental Health Workforce

The mental health workforce in the United States is struggling to meet the increasing need for its services. While estimates of the number of providers vary by organization, according to the most recent Department of Labor's Bureau of Labor Statistics (BLS) [11], there are almost 600,000 mental health professionals practicing in the U.S. whose main focus is the treatment (and/or diagnosis) of mental health or substance abuse conditions. These include:

- Psychiatrists—25,630
- Clinical and counseling psychologists—181,7000
- Mental health and substance abuse social workers—117,700

- Mental health counselors—139,820
- Substance abuse counselors—91,040
- Marriage and family therapists—55,300

In addition to the the mental healthcare providers listed above, another 324,500 people serve as educational, vocational, or school counselors; 119,700 as rehabilitation counsellors; and an additional 707,400 social workers report that, while their primary responsibility is not the treatment or diagnosis of mental health condtions, they often assist families in a mental health capacity as part of their professional role.

While at first glance, these numbers may seem large enough to meet the mental healthcare needs in the US, they are not. In fact, according to Mental Health America roughly 22.3% of Americans are unable to obtain needed care in part because of a lack of providers or a lack of insurance ("Mental Health in America—Access to Care Data" 2020). This disparity is expected grow. The Health Resource and Services Administration (HRSA) estimates a significant decline in the number of psychiatrists in the country by 2030 [5]. Based on current consumer demand characteristics this translates to an unmet need of 21,000 psychiatrists by 2030 [5]. HRSA estimates also project a 12,000 person deficit in the psychologist workforce by 2030 [6]. While these deficits may in part by remedied by advanced practice practitioners, such as physicians assistants and nurse practitioners, or clinical social workers, with both groups estimated to grow in excess of demand by 2030 [5, 7], that simply will not be enough.

America is not the only nation with a mental healthcare workforce disparity. Data from the Global Health Observatory, supported by the World Health Organization, suggests more mental healthcare providers of all types are needed across the world. The need for more psychiatrists is particularly acute. It is estimated that mental healthcare requires an average of 25.9 psychiatrists per 100,000 people. While this can vary slightly by country, it should be noted that in low and middle income countries the average provider:population ratio is 1 psychiatrist and 3 psychiatric nurses for every million individuals. In the United States, there are just under 30,000 psychiatrists currently practicing, which is roughly 10 psychiatrists per 100,000 people [12].

While the deficit of providers in the mental healthcare workforce contributes to the long standing disparity between in mental and physical healthcare around the world, it is not the only cause. In the United State, disparities in insurance coverage for mental and physical healthcare also plays a role. The Affordable Care Act saw an initial decline in the uninsured in the United States, from 17.8% in 2010 to 10.0% in 2016 [13]. These numbers, however, have since started to climb [13]. Furthermore, even for those who covered, coverage is often inadequate. In fact, a 2017 Substance Abuse and Mental Health Services Administration (SAMHSA) report found that 9–11% of those needing, but not receiving, mental healthcare services cited inadequate coverage by their insurance provider as the primary reason for not obtaining care [2].

The disparity in mental and physical healthcare will not be solved solely by increasing the number of mental healthcare providers, nor is it anticipated that large financial investments will be made to improve access. Rather, this problem will require innovative strategies that marry robust state of the art technological solutions for the prevention, diagnosis, and treatment of mental health conditions to a tiered healthcare delivery system leveraging the full expertise of the available mental healthcare workforce.

4.5   Mental Healthcare Payment Models

In order to understand access to care, one must understand how mental healthcare is funded. Traditionally there have been three systems of mental healthcare in the US, organized primarily around funding source: private insurance, public insurance, and block grant funding for the uninsured. As of 2018, 65.1% of the US population had private insurance, 25.5% had public insurance, and 11.1% had no insurance [14].

4.5.1   Privately-Funded Insurances

Private mental healthcare is healthcare funded either by the person seeking care or by private health insurance. In general, this system serves the less severely mentally ill. Up until the mid-twentieth century, most mental healthcare (and physical healthcare also) had been by private pay. One would pay for the either the amount of healthcare needed or the amount that one could afford. Even the large state hospitals that became widespread in the 1800s – and were the primary source of care for those suffering with mental health conditions until the mid-1900s – were initially funded by private pay. Because healthcare was not provided by the government, companies in the early twentieth century began offering healthcare plans (insurances) as a way of attracting and keeping a highly trained employee workforce. Eventually, as medical treatments for mental health conditions were discovered in the mid-twentieth century, the insurance plans began offering coverage for some mental health services as well.

Private health insurance plans usually cover both inpatient and outpatient costs, including physician fees, diagnostic procedures and laboratory testing. Self-pay patients in a health plan pay a premium, in which the plan's cost is divided equally among group members. Before the rise of managed care, most health insurance used a "fee-for-service" model in providers are paid based solely on the services rendered and the insurance holder pays a predetermined percentage of the cost of services.

In the latter part of the twentieth century, healthcare plans began migrating to a "managed care" system in which a healthcare insurer works directly with providers to ensure cost containment. Expense control was focused on restrictions to the coverage of certain kinds of care, limiting formulary options (e.g., expensive medications or procedures), and limiting hospitalizations (or hospital days) by emphasizing outpatient care and health promotion. *Health Maintenance Organizations* (HMOs) developed as organized systems providing comprehensive care. There are three primary types of HMOs. The staff model is one in which physicians are salaried employees of the HMO and provide care in the HMO facility. The group model is one in which healthcare is furnished by one or more groups of doctors who are contracted to provide full coverage for a predetermined rate. Finally, the individual practice association network (IPA) is a group of individual physicians with whom the HMO negotiates a capitated fee to provide services.

A final private insurance option is the *Preferred Provider Organizations* (PPOs). In this model, an insurance company contracts with a particular group of community hospitals, doctors, and other healthcare providers to supply health services to members at a determined discounted rate. This has become the most common type of managed care practice over the past twenty years.

As can be seen by these multiple types of insurance products, mental healthcare has the potential to be handled quite differently, and cost the individual different amounts depending on the model of care. In fact, even for those with insurance coverage, mental health treatment was not consistently covered across insurers. That prompted the *2008 Mental Health Parity and Addiction Equity Act* which attempted to drive insurers to cover mental health treatment comparably to medical and surgical treatment. Despite the act, however, full parity has not been realized. For instance, the act does not apply to companies with fewer than 50 employees. This has resulted in many individuals seeking insurance on the open marketplace to access plans with appropriate coverage benefits. More recently, the enactment of the *Affordable Care Act* (ACA, also known as "Obamacare") increased the insurance availability for purchase outside of one's employer, offering federally regulated and (often) subsidized healthcare insurance through the health insurance marketplace. While the ACA sets minimum standards for benefits, these still may vary widely (especially mental health coverage) depending on the policy purchased.

4.5.2 Publicly-Funded Insurances

Public mental healthcare is funded by government monies provided at the federal, state, or local level. It usually serves those with chronic or difficult mental health problems (often referred to as "severe and persistently mentally ill (SPMI)" [x]). Access to care, quality of care, type of care, and even philosophy of care is often greatly influenced by the different systems. Because individuals with severe mental illnesses usually require long-term treatment and may have only limited response to current treatment options, public based insurances can disagree widely over what services should be offered to provide the "best quality of life." Further, a review of the evolution of public mental healthcare [15] noted that though most of the care is now provided in the community (rather than in state hospitals), there is a large diversity in treatment options and quality available across the country. This has often resulted in only very limited treatment and support options are actually available to mentally ill individuals. Increasingly, it is being seen that mentally ill often end up in jail or prison, which has become "the de facto system of public care."

Government supported state hospitals or community mental health centers are primarily organized at the state level (with large block grants from the federal government). From the 1950s to 1970s, most states focused on de-institutionalization. This was the mental healthcare philosophy that attempted to deemphasize state mental hospitals while encouraging more community-based care (see Box 4.2). In the 1980s to early 1990s, the focus of mental healthcare shifted toward a coordination and integration of community mental health services, developing centralized authorities, and extending services to those most in need. Since the 1990s, publicly funded mental healthcare has been provided through semi-privatized, government-directed managed care services. State mental health authorities contract with managed mental healthcare vendors who then contract out services to private organizations previously controlled by community health centers.

In addition to block grant funding, the government also provides mental healthcare through Medicare (Title 18) and Medicaid (Title 19) funding.

Medicare is a federally funded health insurance program, established by the Federal Social Security Act of 1965. It provides both hospital and medical coverage for people 65 years and older, as well as for people with certain disabilities (e.g., renal disease, blindness). Medicare consists of four parts. Part A covers inpatient hospital care, dialysis, skilled nursing facilities (only after being formally admitted to a hospital for three days and not for custodial care), and hospice care. Part B is an optional medical insurance that can be purchased. It covers services such as physicians' fees, medical supplies, diagnostic tests, outpatient hospital care, and therapy. Part D covers mostly self-administered prescription drugs. Part C is an alternative called Managed Medicare which allows people to choose health plans that provide at least the same service coverage as Parts A and B, and often the benefits of Part D as well. In 2018, Medicare provided health insurance for over 59.9 million individuals—more than 52 million people aged 65 and older and about 8 million younger people. According to the annual Medicare Trustees report, Medicare covers about half of healthcare expenses of those enrolled. Enrollees almost always cover most of the remaining costs by taking additional private insurance and/or by joining a public Part C or Part D Medicare health plan.

Medicaid is a government assistance program for certain high need groups and low-income persons. Also established in 1965, it is financed by both federal and state governments. In contrast to the Medicare program, which is administered federally, Medicaid eligibility and administration is defined by each individual state. Although benefits vary from state to state, federal rules require Medicaid cover inpatient and outpatient hospital care (including psychiatric care), outpatient care, and laboratory services. Medicaid, unlike Medicare, also covers prescription medications. In 2017, more than 74 million people were covered by Medicaid. The majority of states have contracts with managed care organizations (MCOs) to manage their Medicaid programs. Nationwide, roughly 80% of enrollees in Medicaid are enrolled in a managed care plan.

4.6   Summary

This chapter focused on the basic building blocks of the mental healthcare system and how they are accessed. These components include the various types of mental healthcare providers, various settings in which services are delivered, and the funding that enables or limits access to mental healthcare. Each of these elements represents a structural filter in the pathway to care and must be understood in order to interpret data that will inform a mental health informatician's analyses.

References

1. Mark TL, Levit KR, Vandivort-Warren R, Buck JA, Coffey RM. Changes in US spending on mental health and substance abuse treatment, 1986-2005, and implications for policy. Health Affairs (Project Hope). 2011;30(2):284–92. https://doi.org/10.1377/hlthaff.2010.0765.
2. Substance Abuse and Mental Health Services Administration. Key substance use and mental health indicators in the United States: Results from the 2017 National Survey on Drug Use and Health (HHS Publication No. SMA 18–5068, NSDUH Series H-53). Rockville, MD: Center for Behavioral Health Statistics and Quality, Substance Abuse and Mental Health Services Administration; 2018. Retrieved from https://www.samhsa.gov/data/
3. Schulze B. Stigma and mental health professionals: a review of the evidence on an intricate relationship. International Review of Psychiatry (Abingdon, England). 2007;19(2):137–55. https://doi.org/10.1080/09540260701278929.
4. Mojtabai R. Americans' attitudes toward mental health treatment seeking: 1990-2003. Psychiatric Services (Washington, DC). 2007;58(5):642–51. https://doi.org/10.1176/ps.2007.58.5.642.
5. Health Resource and Services Administration. Behavioral health workforce projections, 2016–2030: psychiatric nurse practitioners, psychiatric physician assistants; 2019b. https://bhw.hrsa.gov/sites/default/files/bhw/nchwa/projections/psychiatric-nurse-practitioners-physician-assistants-2018.pdf
6. Health Resource and Services Administration. Behavioral health workforce projections, 2016–2030: clinical, counseling and school psychologists; 2019a. https://bhw.hrsa.gov/sites/default/files/bhw/nchwa/projections/psychologists-2018.pdf
7. Health Resource and Services Administration. Behavioral health workforce projections, 2016–2030: psychiatrists (adult), child and adolescent psychiatrists; 2019c. https://bhw.hrsa.gov/sites/default/files/bhw/nchwa/projections/psychiatrists-2018.pdf
8. Health Resource and Services Administration. Behavioral health workforce projections, 2016–2030: social workers; 2019d. https://bhw.hrsa.gov/sites/default/files/bhw/nchwa/projections/social-workers-2018.pdf
9. Kramer M. Long-Range Studies of mental hospital patients: an important area for research in chronic disease. The Milbank Quarterly. 2005;83(4). https://doi.org/10.1111/j.1468-0009.2005.00422.x.
10. One-Third of U.S. Adults Have Now Tried Telemedicine, But Many Remain Skeptical. (2020, June 24). CivicScience. https://civicscience.com/one-third-of-u-s-adultshave-now-tried-telemedicine-but-many-remain-skeptical/.
11. Bureau of Labor Statistics. Occupational outlook handbook; 2019. Retrieved from bls.gov on May 16, 2020.
12. World Health Organization. Global Health Observatory data I psychiatrists and nurses (per 100 000 population); 2014. WHO. Accessed January 17, 2020.
13. Tolbert J, Orgera K, Singer N, Damico A Published: Dec 13, and 2019. "Key facts about the uninsured population." The Henry J Kaiser Family Foundation (blog), 2019. https://www.kff.org/uninsured/issue-brief/key-facts-about-the-uninsured-population/
14. Cohen RA, Terlizzi EP, Martinez ME. Health insurance coverage: Early release of estimates from the National Health Interview Survey, 2018. National Center for Health Statistics. May 2019. Available from: https://www.cdc.gov/nchs/nhis/releases.htm.
15. Mechanic D. Better but Not Well: Mental Health Policy in the United States since 1950. By Richard G. Frank and Sherry A. Glied. 183 pp. Baltimore, Johns Hopkins University Press, 2006. 21.95 (paper). ISBN 0-8018-8442-X (cloth); 0-8018-8443-8. The New England Journal of Medicine. 2006;355(21):2263–4.

Chapter 5
The Mental Health System: Access, Diagnosis, Treatment, and Monitoring

Mina Boazak and John L. Beyer

Abstract This chapter reviews the mental healthcare cycle—the process that takes an individual from problem recognition to treatment. The mental healthcare cycle is multi-faceted and rarely straightforward. It involves creating access to care, conducting a professional assessment/diagnostic evaluation, selecting appropriate interventions from the wide variety of treatment options, and finally monitoring the individual for both treatment response as well as maintenance of care. Understanding each part of the cycle is important to the informatician, so that they can best identify the components that provide data points for their work. In order to do so, each part of the cycle will be reviewed, beginning with the various pathways to mental healthcare through the meeting between a person and a mental health provider.

Keywords Mental health · Mental wellbeing · Diagnostic standards · DSM-5 ICD-10 · Theories of psychopathology

5.1   Introduction

This chapter is a broad introduction to the mental healthcare system in the United States. It provides a view of the system from both the care seeker and care provider perspectives. As you review the content please note that there are significant differences between the mental healthcare system and medical

M. Boazak (✉) · J. L. Beyer
Duke University School of Medicine, Department of Psychiatry and Behavioral Sciences, Durham, NC, USA
e-mail: mina.boazak@duke.edu; john.beyer@duke.edu

© Springer Nature Switzerland AG 2021   97
J. D. Tenenbaum, P. A. Ranallo (eds.), *Mental Health Informatics*, Health Informatics, https://doi.org/10.1007/978-3-030-70558-9_5

healthcare system at large. For example, while there is a dynamic interplay between social determinants of health and health in general, that relationship is magnified in the case of mental health. Consequently, there exists a strong bond between mental healthcare and social care. In fact, social workers make up a large proportion of the mental health work force. Thus, good mental healthcare requires regular interactions among providers of different skillsets in order to connect the various care delivery environments. Unfortunately, that is often not the case. As you review the content of this chapter, which attempts to honestly address the current process flow of mental healthcare delivery, ask yourself how informatics can contribute to the growth and development of the mental health-care system.

We have arranged our discussion of the delivery of mental health based on mental healthcare cycle (Fig. 5.1). We have divided the mental healthcare delivery cycle into its four major components: initial problem detection and pathways to care, formal assessment and diagnosis, treatment, and monitoring. Naturally, this cycle does not comprehensively cover the care delivery process, but rather aims to address those elements most pertinent for your success as a mental health informatician.

Fig. 5.1 The mental healthcare cycle is comprised of four primary processes: access to care, the diagnostic assessment, treatment, and outcome monitoring

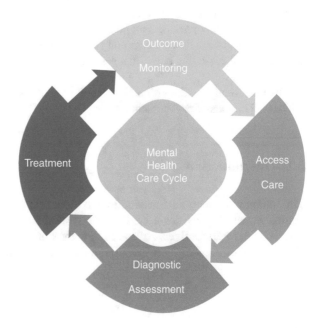

5.2   Access to Mental Healthcare

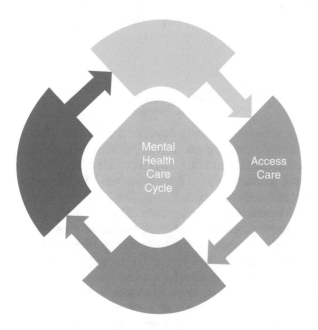

The pathway to mental healthcare begins with the identification of a problem. While this may appear to be an overly simplistic statement, identifying a problem is often the most difficult step in access to care. Not all people with a mental health condition will receive treatment. In fact, up to 50% may never receive mental health services [1]. We will discuss barriers to healthcare more fully later, but the first great challenge in the mental healthcare cycle is that an individual must recognize that there is a problem and decide to seek care. Identifying a problem is not the same as identifying a treatable condition. For example, an individual who has hurt their arm may feel pain or recognize that it does not move normally, but they would not necessarily know if those problems are due to a bruise, a sprain, or a broken bone. In order to determine whether there is an underlying condition, they must be evaluated. Once a condition is diagnosed, then treatment can be given. Similarly, in mental healthcare, an individual may experience distress associated with a mental health condition, or recognize that they are not functioning as they previously have, but they may not know whether the distress and dysfunction are due to an underlying condition that the mental healthcare system may be able help with.

As discussed in Chap. 3, mental health and illness are not clear-cut concepts. What may appear to some to be a mental health problem, may be perceived as just "eccentric" to others. Further, complicating the process is that mental health conditions most often do not occur suddenly, with an obvious break between "pre-mental health problem" experiences and "post-mental health problem" experiences. Usually symptoms of mental health conditions develop gradually over time, and may only be noted when they at last cause some significant level of distress, either to the individual or others within his or her social network (whether it is loved ones, acquaintances, co-workers, community leaders, or even the criminal justice system). Because of this, recognition of a problem and access to care may vary widely.

5.2.1 Pathways to Care: Primary Care

Much of the work evaluating pathways to care is based on the original work of Goldberg and Huxley [2]. These researchers were interested in what barriers inhibited (or factors enabled) access to mental healthcare. They identified "filters" at each transition point of the mental healthcare cycle that determined whether a person would seek or obtain care at the next appropriate level. The first of the filters is at the level of the individual—representing the proportion of those in the community who experience a mental health problem and eventually seek care. One of their most important observations was that despite the need, not every person experiencing a mental health problem sought care. While it is difficult to identify who "needs" care in the general population, in Goldberg and Huxley's model about 8% of people never sought treatment. This assessment may be an underestimate. A 2018 SAMHSA survey of the US general population found that of those meeting diagnostic criteria for depression within the previous year, 35% did not access care [3]. Further, even for those adults identified as experiencing depression that resulted in "severe" impairment within the previous year, 32% did not access care [3] (Fig. 5.2).

Inside the first filter, there are a variety of factors which may contribute to not seeking mental healthcare. These include factors related to the mental health condition itself (the impact the condition may have in making the decision to access care),

Fig. 5.2 Goldberg and Huxley's reported proportions of those who experience a mental health condition who are eventually referred to mental healthcare through the primary care pathway

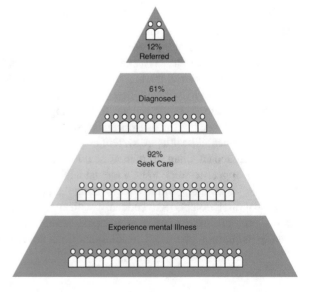

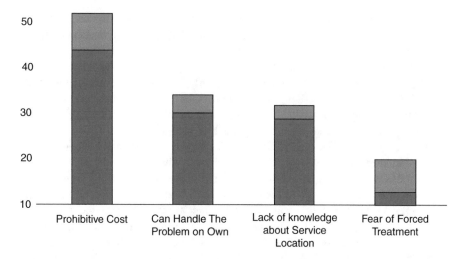

Fig. 5.3 Lower to upper end values of reported reasons for not seeking mental healthcare in 2017 SAMHSA survey

the role of stigma toward mental health problems (in the person him or herself and/ or in friends and family), availability of care, and the cost of care. In the 2017 SAMHSA survey mentioned earlier, the most common reasons reported for not accessing care were prohibitive cost (44–52%), lack of knowledge about where to access services (29–32%), belief that they could handle the problem by themselves (30–34%), fear of forced hospitalization or forced treatment (13–20%), as well as fear of taking a medication, lack of time, and stigma [1] (Fig. 5.3).

One of the most prominent reasons for either seeking or rejecting care is the attitudes of loved ones toward mental health conditions and mental healthcare. The role of relatives and loved ones is vital in the mental healthcare cycle. Their stigma (or lack of it) toward mental health conditions is often a key determinant in not only how a person seeks care, but also when that may occur. The role of relatives and loved ones is particularly important in adolescence and children. One literature review of children and young adults, aged 11–30, found that more than 70% of those who sought care did so on the encouragement of relatives [4]. Other variables that lead to a higher likelihood of accessing care include the presence of low cultural stigma, female gender, and recognition of a problem at a younger age [5].

Box 5.1 A Note to the Informatician

Having read about the filters to mental healthcare, you might ask yourself how each of these filters can be evaluated. At the first filter, for instance, data can be gathered from surveys of the incidence of mental health conditions across large populations (such as the SAMHSA data previously presented, or the NCS-R data noted in Chap. 3). The second and third filter can be represented by studies of the incidence of mental health conditions in primary care populations, either through the use of health system electronic health record data, or information from health information exchange. How else can this data be gathered?

Once a person seeks care, the primary goal of the treatment process is to cor-rectly identify the presence or absence of an underlying mental health condition. Unfortunately, this does not always occur. Here is the second "filter" noted by Goldberg and Huxley: accurate identification of an underlying mental health condi-tion by a healthcare provider. In their model, only 61% of those with mental health condition who presented to a primary care provider (PCP) were correctly identified as having some type of a mental health condition by the PCP. This finding is consis-tent with several other studies that note a low recognition rate of mental health conditions by PCPs. For example, in a 2003 study, Hirschfeld and colleagues used a questionnaire to screen over 85,000 community dwelling adults in the United States for symptoms of bipolar disorder [6]. The survey found that 3.7% (more than 3000 people) screened positive for the criteria of a bipolar disorder. Of those who screened positive, Hirschfeld and colleagues then asked how many had been diag-nosed by their doctor with a bipolar disorder. They found that less than 20% of people who had screened positive for bipolar disorder had ever been diagnosed with the disorder. Interestingly, about 50% of people who screened positive did actually receive a diagnosis from their PCP, but that diagnosis was not bipolar disorder. Rather it was major depressive disorder (a diagnosis that requires a different treat-ment pathway).

There are several reasons why mental health conditions may be missed by health-care professionals. For primary care providers, these may include an inadequate knowledge about mental health, discomfort diagnosing mental health conditions, an inability to recognize nuanced symptoms (often due to limited time available to spend with people seeking care), or an inadequate referral network. For people seeking healthcare services, factors leading to missed diagnoses may include an unwillingness to seek treatment or share symptoms due to the stigma associated with receiving a mental health diagnosis, focus on alternative concerns over mental health concerns (presenting complaints may not include symptoms of mental health conditions), or even interpersonal factors (such as poor communication between the health professional and the person seeking healthcare services, or embarrassment in discussing symptoms). In order to address the challenges of recognizing mental health conditions, PCPs are increasingly using "Patient Reported Outcome" (PRO) measures to track mental health symptoms. These are usually short, structured sur-veys that can sensitively identify mental health problems. However, the introduction of these surveys into daily practice has not been without challenges. Concern has been expressed about liability of asynchronous evaluations of potentially urgent symptoms (such as suicidal ideation or behaviors), or how the increased amount of data from the various scales and surveys may exceed the PCPs ability to monitor the results.

Finally, while not all people with mental health concerns require a referral to a mental health professional, Goldberg and Huxley found that only 12% of their sam-ple were eventually referred for specialty care [7]. This is the third "filter" to mental healthcare. While multiple factors contribute to this drop in the escalation of the care pathway (including the PCP's comfort in treating mental health conditions and the person's interest in seeking mental healthcare), a large contributor is the referral process itself (see Box 5.2). The referral process to a mental health provider has no clear standard and is riddled with variabilities that often leave both care seekers and care providers with much uncertainty.

The challenges of engaging the mental health system found in Goldberg and Huxley's study have also been seen in larger epidemiologic studies which reported that as many as 35–50% of people experiencing a serious mental health condition in developed countries may never receive treatment [8]. The statistics are even worse in developing countries where 76–85% of perople experiencing a serious mental health condition may never receive treatment [8].

Box 5.2 A Note on Referrals

Primary Care Providers (PCPs) are often the first contact or main provider for mental healthcare. In our healthcare system, they often have been vested through the broad social contract (or insurance company policies) as the "gatekeeper" for specialized mental healthcare. Access to a "specialized" mental healthcare provider then is often accomplished through a process of "referrals".

There are few criteria regulating clinical referrals and none have been established as an industry standard. Therefore, provider referrals are generated in multiple ways. These include electronic orders or requests sent to another provider (generally those individuals within the same health system and on the same electronic health record platform), a fax request to a mental health provider's office, a telephone request to a mental health provider's office requesting a consultative appointment, or (still most commonly) a printed document outlining the PCP's recommendation for the person to find a mental health provider. Because of the informal relationships in the larger healthcare system, referrals are often made to providers with whom the referring PCP has had limited contact or experience. Often there is no feedback to the PCP from the mental health provider after referral either confirming the contact or treatment plan. Given the lack of standardization in method and content related to referrals, a substantial number of people do not end up receiving an appointment after a referral is made, and fewer actually keep the appointment when one is made. To address the lack of standardization in the referral process, the Department of Health and Human Services (DHHS) introduced a requirement in their meaningful use incentive program for transition of care summaries. The transition of care measure requires providers to transmit a summary of care records in at least 50% of cases of referrals. While the requirement does not ease the referral process flow, it certainly stands to improve care outcomes by setting baseline expectations for communication between providers in the referral process.

5.2.2 Alternate Pathways to Care

While the Goldberg and Huxley model described the pathway to mental healthcare through a PCP, it represents just one of a multitude of pathways for mental health access. McDonald and colleagues conducted a systematic study of the most common pathway agents and specific first contacts for children and young adults who were eventually diagnosed with a mental health condition (Table 5.1) [4]. They identified a dizzying array of contacts in the person's pathway to care. These contacts included medical professionals (general practitioners, psychiatrists); non-medical professionals (psychologists, social workers, counsellors, school teachers, rural healthcare workers); informal sources of help (family, friends, employers, colleagues); healthcare institutions (emergency services, inpatient units, walk-in clinics); the criminal or justice system (police, prisons, lawyers, courts); traditional or faith-based healers (prayer houses, priests, herbalists, clergy); and technology-enabled contacts (websites, helplines, crisis lines). They also found that the actual "first contact" for mental healthcare were usually PCPs, psychiatric or specialized services (often through an emergency room), and faith-based providers [4]. The authors concluded that pathways to mental healthcare were often complex and multi-faceted. Further, they noted that first contacts for care often did not necessarily represent the best nor the easiest route to *appropriate* care. In fact, the most common successful referral source to care was the Emergency Room [4]. Unfortunately, this suggests that for many people, problem severity may reach dangerous levels before the care pathway is initiated and appropriate referrals are made.

While there are pathways to care that are preferred, including pathways through general practitioners or social workers, there are others that are considered "negative" pathways and signify failings of the mental healthcare system. These include introduction to mental healthcare through contact with the police or judicial system, and often involve compulsory/involuntary care (see Box 5.3). Unfortunately, many still have their first contact with mental healthcare through the negative pathways. Livingston and colleagues [9] have estimated that 10% of individuals' first contact with a mental healthcare provider involves interactions with police [9]. Though there is only limited literature on negative pathways, it is clear this

Table 5.1 Findings of pathway agents, first contacts, and successful referral sources to care in young adults [4]

General Pathway Agents	Top First Contacts	Successful Referral Source (last contact)
• Medical professional • Non-medical professional • Informal sources • Healthcare institution • Crimal justice system • Technology-enabled contacts	• General practitioners • Psychiatrists • Faith-based healer/clergy • Emergency rooms and inpatient units • Family or friends • Social workers	• Emergency room and inpatient unit • Self or family-referrals • General practitioners • Helplines

disproportionately impacts ethnic minorities, particularly African Americans [4]. In one systematic review of the literature in the United Kingdom, it was found that black people suffering from a mental health condition not only had more contacts with police, but also were disproportionately admitted to hospitals against their will as compared to white counterparts (45% vs 21%) [10]. These "negative" pathways to care are important to track as they represent delays in detection of mental health conditions and may result in psychological trauma to people who are already vulnerable. Such trauma can create a negative associative connection between the mental health system and the criminal justice system, leading many to abandon care.

Box 5.3 A Note on Voluntary and Involuntary Care

In addition to the elements highlighted in this section the reader should be aware that the discussion has primarily focused on pathways to mental health-care in which individuals voluntarily seek treatment. While most individuals do access care through voluntary pathways, in the United States, each state has its own regulations that may provide a involuntary pathway for care. Provision of involuntary care is usually constrained to three extreme circumstances: situations where a person's mental health status makes them a danger to self, a danger to others, or renders them unable to care for their basic survival needs. Note that these are legal processes within the mental healthcare system. The use of involuntary commitment procedures has fluctuated over time, especially since one of the primary principles of healthcare ethics is that of *autonomy*—the belief that an individual has the right to make their own healthcare decisions. This often creates a tension between a person experiencing a mental health condition that prevents them from perceiving the problem or accepting treatment, and society (represented often by mental healthcare providers, law enforcement, and families) who perceive the problem and the need for treatment as part of the "greater good" for both the individual and the community.

5.2.3   Delays in Care

Not specifically mentioned in the above section is that fact that access to care often does not transition smoothly to recognition and treatment. In their review of studies evaluating pathways of care for children and young adults, MacDonald et al. [4] found that on average 2.9 contacts (range 1–15) with professional services occurred before a referral was made to mental healthcare [4]. Similarly, for adults that seek care, Steel et al. [11] noted an average of 3 professional contacts occurred prior to a mental health referral [11]. In that study, the median time to care was found to be 6.3 months. Even then, over 25% of individuals did not receive care for more than 2 years [11]. MacDonald and colleagues, on the other hand, found that time between the onset of a mental health condition and initiation of treatment ranged from

1 week to 45 years. However, the three studies that focused on care in the United States found mean duration of illness (DOI) ranged from 27.7 [12] to 146.4 [13] weeks. While such delays are concerning, the numbers may actually be optimistic estimations of real-world experience. The World Health Organization's World Mental Health Survey Initiative, found that in the United States only a small subset of individuals experiencing anxiety disorders (11.3%), mood disorders (35.4%), and substance use disorders (10%) received care within a year of onset [5].

These delays are not inconsequential. A growing body of literature has demonstrated that early intervention leads to better outcomes. Evidence suggests that an increased DOI, particularly in the case of serious mental health conditions, contributes to poorer response to treatment and increased morbidity and mortality [14, 15].

5.3 Mental Health Assessment and Diagnosis

In the previous section, we reviewed how people access mental healthcare and discussed barriers to access. Once a person engages a mental healthcare professional, what is the process by which a mental health condition is either identified or ruled out, and, if identified, treatment selected?

In Chap. 3, we reviewed the current nosologies used by most mental health professionals around the world, the DSM-5 and ICD-11. Diagnostic standards alone, however, do not diagnose illness; rather, they are the tools that providers employ to guide their clinical assessments. In practice, the application of these standards can vary significantly by provider type and setting. An emergency room psychiatrist will employ different tactics than an office-based cognitive-behavioral therapist; yet, each will also employ some basic common components to the diagnostic process. The following discussion is presented so that informaticians may understand the basic process leading to a DSM-5 or ICD-11 diagnosis, and what data points may be consistently documented in, or extracted from, a person's medical record.

5.3.1 The Assessment of Illness

During a mental health examination, a provider performs a **diagnostic clinical interview**. This is most commonly conducted as an unstructured conversation. Questions clarifying symptoms or experiences are usually asked in an open-ended, flexible format that allows the provider to develop an understanding of what the person is experiencing and the impact the problems have had on his or her life. Throughout the interview, providers are taught to not only focus on the person's words, but also on his or her body language, eye contact, and expressions. The flexible, relaxed structure of the interview (as opposed to a more rigid series of questions) has been found to promote the development of trust and openness. For example, people experiencing delusions (fixed and false beliefs) often do not openly share the content of their thoughts, particularly if asked in a closed ended manner ("Do you believe people are out to get you?"). Rather, it is often in responses to open ended questions ("Tell me about a time when you did not feel safe?") that a person may share content that could identify an underlying delusion. It should be noted that despite the more casual, conversational nature of the interview, referring to it as an "unstructured" interview is a misnomer. Providers are trained to collect specific information during a clinical interview and most utilize an underlying organized approach for data collection. Common elements of the diagnostic interview include: the presenting complaint, an extensive history of the symptoms (history of present illness), and past psychiatric, medical, family, and relevant social history.

The **history of present illness (HPI)** includes information about a person's current symptoms, their intensity, and the impact they have had on functioning. As the person describes his or her symptoms and the events leading to the evaluation, the provider develops a deeper understanding of the person's experience by focusing the questions on increasingly more specific information. A provider may ask "rule-in" questions focused on confirming the presence of symptoms of a specific condition, but they will also ask "rule-out" questions that evaluate possible alternative conditions that may cause similar symptoms or experiences. For example, during an evaluation focused on anxiety symptoms, the provider will ask "rule-in" questions about specific symptoms included in a list of diagnostic criteria for an anxiety disorder (such as the presence of worry, irritability, insomnia, or other physical symptoms suggestive of panic), in addition to "rule-out" questions that help distinguish an anxiety disorder from other conditions (such as depression, thyroid abnormalities, or excessive caffeine use).

Providers will also collect information about the person's history. Information about a person's **past psychiatric history** helps the provider understand the course of the current problem, whether the person sought or received healthcare services related to the problem in the past, and, if so, what treatments were successful or unsuccessful in the past. The person's **medical history** may help identify a physical condition or medical treatment that may be causing or contributing to current symptoms. Information about substance use is also typically collected as part of the medical history. A **family history**, with special emphasis on mental health conditions or treatments in close relatives, is also collected since many mental health conditions are highly correlated with genetic predisposing factors [16]. A **social history** which broadly outlines the person's childhood experiences, developmental milestones, important relationships, educational background, current living circumstances, work history, and strengths/challenges is also collected. Finally, during the interview, the provider conducts the mental health equivalent of a physical exam, the **mental status exam** (See Table 5.2). All this information allows the provider to develop a working differential of what condition(s) the person may have, and what conditions they do not have.

Clearly the diagnostic interview is a complex and very personal conversation that covers a broad range of topics and details essential for the provider to make a well informed and accurate diagnosis. The breadth of the interview means that without extensive training, a provider could potentially miss important details that may

Table 5.2 Domains of the mental status exam

Domain	Description
Appearance	Observations about physical characteristics of the person such as apparent age, height, weight, and manner of dress and grooming.
Attitude	Observations about the person's general attitude during the interview, as well as the level of rapport and cooperation between the person and the provider during the interview process.
Behavior	Observations about the person's activity level, eye contact, gait, and the presence of abnormal movements.
Mood and affect	Observations about the person's apparent emotional state as conveyed by his or her nonverbal behavior (affect) and the person's own description of his or her internal emotional state.
Speech	Observations about vocal and linguistic characteristics of speech including spontaneity, paucity, volume, and structure of language
Thought process	Observations about the quantity, tempo and form (logical coherence) of thought, inferred from a person's speech.
Thought content	Observations about the content (subject or topic) of the person's thought including delusions, obsessions, phobias, suicidal ideations, overvalued ideas, etc.
Perceptions	Observations about the person's perceptual experiences such as hallucinations, pseudo-hallucinations, and illusions.
Cognition	Observations about the person's level of alertness, orientation, attention, memory, visuospatial functioning, language functions, and executive functions.
Insight	Observations about the person's understanding of their current mental health as expressed in their explanation of the problem and understanding of treatment options.

differentiate between two or more mental health conditions with overlapping symptoms. For example, psychotic symptoms may be present in schizophrenia, depressive disorders, bipolar disorders, dementias, or physical conditions such as delirium and thyroid disease. Thus, just knowing a person is experiencing symptoms of "psychosis" does not by itself indicate that he or she is suffering from a specific underlying condition. Even with training, important details may be missed due to time constraints or the person's misidentification of history or experiences.

In order to increase diagnostic reliability, semi-structured and structured interviews have been developed to ensure that key diagnostic questions are not missed. Semi-structured and structured interviews provide a script of pre-developed questions that a provider may use to guide his or her clinical evaluation, either partially or completely. With appropriate training these interviews have been demonstrated to reliably identify people who meet diagnostic criteria various mental health conditions (see Table 5.3). An advantage of semi-structured and structured interviews is that the provider employing the tools generally needs less training. However, structured interviews tend to vary in their diagnostic reliability, often under-diagnosing certain conditions, and over-diagnosing others. Furthermore, while structured interviews comprehensively evaluate for gross symptomatology, few are apt to pick up on individual-specific nuances which may influence treatment strategies.

Table 5.3 Examples of semi-structured and structured diagnostic interviews

Questionnaire	Details
MINI international neuropsychiatric interview (MINI)	A short, structured interview used to assess for 17 common mental health conditions defined in the DSM-IV and ICD-10. Administration time: 15–20 minutes [17]
Structured clinical interview for DSM-5 (SCID)	A semi-structured interview, developed by the American Psychiatric Association, used by clinicians and researchers in evaluating common DSM-5 diagnosis. Administration time: Greater than 1–1.5 hours [18].
World mental health composite international diagnostic interview (WMH-CIDI)	A structured, comprehensive interview used to assess for mental health conditions defined in the DSM-IV and ICD-10. The WMH-CIDI was developed by the World Health Organization for use by trained lay interviewers. Administration time: 2 hours [19].

5.3.2   Diagnosis and Case Conceptualization

As mentioned previously, our current theory of mental illness is that it is attributable to a combination of biological, psychological, and social factors, many of which we are still trying to understand. This model of illness is known as the biopsychosocial model of illness, first coined by George Engel in 1977 [20]. In assessing illness, it should therefore be no surprise that providers take each of the biopsychosocial elements into consideration. In fact, earlier versions of the Diagnostic and Statistics Manual (DSM) incorporated a multi-axial system for assessments. Five "axes" of assessment covered (1) mental health conditions other than personality disorders and intellectual disability, (2) personality disorders and intellectual disability, (3) physical conditions, (4) psychosocial and environmental problems, and (5) a global assessment of functioning. While the multiaxial system is no longer in use, it remains a good example of the various domains mental health providers must consider during their evaluation. It is not enough for the provider to come to a diagnosis after having conducted an interview. Instead the provider aims to achieve an understanding of the person's experience with the symptoms that lead to distress, all co-occurring mental health conditions (including personality disorders, substance use disorders, and intellectual disability) and medical conditions contributing to the primary problem, the cognitive and behavioral patterns in which the individual engages that promote and/or prevent illness, and the strengths and weaknesses of the individual's social system that may contribute to or deter recovery. Each of these elements allows the provider to develop a more detailed understanding of the individual. This has often been referred to as the "psychiatric formulation". In assessing each of these elements, the provider then can identify problems, diagnose any conditions, and work with the individual on an appropriate strategy to promote quality of life and relieve suffering. The extent to which the provider focuses on some of these elements as compared to others can vary by the scope of the provider's practice, the provider's theoretical orientation, and the person seeking their care. The latter can be of significant influence, since individuals present for mental healthcare due to variety of reasons ranging from simple interest in promoting their mental wellbeing, to a required intervention because of severe mental illness.

Box 5.4 Biomarkers and Mental Illness

You may be wondering where blood tests, imaging, and additional neurophysiological tests fit into the mental health evaluation? At present, there are relatively few biomarkers that identify a specific mental health condition. Rather, most available biomarker tests are used as tools to rule out physical and substance related illness' that may be contributing to a person's symptoms (See Table 5.4). For example, hypothyroidism may cause loss of energy, weight gain, poor concentration, depressed mood, and anhedonia—symptoms that overlap with the presentation of a major depressive disorder. Therefore, a blood test to check thyroid function is indicated. Similarly, people with certain autoimmune disorders such as the autoimmune encephalitides, may present with symptoms similar to those seen in people experiencing a psychotic disorder. In that case, neuroimaging may be required. Distinction in the underlying cause of symptoms is important as without the appropriate treatment of the underlying dysfunction, the person's symptoms are unlikely to improve.

Table 5.4 Examples of medical illnesses that may be misdiagnosed as mental illness

Physical Condition	Mental Health Condition
Thyroid disease	Anxiety disorders, mood disorders, psychotic disorders
Anemia	Mood disorders
Electrolyte imbalances	Anxiety disorders, mood disorders
Autoimmune disorders	Anxiety disorders, mood disorders, psychotic disorders
Vitamin B12/Folate deficiency	Mood disorders
Neurosyphilis	Mood disorders, anxiety disorders, psychotic disorders
Cardiac arrhythmias	Anxiety disorders, psychosomatic disorder
Seizure disorder	Psychosomatic disorder

5.4 Mental Health Treatment

Having completed the interview and identified a working diagnosis, the provider must develop a treatment plan. This section will focus on two major components of the treatment plan: identification of, and referral to, an appropriate treatment setting, and selection of the optimal treatment. Treatment decisions are influenced by a variety of factors, including the specific diagnosis, severity of the condition, the person's family history, treatment history, concomitant conditions and medications, the available social support network, individual preference, and/or availability of options as influenced by geography and finances. Balancing these often-conflicting factors requires experience, an understanding of the mental health system, knowledge of good clinical practice, and an ability to communicate these well with individuals and families.

5.4.1   The Treatment Setting

One of the first decisions a person and his or her mental healthcare provider make is about the setting in which treatment may be provided. The provider must determine if the individual's condition can be adequately treated using their expertise and site, or if they would be better served through referral to an alternative setting or provider expertise. This decision is most often driven by the acuity of the condition and the accessibility of options. The optimal treatment setting is the one that provides the appropriate level of care in the least restrictive environment. Options are usually grouped in the following five categories: (listed in a rough approximation of the intensity of care) outpatient office-based care, intensive outpatient programs, partial hospital programs, residential programs, and inpatient hospitalization. These and other settings were reviewed in more detail in Chap. 4.

Outpatient mental healthcare is delivered in a wide variety of clinical settings, with varying frequency of treatment contacts. Settings include PCP offices, psychiatric clinics (either solo or group practices), psychotherapy clinics (also solo or group practices), and community mental health centers (see Box 5.5). For people with chronic or recurrent mental health conditions, the focus of outpatient care may be on long-term management and recovery. In these cases, for an individual whose health has been stabilized and are in the maintenance phase of treatment, the provider managing medications may only meet with them once every few months or even annually; the therapist/counselor though may meet with them monthly. Alternatively, an individual in the active phase of treatment may need to be seen more frequently for medication management and up to multiple times a week by their therapist/counselor. Decision-making for the frequency of treatment contact include individual stability (symptomatology), management of potential side effects/treatment monitoring, type of psychotherapy, and level of social support.

Box 5.5 A Note on Telepsychiatry

Each of the outpatient care settings mentioned above may also be available via telehealth care (telepsychiatry). Telepsychiatry services has the potential to significantly improve access to mental healthcare in under resourced settings, rural setting, or areas where travel burden may contribute to stress on individual's requiring frequent monitoring [21, 22]. Unfortunately, despite evidence demonstrating comparable efficacy to in-person care [23], telehealth care access had classically been limited by payor non-parity (it did not pay the same as in-person care) and variations in state board regulations [24]. In March of 2020, the COVID-19 epidemic resulted in the declaration of a Public Health Emergency. The Department of Health and Human Services (DHHS), the Centers for Medicare and Medicaid Services (CMS), and private insurers increased the parity between telehealth and in-person visits. This allowed the mass adoption of telepsychiatry for the majority of outpatient psychiatric services and a large proportion of acute care services. Since then, CMS has transitioned multiple billing codes from temporary use for telehealth services to permanent status. As of the writing of this chapter the COVID-19 epidemic remains an active problem, but many believe that the increase in the utilization of telehealth services will persist well past the pandemic's end.

More intensive **outpatient** care is provided through intensive **outpatient** programs (IOP) or partial hospitalization programs (PHP). IOPs/PHPs can either be programs that treat a wide variety of mental health conditions, or that target specific conditions, such as substance use disorders or eating disorders. Both IOP and PHP programs incorporate elements of group therapy, individual therapy, skills training and psychoeducation, and medication management. They may vary in the frequency of care contact. In the case of IOP, programs are part time and generally do not exceed 15 hours each week. PHP programs, on the other hand, are more intensive, and usually are attended 5–7 days a week.

Residential care programs represent a more intensive care setting than PHP. People attending PHP programs live in their own homes while they receive care in the hospital facility during the day. For residential care programs, people live at the care facility while undergoing treatment. However, the facility is usually not closely secured. In most cases, people have the ability to come and go as they please, as long as they are engaged in the treatment program.

An inpatient psychiatric hospital is the highest level of care in mental health. A person is typically admitted to an inpatient setting when intensive medical or mental health support and monitoring is required to stabilize an acute condition, or when a person's current state creates a risk to his or her physical safety or the safety of others. Inpatient hospitals are highly secured settings that seek to minimize risk of phsyical injury by restricting access to objects that may pose a danger. These facilities also allow for direct and (if necessary) continuous observation, as well as more intensive treatment interventions. Because inpatient care provides the highest acuity of care and is the most restrictive in its environment, it is also the costliest. Generally, inpatient care is reserved as a final option of care, only used when necessary.

5.4.2 Selecting the Right Treatment

The second major decision a person and his or her mental healthcare provider make is about which intervention or treatment regimen to pursue. Similar to the wide variety of mental health treatment providers noted in Chap. 4, there are also a wide variety of treatment options. Here, we divide these treatments into 4 broad categories: psychotherapy and social interventions, pharmacotherapy, neuromodulation, and surgical intervention (Table 5.5).

Table 5.5 Broad categories of mental health treatments, their subtypes, and types of trained providers

Treatment Category	Training Required	Treatment Subtypes
Psychotherapy and Social Interventions	Licensed Clinical Social Workers, Advanced Practice Providers, Psychologists, Psychiatrists	The most commonly used psychotherapeutic techniques include cognitive behavioral therapy (CBT), exposure therapy, behavioral therapy, acceptance and commitment therapy (ACT), dialectic behavior therapy (DBT), psychodynamic psychotherapy, and psychoanalysis among a wide assortment of other treatments or variations of interventions. Social interventions range widely, but can include assistance with housing, seeking employment, or seeking disability.
Pharmacotherapy	Advanced Practice Provider, Primary Care Providers, Psychiatrists	There are multiple different categories and numerous subcategories of medication utilized by mental health providers. Broadly the most well-known categories are the antidepressants, the antipsychotics, mood stabilizers, anxiolytic, and stimulant medications.
Neuromodulation	Physicians	Neuromodulation is split into non-invasive and invasive treatments; these can range from transcranial magnetic stimulation through to neurosurgical techniques including deep brain stimulation.
Surgical techniques	Trained Physicians	At the highest level of invasiveness are techniques that include resection, either through radiotherapy or surgical resection, of brain regions linked to the pathological development of the disorder at hand.

5.4.3   Psychotherapy and Social Interventions

Psychotherapy. As illustrated in Table 5.5, there are many types of psychotherapies available for the treatment of mental health conditions. Two of the most common interventions in the United States are cognitive behavioral therapy (CBT) and psychodynamic therapy. CBT is a technique that promotes changes in unwanted thoughts and behaviors with the goal of reducing distress and suffering. As a therapy, CBT distinguishes itself from psychodynamic psychotherapy in that it is highly structured, analytical and problem focused. As a part of the frame of CBT the therapist and individual confront unhelpful thoughts and beliefs (such as "no one likes me" or "I am not a good enough") using techniques such as reframing, guided discovery, and Socratic questioning. CBT also utilizes "homework" or home exercises to promote change. Most often, CBT is performed in outpatient office sessions. Other examples of structured therapeutic interventions include Behavior Therapy and Dialectic Behavior Therapy (DBT).

While CBT is problem focused and highly structured, psychodynamic psychotherapy is unstructured and focused on the interpersonal dynamic. Psychodynamic therapy was the predominant form of therapy prior to the rise in CBT, and is often the type of therapy pictured when lay people talk about psychotherapy. The key principal underlying psychodynamic psychotherapy is that unconscious conflicts cause an individual's mental suffering;

those unconscious conflicts manifest themselves in the therapeutic interaction; and exposing those conflicts to awareness results in the reduction of suffering. During sessions the therapist and person "work through" session content, particularly the person's thoughts and feelings. The therapist directs the session toward material he or she believes is representative of a more deeply rooted unconscious process. With time this exploration of thoughts and feelings is believed to improves the individual's awareness of unconscious conflicts and, in so doing, to reduce intrapsychic tensions and suffering.

The evidence for the effectiveness of psychotherapy has been a subject of debate over the past several decades, often between the practitioners of various (sometimes competing) types of therapy, or between therapy providers and psychopharmacologists (most often represented by psychiatrists). In the past decade, the rise of manual-based therapies (such as CBT or DBT) has improved the evidence base for efficacy and increased the acceptance of these interventions in treatment guidelines. However, given the nature of therapy and the variations that can introduce difficulties in standardization, the evidence is often subject to confounding [25]. Increasingly, certifications have been developed for the manualized treatments, yet the practice of these treatments is not limited to those with certification. When psychotherapy is recommended for treatment, many practitioners rely more on the art of medicine (adapting their treatment to fit the patient, the problem, or their own comfort level with various therapy interventions) rather than the applied science of medicine. Given limitations in the evidence and inconsistent reliance on guidelines, clinical decisions about which therapy to utilize for which indication are most often influenced by the provider's own theoretical leaning, training, and/or experience.

Social Interventions. While psychotherapy aims to promote positive change in the person engaging in therapy, social interventions aim to promote change in the environment. Mental health conditions both impact and are impacted by a person's environment. Experiencing a mental health condition, particularly a serious condition, may result in isolation, lack of employment, or housing and food insecurity. Each of these factors, in turn, can contribute to declining health. As such, high quality mental healthcare includes social interventions to address these basic human needs. These include psychosocial intervention programs, group-based programs that may also focus on social skills training, basic employment search training, and access to support groups, amongst other social interventions or support systems. Social interventions may also include focused assistance in helping the person find employment, obtain disability support, locate housing, or even in some instances acquire government identification so that services can be accessed. Sadly, while these services are extremely useful and practical in supporting persons suffering with serious mental health conditions, they are also often underfunded or not consistently available in many areas.

5.4.4 Pharmacotherapy

Medication treatment represents a more invasive approach to mental healthcare than psychotherapy and social interventions. As in physical healthcare, the decision to prescribe or take use medications must include an evaluation of the individual's illness severity, the sufficiency of available alternatives, and the individual's personal preference. The provider also utilizes the content obtained during their clinical interview to select a medication that is likely to be efficacious and least likely to cause side effects. This process is often imprecise, also requiring more of the "art" of medicine when the "science" is limited. Guidelines have been developed in an effort to ensure clinicians utilize evidence-based approaches for care. However, due to inconsistencies among guidelines, many providers do not directly rely on guidelines in making medication management decisions. This often leads to variability in practice, delays in the initiation of appropriate medications, and possibly increased morbidity.

5.4.5   Neuromodulation and Surgical Interventions

Finally, while psychotherapy and pharmacotherapy are the primary intervention strategies, other treatment options have also been developed. These include effective and long-practiced interventions such as electroconvulsive therapy (ECT), or the newer neuromodulation techniques such as transcranial magnetic stimulation (TMS) or vagal nerve stimulation (VNS). For more severe illnesses that have been very resistant to other less invasive treatment, new techniques have been developed and refined that involve resection or stimulation of certain brain regions or nerve bundles using surgical intervention or implanted electrodes (deep brain stimulation) in order to interrupt the pathological pathways contributing to the mental health condition. These techniques are reserved for severe, treatment refractory conditions, and for some they can be highly effective for the alleviation of suffering. In fact, the most publicly recognized and misunderstood of the neuromodulating techniques, electroconvulsive therapy (ECT), remains one of the most efficacious treatment strategies for treatment resistant depression [26].

5.5   Treatment Monitoring

Having initiated treatment, the mental health provider must monitor the individual's response. Consistent across all practice settings and providers, treatment outcome monitoring incorporates regular to semi-regular clinical evaluations. As with the diagnostic interview, follow up interviews may be performed along the continuum from unstructured to structured approaches. Follow up interviews, however, differ from the initial interview in that they are less comprehensive in scope and more problem focused. For psychotherapists, monitoring can range from subtle evaluations of symptoms during the therapy interaction to more direct symptom tracking using scales such as those listed in Table 5.6. For medication management providers, monitoring may also be done in conversation over an individual's experience since the last visit, or with a structured scale. Their goal is to identify symptomatic change, level of functioning, and potential side effects. Since the most common symptom monitoring approach in mental health remains the clinical interview, providers often obtain

Table 5.6 Commonly used patient reported outcome measures in mental healthcare

Measure	Description
Patient health questionnaire (PHQ-9)	A 9-item, self-administered, questionnaire that screens for the presence of depression.
Generalized anxiety disorder 7 (GAD-7)	A 7-item, self-administered, questionnaire that screens for the presence of anxiety.
Alcohol use disorder identification test (AUDIT-C)	A 3-item, self-administered, questionnaire that screens for alcohol use disorder.
Edinburgh postnatal depression scale (EDPS)	A 10-item, self-administered, questionnaire that screens for postpartum depression.

information of the person's progress based on the content they collected during relatively brief interactions. To address the time restriction of the clinical interview many providers are starting to use Patient Reported Outcome measures (PROs).

5.5.1 Patient Reported Outcome Measures

PROs are generally domain specific validated questionnaires that can be completed by an individual to measure their wellbeing for the domain being evaluated. While PROs (Table 5.6) have been in use for decades, recent regulatory efforts have both supported and encouraged their use in clinical practice. There are several benefits for the use of PROs. First, they allow providers and care seekers to objectively evaluate and track illness symptoms consistently over time. Second, they may be self-administered (meaning the person can fill them out prior to the visit) allowing the clinician to review responses and focus on addressing the pertinent issues at hand. Third, their use is not limited just to the clinic appointment but may also be completed at any time allowing for better tracking of symptoms.

PROs do have some limitations. Creating a usable PRO requires that they be brief and focused. Because of this, sensitivity to presence of illness or symptom change may be decreased. Furthermore, their sensitivity is directly affected by the user's understanding of the questions and the terminology used. Nonetheless, PROs have become increasingly more precise, and the majority adequately capture the presence of disease and track symptoms.

5.5.2 Side Effect Monitoring

Medications used for the treatment of mental health conditions are powerful tools. When appropriately employed, they can effectively and significantly improve a person's functioning and quality of life. However, they are relatively non-specific in their actions, since they affect certain neurotransmitters that often influence multiple biological functions. Consequently, medications can cause side effects. Furthermore, these side effects may occur either suddenly or through the course of long-term treatment. Because of this, monitoring for side effects is an essential part of treatment. First, monitoring ensures that the provider is attentive to the person and allows them to quickly adapt the treatment to limit unwanted side effects. This good clinical practice often results in improved confidence in the provider, improved medication utilization, and thus improved outcomes. Second, monitoring for adverse events helps decrease morbidity, or in the case of some adverse events, can prevent mortality.

Monitoring for side effects is usually focused on short-term and long-term events. For short-term assessments, providers focus on the most common side effects, the most dangerous side effects, and black box warnings provided with the medication profile. For long term treatment, some medications may induce adverse events only after protracted use. For example, antipsychotics often cause short term side effects such as weight gain, muscle stiffness, or blurred vision; however, they may also cause long term side effects, such as increasing the risk of diabetes or inducing movement disorders. In those instances, where the adverse event takes months, or years to develop, the provider must monitor symptoms on a semi-regular basis, in accordance with the appropriate guidelines. Medications and neuromodulation procedures (such as electroconvulsive therapies) are typically what is thought of when it comes to adverse events of mental health treatment, however, psychotherapy has also been shown to result adverse events. Exact adverse events secondary to psychotherapy are less well understood in terms of their frequencies, however, they have been shown to include worsening symptoms and the development of new symptoms. While psychotherapy can cause some adverse events, monitoring adverse events in psychotherapeutic care is less well defined and less consistently practiced than for pharmacotherapy or neuromodulation. The reasons for this variability are more nuanced than what one may initially expect. Core to the practice of psychotherapy is the underlying premise that the focus of the clinical interaction will have an influence on the person. Thus, for some a focus on adverse event during psychotherapy encounters may in and of itself result in adverse outcomes, such as decreased participation in therapeutic exercises.

5.6   Conclusion

The flow of mental healthcare is clearly not without complexities. Having learned about the various pathways of care, the assessment and diagnosis of illness, and the treatment of illness we hope you have gleaned enough information to better recognize the fit and role of the informatician in the mental healthcare system. From improving approaches to population level prevalence assessments, understanding the available data and its limitations, through to promoting the development of standards in care, much needs to be done in the mental healthcare system. As you go through the next chapters, be sure to regularly reflect on those elements of the mental healthcare system we discussed here, asking often how it is that the processes, policies, and techniques you learn about directly apply to the practice of mental healthcare.

References

1. Substance Abuse and Mental Health Services Administration. Key substance use and mental health indicators in the United States: results from the 2017 national survey on drug use and health (HHS Publication No. SMA 18–5068, NSDUH Series H-53). Rockville, MD: Center for Behavioral Health Statistics and Quality, Substance Abuse and Mental Health Services Administration; 2018. Retrieved from https://www.samhsa.gov/data/
2. Goldberg D, Huxley P. Mental illness in the community: the pathways to psychiatric care. New York: Tavistock; 1980.
3. Substance Abuse and Mental Health Services Administration. Key Substance Use and Mental Health Indicators in the United States: Results from the 2018 National Survey on Drug Use and Health (HHS Publication No. PEP19–5068, NSDUH Series H-54). Rockville, MD: Center for Behavioral Health Statistics and Quality, Substance Abuse and Mental Health Services Administration; 2019. Retrieved from https://www.samhsa.gov/data/
4. MacDonald K, Fainman-Adelman N, Anderson KK, Iyer SN. Pathways to mental health Services for Young People: a systematic review. Soc Psychiatry Psychiatr Epidemiol. 2018;53(10):1005–38. https://doi.org/10.1007/s00127-018-1578-y.
5. Wang PS, Angermeyer M, Borges G, Bruffaerts R, Chiu WT, De Girolamo G, Fayyad J, et al. Delay and failure in treatment seeking after First onset of mental disorders in the World Health Organization's world mental health survey initiative. World Psychiatry. 2007;6(3):177–85.
6. Hirschfeld RMA, Calabrese JR, Weissman MM, Reed M, Davies MA, Frye MA, Paul E. Keck, et al. Screening for bipolar disorder in the community. J Clin Psychiatry. 2003;64(1):53–9. https://doi.org/10.4088/jcp.v64n0111.
7. Huxley P. Mental illness in the community: the Goldberg-Huxley model of the pathway to psychiatric care. Nord J Psychiatry. 1996;50(sup37):47–53. https://doi.org/10.3109/08039489609099730.
8. Demyttenaere K, Bruffaerts R, Posada-Villa J, Gasquet I, Kovess V, Lepine JP, Angermeyer MC, et al. Prevalence, severity, and unmet need for treatment of mental disorders in the World Health Organization world mental health surveys. JAMA. 2004;291(21):2581–90. https://doi.org/10.1001/jama.291.21.2581.
9. Livingston JD. Contact between police and people with mental disorders: a review of rates. Psychiatr Serv. 2016;67(8):850–7. https://doi.org/10.1176/appi.ps.201500312.
10. Morgan C, Mallett R, Hutchinson G, Leff J. Negative pathways to psychiatric care and ethnicity: the bridge between social science and psychiatry. Social Science & Medicine, Heresy and orthodoxy in medical theory and research. 2004;58(4):739–52. https://doi.org/10.1016/S0277-9536(03)00233-8.
11. Steel Z, Mcdonald R, Silove D, Bauman A, Sandford P, Herron J, Harry Minas I. Pathways to the First contact with specialist mental health care. Australian & New Zealand Journal of Psychiatry. 2006;40(4):347–54. https://doi.org/10.1080/j.1440-1614.2006.01801.x.
12. Chien VH, Compton MT. The impact of mode of onset of psychosis on pathways to Care in a Hospitalized, predominantly African-American, First-episode sample. Early Interv Psychiatry. 2008;2(2):73–9. https://doi.org/10.1111/j.1751-7893.2008.00061.x.
13. Compton MT, Esterberg ML, Druss BG, Walker EF, Kaslow NJ. A descriptive study of pathways to care among hospitalized urban African American First-episode schizophrenia-Spectrum patients. Soc Psychiatry Psychiatr Epidemiol. 2006;41(7):566–73. https://doi.org/10.1007/s00127-006-0065-z.
14. Altamura AC, Dell'Osso B, Berlin HA, Buoli M, Bassetti R, Mundo E. Duration of untreated illness and suicide in bipolar disorder: a naturalistic study. Eur Arch Psychiatry Clin Neurosci. 2010;260(5):385–91. https://doi.org/10.1007/s00406-009-0085-2
15. McGlashan TH. Duration of untreated psychosis in First-episode schizophrenia: marker or determinant of course? Biol Psychiatry. 1999;46(7):899–907. https://doi.org/10.1016/S0006-3223(99)00084-0.

16. Merikangas KR, Merikangas AK. Harnessing Progress in psychiatric genetics to advance population mental health. Am J Public Health. 2019 Jun;109(S3):S171–5. https://doi.org/10.2105/AJPH.2019.304948.
17. Sheehan DV, Lecrubier Y, Sheehan KH, Amorim P, Janavs J, Weiller E, Hergueta T, Baker R, Dunbar GC. The mini-international neuropsychiatric interview (M.I.N.I.): the development and validation of a structured diagnostic psychiatric interview for DSM-IV and ICD-10. J Clin Psychiatry. 1998;59(Suppl 20):22–33. quiz 34-57
18. First MB. Structured clinical interview for the DSM (SCID). In: The encyclopedia of clinical psychology: American Cancer Society; 2015. p. 1–6. https://doi.org/10.1002/9781118625392.wbecp351.
19. Kessler RC, Bedirhan Üstün T. The world mental health (WMH) survey initiative version of the World Health Organization (WHO) composite international diagnostic interview (CIDI). Int J Methods Psychiatr Res. 2004;13(2):93–121. https://doi.org/10.1002/mpr.168.
20. Engel GL. The need for a new medical model: a challenge for biomedicine. Science (New York, NY). 1977;196(4286):129–36. https://doi.org/10.1126/science.847460.
21. Stingley S, Schultz H. Helmsley trust support for Telehealth improves access to care in rural and frontier areas. Health Aff. 2014;33(2):336–41. https://doi.org/10.1377/hlthaff.2013.1278.
22. Hughes MC, Gorman JM, Ren Y, Khalid S, Clayton C. Increasing access to rural mental health care using hybrid care that includes Telepsychiatry. J Rural Ment Health. 2019;43(1):30–7. https://doi.org/10.1037/rmh0000110.
23. Hubley S, Lynch SB, Schneck C, Thomas M, Shore J. Review of key Telepsychiatry outcomes. World J Psychiatr. 2016;6(2):269–82. https://doi.org/10.5498/wjp.v6.i2.269.
24. Harvey JB, Valenta S, Simpson K, Lyles M, McElligott J. Utilization of outpatient Telehealth Services in Parity and Nonparity States 2010–2015. Telemedicine and E-Health. 2018;25(2):132–6. https://doi.org/10.1089/tmj.2017.0265.
25. Goldstone D. Cognitive-Behavioural therapy versus psychodynamic psychotherapy for the treatment of depression: a critical review of evidence and current issues. S Afr J Psychol. 2017;47(1):84–96. https://doi.org/10.1177/0081246316653860.
26. Husain MM, John Rush A, Fink M, Knapp R, Petrides G, Rummans T, Melanie M. Biggs, et al. Speed of response and remission in major depressive disorder with acute electroconvulsive therapy (ECT): a consortium for research in ECT (CORE) report. J Clin Psychiatry. 2004;65(4):485–91. https://doi.org/10.4088/jcp.v65n0406.

Chapter 6
Mental Health Informatics

Piper A. Ranallo and Jessica D. Tenenbaum

Abstract Mental health informatics (MHI) is a relatively new specialty within the field of biomedical informatics. MHI seeks to develop, enhance, and apply informatics theories, paradigms, and technologies to optimize the mental health of individuals and communities. In this chapter we define the scope of the field and discuss its relationship not only to the larger field of biomedical and health informatics, but also to work occurring natively within the field of mental health. We introduce the three primary fields of science within which our basic scientific knowledge of mental health and illness is produced: the biological sciences, the behavioral sciences, and the social sciences. We describe the opportunities and challenges inherent in developing and using informatics technologies in a field in which knowledge is acquired in the context of three different fields in two different branches of science, each with its own unique epistemology, or way of knowing. We describe some of the unique features of the behavioral and social sciences that call for novel informatics paradigms and that highlight the need for significant enhancements in existing informatics technologies.

Keywords Mental health · Informatics · Behavioral health · Psychiatry · Psychology

6.1 Mental Health Informatics as an Informatics Subdiscipline

Mental Health Informatics (MHI) is a subdiscipline within the field of informatics. As described briefly in Chaps. 1 and 2, and exhaustively in Shortliffe and Cimino's textbook on Biomedical Informatics [1], the science of informatics is concerned

P. A. Ranallo (✉)
Six Aims for Behavioral Health, Minneapolis, MN, USA
e-mail: pranallo@sixaims.org; sven0018@umn.edu

J. D. Tenenbaum
Duke University, Durham, NC, USA
e-mail: jessie.tenenbaum@duke.edu

© Springer Nature Switzerland AG 2021
J. D. Tenenbaum, P. A. Ranallo (eds.), *Mental Health Informatics*, Health
Informatics, https://doi.org/10.1007/978-3-030-70558-9_6

with developing and applying theories, methods, and paradigms for transforming data into actionable knowledge to improve human health [1–3]. Informatics is inherently interdisciplinary, drawing upon theories and methods from many fields, including computer science, statistics, cognitive science, and information technology. Informatics integrates theories of human knowledge acquisition and the paradigms and technologies developed organically with the field of informatics with the theories, paradigms and technologies natively developed within the scientific domain to which it is applied. Just as bioinformatics builds on technologies developed natively within the field of molecular biology for detecting, defining, and measuring molecular entities and processes, MHI builds on technologies developed natively within the behavioral and social sciences for detecting, defining, and measuring mental and behavioral phenomena.

Mental health informatics is unique among health informatics specialties in that it seeks to acquire and integrate knowledge across all levels of the biopsychosocial model of health [4] (Fig. 6.1) with the goal of elucidating the complex interconnections between biological, mental, interpersonal, and socio-environmental phenomena. In other words, mental health informatics addresses the entire spectrum of functional systems, from physiological systems, such as the nervous system, immune system, digestive system, to those functional systems studied primarily by behavioral and social scientists such as the mind (emotion, cognition), behavior, and human communities. The entities and phenomena of interest and a few examples, are enumerated in Table 6.1.

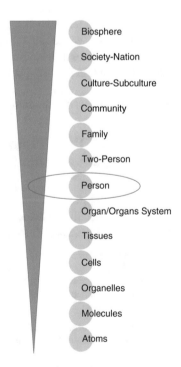

Fig. 6.1 Engel's biopsychosocial model of health. Adapted from [4]

Table 6.1 Phenomena of interest in mental health informatics

Level of analysis	Primary phenomena of interest	Constructs commonly referenced in the scientific literature
Body The anatomic entities and physiologic processes comprising the entire human body • The biological part of Engel's "Person" level and all levels below it [4] • The *genes*, *molecules*, *cells*, *circuits*, and *physiology* units of analysis defined in the National Institute of Mental Health's Research Domain Criteria (RDoC) framework [5, 6]	Mental health informatics is particularly concerned with physiologic processes that influence one's own or another's brain, e.g., how the microbiome of a person's digestive system influences his or her brain, or how pheromones produced by one person influence the brain of another person.	Anatomic entities and processes comprising physiological systems, including (but not limited to) the: • Nervous system • Endocrine system • Immune system • Integumentary system • Digestive system The molecules (including genes), cells, circuits, and physiological phenomena defined in the RDoC framework [5, 6].
Person The body, mind, and behavior of a single human being • The psychological (mental, cognitive, behavioral) part of Engel's "Person" level of analysis • The *behavior* and *self-report* units of analysis defined in RDoC [5, 6]	The phenomenological experiences, and mental and cognitive functions occurring *within* a single person. The behaviors—ranging from simple motor behavior to complex social behavior—that an individual selects and executes. The attributes of the relevant contexts in which each of these phenomena occur, and the relationship *between* these "intrapersonal" phenomena and the context.	Mind • Mental functions, e.g., consciousness [7–11], motivation and drive [12–18], emotion [19–24], and sensation [25] • Cognitive functions [5, 26–28], e.g., perception [5, 25, 29–31], memory [5, 32], attention [33–36], thinking [37, 38], learning [39–41], language [42], reasoning [43–47] • The component and integrative functions that comprise the "gestalt" construct mind [48–51] Self • Agentic self [52–54] • Objective self [5, 55], self-concept [56–61], self-efficacy [62], self-esteem [57, 63] • Personality [64–68], identity [69–71], moral development [72–74] Behavior • Affect (expression of emotion) [75, 76] • Posture, motor behavior, and symbolic communication [5, 77, 78] • Complex social behavior [39, 79–81]

(continued)

Table 6.1 (continued)

Level of analysis	Primary phenomena of interest	Constructs commonly referenced in the scientific literature
Dyad Two people co-located in the same space and time, interacting in ways that range from nothing more than awareness of co-location to ongoing and extensive interaction. • Engel's "Two-Person" level [4]	The novel physiological and behavioral phenomena that emerge *between* two people when they interact and the unique physiological, mental, and behavioral phenomena that emerge *within* each person as a participant in a dyad. The attributes of both the dyad, e.g., nature of relationship, and the individual people, e.g., social class, gender, personality traits, that influence these phenomena.	Types of Dyads • Parent-child relationships [82] • Close [83–86] and romantic [87] relationships Interpersonal functions and processes • The component and integrative functions comprising the "gestalt" of interpersonal process [84, 88] • Attachment [5, 89–93]
Group Three or more people co-located in the same space and time, interacting in ways that range from nothing more than awareness of co-location to ongoing and extensive interaction. • Engel's "Two-Person" level [4]	The novel physiological and behavioral phenomena that emerge *between* people when they interact in groups of three or more, as well as the unique physiological, mental, and behavioral phenomena that emerge *within* each person (and each dyad) in this context. The attributes of the group, the component dyads, and the individual people that influence these phenomena.	Types of Groups • The Family [94, 95] • Community and tribe [96–98] Group functions and process [99–104] • Affiliation [5, 105–107] • Alliance formation [108–110] • Social identification [103, 111–114] • Competition, cooperation, and compliance [115–117] • Dominance hierarchies [118, 119]
Society, Culture A group of people co-located in the same sociocultural and geospatial context (a peer group, organization, neighborhood, community, country, world), interacting in ways that range from simple temporal co-location to extensive interaction.	The novel physiological and behavioral phenomena that emerge *between* people when they interact in some larger sociocultural and geospatial context, as well as the unique physiological, mental, and behavioral phenomena that emerge *within* each subgroup and person in this context. The attributes of the group, subgroups, and individual people that influence these phenomena.	Types of cultures and social communities: • Organizational (educational, employment, or living environment-based) and peer cultures [120–122] • Geographic, political, religious, racial, ethnic groups and cultures [123, 124] Social functions and processes: • Social structuralism [125] and social agency [126] • Social norms [117, 127] • Social cognition [128–130] and social identification [103, 111–114] • Acculturation [124, 131]

Table 6.1 (continued)

Level of analysis	Primary phenomena of interest	Constructs commonly referenced in the scientific literature
Physical Environments The biological and non-biological entities and processes within a defined geospatial context	The novel phenomena that emerge *between* and *within* people in the context of specific physical environments. The novel phenomena that arise within the physical environment when people spend time in the environment (with an emphasis on phenomena that in turn impact human mental health). The attributes of the environments and the people that influence these phenomena.	Types • Spaces, buildings, neighborhoods, larger ecological environments Phenomena • Amount and configuration of space [132–135] • Light [136–138], noise [139, 140] other sensory stimuli in the environment

6.2   Contrasting Mental Health Informatics with Related Disciplines

The field of MHI overlaps significantly both with mainstream informatics special-ties and with work being done in several mental health specialties. In this section we focus on the ways in which MHI is similar to, and differs from, mainstream bio-medical and health informatics. We go on to describe how MHI aligns with, and builds upon, informatics paradigms being developed and use natively within mental health disciplines, as well as how it differs. We end this section by providing a brief overview the ways in which mainstream biomedical and health informatics has addressed mental, behavioral and social phenomena.

6.2.1   How Mental Health Informatics Differs from Mainstream Biomedical and Health Informatics

While there is significant overlap between MHI and other informatics specialties, there are several things that make MHI unique. First, MHI deals with phenomena not typically encountered by informaticians working in other domains of health. Second, because the phenomena of interest in mental health are fundamentally dif-ferent from those of interest in medicine, the paradigms used to isolate, define, and quantify them are also different. Consequently, there are important differences in how we approach the core informatics knowledge acquisition cycle in MHI com-pared to mainstream health informatics.

6.2.1.1   Differences in the Phenomena of Interest

Mental and psychological phenomena (the "mind" and "self") as well as interper-sonal, social, and cultural phenomena, all play a central role not only in theories of mental health and illness, but also in interventions designed to optimize health and treat illness. This is not to say that these phenomena are not relevant in mainstream theories of physical health. Rather, they are generally not part of the core epistemol-ogy (see definition in Table 6.2) of the biological sciences upon which knowledge of physical health and illness is based.

Because the phenomena of interest in mental health are fundamentally different kinds of things from the phenomena of interest in physical healthcare, there are fundamental differences in the way these phenomena are named, defined, and quan-tified. Compared to physiologic phenomena, such as temperature, blood pressure, or weight, "psychological" phenomena such as level of introversion, depth of sadness, ability to detect social cues, and cognitive capacities are much more difficult to clearly define, isolate, sample, and quantify. Interpersonal phenomena, such as quality of attachment, manifestations of racial contempt, or level of interpersonal

Table 6.2 Key terms defined

Brain	The physical organ inside the skull that controls and coordinates physical, mental and behavioral functions.
Mind	The conceptual entity used to describe entities, functions, processes, and states underlying observable physical and phenomena being attributed to something occurring in the brain. For example, memory is typically described in terms of things that happen in the mind (v. the brain), such as 'storing', 'retrieving', and 'representing' information. Phenomena that cannot be fully and explicitly defined in terms of biological entities or processes in the brain are typically defined in terms of entities or processes attributed to the mind.
Biological sciences	The science concerned with the study of living organisms.
Behavioral sciences	The science concerned with the study of human and animal behavior.
Social sciences	The science concerned with the study of groups and social relationships.
Epistemology	The field of philosophy concerned with the study of human knowledge. In the context of a specific scientific discipline, the field's "epistemology" is the set of theories, paradigms, and methodologies the field uses to determine what constitutes valid knowledge (sometimes defined as "justified, true belief") [141–145].
Construct	A real-world thing that has no tangible manifestation in the physical world, but rather, is inferred on the basis of other observations. For example, 'memory' is a construct, because we can't directly observe memory, we can only infer its existence based on observations (i.e., we can recall the name of a person we met last week) along with theories about observations (there is some 'thing' called memory within the brain that captures and saves information about people we meet, when we see the person again, we can pull information back out of this 'thing'). The existence of—and accuracy of any definition of—the construct can only be assessed in the context of both the observations and the associated theory [146].
Mental phenomena	Functions, processes, and states that can be *fully* defined only by referring to entities or processes attributed to the mind, rather than to entities or processes attributes to the body (brain). Examples include one's visual perception of an image or auditory perception of a song; a thought, a belief, or an attitude; an emotion, a memory, or an intuition; reasoning, planning, comprehending, and calculating.
Psychological phenomena	A commonly used, but poorly defined term. The American Psychological Association (APA) defines psychological phenomena as including "all aspects of the human experience—from the functions of the brain to the actions of nations" [147]. To the APA, psychological phenomena are the superset of functions, processes, and states that comprise human existence—biological, mental, behavioral, interpersonal, social, and cultural. Many behavioral scientists and clinicians, including psychologists, use the term "psychological" more narrowly to refer to the things that occur within an person's mind.
Behavior	We defined behavior here as observable physical activities ranging from simple physical and motor behavior to complex interpersonal and social behavior. The term is sometimes used to more broadly to refer to any function, process, or state that can be objectively observed or measured [147].

(continued)

Table 6.2 (continued)

Social phenomena	The entities (e.g., dyads, groups, organization structures, social norms, laws, etc.) and processes that emerge when two or more people co-exist or interact in the same place and time [148].
Psychometrics	The field of study concerned with measurement of psychological phenomena (defined in the broad sense of the term). It includes the set of theories, paradigms, instruments, and quantitative methods used to identify and define latent (underlying, unobservable) constructs based on samples of observable behavior [147].

respect between members of a family, team, or community are equally difficult to clearly define, isolate, sample, and quantify. Consequently, in mental health, there is less consistency in the naming of major clinical concepts, and less consensus about their explicit definitions and relationships to other concepts. For example, the terms "mental model" [149], "schema" [150], and "working model" [151] are used by various researchers and clinicians to describe the mental representation a person has of some person, situation, or event. While there is some overlap in the definition of these terms, the theoretical model in which each construct is defined posits nuanced differences between the construct and its relationships to other constructs. There are also different paradigms and methods (including instruments) used to measure this construct in both research and practice, with different paradigms and methods developed and used by those belonging to each theoretical camp in which the construct is articulated.

This is different from physical health where major concepts such as blood pressure, inflammation, and platelet count are named and defined the same way across the entire field. There is general consensus among health professionals not only about the definitions of, but also about optimal methods for measuring, each of these things. In contrast to mental health, the definitions and methods do not vary based on the school the healthcare professional attended, the institution where she or he trained, or whether she or he specialized in oncology, cardiology, or pediatrics. Moreover, there is widespread consensus about the relationship each of these entities or processes has to other biomedical entities and processes.

In traditional biomedicine, then, the instruments and methods used to measure most biomedical phenomena are universal and readily available, and the same kinds of instruments used in research are used in routine healthcare. This is not the case in mental healthcare. In mental healthcare, while formal methods and instruments for measuring clinical phenomena are used in research paradigms, these instruments are rarely used in routine clinical practice. For example, with the exception of a few instruments, such as the PHQ-9, the standardized assessment and imaging technologies used in research are rarely used in practice. Moreover, while increasingly sophisticated and reliable technologies that allow researchers and clinicians to visualize, measure, and quantify biological entities and processes are continuously developed and widely disseminated, most of the instruments and methods currently in use in physical healthcare have been vetted over a long period of time. The data generated using these instruments and methods are assumed to be valid and reliable representations of the phenomena of interest. A neutrophil count generated by a CBC machine in one part of the world in 1980 is assumed to be comparable to a neutrophil count generated by a CBC machined in another part of the world in 2020. A measure of the existence or severity of depression generated by the available version of the Beck Depression Inventory (BDI) in 1980 (the BDI-I [152]) however, may not be comparable to a measure of the existence or severity of depression generated based on a clinical interview, another depression assessment, or even based on the version of the Beck Depression Inventory available in 2020 (BDI-II [153]).

This consistency in terminology, operational definitions, and instrumentation makes it possible to perform meta-analyzes of research findings and to pool and analyze clinical data across researchers and clinicians. In mental health, on the other hand, the inconsistency in terminology, the variation in operational definitions of core constructs, and the variety of instrumentation makes it difficult to pool data or perform meta-analyzes across theoretical and philosophical boundaries.

6.2.1.2   Differences in the Knowledge Acquisition Cycle

The aspiring mental health informatician will need to be aware that the unique types of phenomena of interest in mental health—and the many challenges inherent in unambiguously defining and quantifying them—create a different kind of relationship between the *data* an informatician has to work with and the underlying real-world "thing" the data represents. Despite the widespread existence of empirically validated methods and instruments for measuring the behaviors, internal experiences, and interpersonal and social phenomena relevant to mental health, not all instruments that purport to measure the same underlying construct, e.g., impulsivity, introversion, racism, etc., are actually measuring precisely the same thing [154]. Unlike in physical healthcare, where we can be relatively confident that two tests claiming to measure some biological entity—say, antibodies to COVID19—are fact measuring the same thing, i.e., one test is not measuring, for example, a mix of COVID19 and Flu antibodies, we cannot always be certain that two validated instruments claiming to measure the same psychological construct—say, impulsivity—are in fact measuring the same thing. Observations ("data") about the phenomena of interest in mental health are much more sensitive to the paradigms and instruments used to sample and measure them than are the biological phenomena commonly measured in physical health. Moreover, each paradigm and instrument may actually be measuring different aspects of the same construct, or completely different constructs altogether [154–156]. Consequently, data about mental, social, and behavioral phenomena must be accompanied by much more data about the context of measurement in order to be useful in knowledge acquisition paradigms. Moreover, in routine mental healthcare, the method used as the basis for a clinical observation is often not explicitly captured with the data, and in those cases, it is important for the informatician to understand that gaps in context may imply a method was "clinical impression' and the instrument used was "none". This distinction between observation and context of observation that is not typically made in medical informatics paradigms—probably because it is tacitly accepted as "redundant"— must be explicitly acknowledged in mental health informatics paradigms.

As described in Chap. 2, data are the primary inputs to the *data to information to knowledge to action cycle* (the "DIKA Cycle") that defines informatics. Implied in the data acquisition step is a "signal to data" step, where the observable signals generated by the real-world phenomena are captured, quantified, and represented as "data" (Fig. 6.2) from which information can be generated and knowledge subsequently acquired.

This "signal to data" step (Fig. 6.3) presents a challenge to many informaticians working in mental health because the paradigms, methods and instruments used to isolate, acquire, and quantify these mental, behavioral, and social "signals" differ

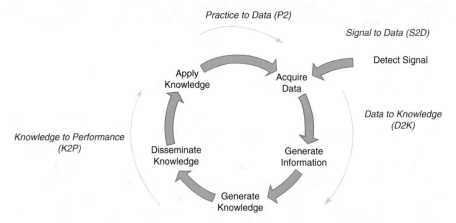

Fig. 6.2 The core *data to information to knowledge to action* (DIKA) cycle with an emphasis on the prerequisite process of detecting and quantifying observable signals of the phenomena of interest

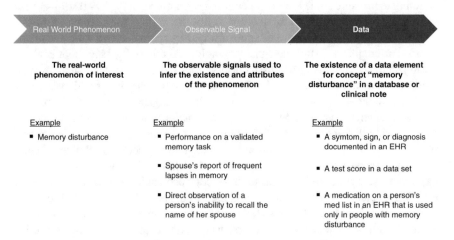

Fig. 6.3 Data as representations of the observable signals used to infer the existence of some real-world phenomenon

significantly from those used to acquire basic knowledge about physiological phenomena (see Chap. 9). Similarly, the instruments and methods used in clinical practice to detect, diagnose, prevent, and treat mental health conditions differ in important ways from those used in traditional medical practice. While they may not provide the same certainty of insight into, and comparability of results about, the phenomena they measure as the medical instruments we, as informaticians, have come to know and trust, they are, nonetheless, developed using robust scientific methods that have been empirically demonstrated to produce high quality representations of the phenomena they seek to measure. In fact, there is an entire subspecialty in the behavioral and social sciences dedicated to developing these measurement technologies. This is the science of *psychometrics*, described in detail in Chap. 9. Here, we simply point out that there is a fundamental difference between mental and physical health in how the raw "signals" underlying the phenomena of interest are detected and measured, and how these signals become "data" in the knowledge acquisition (DIKA) lifecycle. Because most experienced informaticians tend to have far less knowledge about, and experience with, psychometric theory and methods than they do with the biological theories and methods, this is an important domain of study for any aspiring mental health informatician.

While many of the methods and paradigms used to derive meaningful information and knowledge from physiologic observations can be applied to mental, behavioral, and social observations and data, many methods are specific to the phenomena being observed. Chapters 10, 13, and 14 describe informatics methods that can be applied universally across virtually all types of observable phenomena, given that the phenomena in question are accurately represented and quantified. These methods include computational and analytic methods (Chap. 10), natural language processing (NLP) methods (Chap. 13), and data visualization methods (Chap. 14). Chapters 9 and 12 describe methods used to derive actionable knowledge from data points representing signals derived from fundamentally different types of phenomena. While Chaps. 8 and 11 describe methods for knowledge acquisition given data points representing physiologic signals, Chap. 12 describes methods for knowledge acquisition given data points representing mental, behavioral, and social signals.

In addition to differences between the scientific paradigms used to derive knowledge about mental versus physical health, there are also significant differences in the overall landscape of theories of pathology and approaches to treatment used in mental versus physical health. As described in Chaps. 3, 9, and 12, there are many widely accepted—sometimes contradictory—theories of the mechanism underlying not only mental illness but also normative psychological development. This plethora of etiological theories of psychopathology, combined with the number of different clinical treatment models (even for a single, shared etiological conceptualization of one disorder) is common in mental healthcare, yet far less frequently seen in biomedical healthcare. This creates an added layer of complexity to the information and knowledge acquisition process. Specifically, the aspiring mental health informatician will need to build multiple models—each one incorporating assumptions from each of the multiple theoretical models of pathology—into the paradigms and methods used in the initial processing of the data, and find a way to integrate these models as she or he applies analytic methods to derive information and knowledge from raw data.

6.2.1.3 How Mental Health Informatics Differs from Other Informatics Work in Mental Health

Mental health informatics differs not only from traditional health informatics, but also from other informatics subdisciplines working to explicitly address mental health and illness, such as computational psychiatry, neuroinformatics, and behavioral health informatics. In the past several years, an increasing body of work [157–163] has begun to emerge describing informatics efforts applied to mental health. These works demonstrate how researchers in the basic behavioral sciences are applying informatics methods to better understand phenomena related to the brain, mind, and behavior. They also demonstrate how clinicians and healthcare administrators are addressing the use of informatics technologies to improve care delivery and accelerate the rate of knowledge acquisition based on data captured during the routine delivery of care. These efforts—and the similarities and differences between them—are described in Table 6.3.

Table 6.3 Informatics applied to mental and behavioral health

Terms	Primary phenomena of interest[a]	Objective
Neuroinformatics	The structure and function of nervous system molecules, cells and tissue, and neural circuits.	Improve physical and mental health by building a robust informatics infrastructure to support the acquisition and dissemination of knowledge required to optimize the structure and function of the nervous system [157, 160, 162].
Computational psychiatry	Mental functions, processes, and states and their relationships the brain functions, processes, and states.	Improve mental health by building an integrated scientific and clinical infrastructure capable of acquiring and applying knowledge required to optimize mental and behavioral functions and processes [163, 164].
Behavioral health informatics, mental health informatics	The development and application and development of computer-based technologies to support knowledge acquisition and delivery of mental healthcare.	Improve mental health by optimizing the scientific and clinical workflows used to prevent and treat mental, behavioral, interpersonal, and social dysfunction [165, 166]
Mental health informatics (as defined in this text)	The complex interactions between mental, behavioral, interpersonal, social, and environmental entities, functions, processes, and states, and the informatics paradigms	Improve mental health by building a robust LHS capable of acquiring, disseminating, and skillfully applying precision knowledge to prevent and treat mental, behavioral, interpersonal, and social dysfunction.

[a]Primary phenomena are those that appear to be the focus of research and implementation paradigms; that is, while other phenomena may be studied in relation to one or more of the primary phenomena of interest, it appears to be primarily with the goal of understanding their relationship to the primary phenomena

6.2.2 Mental, Behavioral, and Social Phenomena in Mainstream Health Informatics

While mainstream medicine has traditionally focused primarily on physiological phenomena, it is increasingly recognizing the intricate relationships between mind and body, as well as the significant role that social and physical environments play in overall health. Moreover, both researchers and clinicians are increasingly emphasizing the role of non-physiological variables in physiologic health and illness. This shift in emphasis to an integrated, whole-person approach to health is clearly reflected in developments in the field of informatics. In the past several years, there have been many studies describing the application of informatics technologies not only to research on mental health conditions [165, 167, 168], but also more generally to the mental, behavioral, social, cultural, and environmental aspects of human health [169–171].

Researchers in bioinformatics have performed genome-wide association studies (GWAS) for many mental health conditions in an effort to learn more about the genetic basis of these conditions [172–175]. They have studied the genetic basis of various anatomic and physiologic phenotypes associated with mental health conditions [176–178] and to a lesser extent, the genetic basis of behavioral phenotypes associated with the same [179]. Researchers in pharmacogenomics have moved this basic bioinformatics research down the translational spectrum by performing clinical research to address the problem of predicting which psychiatric pharmacotherapies are most likely to work for which people [180]. Applied clinical informaticians have moved this knowledge even further down the translational spectrum by implementing clinical guidelines for pharmacogenomics testing as clinical decision support for prescribing behavior by front-line clinicians [181, 182]. These and many other examples of the use of bioinformatics research paradigms for knowledge discovery in mental health are described in Chap. 11. Researchers in neuroinformatics have made similar strides in understanding not only the structural and biochemical underpinnings of behavioral phenomena and common mental health syndromes, but also the neurocircuitry [157, 160, 162] underlying the same. Examples of the application neuroinformatics paradigms for knowledge discovery in mental health are described in Chap. 8.

There has also been progress in the development of an important, foundation set of informatics technologies: technologies for concept and knowledge representation which underpin all other informatics technologies (Chap. 7). As the use of electronic health records (EHRs) and other clinical information systems in mental health has increased, there has been increasing demand for robust clinical terminologies that can be used to unambiguously represent clinical observations in mental health research and care. In 2010, for example, the Logical Observations Indentifiers Names and Codes (LOINC) [183] terminology created a way to define and code structured assessment instruments to support the explicit representation of data captured using psychological assessment instruments [184, 185]. Similarly, in

2018, under the auspices of SNOMED International, the Mental and Behavioural Health Clinical Reference Group (MABH-CRG) was established to evaluate and address gaps in SNOMED-CT (the Systematized Nomenclature of Medicine—Clinical Terms [186]) relative to mental health. These activities reflect an urgency to address gaps in frameworks and standard terminologies relative to mental health [187–189] in an era of increasing policy pressure for interoperability of health data [190–192].

Informaticians in collaboration with mental health researchers and practitioners have addressed the need for more robust informatics technologies for mental health at virtually all points in the research and care delivery process (Chap. 5). For example, many technologies have been developed for signal detection at a physiologic (e.g., heart rate and oxygen uptake) [193, 194], mental (e.g. detection of depressive symptoms) [195–197], phenomenological (e.g., sleep) [198], and behavioral level (e.g., Ecological Momentary Assessment, promotion of physical activity and weight loss) [199–201]. These technologies are discussed in detail in Chap. 9. The research framework constructs and subconstructs put forth by the National Institute of Mental Health's (NIMH) Research Domain Criteria (RDoC) [5, 6], including mental, behavioral, and social constructs have also become the focus of much informatics activity [202, 203] (Chaps. 7, 12, and 23).

Biomedical informatics has also addressed mental and behavioral phenomena in work on important topics such as computer-human interaction (HCI) and implementation science. In these cases, the mental and behavioral phenomena of interest are as like to be those occurring within the healthcare practitioner as those occurring within the healthcare recipient (e.g., how a healthcare practitioner processes information presented in various ways in a clinical information system). Electronic health record systems (EHRs) have been one particular area of interest in HCI [204]. A significant body of work takes HCI one step further into the mental/cognitive domain in an interdisciplinary subdomain known as cognitive informatics, which focuses on human information processing [205]. In addition, health information technologies may be deployed at home after patient discharge, emphasizing an entirely different area of study in human factors [206].

6.3 Mental Health Informatics: Bridging the Biological, Behavioral, and Social Sciences

Our current scientific knowledge about mental health and illness comes from two distinct branches of science: the social and behavioral sciences on the one hand, and the biological sciences on the other. In the social and behavioral sciences, in fields such as sociology, psychology, and cognitive science, a diverse range of mental, interpersonal, social, and cultural phenomena play a central role in theories of mental and behavioral functioning. In the biological sciences, in fields such as psychiatry and neuroscience, physiological systems such as the nervous system, endocrine system, and immune system take center stage in theories of mental and behavioral functioning.

Consequently, MHI must be able to accommodate the theories, paradigms, and methods of multiple, distinct branches of science. This is challenging for a number reasons. The first is that traditional biomedical informatics is ill-equipped to handle the kinds of mental, behavioral and social phenomena that dominate theories and clinical models in mental health. The second is that profound differences in epistemology, or "ways of knowing" between the behavioral and biological sciences create obstacles to collaboration between informaticians and behavioral and social scientists. Lastly, the vast number of competing, and often contradictory theories within the behavioral and social sciences [189] places unique demands on informaticians (or indeed any reseachers) working in the domain.

6.3.1   Mainstream Health Informatics Has Not Fully Embraced Social and Behavioral Phenomena

Because health informatics has its historical roots in the biological sciences, many of the informatics technologies required to address social and behavioral phenomena are not part of the standard informatician's toolkit. Moreover, the informatics technologies developed over the first several decades of the field's existence have been developed and optimized for acquiring and applying knowledge about physiological, rather than mental, behavioral, or social phenomena. Consequently, many of these technologies are not well suited for use in mental health informatics paradigms. Let's take a look at how these historical blinders impact the work of the mental health informatician at each stage in the knowledge acquisition process.

As previously discussed, all informatics paradigms consist of the same core goal of acquiring actionable knowledge from data about some underlying health-related entity or process. The same core steps occur in all informatics paradigms. First, the relevant underying real-world entities and processes of interest are identifed. Next, the observable signals produced by these entities and processes are captured and quantified (measured). Third, these observed signals are described in the form of "data" that can be manipulated both by the human brain and computer based system. Fourth, these data are transformed into information. Next, the information is transformed into actionable knowledge. Finally, as the ultimate goal, actions are taken to implement the aquired knowledge into research and clinical workflows to improve human health (Fig. 6.4).

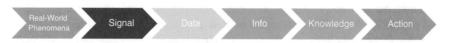

Fig. 6.4 Informatics technologies are developed and applied for each of several core steps in the knowledge acquision process

Differences between paradigms for signal detection and data catpure in the bio-medical versus the social and behavioral sciences were discussed in the previous section, and are described in more detail in Chap. 9. The process by which both the real world phenomena of interest in healthcare and the observable signals used to isolate, identify and measure them are transformed into data is described in infor-matics as "concept and knowledge representation" [89, 187, 188] and is discussed in detail in Chap. 7. Because data is the foundational input to all informatics para-digms and methods, there is arguably no area of informatics that is most critical to enabling an LHS for mental health than ensuring that technologies for concept and knowledge reqpresentation are both adequate for representing mental health con-tent, and fully cover the domain.

Two clinical terminologies essential to a building an LHS in mental health health—Logical Observation Identifiers Names and Codes (LOINC) and the Systematized Nomenclature of Medicine-Clinical Terms (SNOMED CT)—not only have significant gaps in content relative to mental and behavioral health [187, 188], but are also designed in such a way that they cannot capture the meaning of concepts relevant to mental health as completely as they represent the meaning of concepts relevant to biomedical health. This is because the terminologies them-selves have been designed based on assumptions inherent in the biological sciences. An unpublished evaluation of the attributes used to define clinical finding concepts in SNOMED-CT, for example, revealed an implicit assumption that the universe of health findings and diseases can be fully defined in terms of physical, biological, and morphological entities. This is evidenced by a conceptual world view that defines clinical findings in terms of the functional systems, body structures, mor-phological alterations, and processes involved, and that restricts the range of func-tional systems and processes to those outside of mental, interpersonal, or social systems (See Chap. 7). Similarly, MeSH (Medical Subject Headings), the terminol-ogy used to index publications in PubMed, contains far fewer, and far less detailed, index terms for retrieving research about mental, behavioral, and social phenomena, diseases, and treatments, than for retrieving research about biological phenomena, diseases, and treatments [188]. Where terminologies do exist with a detailed and accurate representation of mental, behavioral, and social phenomena, they tend to have been developed natively within the behavioral sciences, without the benefit of informatics best practices for terminology development [87]. Moreover, these ter-minology products are less likely to be included in systems that manage and publish inventories of national industry standards (see Chap. 7).

Knowledge dissemination is another part of the process not well addressed by traditional informatics technologies in the context of mental health. Knowledge dis-semination is a critical step in moving from knowledge to action. Methods for bio-medical knowledge dissemination include those commonly used in medical schools and medical healthcare settings, as well as those used by medical boards and medi-cal professional societies. Examples include publishing clinical guidelines, imple-menting those guidelines through order sets in EHRs, ongoing continuing education and maintenance of certification requirements, and other forms of education includ-ing journal articles and professional conferences. Knowledge dissemination in mental health is more complex, primarily because of the number and variety of educational programs and settings, as well as professional boards and societies.

As discussed in Chap. 4, there are several times as many psychologists as psychiatrists in the United States, in addition to the ranks of case workers, social workers, etc. As a result, primary dissemination is not through a small, relatively homogenous group of medical schools, settings, boards, and societies, but rather through a complex system of training and licensure programs. Moreover, complete knowledge about mental health is often shared across scientific and disciplinary boundaries. Physicians and advanced practice nurses typically do not have the same depth of psychological, behavioral, and social science training that mental health professionals trained in the behavioral and social sciences do. Similarly, mental health practitioners trained in the behavioral sciences typically do not have the same depth of biomedical training that physicians and advanced practice nurses do. Each group has limited insight into not only the complete knowledge base, but also the theoretical models and knowledge discovery paradigms of the other. Consequently, neither group is fully equipped to integrate relevant knowledge from the discipline in which they were not trained.

In addition, mental healthcare is often delivered in a small or solo practice setting rather than in a hospital or large clinic setting. These smaller settings are less likely to have deployed EHRs than hospitals and clinical settings providing biomedical healthcare services (see Chap. 16). While there has been a significant uptick in EHR adoption since the HITECH Act in 2009 due to financial incentives for demonstrating "meaningful use" of electronic systems [207], due to the initial exclusion of mental health providers from these incentive programs, EHR adoption in mental health has lagged behind [208]. Thus, knowledge dissemination through EHR-enabled clinical decision support is not feasible in many common mental health care settings.

6.3.2 Epistemological Differences Between the Behavioral and Biological Sciences

Arguably the biggest challenge facing informaticians working in mental health informatics is that the biological, behavioral, and social sciences are based on profoundly different assumptions about the nature and relevance of mental, behavioral, social, and biological phenomena in health and illness. In addition, the biological and behavioral sciences differ in the scope of phenomena about which they believe knowledge can be legitimately acquired. In the biological sciences, the scope is physical phenomena that can—at least theoretically—be directly observed. The behavioral and social sciences, on the other hand, focus on phenomena that cannot be directly observed, such as thoughts, emotion, and social norms. As a result of differences in objects of study, the biological and behavioral sciences have different ideas about the methods by which they believe the objects of scientific study can be

Fig. 6.5 Knowledge as justified true beliefs (adapted from https://en.wikipedia.org/wiki/Epistemology)

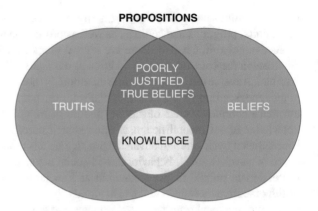

legitimately known. In other words, the behavioral and biological sciences have fundamentally different *epistemologies* (Fig. 6.5).

The term *epistemology*, from the Greek words for 'knowledge' and 'discourse', refers to the study of the nature of human knowledge [49, 209]. As a field of study, epistemology is concerned with answering the question: "How we can legitimately claim to know something?". That is, how can we make the leap from believing something to be true, to "knowing" something to be true? When used in the context of a field of science, *epistemology* refers to the criteria a scientific field uses to determine that sufficiently valid evidence has been produced to say that a hypothesis (a belief) has achieved the status of knowledge. It refers to the rules (or criteria) the field has about what a scientist must do to justify a belief. These criteria are typically defined in terms of the paradigms, methodologies, and instruments the field believes are capable of reliably producing valid observations. A neuroscientist, for example, may say that only emotional states that can be reliably distinguished based on neural signals measured using brain imaging technologies can be known. She might say that the names we give to more nuanced emotional states measured using psychometric methods are hypothetical (beliefs), but cannot be known, because to the neuroscientist, psychometric methods and instruments are not valid methods for identifying or measuring emotional states. A field's epistemology also defines *what* can be known [144, 145]. That is, *what* classes of phenomena are capable of producing a valid, observable signal capable of detection, and what classes of phenomena can be detected using the tools and technologies available in the field. Finally, an epistemology defines *who* can be knowers [144, 145, 209]—what skills or training are required to be capable of "knowing" in the specific field. Each field develops, validates, and iteratively refines a set of tools and technologies to "come to know" the entities and phenomena the field believes can be known.

Previously, we described how the entities and phenomena of interest, as well as the methods and paradigms used to acquire actionable knowledge from these phenomena vary accross the biological, behavioral, and social sciences. Epistemology gives us a framework for thinking more systematically about the differences between the fields. Importantly, it allows us to explicity represent and proactively identify potential obstacles to knowledge acquisition in a field grounded in more than one branch of science. It also helps us operalize strategies for addressing these obstacles.

Neuroscientists tend to define mental and behavioral phenomena in terms of the brain [160, 163, 164], or an 'embodied mind' [50]. The constructs, theories, tools, and technologies they develop and use are designed to elucidate the relationship between biological (non-brain), mental, behavioral, interpersonal, social, and environmental phenomena on the one hand, and brain phenomena on the other. The empirical questions they ask are aimed at understanding ways in which both non-biological (mental, social, environmental) and biological (immune, digestive, integumentary, etc.) phenomena influence—or are influenced by—structural and physiological aspects of the brain. For example, a neuroscientist studying racial descrimination might use fMRI imaging to understand the circuitry and biological processes underlying differences in emotional responses to, and reasoning about, an injustice perpetrated upon a member of the same versus a different racial group. She or he might compare systematic differences in neural activity between a cohort of individuals who self identify as racial separatists, and those who self-identify as anti-racist.

In contrast, behavioral scientists tend to define mental and behavioral phenomena in terms of a mind, agnostic about the relationship between mental phenomena and the brain [160, 163, 164]. The constructs, theories, tools, and technologies they develop and use are designed to elucidate the relationships between and among various mental, behavioral, interpersonal, and social phenomena. Social scientists address a slightly different range of phenomena, interested primarily in relationships between individual people, groups of people, and phenomena that arise in the context of the interaction between them. Like the pure behavioral scientist, the pure social scientist is agnostic about the relationship between social phenomena and the brain. Whereas the neuroscientist described above studied racial discrimination by looking at the biological correlates of racism, a behavioral scientist is more likley to examine the relationship between internal beliefs and attitudes and emotionally charged experiences with members of the same and different racial groups. A social scientist, on the other hand, might examine the relationship between a person's attitudes towards people of a different racial group and the attitudes and behavior of peers and authority figures. Alternatively, she or he may study the relationshipo between a person's attitutes towards people of a different racial groups and the types and prevalence of various images of that racial groups in the media.

This is not to say that pure biological scientists do not 'believe in', or care about, more abstract aspects of the mind and social phenomena, or that pure behavioral and social scientists do not 'believe in', or care about, the biological basis of the mind and social phenomena. In fact, there is significant overlap between these fields and a number of interdisciplinary sciences have emerged at their intersections (Fig. 6.6).

There are fundamental epistemological challenges inherent in acquiring knowledge by integrating theories within and across each of the three branches of science most relevant to MHI. These challenges are embraced, and explicitly addressed by the NIMH's Research Domain Criteria (RDoC) framework, discussed in detail in Chap. 12. Here, we want to briefly touch on the fundamental challenge of defining the relationships between brain and behavior.

Fig. 6.6 Interdisciplinary knowledge base underlying mental healthcare

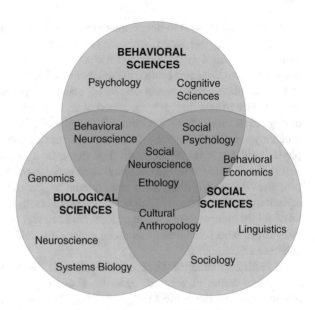

6.3.3 A Primary Epistemological Challenge for Informaticians: The Relationship Between the Mind and Brain

One of the primary challenges for informaticians working in MHI Is developing paradigms and technologies that integrate the disparate theories of mental functions and human behavior espoused by scientists working in the biological and behavioral sciences, and the often-passionate belief in the unique legitimacy of one perspective. Thanks to our more philosophically oriented colleagues in the field of Neurophilosophy (see [49]), we can operationally define the root cause of this inter-scientific conflict. Neurophilosophy tell us our conflict is not new and that this difference of opinion about the relationship between mind and brain has deep historical roots [49, 51, 209]. While a comprehensive review of the philosophical literature on the mind-brain question is beyond the scope of this book,[1] a core distinction can be made between 'monism' and 'dualism' (Table 6.4). The monist's stance is that the brain and mind are not distinct entities and that there is only one entity—the brain. Monism does not deny the existence of the mind. Rather, it views it as an epiphenomenon of brain functioning. The dualist stance is that the brain and the mind are, in fact, distinct conceptual entities. Dualism argues that the brain directly influences the mind, and the mind directly influences the brain, but that even with the most sophisticated tools and technologies, science will never be able to reliably and fully define complex mental phenomena in terms of specific physiologic brain phenomena.

---

[1] See *Neurophilosophy: Towards a Unified Science of the Mind/Brain* by Patricia Smith Churchland for a thorough and accessible discussion of the historical foundations of the issue.

Table 6.4 Philosophical approaches to defining the relationship between the brain and mind

Model	Description
Monism	The brain and the mind are not distinct entities—the brain is the one true ontological[a] entity and the mind is a conceptual entity that allows us talk about functions of the brain that we cannot (yet) describe at the neuronal level
Physicalism	Each mind function is synonymous with some brain function
Reductionism	Each mind function can be reduced to some brain function
Dualism	The brain and mind are distinct entities
Interactionism	The brain influences the mind and the mind influences the brain
Parallelism	The mind and brain do not directly influence each other, although they operate in parallel

[a]Ontological: something that really exists in the world, not just a concept or idea

For example, a dualist might argue that while much is known about the neuro-anatomic and biochemical correlates of emotion, including some of the very specific brain circuits involved, it is currently not possible to reliably define specific emotional states (emotion 'quality') in terms of specific neurophysiologic states (see [210]). That is, a neuroscientist cannot accurately "measure" the quality of emotion a person is experiencing based on patterns of activity in specific brain circuits. A monist would counter that our inability to define (i.e., reduce) highly specific phenomenological emotional qualities (e.g., joyful surprise versus fearful surprise) in terms of specific neurophysiologic states is due only to the limitations of current technologies for detecting these states. She would argue that once we have sufficiently refined technologies, we will be able to accurately describe all aspects of a person's emotional state (quality and intensity) based solely on patterns of neuroactivity. The dualist, in turn, would counter that there is no such future technology—that there is something fundamentally (ontologically) different between the way the mind manifests emotional qualities and the way the brain manifests them.

6.3.4   *Epistemological Differences within the Behavioral and Social Sciences: A Multiplicity of Theories of 'Mind' and Behavior*

If the theoretic and epistemic differences between the behavioral and biological sciences don't make your head spin, the multiplicity of theories within the behavioral and social sciences certainly will! Whereas disagreements between scientists and clinicians working in the biomedical domain tend to be primarily about nuanced mechanisms, and directions of causal relationships, scientists and clinicians working within the behavioral and social sciences often disagree about the fundamental entities and mechanisms themselves. Imagine working in research informatics in cardiology in a time before the existence of modern tools and technologies for visualizing the structures and function of the heart in a living human. Imagine two scientific camps within the field of cardiology—each one having a fundamentally different model of the structure and function of the heart. Imagine the number of competing entities, processes, and theories that scientists could justify based only on phenomena that could be directly observed. This is the current state of the behavioral sciences. The primary entity of interest—the mind—cannot be directly observed. Consequently, the functional properties of this key entity are defined in radically different ways within the behavioral sciences.

For informaticians working in MHI, the significance of these philosophical (theoretic) distinctions cannot be overstated. MHI embraces the spirit of the vision put forth by NIMH in the RDoC framework which strives to improve the process of acquiring knowledge across the diverse branches of science in which knowledge is being generated. To do this, informaticians working in MHI must be fluent in the many theoretical languages of the biological, behavioral, and social sciences. At minimum, this means understanding the nuances of the data-to-knowledge process employed by each field. This includes understanding how the field defines and models the real-world phenomena of interest as well as how the field identifies, captures, and represents these phenomena (signals) in the form of quantifiable data points. It includes understanding the paradigms and computational (statistical, analytic) methods the field uses to transform these data into meaningful information, and then into actionable knowledge.

6.3.5 Points of Intersection Between the Biological, Behavioral, and Social Sciences

Despite the many challenges inherent in bridging the gap between the biological and behavioral sciences, over time we are seeing increasingly more overlap between the sciences (Fig. 6.7). This impetus is coming from within each of the sciences

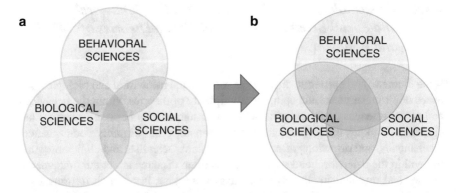

Fig. 6.7 (**a**) Relationship between phenomena of interest in the biological, behavioral, and social sciences. (**b**) Increasing overlap between phenomena of interest in the biological, behavioral, and social sciences as more is understood about the interrelationships among them

themselves and there has been great progress in understanding the complex, reciprocal ways in which biological, behavioral, and social phenomena mutually influence each other. Increasingly, behavioral and social scientists are asking sophisticated questions about the mechanisms by which biological, mental, behavioral, and social phenomena influence each other [211–214]. Similarly, biological scientists are developing novel methods for investigating not only the ways that biological functions drive mental and behavioral functions, but conversely, the ways that mental, behavioral, interpersonal and social functions drive biological functions [157, 159, 160, 163]. This knowledge is being generated by interdisciplinary scientists working explicitly at the intersections of the biological, behavioral, and social sciences (Fig. 6.6).

While there is strong consensus that biological underpinnings of many, if not most, mental and behavioral phenomena will undoubtedly be discovered as technologies for assessing both neurobiological and mental phenomena become more sophisticated [100, 110, 112], the real challenge lies in identifying the causal direction and mediating variables in these relationships. In some cases, as we understand more about the brain and the physiological underpinnings of the associated mental and behavioral phenomena, the differences between mental and biomedical disorders may begin to fade [100, 110, 112]. Those psychiatric disorders discovered to have a clear, primary biologic etiology may be re-categorized as biomedical disorders, e.g., as neurological or endocrine disorders [98]. In other cases, discovery of the biological underpinnings of mental health conditions may provide insight into ways that different social and interpersonal experiences shape our brains in ways that lead to long term dysfunction or distress.

6.4 How Mental Health Informatics Extends Informatics

Above we focus on the differences between MHI and other informatics subdisciplines, and on ways in which mainstream biomedical and health informatics has neglected the behavioral and social sciences. However, several mainstream informatics technologies are being heavily utilized in the field of mental health. For example, the use of mobile health technology (mHealth) has been an area of increasing interest in medicine in recent years due to both the ubiquity of smartphones and the development of new technologies such as activity trackers and smartwatches [215]. Given the importance of activity-related behavior in risk, diagnosis, and treatment for mental health conditions, this technology has been game-changing for data-driven study and treatment in mental health [196, 216, 217] (see Chap. 17).

Natural language processing (Chap. 13) is a major subfield of informatics with NLP paradigms routinely applied across scientific literature, clinical text, and social media alike [218–222]. It is particularly useful in the context of mental health, where symptoms and environmental factors) are often recorded only in free text and rarely as structured data or as results of quantitative assessments. Social media in particular is a rich source of the kinds of information of interest to behavioral and social scientists (e.g., emotion, thoughts, behavior, social interaction, and environments). Moreover, social media can be an outlet for people struggling with mental health concerns, whether to vent privately to friends on Facebook, or to share their distress with the world through Twitter [221, 223, 224]. Information shared in these places may rarely make it to a healthcare provider's radar but can be invaluable for tracking a person's mental health over time.

Ethical, legal, and social issues (Chap. 18), particularly around data privacy and security, are important in informatics at large, but particularly so for mental health data due to the stigma that is unfortunately still attached to these conditions. Substance use disorder (SUD) information is even more sensitive, protected under its own legislation, 42 CFR (Code of Federal Regulations) Part 2 prohibiting unauthorized disclosures of health records except in limited circumstances [225].

Arguably the most important way in which MHI extends traditional informatics is by focusing our attention on the many implicit assumptions we make, and the beliefs we hold, about the nature of the relationship between the underlying entities and processes about which we seek knowledge, and the concrete data that serves as their proxies in our knowledge acquisition paradigms. Because informaticians working in mental health deal with fundamentally different kinds of things than those working in biomedicine, and because the paradigms used to isolate and measure these phenomena are fundamentally different from the paradigms used in biomedicine, mental health informaticians cannot take for granted that the data generated from traditional sources accurately and complete represents the underlying phenomena of interest. Consequently, mental health informaticians will likely elucidate critical aspects of the early phases of the DIKA process: the process by which the observable signals produced by real world phenomena become concrete data—linguistic representations with associated quantitative and qualitative metrics.

6.5   Summary

The relatively young field of Mental Health Informatics overlaps significantly with the broader field of Biomedical and Health Informatics, but also extends some existing aspects of the field, and introduces new complexity and challenges derived from its unique position at the confluence of several different branches of science: the biological, social, and behavioral sciences. Complexity within the social and behavioral sciences in terms of the multiplicity, and sometimes inconsistency among, models of mental and behavioral function further contribute to the challenges. As described in detail in the discussion of epistemological differences between the social and behavioral sicences on the one hand and the biological sciences on the other, as well as the discussion about the historical roots of informatics in the biological sciences, mental health informaticians will be required to adopt new paradigms for knowledge discovery. One important areas of work will be reconciling different approaches to concept and knowledge representation (Chap. 7). Another will reconciling different approaches to knowledge acquisition itself (see Chap. 12). Finally, significant advances in technologies for signal detection, the acquisition of data, methods for transforming data into knowledge, and opportunities to apply that new knowledge in both standard and novel avenues for mental healthcare pose tremendous opportunities for students, researchers, and practitioners in this exciting field.

References

1. Shortliffe EH, Cimino JJ. Biomedical informatics. Berlin: Springer; 2006.
2. Kulikowski CA, Shortliffe EH, Currie LM, et al. AMIA Board white paper: definition of biomedical informatics and specification of core competencies for graduate education in the discipline. J Am Med Inform Assoc. 2012;19(6):931–8.
3. Warner HR. Medical informatics: a real discipline? J Am Med Inform Assoc. 1995;2(4):207.
4. Engel GL. The need for a new medical model: a challenge for biomedicine. Science. 1977;196(4286):129–36. https://doi.org/10.1126/science.847460. [published Online First: Epub Date]
5. National Institute of Mental Health. Research Domain Criteria (RDoC). Secondary Research Domain Criteria (RDoC) November 9 2012. http://www.nimh.nih.gov/research-funding/rdoc/index.shtml.
6. Insel TR. The NIMH research domain criteria (RDoC) project: precision medicine for psychiatry. Am J Psychiatry. 2014;171(4):395–7. https://doi.org/10.1176/appi.ajp.2014.14020138. [published Online First: Epub Date]
7. Baars BJ. A cognitive theory of consciousness. Cambridge, MA: Cambridge University Press; 1993.
8. Carruthers P. Phenomenal consciousness: a naturalistic theory. Cambridge: Cambridge University Press; 2003.
9. Crick F, Koch C. Towards a neurobiological theory of consciousness. Semin Neurosci. 1990;2:263–75.
10. Tononi G. An information integration theory of consciousness. BMC Neurosci. 2004;5(1):42.
11. Edelman GM. The remembered present: a biological theory of consciousness. New York: Basic Books; 1989.
12. Holt RR. Drive or wish? A reconsideration of the psychoanalytic theory of motivation. Psychol Issues. 1976;9(4):158–97.
13. Geen RG, Gange JJ. Drive theory of social facilitation: twelve years of theory and research. Psychol Bull. 1977;84(6):1267.
14. Mitchell SA. Hope and dread in psychoanalysis. New York: Basic Books; 1993.
15. Guerin B. Social facilitation. In: Weiner IB, Craighead WE, editors. The Corsini encyclopedia of psychology. Hoboken, NJ: Wiley; 2010. p. 1–2.
16. Di Domenico SI, Ryan RM. The emerging neuroscience of intrinsic motivation: a new frontier in self-determination research. Front Hum Neurosci. 2017;11:145.
17. Dweck CS. From needs to goals and representations: foundations for a unified theory of motivation, personality, and development. Psychol Rev. 2017;124(6):689.
18. Berridge KC. Evolving concepts of emotion and motivation. Front Psychol. 2018;9:1647.
19. Cannon WB. The James-Lange theory of emotions: a critical examination and an alternative theory. Am J Psychol. 1927;39(1/4):106–24. https://doi.org/10.2307/1415404. [published Online First: Epub Date]
20. James W. The physical bases of emotion. 1894. Psychol Rev. 1994;101(2):205–10. https://doi.org/10.1037/0033-295x.101.2.205. [published Online First: Epub Date]
21. Lazarus RS. Progress on a cognitive-motivational-relational theory of emotion. Am Psychol. 1991;46(8):819–34. https://doi.org/10.1037//0003-066x.46.8.819. [published Online First: Epub Date]
22. Moors A. Theories of emotion causation: a review. Cognit Emot. 2009;23(4):625–62. https://doi.org/10.1080/02699930802645739. [published Online First: Epub Date]

23. Schachter S, Singer JE. Cognitive, social, and physiological determinants of emotional state. Psychol Rev. 1962;69:379–99. https://doi.org/10.1037/h0046234. [published Online First: Epub Date]
24. Zajonc RB, Murphy ST, Inglehart M. Feeling and facial efference: implications of the vascular theory of emotion. Psychol Rev. 1989;96(3):395–416. https://doi.org/10.1037/0033-295x.96.3.395. [published Online First: Epub Date]
25. Goldstein EB. Sensation and perception. Boston, MA: Cengage Learning; 2009.
26. Newell A. Unified theories of cognition. Cambridge, MA: Harvard University Press; 1990.
27. Johnson-Laird PN. Mental models. Cambridge: Cambridge University Press; 1989.
28. Gentner D, Stevens AL. Mental models. New York: Psychology Press; 2014.
29. Ahissar E, Assa E. Perception as a closed-loop convergence process. elife. 2016;5:e12830.
30. Gibson JJ. The perception of the visual world. Houghton Mifflin: Oxford; 1950.
31. Hurley SL. Consciousness in action. Cambridge, MA: Harvard University Press; 2002.
32. Baddeley AD. Human memory: theory and practice. Hove: Psychology Press; 1997.
33. Deutsch JA, Deutsch D. Attention: some theoretical considerations. Psychol Rev. 1963;70(1):80.
34. Norman DA, Shallice T. Attention to action. In: Consciousness and self-regulation. New York: Springer; 1986. p. 1–18.
35. Knudsen EI. Fundamental components of attention. Annu Rev Neurosci. 2007;30:57–78.
36. Wells A, Matthews G. Attention and emotion (classic edition): a clinical perspective. New York: Psychology Press; 2014.
37. Simon HA. Models of thought. New Haven: Yale University Press; 1979.
38. Holyoak KJ, Spellman BA. Thinking. Annu Rev Psychol. 1993;44(1):265–315.
39. Mowrer O. Learning theory and behavior. New York: Wiley; 1960.
40. Skinner BF. Are theories of learning necessary? Psychol Rev. 1950;57(4):193.
41. Bandura A, McClelland DC. Social learning theory. Englewood cliffs: Prentice Hall; 1977.
42. Fromkin V, Rodman R, Hyams N. An introduction to language. Boston, MA: Cengage Learning; 2018.
43. Sloman SA. The empirical case for two systems of reasoning. Psychol Bull. 1996;119(1):3.
44. Evans JSB. In two minds: dual-process accounts of reasoning. Trends Cogn Sci. 2003;7(10):454–9.
45. Starkey P, Spelke ES, Gelman R. Numerical abstraction by human infants. Cognition. 1990;36(2):97–127.
46. Dehaene S. Varieties of numerical abilities. Cognition. 1992;44(1–2):1–42.
47. McCloskey M, Macaruso P. Representing and using numerical information. Am Psychol. 1995;50(5):351.
48. Redish AD. The mind within the brain: how we make decisions and how those decisions go wrong. New York: Oxford University Press; 2013.
49. Churchland PS. Neurophilosophy : toward a unified science of the mind-brain. Cambridge, MA: MIT Press; 1986.
50. Varela FJ, Thompson E, Rosch E. The embodied mind : cognitive science and human experience. Revised edition. Cambridge, MA: MIT Press; 2016.
51. Chalmers D. Guide to the philosophy of mind. New York: New York University; 2017.
52. Epstein S. Cognitive-experiential self-theory of personality. Handb Psychol. 2003;10:159–84.
53. Samsonovich AV, Ascoli GA. The conscious self: ontology, epistemology and the mirror quest. Cortex. 2005;41(5):621–36.
54. Bandura A. Toward an agentic theory of the self. Adv Self Res. 2008;3:15–49.
55. Sui J, Gu X. Self as object: emerging trends in self research. Trends Neurosci. 2017;40(11):643–53.
56. Epstein S. The self-concept revisited: Or a theory of a theory. Am Psychol. 1973;28(5):404.
57. Greenwald AG, Banaji MR, Rudman LA, Farnham SD, Nosek BA, Mellott DS. A unified theory of implicit attitudes, stereotypes, self-esteem, and self-concept. Psychol Rev. 2002;109(1):3.

58. Harter S. The construction of the self: a developmental perspective. London: Guilford Press; 1999.
59. Haslam SA. Stereotyping and social influence: foundations of stereotype consensus. In: Spears R, Oakes PJ, Ellemers N, Haslam SA, editors. The social psychology of stereotyping and group life. Oxford: Blackwell; 1997. p. 119–43.
60. Marsh HW. A multidimensional, hierarchical model of self-concept: theoretical and empirical justification. Educ Psychol Rev. 1990;2(2):77–172.
61. Marsh HW, Hattie J. Theoretical perspectives on the structure of self-concept. In: Bracken BA, editor. Handbook of self-concept: developmental, social, and clinical considerations. New York: Wiley; 1996.
62. Bandura A. Self-efficacy. In: The Corsini encyclopedia of psychology. Hoboken, NJ: Wiley; 2010. p. 1–3.
63. Leary MR, Baumeister RF. The nature and function of self-esteem: sociometer theory. In: Advances in experimental social psychology. New York: Elsevier; 2000. p. 1–62.
64. Hogan R. A socioanalytic theory of personality. In: Page MM, editor. Nebraska Symposium on Motivation: Vol. 30 Personality: current theory and research. Lincoln: University of Nebraska Press; 1982. p. 55–89.
65. Pincus AL, Ansell EB. Interpersonal theory of personality. In: Handbook of psychology. Hoboken, NJ: Wiley; 2003. p. 209–29.
66. McCrae RR, Costa PT Jr. The five-factor theory of personality. In: Pervin LA, John OP, editors. Handbook of personality: theory and research. 2nd ed. New York: Guilford; 2008.
67. John OP, Robins RW, Pervin LA. Handbook of personality: theory and research. New York: Guilford Press; 2010.
68. Cervone D, Pervin LA. Personality: theory and research. Hoboken, NJ: Wiley; 2015.
69. Helms JE. Black and White racial identity: theory, research, and practice. Westport: Greenwood Press; 1990.
70. Stets JE, Burke PJ. Identity theory and social identity theory. Soc Psychol Q. 2000;63:224–37.
71. Turner JC, Oakes PJ. The significance of the social identity concept for social psychology with reference to individualism, interactionism and social influence. Br J Soc Psychol. 1986;25(3):237–52.
72. Gilligan C. Moral orientation and moral development [1987]. In: Justice and care. London: Routledge; 1995. p. 31–46.
73. Eisenberg N. Emotion, regulation, and moral development. Annu Rev Psychol. 2000;51(1):665–97.
74. Gibbs JC. Moral development and reality: beyond the theories of Kohlberg, Hoffman, and Haidt. New York: Oxford University Press; 2019.
75. Ekman P, Sorenson ER, Friesen WV. Pan-cultural elements in facial displays of emotion. Science. 1969;164(3875):86–8.
76. Ekman P, Freisen WV, Ancoli S. Facial signs of emotional experience. J Pers Soc Psychol. 1980;39(6):1125.
77. Mohr J, Spekman R. Characteristics of partnership success: partnership attributes, communication behavior, and conflict resolution techniques. Strateg Manag J. 1994;15(2):135–52.
78. Mehrabian A. Communication without words. In: Communication theory. London: Routledge; 2017. p. 193–200.
79. Skinner BF. Science and human behavior. New York: Simon and Schuster; 1965.
80. Goffman E. Behavior in public places. New York: Simon and Schuster; 2008.
81. Miller GA, Eugene G, Pribram KH. Plans and the structure of behaviour. London: Routledge; 2017.
82. Bowlby J. A secure base: parent-child attachment and healthy human development. New York: Basic Books; 2008.
83. Kelley HH. Personal relationships: their structures and processes. New York: Psychology Press; 2013.

84. Kiesler DJ. Contemporary interpersonal theory and research: personality, psychopathology, and psychotherapy. New York: Wiley; 1996.
85. Pietromonaco PR, Uchino B, Dunkel SC. Close relationship processes and health: implications of attachment theory for health and disease. Health Psychol. 2013;32(5):499.
86. Underwood LG. Compassionate love: a framework for research. In: Fehr B, Sprecher S, Underwood LG, editors. The science of compassionate love: theory, research, and applications. Oxford: Wiley Blackwell; 2009. p. 3–25.
87. Hendrick SS, Hendrick C. Romantic love. New York: Sage Publications; 1992.
88. Horowitz LM, Strack S. Handbook of interpersonal psychology: theory, research, assessment and therapeutic interventions. Hoboken, NJ: Wiley; 2010.
89. Bowlby J. Attachment and loss: volume I: attachment. Attachment and loss: volume I: attachment. London: The Hogarth Press and the Institute of Psycho-Analysis; 1969. p. 1–401.
90. Carlson EA, Sroufe LA. Contribution of attachment theory to developmental psychopathology. In: Cicchetti D, Cohen DJ, editors. Developmental psychopathology: theory and method. Hoboken, NJ: Wiley; 1995.
91. Cassidy J, Shaver PR. Handbook of attachment: theory, research, and clinical applications. New York: Rough Guides; 2002.
92. Bowlby J. Attachment. New York: Basic Books; 2008.
93. Feldman R, Gordon I, Zagoory-Sharon O. Maternal and paternal plasma, salivary, and urinary oxytocin and parent–infant synchrony: considering stress and affiliation components of human bonding. Dev Sci. 2011;14(4):752–61.
94. Cummings EM, Davies PT, Campbell SB. Developmental psychopathology and family process: theory, research, and clinical implications. New York: Guilford Press; 2002.
95. Szapocznik J, Kurtines WM. Family psychology and cultural diversity: opportunities for theory, research, and application. Am Psychol. 1993;48(4):400.
96. Fiske AP. Structures of social life: the four elementary forms of human relations: communal sharing, authority ranking, equality matching, market pricing. New York: Free Press; 1991.
97. Fiske ST. Social beings: Core motives in social psychology. Hoboken, NJ: Wiley; 2018.
98. Warner BD, Fowler SK. Strain and violence: testing a general strain theory model of community violence. J Crim Just. 2003;31(6):511–21.
99. Borgatti SP, Mehra A, Brass DJ, Labianca G. Network analysis in the social sciences. Science. 2009;323(5916):892–5.
100. Griffin EA. A first look at communication theory/Em Griffin. New York: McGraw-Hill; 2012.
101. Hargie O. Skilled interpersonal communication: research, theory and practice. New York: Routledge; 2016.
102. Turner JC. Social categorization and the self-concept: a social cognitive theory of group behavior. In: Postmes T, Branscombe NR, editors. Rediscovering social identity. New York: Routledge; 2010.
103. Abrams D, Hogg MA. Social identifications: a social psychology of intergroup relations and group processes. London: Routledge; 2006.
104. Brown R, Pehrson S. Group processes: dynamics within and between groups. Hoboken, NJ: Wiley; 2019.
105. Faust K. Centrality in affiliation networks. Soc Networks. 1997;19(2):157–91.
106. Hill CA. Affiliation motivation: people who need people… but in different ways. J Pers Soc Psychol. 1987;52(5):1008.
107. Koestner R, McClelland DC. The affiliation motive. In: Smith CP, Atkinson JW, McClelland DC, Veroff J, editors. Motivation and personality: handbook of thematic content analysis. Cambridge: Cambridge University Press; 1992. p. 393–400.
108. Cranmer SJ, Desmarais BA, Kirkland JH. Toward a network theory of alliance formation. Int Interact. 2012;38(3):295–324.
109. Harcourt AH, de Waal FB. Coalitions and alliances in humans and other animals. Oxford: Oxford University Press; 1992.
110. Mitsuhashi H, Greve HR. A matching theory of alliance formation and organizational success: complementarity and compatibility. Acad Manag J. 2009;52(5):975–95.

111. Abrams D, Hogg MA. Social identification, self-categorization and social influence. Eur Rev Soc Psychol. 1990;1(1):195–228.
112. Brewer MB, Silver MD. Group distinctiveness, social identification, and collective mobilization. In: Stryker S, Owens TJ, White RW, editors. Self, Identity, and Social Movements, vol. 13. Minneapolis: University of Minnesota Press; 2000. p. 153–71.
113. Deaux K, Reid A, Mizrahi K, Cotting D. Connecting the person to the social: the functions of social identification. In: The psychology of the social self. New York: Psychology Press; 2014. p. 99–122.
114. Ellemers N, Van Knippenberg A, De Vries N, Wilke H. Social identification and permeability of group boundaries. Eur J Soc Psychol. 1988;18(6):497–513.
115. Stapel DA, Koomen W. Competition, cooperation, and the effects of others on me. J Pers Soc Psychol. 2005;88(6):1029.
116. Tauer JM, Harackiewicz JM. The effects of cooperation and competition on intrinsic motivation and performance. J Pers Soc Psychol. 2004;86(6):849.
117. Cialdini RB, Trost MR. Social influence: social norms, conformity and compliance. In: Gilbert DT, Fiske ST, Lindzey G, editors. The handbook of social psychology. London: Routledge; 1998.
118. De Vries H, Stevens JM, Vervaecke H. Measuring and testing the steepness of dominance hierarchies. Anim Behav. 2006;71(3):585–92.
119. Shizuka D, McDonald DB. A social network perspective on measurements of dominance hierarchies. Anim Behav. 2012;83(4):925–34.
120. Coie JD, Dodge KA, Kupersmidt JB. Peer group behavior and social status. In: Asher SR, Coie JD, editors. Peer rejection in childhood. New York: Cambridge University Press; 1990. p. 17–59.
121. Evans WN, Oates WE, Schwab RM. Measuring peer group effects: a study of teenage behavior. J Polit Econ. 1992;100(5):966–91.
122. Salmivalli C. Bullying and the peer group: a review. Aggress Violent Behav. 2010;15(2):112–20.
123. James P. Globalism, nationalism, tribalism: bringing theory back in. London: Pine Forge Press; 2006.
124. Berry JW. Globalisation and acculturation. Int J Intercult Relat. 2008;32(4):328–36.
125. Glucksmann M. Structuralist analysis in contemporary social thought (RLE social theory): a comparison of the theories of Claude Lévi-Strauss and Louis Althusser. Hoboken, NJ: Routledge; 2014.
126. Eisenhardt KM. Agency theory: an assessment and review. Acad Manag Rev. 1989;14(1):57–74.
127. Bicchieri C, Muldoon R. Social norms. Cambridge: Cambridge University Press; 2011.
128. Fiske ST, Taylor SE. Social cognition. New York: McGraw-Hill; 1991.
129. Greenwald AG, Banaji MR. Implicit social cognition: attitudes, self-esteem, and stereotypes. Psychol Rev. 1995;102(1):4.
130. Adolphs R. The neurobiology of social cognition. Curr Opin Neurobiol. 2001;11(2):231–9.
131. Berry JW. Acculturation: living successfully in two cultures. Int J Intercult Relat. 2005;29(6):697–712.
132. Mehrabian A, Russell JA. An approach to environmental psychology. London: MIT Press; 1974.
133. Schreuder E, van Erp J, Toet A, Kallen VL. Emotional responses to multisensory environmental stimuli: a conceptual framework and literature review. SAGE Open. 2016;6(1):2158244016630591.
134. Graham LT, Gosling SD, Travis CK. The psychology of home environments: a call for research on residential space. Perspect Psychol Sci. 2015;10(3):346–56.
135. Bell PA, Green T, Fisher JD. In: Baum A, editor. Environmental psychology. New York: Psychology Press; 2001.

136. Stevens RG, Blask DE, Brainard GC, et al. Meeting report: the role of environmental lighting and circadian disruption in cancer and other diseases. Environ Health Perspect. 2007;115(9):1357–62.
137. Dunn R, Krimsky JS, Murray JB, Quinn PJ. Light up their lives: a review of research on the effects of lighting on children's achievement and behavior. Read Teach. 1985;38(9):863–9.
138. Flynn JE, Spencer TJ, Martyniuk O, Hendrick C. Interim study of procedures for investigating the effect of light on impression and behavior. J Illum Eng Soc. 1973;3(1):87–94.
139. Kryter K. The handbook of hearing and the effects of noise: physiology, psychology, and public health. Bingley: Emerald; 1994.
140. Mathews KE, Canon LK. Environmental noise level as a determinant of helping behavior. J Pers Soc Psychol. 1975;32(4):571.
141. Goldman AI. Epistemology and cognition. Cambridge, MA: Harvard University Press; 1986.
142. Conee E, Feldman R. Evidentialism: essays in epistemology. Oxford: Clarendon Press; 2004.
143. Steup M, Neta R. Epistemology. Cambridge, MA: Harvard University Press; 2005.
144. Harding SG. The science question in feminism. Ithaca, NY: Cornell University Press; 1986.
145. Harding SG. Whose science? Whose knowledge? : Thinking from women's lives. Ithaca, N.Y: Cornell University Press; 1991.
146. Cronbach LJ, Meehl PE. Construct validity in psychological tests. Psychol Bull. 1955;52(4):281–302. https://doi.org/10.1037/h0040957. [published Online First: Epub Date]
147. Association AP. APA dictionary of psychology. Washington, DC: Association AP; 2021.
148. Markey J. A redefinition of social phenomena: giving a basis for comparative sociology. Am J Sociol. 1925-26;31:733–43.
149. Westbrook L. Mental models: a theoretical overview and preliminary study. J Inf Sci. 2006;32(6):563–79. https://doi.org/10.1177/0165551506068134. [published Online First: Epub Date]
150. Hawke LD, Provencher MD. Schema theory and Schema therapy in mood and anxiety disorders: a review. J Cogn Psychother. 2011;4:257–76. https://doi.org/10.1891/0889-8391.25.4.257. [published Online First: Epub Date]
151. Pietromonaco PR, Barrett LF. The internal working models concept: what do we really know about the self in relation to others? Rev Gen Psychol. 2000;4(2):155–75. https://doi.org/10.1037/1089-2680.4.2.155. [published Online First: Epub Date]
152. Beck AT, Ward CH, Mendelson M, Mock J, Erbaugh J. An inventory for measuring depression. Arch Gen Psychiatry. 1961;4(6):561–71.
153. Beck AT, Steer RA, Brown G. Beck depression inventory–II. Psychol Assess. 1996;25:136–45.
154. Eisenberg IW, Bissett PG, Enkavi AZ, et al. Uncovering the structure of self-regulation through data-driven ontology discovery. Nat Commun. 2019;10(1):1–13.
155. O'Leary-Kelly SW, Vokurka RJ. The empirical assessment of construct validity. J Oper Manag. 1998;16(4):387–405.
156. Lissitz RW. The end of construct validity. The concept of validity: revisions, new directions and applications, Oct, 2008. Charlotte, NC: IAP Information Age Publishing; 2009.
157. Kasabov NK. Springer handbook of bio–/neuroinformatics. 1st ed. New York: Springer; 2013.
158. Levin BL, Hanson A. Mental health informatics. New York: Springer; 2013.
159. Cipresso P, Serino S, Villani D. Pervasive computing paradigms for mental health. New York: Springer; 2016.
160. Crasto CJ. Neuroinformatics. Totowa, NJ: Humana; 2007.
161. Dewan NA, Luo JS, Lorenzi NM. Information technology essentials for behavioral health clinicians. London: Springer; 2010.
162. Jagaroo V. Neuroinformatics for neuropsychology. New York: Springer; 2009.
163. Wallace R. Computational psychiatry : a systems biology approach to the epigenetics of mental disorders. New York: Springer Science+Business Media; 2017.

164. Insel TR, Cuthbert BN. Medicine. Brain disorders? Precisely. Science. 2015;348(6234):499–500. https://doi.org/10.1126/science.aab2358. [published Online First: Epub Date]
165. Hanson A, Levin BL. Mental health informatics. Berlin: Oxford University Press; 2013.
166. Dewan NA. Behavioral healthcare informatics. New York: Springer; 2002.
167. Goldmann H. Behavioral healthcare informatics. New York: Springer Science & Business Media; 2014.
168. Laranjo L, Lau A, Coiera E. Design and implementation of behavioral informatics interventions. In: Cognitive informatics in health and biomedicine. London: Springer; 2017. p. 13–42.
169. Manrai AK, Cui Y, Bushel PR, et al. Informatics and data analytics to support exposome-based discovery for public health. Annu Rev Public Health. 2017;38:279–94.
170. Witham MD, Frost H, McMurdo M, Donnan PT, McGilchrist M. Construction of a linked health and social care database resource–lessons on process, content and culture. Inform Health Soc Care. 2015;40(3):229–39.
171. Carney TJ, Kong AY. Leveraging health informatics to foster a smart systems response to health disparities and health equity challenges. J Biomed Inform. 2017;68:184–9.
172. Polimanti R, Kaufman J, Zhao H, et al. Trauma exposure interacts with the genetic risk of bipolar disorder in alcohol misuse of US soldiers. Acta Psychiatr Scand. 2018;137(2):148–56. https://doi.org/10.1111/acps.12843. [published Online First: Epub Date]
173. Sun J, Jia P, Fanous AH, et al. A multi-dimensional evidence-based candidate gene prioritization approach for complex diseases-schizophrenia as a case. Bioinformatics. 2009;25(19):2595–6602. https://doi.org/10.1093/bioinformatics/btp428. [published Online First: Epub Date]
174. Liu X, Bipolar Genome S, Kelsoe JR, Greenwood TA. A genome-wide association study of bipolar disorder with comorbid eating disorder replicates the SOX2-OT region. J Affect Disord. 2016;189:141–9. https://doi.org/10.1016/j.jad.2015.09.029. [published Online First: Epub Date]
175. Johnson C, Drgon T, McMahon FJ, Uhl GR. Convergent genome wide association results for bipolar disorder and substance dependence. Am J Med Genet B Neuropsychiatr Genet. 2009;150B(2):182–90. https://doi.org/10.1002/ajmg.b.30900. [published Online First: Epub Date]
176. Woudstra S, Bochdanovits Z, van Tol MJ, et al. Piccolo genotype modulates neural correlates of emotion processing but not executive functioning. Transl Psychiatry. 2012;2:e99. https://doi.org/10.1038/tp.2012.29. [published Online First: Epub Date]
177. Yao X, Yan J, Liu K, et al. Tissue-specific network-based genome wide study of amygdala imaging phenotypes to identify functional interaction modules. Bioinformatics. 2017;33(20):3250–7. https://doi.org/10.1093/bioinformatics/btx344. [published Online First: Epub Date]
178. Arnold PD, Hanna GL, Rosenberg DR. Imaging the amygdala: changing the face of gene discovery in child psychiatry. J Am Acad Child Adolesc Psychiatry. 2010;49(1):7–10.
179. Ebejer JL, Duffy DL, van der Werf J, et al. Genome-wide association study of inattention and hyperactivity-impulsivity measured as quantitative traits. Twin Res Hum Genet. 2013;16(2):560–74. https://doi.org/10.1017/thg.2013.12. [published Online First: Epub Date]
180. Perlis RH. Psychiatric pharmacogenomics: translating genomics. In: Genomics, circuits, and pathways in clinical neuropsychiatry. Amsterdam: Elsevier; 2016. p. 727–47.
181. Brown L, Eum S, Haga SB, Strawn JR, Zierhut H. Clinical utilization of pharmacogenetics in psychiatry – perspectives of pharmacists, genetic counselors, implementation science, clinicians, and industry. Pharmacopsychiatry. 2019;53:162–73. https://doi.org/10.1055/a-0975-9595. [published Online First: Epub Date]
182. Goodspeed A, Kostman N, Kriete TE, et al. Leveraging the utility of pharmacogenomics in psychiatry through clinical decision support: a focus group study. Ann General Psychiatry. 2019;18:13. https://doi.org/10.1186/s12991-019-0237-3. [published Online First: Epub Date]

183. Regenstrief Institute. Logical observation identifiers names and codes (LOINC®). Indiana, IN: Regenstrief Institute, Inc.; 2021.
184. White TM, Hauan MJ. Extending the LOINC conceptual schema to support standardized assessment instruments. J Am Med Inform Assoc. 2002;9(6):586–99.
185. Bakken S, Cimino JJ, Haskell R, et al. Evaluation of the clinical LOINC (logical observation identifiers, names, and codes) semantic structure as a terminology model for standardized assessment measures. J Am Med Inform Assoc. 2000;7(6):529–38.
186. International S. Systematized nomenclature of medicine-clinical terms. 2021.
187. Ranallo PA, Adam TJ, Nelson KJ, Krueger RF, LaVenture M, Chute CG. Psychological assessment instruments: a coverage analysis using SNOMED CT, LOINC and QS terminology. AMIA Annu Symp Proc. 2013;2013:1333–40.
188. Ranallo PA, Kilbourne AM, Whatley AS, Pincus HA. Behavioral health information technology: from Chaos to clarity. Health Aff (Millwood). 2016;35(6):1106–13. https://doi.org/10.1377/hlthaff.2016.0013. [published Online First: Epub Date]
189. Hastings J. Data disintegration and the ontology of mental health: how we talk about mental health, and why it matters in the digital age. Exeter: University of Exeter Press; 2020.
190. ONC. Trusted Exchange Framework and Common Agreement, 2019.
191. Blumenthal D. Launching hitech. N Engl J Med. 2010;362(5):382–5.
192. Hudson KL, Collins FS. The 21st century cures act—a view from the NIH. N Engl J Med. 2017;376(2):111–3.
193. Bouts AM, Brackman L, Martin E, Subasic AM, Potkanowicz ES. The accuracy and validity of iOS-based heart rate apps during moderate to high intensity exercise. Int J Exerc Sci. 2018;11(7):533–40.
194. Kwon SB, Ahn JW, Lee SM, et al. Estimating maximal oxygen uptake from daily activity data measured by a watch-type fitness tracker: cross-sectional study. JMIR Mhealth Uhealth. 2019;7(6):e13327. https://doi.org/10.2196/13327. [published Online First: Epub Date]
195. Kim J, Lim S, Min YH, et al. Depression screening using daily mental-health ratings from a smartphone application for breast cancer patients. J Med Internet Res. 2016;18(8):e216. https://doi.org/10.2196/jmir.5598. [published Online First: Epub Date]
196. Knight A, Bidargaddi N. Commonly available activity tracker apps and wearables as a mental health outcome indicator: a prospective observational cohort study among young adults with psychological distress. J Affect Disord. 2018;236:31–6. https://doi.org/10.1016/j.jad.2018.04.099. [published Online First: Epub Date]
197. Matcham F, Barattieri di San Pietro C, Bulgari V, et al. Remote assessment of disease and relapse in major depressive disorder (RADAR-MDD): a multi-Centre prospective cohort study protocol. BMC Psychiatry. 2019;19(1):72. https://doi.org/10.1186/s12888-019-2049-z. [published Online First: Epub Date]
198. Cook JD, Prairie ML, Plante DT. Utility of the Fitbit flex to evaluate sleep in major depressive disorder: a comparison against polysomnography and wrist-worn actigraphy. J Affect Disord. 2017;217:299–305. https://doi.org/10.1016/j.jad.2017.04.030. [published Online First: Epub Date]
199. Cheatham SW, Stull KR, Fantigrassi M, Motel I. The efficacy of wearable activity tracking technology as part of a weight loss program: a systematic review. J Sports Med Phys Fitness. 2018;58(4):534–48. https://doi.org/10.23736/S0022-4707.17.07437-0. [published Online First: Epub Date]
200. Martin SS, Feldman DI, Blumenthal RS, et al. mActive: a randomized clinical trial of an automated mHealth intervention for physical activity promotion. J Am Heart Assoc. 2015;4(11):e002239. https://doi.org/10.1161/JAHA.115.002239. [published Online First: Epub Date]
201. Burke LE, Shiffman S, Music E, et al. Ecological momentary assessment in behavioral research: addressing technological and human participant challenges. J Med Internet Res. 2017;19(3):e77. https://doi.org/10.2196/jmir.7138. [published Online First: Epub Date]

202. Clark C, Wellner B, Davis R, Aberdeen J, Hirschman L. Automatic classification of RDoC positive valence severity with a neural network. J Biomed Inform. 2017;75S:S120–S28. https://doi.org/10.1016/j.jbi.2017.07.005. [published Online First: Epub Date]|

203. Li F, Rao G, Du J, et al. Ontological representation-oriented term normalization and standardization of the research domain criteria. Health Informatics J. 2019;26(2):726–37. https://doi.org/10.1177/1460458219832059. [published Online First: Epub Date]|

204. Clarke MA, Steege LM, Moore JL, Belden JL, Koopman RJ, Kim MS. Addressing human computer interaction issues of electronic health record in clinical encounters. International conference of design, user experience, and usability. Cham: Springer; 2013.

205. Patel VL, Kannampallil TG. Cognitive informatics in biomedicine and healthcare. J Biomed Inform. 2015;53:3–14. https://doi.org/10.1016/j.jbi.2014.12.007. [published Online First: Epub Date]

206. Or CK, Valdez RS, Casper GR, et al. Human factors and ergonomics in home care: current concerns and future considerations for health information technology. Work. 2009;33(2):201–9. https://doi.org/10.3233/WOR-2009-0867. [published Online First: Epub Date]

207. Adler-Milstein J, Jha AK. HITECH act drove large gains in hospital electronic health record adoption. Health Aff. 2017;36(8):1416–22.

208. Cohen D. Effect of the exclusion of behavioral health from health information technology (HIT) legislation on the future of integrated health care. J Behav Health Serv Res. 2015;42(4):534–9. https://doi.org/10.1007/s11414-014-9407-x. [published Online First: Epub Date]

209. Zalta EN. Center for the Study of language and information (U.S.). Metaphysics research lab. Stanford encyclopedia of philosophy. Stanford, CA: Metaphysics Research Lab, Center for the Study of Language and Information, Stanford University; 2004.

210. Kassam KS, Markey AR, Cherkassky VL, Loewenstein G, Just MA. Identifying emotions on the basis of neural activation. PLoS One. 2013;8(6):e66032. https://doi.org/10.1371/journal.pone.0066032. [published Online First: Epub Date]

211. Colibazzi T. Journal watch review of research domain criteria (RDoC): toward a new classification framework for research on mental disorders. J Am Psychoanal Assoc. 2014;62(4):709–10. https://doi.org/10.1177/0003065114543185. [published Online First: Epub Date]

212. Cuthbert BN, Insel TR. Toward the future of psychiatric diagnosis: the seven pillars of RDoC. BMC Med. 2013;11:126. https://doi.org/10.1186/1741-7015-11-126. [published Online First: Epub Date]

213. Gordon J. RDoC: outcomes to causes and back. Bethesda: National Institute of Mental Health; 2017.

214. Insel T, Cuthbert B, Garvey M, et al. Research domain criteria (RDoC): toward a new classification framework for research on mental disorders. Am J Psychiatry. 2010;167(7):748–51. https://doi.org/10.1176/appi.ajp.2010.09091379. [published Online First: Epub Date]

215. Luxton DD, McCann RA, Bush NE, Mishkind MC, Reger GM. mHealth for mental health: integrating smartphone technology in behavioral healthcare. Prof Psychol Res Pract. 2011;42(6):505.

216. Seppälä J, De Vita I, Jämsä T, et al. Mobile phone and wearable sensor-based mHealth approaches for psychiatric disorders and symptoms: systematic review. JMIR Ment Health. 2019;6(2):e9819.

217. Torous J, Firth J, Mueller N, Onnela J-P, Baker JT. Methodology and reporting of mobile heath and smartphone application studies for schizophrenia. Harv Rev Psychiatry. 2017;25(3):146.

218. Chandran D, Robbins DA, Chang CK, et al. Use of natural language processing to identify obsessive compulsive symptoms in patients with schizophrenia, schizoaffective disorder or bipolar disorder. Sci Rep. 2019;9(1):14146. https://doi.org/10.1038/s41598-019-49165-2. [published Online First: Epub Date]

219. Viani N, Kam J, Yin L, et al. Annotating temporal relations to determine the onset of psychosis symptoms. Stud Health Technol Inform. 2019;264:418–22. https://doi.org/10.3233/SHTI190255. [published Online First: Epub Date]

220. Tran T, Kavuluru R. Predicting mental conditions based on "history of present illness" in psychiatric notes with deep neural networks. J Biomed Inform. 2017;75S:S138–S48. https://doi.org/10.1016/j.jbi.2017.06.010. [published Online First: Epub Date]
221. Sarker A, O'Connor K, Ginn R, et al. Social Media Mining for Toxicovigilance: automatic monitoring of prescription medication abuse from twitter. Drug Saf. 2016;39(3):231–40. https://doi.org/10.1007/s40264-015-0379-4. [published Online First: Epub Date]
222. Rosemblat G, Fiszman M, Shin D, Kilicoglu H. Towards a characterization of apparent contradictions in the biomedical literature using context analysis. J Biomed Inform. 2019;98:103275. https://doi.org/10.1016/j.jbi.2019.103275. [published Online First: Epub Date]
223. Karmen C, Hsiung RC, Wetter T. Screening internet forum participants for depression symptoms by assembling and enhancing multiple NLP methods. Comput Methods Prog Biomed. 2015;120(1):27–36. https://doi.org/10.1016/j.cmpb.2015.03.008. [published Online First: Epub Date]
224. Conway M, Hu M, Chapman WW. Recent advances in using natural language processing to address public health research questions using social media and consumer generated data. Yearb Med Inform. 2019;28(1):208–17. https://doi.org/10.1055/s-0039-1677918. [published Online First: Epub Date]
225. HHS. Fact sheet: SAMHSA 42 CFR Part 2 Revised Rule, 2020.

Chapter 7
Technologies for the Computable Representation and Sharing of Data and Knowledge in Mental Health

Piper A. Ranallo and Jessica D. Tenenbaum

Abstract Mental health as a domain is in dire need of more efficient, cost effective methods for acquiring and disseminating new knowledge. We need new methods not only to efficiently develop the knowledge base upon which precision mental healthcare can be based, but also reliable methods to put this knowledge in the hands of consumers, front-line researchers, and providers. More than two decades of experience in general biomedical healthcare has demonstrated that computerized information systems are essential for achieving these goals. Our ability to acquire and disseminate high quality knowledge using health information systems, however, depends on our ability to both represent and exchange data in ways that computerized systems understand. In this chapter we introduce the foundational informatics technologies upon which this knowledge acquisition and dissemination depends—technologies for standardizing the representation and exchange of data, information, and knowledge. We introduce technologies for data and knowledge representation, such as terminologies, ontologies, and information models. We describe methods for specifying the kinds of information required as inputs for a specific purpose, such as *minimum clinical data sets* (MCDSs) and *common data elements* (CDEs), with an emphasis on those used in the context of mental health. Next, we introduce the concept of "standards" and describe three basics types of standards and their critical role in enabling both technical and semantic interoperability. Finally, we highlight the substantial gaps in systems for both concept and knowledge representation in mental health and outline a preliminary foundation for the systematic enhancement of technologies for the computable representation of mental health data and knowledge.

P. A. Ranallo (✉)
Six Aims for Behavioral Health, Minneapolis, MN, USA
e-mail: pranallo@sixaims.org; sven0018@umn.edu

J. D. Tenenbaum
Duke University, Durham, NC, USA
e-mail: jessie.tenenbaum@duke.edu

© Springer Nature Switzerland AG 2021
J. D. Tenenbaum, P. A. Ranallo (eds.), *Mental Health Informatics*, Health Informatics, https://doi.org/10.1007/978-3-030-70558-9_7

Keywords Concept representation · Knowledge representation · Interoperability Standards · Data standards · Precision mental health

7.1 Introduction

More than any other domain of healthcare, mental health needs more efficient, cost effective methods for acquiring and disseminating knowledge. Not only do we need new methods for efficiently developing the knowledge base upon which precision mental healthcare can be built, we also need reliable methods for putting this knowledge in the hands of front-line providers. More than two decades of experience in biomedical healthcare has demonstrated that computerized information systems are essential for achieving these goals. Researchers working not only in the biomedical, behavioral, and social sciences, but also those working in health services research, depend on information systems to perform their work efficiently and cost-effectively. Similarly, front line care providers, payers, policy makers, and developers of clinical practice guidelines and quality measures also depend on information systems to acquire and apply new knowledge. The ability of any of these groups to use clinical information systems to achieve their goals depends on the ability not only to fully represent both data and knowledge within them, but also the ability to exchange it among them. In this chapter we introduce informatics technologies for *concept and knowledge representation* (broadly described here as *terminologies* and *ontologies*) as well as technologies for the *exchange* of information (broadly defined here as *interoperability standards*).

In the discussion of concept and knowledge representation, we describe the sometimes-confusing landscape of terms used to describe such technologies, such as *controlled vocabulary, nomenclature, nosology, classification, terminology, ontology,* and *information model*. We also introduce methods for specifying the kinds of data required as inputs for a specific purpose, such as *minimum clinical data sets* (MCDSs) and *common data elements* (CDEs) . We provide a broad overview of the major standards and technologies used across the healthcare enterprise with an emphasis on those relevant to mental health.

Next, we introduce the concept of *standards* and present a rubric for thinking about them in terms of what exactly the standard is designed to standardize: *content, syntax,* or *semantics*. By addressing "standards" separately from technologies for concept, information, and knowledge representation we are distinguishing between the technologies themselves and the context in which the technologies are used, i.e., whether the technologies are used as a proprietary method of representing and exchanging data with a particular health system, a broadly shared method that has not been formally endorsed, a method endorsed by a formal standard making body, or a method mandated by some governing agency for a particular use. Finally, we highlight substantial gaps in technologies for concept and knowledge representation in mental health and outline a preliminary foundation from which the systematic enhancement of computational representations of mental health data and knowledge can occur.

7.2 Technologies for Representing Data, Information, and Knowledge

Any discussion of representation and standardization must begin with an understanding of the kinds of things we intend to standardize. In Chap. 3, we provided a broad overview of the types of phenomena of interest in mental health: the entire range of phenomena relevant to the human body and mind as well as the physical and social environments in which we exist. In Chaps. 1 and 2, we talked about these phenomena in terms of the forms in which we interact with them using informatics technologies in knowledge discovery paradigms—as *data*, as *information*, and as *knowledge*. In this chapter we discuss technologies available to us as mental health informaticians for representing the wide variety of phenomena in the various forms in which we encounter them in research and practice—as raw data, as information, and as complex theoretical knowledge.

The point at which data becomes information, and information becomes knowledge is not clear-cut, and the differences in definitions between *data*, *information*, and *knowledge* found in the literature range from subtle and nuanced to inconsistent (see [1–7]). For example, while some authors would consider '32 weeks gestation' a *data* point, others would say that '32' is the data point, and that once we qualify '32' with 'weeks', and '32 weeks' with 'gestation' we have now moved into the realm of *information*. Here we present a simple and practical way of thinking about the differences between data, information, and knowledge with an emphasis on how these might be understood in the context of real-world informatics work in the behavioral and social sciences (Table 7.1).

Let's start with data. Most informaticians describe *data* as observations without context. Data are the most "atomic" elements of information work with and the data of interest in healthcare cover the entire range of real-world entities and processes that are potentially relevant to understanding human health. In the context of clinical observations, data are representations of raw signals we either passively acquire or actively work to elicit or extract from the real world. These signals may be fairly concrete, observable things such as a red blood cell count or the amplitude of a brain wave, or more abstract phenomena such as the quality of an emotional state, or the racial composition of a group. We can think of both the thing (entity or process) being observed, as well as the "value" (i.e., some quantity or quality) of the observation itself as data. We typically represent data in informatics paradigms using concepts or simple combinations of concepts. For example, *red blood cell count* and *amplitude of brain wave* are discrete concepts, as are *quality of emotion,* and *racial composition of group.* Qualitative and quantitative observations about each of these things can also be represented as discrete concepts.

Information is data analyzed with respect to its context. For example, when we analyze data about the quality and intensity of emotional state (e.g., intense fear) along with data about the stimulus immediately preceding the state (e.g., seeing a large truck cross over the double yellow line into your lane) or the types of physiological or mental phenomena associated with the emotional state (e.g., increased

Table 7.1 Defining data, information, and knowledge

Term	Definition
Data	We define data as discrete observations about things that exist. Data are typically acquired through observation and measurement. The quality of an emotional state (i.e., sadness, joy, surprise), and the significant events of a given day are examples of data, as are the intensity of feeling, the duration of a mood, or the number of times a person has a specific thought or engages in a particular behavior in a given period of time. Data may be qualitative or quantitative. Some informaticians and data scientists argue that only the measurement (the quantitative or qualitative observation) are data.
Information	We define information here as most informaticians do as "data in context". Information provides insight into the *meaning* of observations by providing additional context in the form of associated observations. The quality of a person's emotional state (data) in the context of significant events of the day (data), for example, provides information about the kinds of events that commonly evoke specific kinds of emotional states. Information is typically acquired by applying simple statistical or computational methods to raw data, or by simply observing and cognitively reasoning about patterns in data. For example, the frequencies of specific emotional states evoked in a given period of time, or correlations between specific events and specific emotion qualities is information.
Knowledge	In the context of healthcare, knowledge consists of scientifically accepted observations, or assertions, about universal relationships between the things that exist. Formal healthcare knowledge is typically acquired by applying statistical and computational methods to many observations generated in many different contexts, using many different paradigms over a period of time. In addition to formal knowledge, researchers and healthcare professionals have a fund of knowledge acquired knowledge by applying complex cognitive processes to integrate data and information obtained through education, practice, and lived experience. Both kinds of knowledge are often represented in systems for knowledge representation.

heart rate, images being hit head-on), we are able to use the context to generate additional observations. We may observe that specific kinds of stimuli produce specific emotional states (e.g., personal rejection frequently evokes sadness, shame, or anger, and rarely evokes confidence, joy, or gratitude), and that certain kinds of stimuli commonly produce reflexive and intense emotional states (i.e., a large truck crossing over the double yellow line into your lane typically evokes an immediate and intense physiological and motor responses).

Knowledge takes information and evaluates it in the context of our current base of ideas and theories about the relationships between the entities and processes of interest, and allows us to draw additional conclusions based on the information. When we conclude that specific events are nearly universally associated with specific physiological and motor responses, we are drawing on theories about how the human brain processes and responds to environmental stimuli. When we attempt to understand the highly idiosyncratic responses that specific people or cultures have to specific events, we are seeking to acquire knowledge about how the human brain comes to develop mental models of events and how these mental models influence emotional and behavioral predispositions.

In this section we discuss foundational informatics technologies for representing phenomena relevant to mental health in each of these three forms: as data, as information, and as knowledge. We use the term *technology* here not to refer to computerized systems or applications, but rather in the broad sense of the word—as something that solves a problem. *Technologies for concept and knowledge representation solve the problem of defining and describing health data, information, and knowledge in ways that both humans and computer-based systems can understand and manipulate.* They allow us to clearly define what data is relevant in a given healthcare domain and to unambiguously represent and exchange it. Without these technologies we cannot efficiently capture, extract, reason about, or share mental health data, information, or knowledge.

7.2.1 The Terminology Used to Describe "Terminology"

In the literature on concept and knowledge representation in healthcare, the entire range of technologies used are often subsumed under the label 'terminology' [8]. As one pioneer in the development of systems for concept and knowledge representation put it more than two decades ago:

> "It is easier to speak about health terminology than to write about it, since people may read and wonder exactly what is meant by this word or that term. The 'meta-terminology' of terminology is no exception, fraught as it is with notions of concepts, classification, nomenclature, and terminology. The reality is that these words are often used casually, imprecisely, and even interchangeably." [8]

The truth of these words became particularly clear in the writing of this chapter as the authors struggled to find definitive definitions in the literature to clarify differences in their own ways of conceiving each of these technologies. Even the term "data standard" is, perhaps ironically, often used differently by different people. Data.gov [9] defines a data standard as "a technical specification that describes how data should be stored or exchanged for the consistent collection and interoperability of that data across different systems, sources, and users." This definition suggests that it is the technical specification along with its purpose or goal that makes the specification a data standard, whether or not other parties agree to that specification, and whether or not anyone actually uses it. An alternative interpretation is that in order to be considered a "data standard," such a specification must be at best endorsed by an accredited standards-making body, or at minimum agreed to by at least one other party. One could consider the technical specification the "informatics technology" meant to facilitate data capture, storage, and exchange, while reserving the term "standard" to refer only to that subset of those technologies that have been approved by some accredited standards-development body. In this chapter use the term "standard" to refer to the technologies and specifications (or "artifacts") that are used, or even just intended, to facilitate such agreement and exchange, whether or not they are formally endorsed for general use in healthcare.

Table 7.2 Technologies for concept and knowledge representation

Technology	Description
Controlled vocabulary	The expression "controlled vocabulary" was once used to describe the entire class of technologies used for concept representation (see, for example, [10]). We use the term more precisely, in line with our sense of current trends in usage, and define a controlled vocabulary as set of concepts organized as a simple list. Typically controlled vocabularies have no hierarchical relationships defined between concepts, but some have additional "broader" or "narrower" terms supplied (see, for example, [11]).
Classification	A set of concepts organized hierarchically. Classifications range in complexity from simple classifications in which each concept can belong under one and only one other concept (referred to as a "monohierarchical" structure), to complex classifications in which a concept may belong under more than one concept (referred to as a "polyhierarchical" structure) [8, 12].
Taxonomy	Another term for a classification system, traditionally used to refer to a classification of organisms, but used broadly as a synonym for a *classification.*
Nosology	A specific kind of classification system—one used to classify diseases or disorders.
Terminology	The word "terminology" is often used to describe the entire class of technologies used for concept representation (see, for example, [8]). Here we use the term more precisely to describe a set of concepts organized hierarchically, in which each concept can belong under more than one concept (referred to as "polyhierarchical" structure).
Coding system	A set of concepts organized in any structure (controlled vocabulary, classification. Nosology or terminology) designed specifically for assigning codes to the concepts contained within the system.
Ontology	The set of concepts and the relationships among concepts in a given domain. An ontology has been famously described as a "specification of a conceptualization" [13]

Technologies for concept and knowledge representation range from simple technologies for enumerating concepts, such as *controlled vocabularies*, to complex technologies for representing entire domains of knowledge, such as *ontologies* (Table 7.2). It is important to note that while some technologies are designed for representing primarily data, information, or knowledge, many technologies for concept and knowledge representation include some representation of all three.

7.2.2   Concept Representation

Data are represented in informatics paradigms as *concepts*. Just as data are the building blocks of knowledge, technologies for concept representation are the foundation of all technologies for the computable representation of knowledge. A concept is defined as simply an idea—the internal understanding, or mental representation, we have of a thing that exists in the world [14]. A concept is not the real-world thing itself, nor is it the term, or "linguistic label", used to describe it.

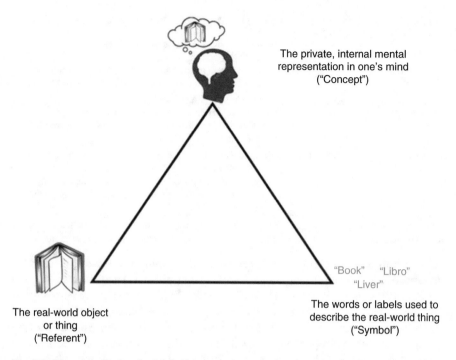

The private, internal mental
representation in one's mind
("Concept")

"Book" "Libro"
"Liver"

The real-world object
or thing
("Referent")

The words or labels used to
describe the real-world thing
("Symbol")

Fig. 7.1 The semiotic triangle, Adapted from Ogden and Richards (1923) [14]

This distinction is an important one, and is depicted nicely in the *semiotic triangle*, proposed by Ogden and Richards in 1923 [14] (Fig. 7.1).

Even among people speaking the same language, many different words are used to refer to the same real-world object or process. Within healthcare, where acronyms and abbreviations are extensively used, the number of linguistic labels for the same clinical idea can be extensive. Not only are many terms used to refer to the same concept (e.g., 'bipolar disorder', 'bipolar affective disorder', 'bipolar depression') the same term or acronym may be used in different contexts to refer to completely different things (e.g., the term 'blue' to describe both mood and skin color). While the human brain can efficiently distinguish between, or *disambiguate*, the meaning of terms based on context, most computer systems cannot do this without the use of complex natural language processing tools.

This is where technologies for concept representation come in. These technologies are designed to solve the problem of making clear the relationship between concepts (meanings) and the linguistic labels (words or acronyms) commonly used to refer to them. Two primary methods for solving this problem are the use of *relationships* and *descriptions*. In fact, one way of thinking about different technologies for concept representation is on the basis of how they use relationships and descriptions (Table 7.3). Most, but not all, technologies for concept representation include relationships between concepts. For example, a terminology may include a

Table 7.3 Contrasting three major technologies for concept representation based on use of *relationships* and *descriptions*

Technology	Relationships	Descriptions
Controlled vocabulary	None or sporadic	Each concept is given a single name; synonyms may be provided as addenda or notes, but they are not linked to the concept via a formal relationship
Classification	Monohierarchical	Each concept is given a single name; synonyms may be provided as addenda or notes, but they are not linked to the concept via a formal relationship
Terminology	Polyhierarchical	Multiple descriptions are typically provided and linked to the concept via a formal relationship; descriptions are often designated as being the fully defined name or a synonym, and synonyms are sometimes designated as being preferred terms or acceptable terms

Note: these are the authors' impressions of how the terms are most commonly used, and how we typically use these terms; there is no consensus definitions for these terms in the literature

relationship between the concept **sad** and the concept **emotion** asserting that **sad** "is a" **emotion**, and a relationship between the concepts **sad affect** and **affect** (expressed emotion) asserting that **sad affect** "is a" **affect**. Defining a relationship between **sad affect** and **affect** (rather than **sad affect** and **emotion**) makes clear that the outward expression of sadness is distinct from the experience of sadness. Similarly, many technologies for concept representation make a distinction between the primary label used to uniquely identify the concept (the concept name) and other labels commonly used to describe the concept (synonyms). For example, a terminology may include both a formal name that clearly describes the idea of feeling blue (e.g., 'sad emotional state') and one or more terms commonly use when referring to the concept (e.g., 'sad mood', 'feeling sad').

7.2.3 Controlled Vocabularies

More than two decades ago, when informaticians began to tackle the problem of healthcare terminology in earnest, the term "controlled vocabulary" was often used a generic term to describe technologies used for representing the observations captured in health records (see, for example, [10]). The term increasingly began being used (and is most commonly used today) to describe a relatively unstructured set of terms that a computerized system will understand. In this sense, a controlled vocabulary is among the simplest technologies for concept representation (Fig. 7.2a). A controlled vocabulary has no—or limited—relationships between concepts and provides only a single term used to describe a concept. It is little more than a list of terms a computerized system will recognize for concepts in some domain. Controlled vocabularies are sometimes seen in publication databases used for searching the literature, such as the American Psychological Association's (APA) *Thesaurus of Psychological Index Terms* [11]. While a controlled vocabulary may include both an overarching concept for bipolar disorder, and a concept for each of two currently

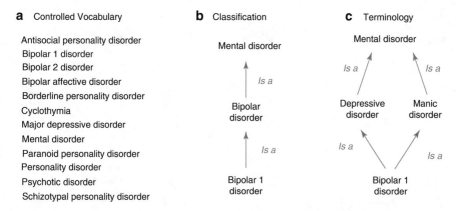

Fig. 7.2 Contrasting use of relationships in controlled vocabularies, classifications, and terminologies

defined subtypes, **bipolar 1 disorder** and **bipolar 2 disorder**, it will not include a relationship representing **bipolar 1 disorder and bipolar 2 disorder** as subtypes of **bipolar disorder**. Consequently, in order to identify all articles related to bipolar disorder, including those addressing specific subtypes (bipolar 1 and bipolar 2), the user of the system will need to search for publications using all three terms.

7.2.4 Classifications

A *classification system* has a simple hierarchical structure, created by adding simple relationships called "is a" relationships, or "parent-child" relationships, between concepts. These relationships assert that a concept as a more specific kind of another concept. For example, in Fig. 7.2b, we see that the concept mental disorder is the *parent* of concept bipolar disorder, and concept bipolar disorder is the *parent* of concept bipolar 1 disorder. These relationships are used to assert that bipolar disorder is a more specific kind of mental disorder, and that bipolar 1 disorder is a more specific kind of bipolar disorder. This type of relationship is also called a *subsumption* relationship, and we say that the concept 'mental disorder' *subsumes* the concept 'bipolar disorder' and that the concept 'bipolar disorder' *is subsumed by* the concept 'mental disorder'. Subsumption, "is a", and parent-child relationships are all ways of defining concepts as more general or more specific types of other concepts.

In a pure classification system, a concept will have one and only one parent [10]. It has a *monohierarchical* structure. In pure classifications, if a concept is a subtype of more than one concept, an arbitrary decision must be made about the hierarchy into which to place the concept. For example, in a classification system, the concept *recurrent suicidal thoughts* would be classified as either kind of *suicidal thought* or a kind of *recurrent thought*, although in the real world it is clearly a subtype of both (Fig. 7.3).

Fig. 7.3 A pure classification
has a *monohierarchical*
structure

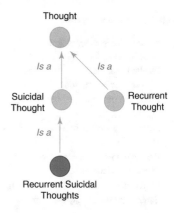

7.2.5   *Terminologies*

A *terminology* is one of the most robust technologies for concept representation. High quality terminologies (see [10, 15–17]) solve the problem of clearly defining concepts and distinguishing between concepts and the terms used to refer to them by including two sophisticated features not included in controlled vocabularies or pure classification systems: *polyhierarchical relationships* and discrete, explicit *descriptions* that are separate from the anchoring name given to the concept. In addition to discrete description terms, many terminologies include a formal, narrative *definition* for each concept. In high quality terminologies, the d.

Polyhierarchical relationships are relationships in which one concept may be a child of more than one concept (Fig. 7.2c). For example, in a terminology, the concept *recurrent suicidal thoughts* discussed above would represent as both a kind of *suicidal thought* and a kind of *recurrent thought* (Fig. 7.4).

A good example of the use of polyhierarchy in a mental health nosology is the way *antisocial personality disorder* (APD) is represented in the latest version of the Diagnostic and Statistical Manual of Disorders, the DSM-5 [18]. This syndrome has essential features of a both personality disorder (i.e., it is a habitual way of thinking, feeling, and behaving across time and situations), and a disruptive, impulse-control, and conduct disorders. Earlier versions of the nosology did not allow for polyhierarchy, so APD was previously classified as only a personality disorder. With the introduction of DSM-5, however, the DSM embraced a polyhierarchical model of disorders, and this disorder is now classified as both a personality disorder and a disruptive, impulse-control, and conduct disorder.

In addition to polyhierarchy, terminologies typically distinguish between the terms or expressions used as the primary linguistic label for the concept, and other terms commonly used when referring to the concept. In most terminologies, a concept has a primary description that is unique within the terminology, and one or more additional descriptions that may or may not be unique within the terminology. For example, in SNOMED-CT, the Systematized Nomenclature for Medicine— Clinical Terms [19], each concept has one primary linguistic label, referred to as the

Fig. 7.4 A terminology has a *polyhierarchical* structure

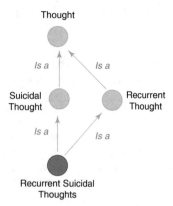

Fig. 7.5 Descriptions associated with the concept *Mood swings (finding)* in SNOMED-CT

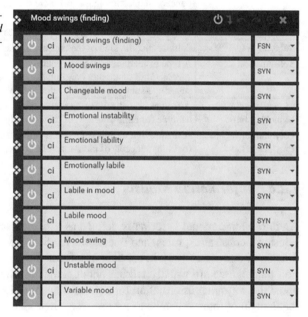

fully specified name, or FSN, and at one or more additional descriptions referred to as *synonyms* (Fig. 7.5).

As previously described, the word "terminology" is often used as a generic term to describe the entire class of technologies for concept representation. For purposes of this discussion, however, we define a terminology more narrowly as those systems that include the features described above. Some of the major terms commonly used to describe technologies for concept representation and their definitions are listed in Table 7.4 below.

Table 7.4 Terms commonly used in describing technologies for concept representation

Term	Definition
Concept	A mental representation of some real-world thing, an idea
Term, description	A word, expression, or "linguistic label" used to describe a concept
Fully specified name	A term or expression designated as the primary linguistic label for a concept in a terminology, typically unique within the terminology
Preferred term	A term designated as the one to be displayed or used by default in a given context; typically, this is the term most commonly used in a specific language or setting
Synonym	A term that is commonly used to describe a concept
Parent concept	A concept that is more general, but of the same kind or type, as the concept in question (e.g., "mood disorder" is parent concept of "depressive disorder")
Child concept	A concept that is more specific, but of the same kind or type, as the concept in question (e.g., "paranoid delusion" is a child concept of "delusion")
Supertype	A more general kind of the concept or class in question, a parent concept
Subtype	A more specific kind of the concept or class in question, a child concept
Subsumption	A type of relationship that defines one concept as a more general or specific kind of another concept; also referred to as parent-child, supertype-subtype, or "is as" relationships
Monohierarchy, Monohierarchic	A feature of a classification that specifies that a concept may be a subtype (or child concept) of one and only one concept.
Polyhierarchy, Polyhierarchic	A feature of a terminology that specifies that a concept may be a subtype (or child concept) of more than one concept

7.2.6 Information Models

An information model is formally defined as a "a representation of concepts, relationships, constraints, rules, and operations to specify data semantics for a chosen domain of discourse" [20]. In the field of informatics, when we talk about information models, we are usually talking about something far simpler. We are talking about the ways that information for a given domain of interest is structured. While the domain of interest can be as narrow as a single clinical finding (for example, a diagnosis) or—theoretically—as broad as an entire longitudinal medical record system capable of capturing clinical information for any patient that walks in the door, most often when we talk about information models, we are talking about defining a fairly narrowly scoped set of information. For example, how we might represent the essential information about a specific condition, diagnostic test, or procedure.

An information model has two core components (Fig. 7.6): the *elements of information* and the *value set*, or the range of allowable values, specified for each information element. The value set for each information element can be a simple controlled vocabulary designed specifically for the information model in question, or it can draw from publicly available industry standards. For example, the allowable values for the element "cause of death" in an information model below could be constrained to diagnostic codes found in the ICD-10-CM. When a value set is constrained to some set of industry standard codes, the information element is said to be "bound" to the terminology from

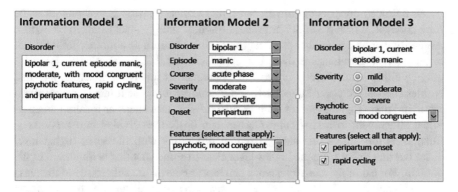

Fig. 7.6 Three different information models for capturing a DSM-5 disorder (Graphic adapted from a graphic for lung cancer created by Linda Byrd)

which the value set comes. It is best practice when creating information models to create them with what we call "bindings to standard terminology". Meaning, each element is bound to a set of values from an industry standard terminology, thus ensuring that the data captured using such models is interoperable (i.e., can be interpreted by systems other than the one in which it was generated).

There are typically many ways to represent the same clinical information. Consequently, many different information models can be created to represent the same information. Figure 7.6, for example, depicts three different information models for capturing the same bipolar I disorder diagnosis. Each of these three models capture the same pieces of information, but each model structures the elements of the diagnosis differently. Information models that contain the same information represented in different ways are referred to as *isosemantic* models [21–23]. One of the tasks commonly involved in working with real-world clinical data—particularly data from multiple sources—is the task of identifying a common model to which all source data can be transformed, and creating the algorithms to perform the transformation to this common model.

7.2.7 Knowledge Representation

In the context of information science, an ontology is a formal way of describing the things that exist in some domain and the ways these things are related to each other. An ontology is often described as "an explicit specification of a conceptualization" [13]. This definition makes clear that an ontology is a technology not only for *concept representation* (defining the things that exist in some domain), but also a technology for *knowledge representation* (defining what we know—or believe—about the things that exists in this domain). In an ontology we not only explicitly define (specify) the entities of interest, we also define how the entities are believed to relate to each other, i.e., how they are conceptualized within our theoretical model.

An ontology consists of *classes*, *roles*, and *axioms*. A *class* is just another name for a concept. It is some entity or process—some "thing"—that exists in the world. An entity can be a concrete, physical thing, like a neuron or a mother-infant dyad, or an abstract, non-tangible thing like an emotion or thought. Similarly, a process may be either some directly observable phenomenon involving concrete, physical entities such as membrane depolarization or smiling, or some inferred phenomenon involving non-tangible entities such as memorizing an address or forming an emotional attachment to a new baby. Classes can be further divided into *subclasses*. Subclasses are things that share essential properties with the same higher-level class, but that differ from the higher-level class in some way that is important in the domain. For example, *sensory neuron* and *motor neuron* are subclasses of the class *neuron*. They differ from each other in many ways, one of which is type of tissue they innervate (or synapse with). A sensory neuron is a neuron that innervates sensory organs and transmits sensory information, whereas a motor neuron is one that innervates muscle tissue and transmits motor information. Similarly, *unipolar neuron*, *bipolar neuron* and *multipolar neuron* are all subclasses of the class *neuron*. These subclasses differ from each other not on the basis of the type of tissue they innervate, but rather on the basis of their morphological (or physical) structure. That is, they differ in the number processes (axon and dendrites) extending from the cell body of the neuron. A class-subclass relationship is no different from the subsumption relationship that we described as an "is a" or parent-child relationship in our discussion of terminologies. Like terminologies, ontologies use subsumption relationships to represent more general and more specific types of the things. Unlike terminologies, however, ontologies include additional kinds of relationships.

A *role* is any relationship between two classes. In our discussion of subclasses, we described sensory and motor neurons as two discrete subclasses of the class 'neuron'. Defining a 'sensory neuron' and a 'motor neuron' as subclasses of 'neuron' using subsumption relationships tells us there is something that makes these two classes of neuron distinct, however, it does not tell us *how* they are distinct. This is where *roles* come in. Roles allow us to define specific kinds of relationships (in addition to subsumption relationships) that one class can have to another. In the case of neurons, we identified a relationship between the class 'neuron' and the class 'tissue'. We represent this relationship in an ontology by creating a role for this relationship (in this case we might name it 'innervates') (Fig. 7.7). For sensory neurons, we would then link the class 'sensory organ tissue' to the role 'innervates', and for motor neurons we would link the class 'muscle tissue'. A role, then, does two things that allow us to more fully represent the meaning of this class of things called 'neuron'. First, it allows us to assert that a defining feature of a neuron is the type of tissue it innervates. Second, it gives us a way to link some other class in our ontology—such as 'sensory organ tissue' or 'muscle tissue'—to this role, thereby defining specifically what it is that makes one subclass different from another.

An *axiom* is a statement about what is true. An axiom is created whenever a relationship (or *role*) is defined for class. A role is an axiom simply because creating it makes

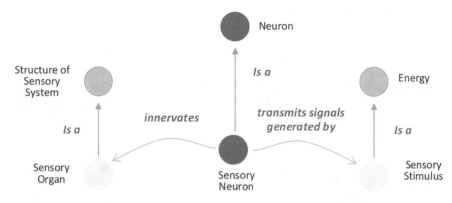

Fig. 7.7 Roles and axioms in an ontology

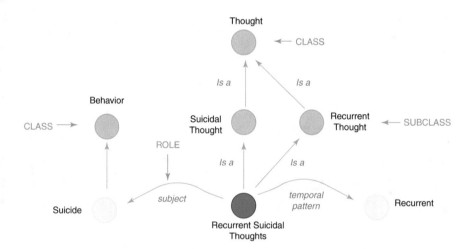

Fig. 7.8 An ontology has explicit defining relationships

an assertion about what is true about the class to which it applies. By defining sensory neuron as a subclass of neuron, for example, we are asserting that a sensory neuron has all the defining features of a neuron. Similarly, by creating a role named 'innervates' for the class 'neuron', we assert that all neurons innervate, or synapse with, some type of tissue. An axiom is also created whenever a class is specified as the value for a relationship (or role) for another class. For example, defining the class of tissue that motor neurons innervate as 'muscle tissue' is asserting what is true about motor neurons.

Returning to our representation of the concept 'recurrent suicidal thoughts', we see that an ontology allows us to more fully define it. Figure 7.8 depicts how adding defining relationships allows us to explicitly define both the subject (a role) and the temporal pattern (a role) of the thought.

7.3 What Is a Standard?

Anyone who has ever traveled internationally and tried to charge a device can appreciate the importance and utility of standards (Fig. 7.9). Every region has a differently shaped outlet, precluding the use of a cord from one region with an outlet in another. Equipment from different regions is therefore not *interoperable*. Standards are a set of informatics technologies designed to prevent this from happening in the context of data and knowledge. Standards are necessary across the translational spectrum, from the storage and exchange of physiological data in a laboratory to diagnostic billing codes in a hospital. They are also used across the spectrum of scale of observations, from molecular profiling to population health. The ability to collect, store, and exchange data in both the research and clinical context is critical to advancing knowledge and improving care.

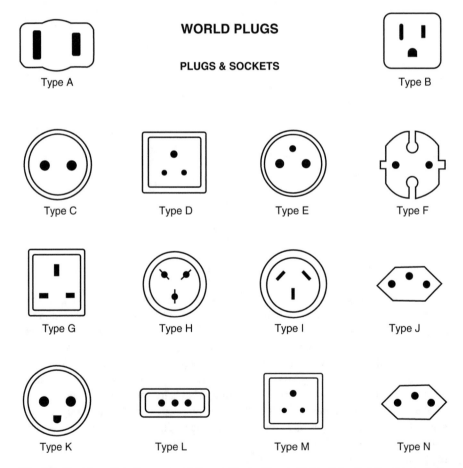

Fig. 7.9 Electric outlets from around the world provide excellent motivation for the need for standards

If standards solve such an important problem, you might wonder, why doesn't everyone just use them? Standards are useful, even powerful, but challenging. For one thing, there's the famous joke (famous among informaticians, anyway) that the great thing about standards is that there are so many to choose from. And as famously depicted in the cartoon xkcd, more all the time (Fig. 7.10). The space of data standards is a dynamic landscape, changing and evolving as the data types themselves, and the technologies used to capture them, continue to advance. It can be challenging to know which of those many standards is the right one to use in a given context [24]. Standards are also sometimes seen as too constraining—stifling creativity or requiring too much effort for adherence. And yet they are absolutely necessary to achieve the many goals discussed in this book: precision medicine, a LHS, decision support, mHealth, and more.

A standard is, at its core, an agreement to follow certain rules for capturing, storing, or sharing data. While standards are useful in facilitating clear communication between people, they are *essential* for communication between computerized systems. One way of thinking about standards is in terms of what it is they are designed to standardize. From this perspective, we can think of three different types of standards: content standards, syntax standards, semantic standards (Table 7.5). *Content standards* specify what pieces of data or information must be captured about a given subject. These are sometimes referred to as core data elements (CDEs) or minimum information lists. *Syntax standards* specify the format in which data are to be represented, particularly in the context of data exchange between computerized systems. Finally, *semantic standards* specify the meaning of information in some domain.

While some standards in healthcare fit neatly into one of these three categories, many standards are a combination of two or more of these types. Information models, described above, for example, specify both content and semantics. Many standards used for data exchange, commonly called *interoperability standards,* specify

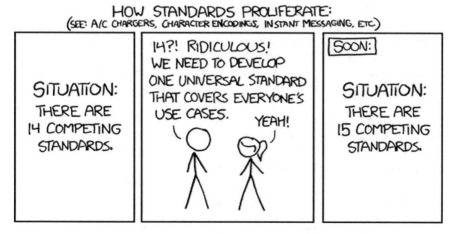

Fig. 7.10 How standards proliferate. Used with permission from https://xkcd.com/927/under Creative Commons License

Table 7.5 Types of standards

Type	Description	Examples
Content	A content standard specifies what data or information to capture about a given subject	Common data elements (CDE) Core data elements Minimum Information lists Minimum clinical data sets Mandatory reporting checklists
Syntax	A syntax standard specifies the format in which data are represented, particularly in the context of data exchange between two computer-based systems	HTML, XML, CSV JSON (JavaScript Object Notation) HL7 Messages
Semantic	A semantic standard defines the concepts in a domain and the relationships between them	SNOMED-CT LOINC FHIR

not only content and semantics, but also syntax. Some examples of these, including HL7 messages and FHIR resources are described later in the chapter.

7.3.1   Content Standards

Regardless of *how* clinical information is stored or exchanged, when using any kind of computer-based system in healthcare, we first need to decide *what* information is relevant. This is as true for the biomedical or behavioral scientist performing basic research in the lab as it is for the front-line health provider diagnosing and treating people seeking mental healthcare services. (Or for the EHR vendor designing the system, or the clinical department configuring the EHR deployment for its staff.) A *content standard* defines the specific elements of data or information that must be captured to fully describe some entity, process, or event. The entity, process or event can be as simple as a diagnosis, or as complex as a study protocol for a clinical trial.

In the basic research context, these are often referred to as *minimum information lists* or *mandatory reporting checklists*. These standards specify *what* must be captured—but not how or in what format. These minimum checklists have received particular attention in the context of science's so-called reproducibility crisis in recent years [25]. They specify the minimal information required to allow another researcher to understand exactly what was done in a particular study or experiment, and to repeat the experiment and replicate the findings.

An example of a content standard from the biological domain is MINSEQE—Minimum Information about a high-throughput nucleotide SEQuencing Experiment [26]. MINSEQE specifies five different elements that must be captured to fully and appropriately describe a DNA or RNA sequencing assay: 1. The description of the biological system, samples, and the experimental variables being studied; 2. The sequence read data for each assay; 3. The 'final' processed (or summary) data for the set of assays in the study; 4. General information about the experiment and sample-data relationships; and 5. Essential experimental and data processing protocols. Note that although there is a *recommendation* to use the FASTQ format (see Chap. 11) for sequence data in item 2, this list does not dictate how the pieces of information must be captured, expressed, or formatted. It does not stipulate, for example, a specific terminology that must be used, or whether the descriptions must be captured in a Word document, PDF, or .txt file.

In the clinical context, these types of standards often describe an essential or "core" set of data elements related to a specific condition, intervention, event, or process. Sometimes they are used to refer to a comprehensive and inclusive set of set of data elements related to an entire class of conditions or domain of healthcare services. When collections of data elements are identified and defined for specific conditions or interventions, and these elements can be mixed or matched as needed, they tend to be described as common data elements, or CDEs. One example is the sets of common data elements (CDEs) for substance use conditions developed and published by is the US National Institute on Drug Abuse (NIDA) for use in in clinical trials and EHRs [27]. Another example is the sets of CDEs published by the National Institute of Neurological Disorders and Stroke (NINDS) [28]. Developing CDEs has become such a common type of content standard that the National Institutes of Health (NIH) maintains and publishes a CDE repository to assist researchers and healthcare professionals in finding already developed CDEs. The site contains CDEs published by more 14 different organizations, covering 10 broad domains of healthcare, including Psychiatry and Psychology [29].

When robust collections of data elements are compiled and there is an expectation that all data elements are captured as a set, often using a pre-specified process, these collections are often referred to as "minimum data sets" or "minimum clinical data sets" [30]. Examples include the United States' Nursing Minimum Data Set (NMDS) [31], the UK's Mental Health Minimum Data Set (MHMDS) [32], and the Irish Nursing Minimum Data Set for Mental Health (INMDS-MH) [33].

7.3.2 Syntax Standards

A *syntax standard* describes the format in which information is to be captured, stored, or exchanged so a computer knows how to interpret it. At the most basic level, one can think of a tab delimited file with defined columns and rows as representing a *de facto* format standard. For example, such a file might contain rows that represent patients and columns that represent variables related to that patient. Alternatively, rows might represent a given encounter for a patient and columns hold different variables related to that encounter. In that case, each patient could have multiple rows in the file. One or the other of these approaches may be more appropriate for a given use case. The key is to specify the approach to be taken and to make sure the receiver of the data understands what the columns and rows represent.

The reader has probably heard of the formatting standards *HTML* (hypertext markup language) and *XML* (extensible markup language) . These syntactical standards simply specify how data are to be represented in a file. For example, HTML specifies that text on a web page should be rendered in bold if the tag "" comes before that text and "" comes after it. An HTML snippet of "This is HTML." would be rendered by a web browser as "**This** is HTML." XML *extends* this paradigm to enable structured descriptions of a much broader set of entities, not just how a web page is rendered. For example, XML might specify how to exchange information about a patient (Box 7.1). JSON, or JavaScript Object Notation, is another popular standard for data exchange in healthcare. It is touted as being easily readable by both humans and computers—sometimes a tricky balance.

Box 7.1 XML Example

```
<patient>
        <name = "Ruth">
        <dob = 3/15/1933>
        <dx = D02.20>
</patient>
```

This XML snippet describes an entity called a "patient" with three attributes: name, date of birth (dob), and diagnosis (dx). As with HTML, this entity begins with a label or tag inside brackets and ends with that same tag with a "/" between the opening bracket and the tag. Attributes of that entity also appear inside brackets but with an attribute name connected by an equals sign to a value for that attribute.

7.3.3 Semantic Standards

A *semantic standard* addresses the meaning of data, information, or knowledge being exchanged. Semantic standards range from those that define the meaning of individual concepts (such as a controlled vocabulary) to those that define the meaning of all concepts in an entire domain and the complex relationships between them (such as an ontology). There are several semantic standards used in healthcare and research.

While content and syntax standards, and the challenges that accompany them, are relatively consistent between general medicine and mental health, semantic standards are where mental health differentiates itself from the rest of medicine. Because many of the entities and processes of interest in mental health are fundamentally different from those of interest in physical health, and because virtually all existing standards have been developed in the context of biomedical healthcare, there is an immense need to fill gaps in semantic standards for mental health.

7.3.3.1 SNOMED CT

SNOMED-CT, the Systematized Nomenclature for Medicine—Clinical Terms [19], is a clinical terminology designed to include concepts used in the delivery of care across the entire domain of healthcare. SNOMED-CT is organized into nineteen "top level" hierarchies—seventeen hierarchies for clinical content and two hierarchies used to manage the terminology itself (Fig. 7.11). The clinical hierarchies include content ranging from clinical findings, disorders, procedures, events, and social contexts to body structures, organisms, and pharmacological products.

While SNOMED-CT is typically referred to as a terminology, it has many features of an ontology. In addition to having a polyhierarchical structure, for example,

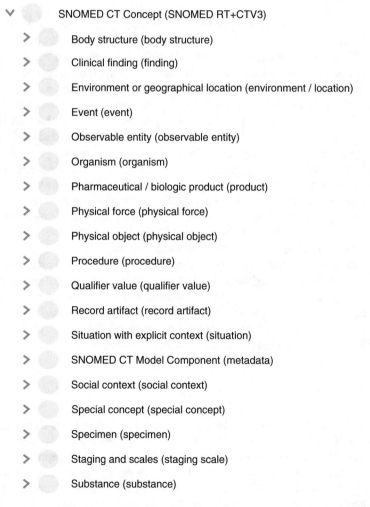

Fig. 7.11 Top level hierarchies in SNOMED-CT

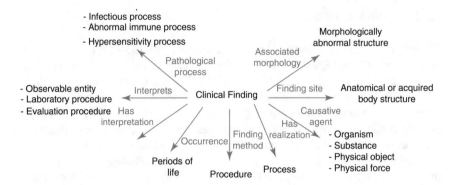

Fig. 7.12 SNOMED CT concept model for clinical findings

SNOMED-CT includes defining attributes for many top-level hierarchies. The set of defining relationships for a given concept hierarchy is referred to as the *concept model* for that hierarchy. Not all hierarchies have a concept model, but for those that do, the concept model is unique to that specific hierarchy. The concept model for the *clinical finding* hierarchy is depicted in Fig. 7.12. As you can see, a clinical finding has a number of defining relationships, such as *finding site*, *associated morphology*, and *pathological process* (depicted in blue). The allowable values for each of these defining relationships is also specified in the concept model (depicted in black at the end of each arrow). The allowable values are defined as the concept hierarchies or sub-hierarchies containing concepts that can be used as to specify the value of the defining attribute. For example, values for the attribute *finding site* can come only from concepts in the *anatomical or acquired body structure* sub-hierarchy. Similarly, values for the attribute *finding method* can come only from concepts in the *procedure* hierarchy. We refer to the set of allowable values for any given defining attribute as the "range" for that particular attribute.

SNOMED-CT is an extremely important terminology for representing mental health concepts. It is one of the few industry-standard terminologies currently available for representing detailed mental health findings and disorders not included in nosologies such as the DSM-5 and ICD-10. It is also the only terminology available for representing granular interventions, treatment regimens, and procedures not included in coding systems such as CPT and ICD-10-PCS.

7.3.3.2 LOINC

LOINC (Logical Observations, Identifiers, Names and Codes) , is a clinical terminology used for encoding clinical observations, measurements, and documents [34]. This includes a range of observations from laboratory tests, imaging studies, and psychological assessment instruments to vital signs, pain assessments and patient discharge summaries. LOINC assigns both a code and a name to each observation. A LOINC code is numeric code followed by a hyphen and a single digit. A LOINC term, or fully specified name, is made up of six parts (Table 7.6).

Table 7.6 Anatomy of a LOINC code

Example:
18262-6:Cholesterol.in LDL:MCnc:Pt:Ser/Plas:Qn:Direct assay

	LOINC Code:	18262-7
●	Component:	**Cholesterol. In LDL**
●	Property:	**MCnc** (mass concentration)
●	Time:	**Pt** (point in time)
○	System:	**Ser/Plasma** (serum/plasma)
●	Scale:	**Qn** (quantitative)
●	Method:	**Direct assay**

LOINC name part	Description	Examples
Component	The entity that is being evaluated or observed	Cholesterol, body weight
Property	The attribute of the entity being evaluated, observed or measures	Mass concentration, presence or identity
Time	Time interval over which observation is being made	Point in time 2-h collection period 14 day look back period
System	The context or specimen type upon which the observation is made	Serum or plasma
Scale	The result type	Quantitative, ordinal, nominal, narrative, etc.
Method	How the component was measured, or the information obtained	Estimated, molecular genetics, computer tomography

Many EHRs and laboratory information systems (LISs) use LOINC codes to transmit both orders for, and results of, laboratory tests. These orders and results are often transmitted using HL7 messages (described in detail in the following section). In these cases, the HL7 v2 message is used to provide context about the patient and other important information, and the LOINC code is used to unambiguously describe the laboratory test that was ordered or resulted. Figure 7.13 depicts a list of LOINC codes, fully specified names, and the six components of a LOINC concept based on a query for LOINC codes containing the term 'PHQ-9'.

7.4 Interoperability Standards

In this section we introduce standards for technical and semantic interoperability, and touch on some of the challenges relative to mental health. Interoperability, when it comes to health information, is generally described at two levels: technical, and semantic. Technical interoperability means that information can be physically transmitted from one system to another. Semantic interoperability means that

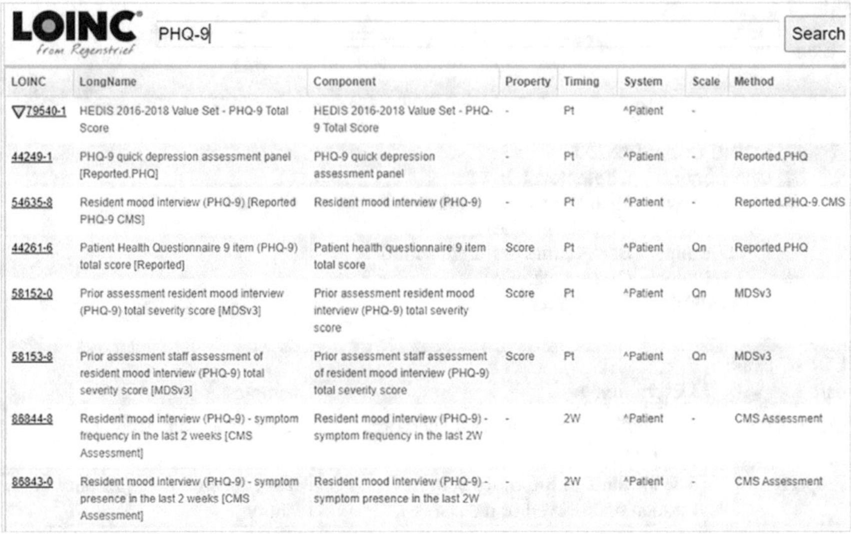

LOINC	LongName	Component	Property	Timing	System	Scale	Method
▽79540-1	HEDIS 2016-2018 Value Set - PHQ-9 Total Score	HEDIS 2016-2018 Value Set - PHQ-9 Total Score	-	Pt	^Patient	-	
44249-1	PHQ-9 quick depression assessment panel [Reported.PHQ]	PHQ-9 quick depression assessment panel	-	Pt	^Patient	-	Reported.PHQ
54635-8	Resident mood interview (PHQ-9) [Reported PHQ-9 CMS]	Resident mood interview (PHQ-9)	-	Pt	^Patient	-	Reported.PHQ-9 CMS
44261-6	Patient Health Questionnaire 9 item (PHQ-9) total score [Reported]	Patient health questionnaire 9 item total score	Score	Pt	^Patient	Qn	Reported.PHQ
58152-0	Prior assessment resident mood interview (PHQ-9) total severity score [MDSv3]	Prior assessment resident mood interview (PHQ-9) total severity score	Score	Pt	^Patient	Qn	MDSv3
58153-8	Prior assessment staff assessment of resident mood interview (PHQ-9) total severity score [MDSv3]	Prior assessment staff assessment of resident mood interview (PHQ-9) total severity score	Score	Pt	^Patient	Qn	MDSv3
86844-8	Resident mood interview (PHQ-9) - symptom frequency in the last 2 weeks [CMS Assessment]	Resident mood interview (PHQ-9) - symptom frequency in the last 2W	-	2W	^Patient	-	CMS Assessment
86843-0	Resident mood interview (PHQ-9) - symptom presence in the last 2 weeks [CMS Assessment]	Resident mood interview (PHQ-9) - symptom presence in the last 2W	-	2W	^Patient	-	CMS Assessment

Fig. 7.13 Web Interface for searching for LOINC codes (loing.org), displaying the six components of a LOINC code: component, property, timing, system, scale and method

Table 7.7 Interoperability standards

System	Description
HL7 Messaging	Health Level Seven (HL7) International is a non-profit ANSI-accredited standards development organization. **HL7 v 2.x** is a *messaging standard* that specifies both the syntax (format) and semantics (meaning) of healthcare information. Special software is installed and configured on both the sender and receiver side to enable transmission of data using HL7 messages.
C-CDA	The Consolidated Clinical Document Architecture (**C-CDA**) is a *document standard* that specifies both the syntax (format) and semantics (meaning) of healthcare information. The C-CDA specification defines required and optional information elements for each type of document and specifies XML for syntax.
FHIR	Fast Health Interoperability Resources (**FHIR**), is a standard developed by HL7. FHIR carves up health information into the small, clinically meaningful pieces of information called "resources", such as *patient, provider, problem,* and *procedure*. FHIR resources are made available and accessed via a FHIR server that allows for exchange of information using simple URL requests, in the same way one would access a website.

information can be transmitted in such a way that there is no loss of meaning from the source system to the destination system. Three major interoperability standards for making health data interoperable are HL7 messaging, C-CDA, and Fast Health Interoperability Resources, or FHIR (Fig. 7.8), (Table 7.7).

7.4.1   HL7 Messages

HL7 messaging is the use of special software along with a number of different HL7 "messages" to transmit health information from one organization to another. An HL7 message is essentially a small bundle of information transmitted as a single unit. Special software must be installed on the sending and receiving systems to transmit the HL7 message, but once it is installed and configured, messages to be triggered by any number of events, such as a patient admission, a lab order, or an immunization. Many EHRs in the United States, for example, are configured to automatically transmit an HL7 vaccination message to a local public health immunization registry whenever a vaccine is administered. In addition to being triggered by some event, systems can be configured to send HL7 messages as an "unsolicited" message. There are many different kinds of HL7 messages, each one designed to transmit specific bundles of clinical information (Box 7.2).

Box 7.2 A Sampling of HL7 Message Types

ADT	ADT (admit, discharge, transfer) message
BPS	Blood product dispense status message
CRM	Clinical study registration message
OMI	Imaging order
PGL	Patient goal message
PPG	Patient pathway message (goal-oriented)
PPR	Patient problem message
REF	Patient referral
RGR	Pharmacy/treatment dose information
RQC	Request clinical information
VXU	Unsolicited vaccination record update
VXQ	Query for vaccination record

While each kind of HL7 message is designed to transmit different kinds of information, each message uses a similar *syntax*. That is, it is organized in a similar way, each message comprised of specific *segments*, and each segment comprised of *fields*. Each segment is designed to transmit a specific kind of information, such as information about the patient, the provider, the healthcare facility, the order, the treatment, or the observed result. In the HL7 message depicted in Fig. 7.14, each line contains one segment, and each segment is defined by the unique 3-character code at the start of the segment. In this example, MSH is the *message header* segment, PID is the *patient identifier* segment, and OBR is the *observation* segment. The *fields* within each segment are specific to the segment itself, and are designed to capture discrete data elements. For example, the patient segment contains fields for first name, last name, and date of birth. Special characters such as the pipe (|), and carrot (^) are used to separate fields and elements within a field.

```
MSH|^~\&|HIS|MedCenter|LIS|MedCenter|20060307110114||ORM^001|MSGID20060307110114|P|2.3
PID|||12001||Wu^Ji^^^Mr||19670824|M|||123 Main St^^Denver^CO^80020^USA|||||||
PV1||O|OP^PAREG^||||2342^Wu^Mi|||OP||||||||||2|||||||||||||||||||||||||||20060307110111|
ORC|NW|20060307110114
OBR|1|20060307110114||003038^Urinalysis^L|||20060307110114
```

Fig. 7.14 An HL7 v2.51 Message

Fig. 7.15 Schematic of CDA Document

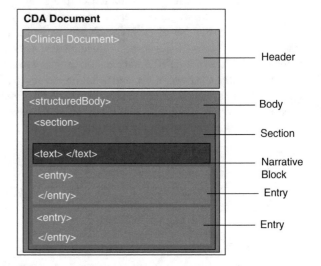

There are two different versions of HL7 message is use around the world today: HL7 version 2 [35] and HL7 version 3 [36]. While Version 3 is used extensively in Europe, in the United States, most organizations continue to use version 2. Version 2 is often written as "**HL7 v 2.x**", because there are multiple versions and releases, each with minor variations.

7.4.2 Consolidated Clinical Document Architecture (C-CDA)

The Consolidated Clinical Document Architecture (C-CDA) is a *specification* describing how to build clinical documents in such a way that they can be easily parsed, or broken into their component parts, by software. The C-CDA standard is based on the earlier Clinical Document Architecture (CDA) standard. The C-CDA standard essentially took components of the CDA (*documents, sections, entries*) and used them to define re-usable templates that could be used in many different CDA documents. Each C-CDA document consists of—at minimum—a header and a body. The header includes document metadata, or data about the document itself. The body of the document contains *sections*, which can include a mix of *narrative blocks* and *entries* (Fig. 7.15).

The C-CDA specification defines several document *templates* along with the rules about which components are required and optional for each document. In specifying the components required for each template, the C-CDA is a content

Table 7.8 Components of a CDA document

Component	Description
Document Header	The **header** of a CDA document contains information required for the receiving system to determine what kind of document is being transmitted, along with other minimum information required for the receiving system to process it.
Document Body	The **body** of a CDA document can be structured into one or more sections or contain an unstructured "blob".
Document Templates	Document templates are essentially "containers" for specific types of clinical information. Templates are designed to communicate specific types of information for specific purposes, but different templates may contain some of the same kinds of information. The following 12 document templates are included in the latest C-CDA standard [37]: • Care Plan including Home Health Plan of Care (HHPoC) • Consultation Note • Continuity of Care Document (CCD) • Diagnostic Imaging Reports (DIR) • Discharge Summary • History and Physical (H&P) • Operative Note • Procedure Note • Progress Note • Referral Note • Transfer Summary • Unstructured Document • Patient Generated Document
Section Templates	Sections define the class of information or observations. Each section contains one narrative block for human readability, and zero or more "entries". There are more than 60 defined section templates, including: • Family History • Allergies • Problem List • Procedures • Plan of Care • Results
Entry Templates	Entries are discrete content structured for machine processing in the receiving system. Zero, one, or many entries may be included in a section.
Narrative Block	Narrative blocks are designed to be rendered for human viewing in the receiving system. Each section must have one narrative block.

standard—it specifies *what* information must be included in each template. The C-CDA specification also a syntax standard. It specifies the format in which the content is to be represented (Table 7.8), specifically, that the document itself is to be formatted as an XML document, with each component defined using XML tags.

The C-CDA standard extends the original CDA standard by defining parts of the document as reusable components that can be mixed and matched across documents.

7.4.3 Fast Health Interoperability Resources (FHIR)

Fast Health Interoperability Resources, or FHIR (pronounced "fire"), is a standard developed by HL7 for exchanging information between health information systems such as EHRs, mobile health devices, laboratory information systems, and imaging information systems. Like other HL7 standards, FHIR specifies not only the content and format of health information, but also a method for transmitting the

AdverseEvent	FamilyMemberHistory Goal	Practitioner
AllergyIntolerance	HealthcareService	Procedure
CarePlan	ImagingStudy	Questionnaire
CareTeam	Medication	QuestionnaireResponse
Communication	MedicationAdministration	RelatedPerson
Condition	MedicationDispense	ResearchElementDefinition
Consent	MedicationStatement	ResearchStudy
Coverage	Observation	ResearchSubject
Device	OperationOutcome	RiskAssessment
DiagnosticReport	Organization	Specimen
Encounter	Patient	Substance

Fig. 7.16 A sampling of HL7 FHIR Resources

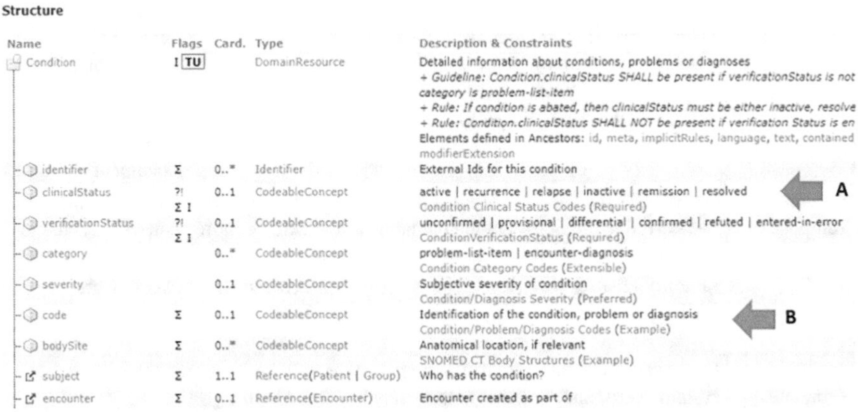

Structure

Name	Flags	Card.	Type	Description & Constraints
Condition	I TU		DomainResource	Detailed information about conditions, problems or diagnoses + Guideline: Condition.clinicalStatus SHALL be present if verificationStatus is not category is problem-list-item + Rule: If condition is abated, then clinicalStatus must be either inactive, resolve + Rule: Condition.clinicalStatus SHALL NOT be present if verification Status is en Elements defined in Ancestors: id, meta, implicitRules, language, text, contained modifierExtension
identifier	Σ	0..*	Identifier	External Ids for this condition
clinicalStatus	?! Σ I	0..1	CodeableConcept	active | recurrence | relapse | inactive | remission | resolved **A** Condition Clinical Status Codes (Required)
verificationStatus	?! Σ I	0..1	CodeableConcept	unconfirmed | provisional | differential | confirmed | refuted | entered-in-error ConditionVerificationStatus (Required)
category		0..*	CodeableConcept	problem-list-item | encounter-diagnosis Condition Category Codes (Extensible)
severity		0..1	CodeableConcept	Subjective severity of condition Condition/Diagnosis Severity (Preferred)
code	Σ	0..1	CodeableConcept	Identification of the condition, problem or diagnosis **B** Condition/Problem/Diagnosis Codes (Example)
bodySite	Σ	0..*	CodeableConcept	Anatomical location, if relevant SNOMED CT Body Structures (Example)
subject	Σ	1..1	Reference(Patient | Group)	Who has the condition?
encounter	Σ	0..1	Reference(Encounter)	Encounter created as part of

Fig. 7.17 FHIR *Condition* resource as an information model with bindings to clinical terminology (https://www.hl7.org/fhir/condition.html)

information. On the content side, FHIR carves out the universe of health information into small, clinically meaningful pieces of clinical information that may need to be exchanged, called "resources". Examples of FHIR resources include *Patient*, *Condition*, *Medication*, *Device*, *Questionnaire*, and *Procedure* (Fig. 7.16).

FHIR resources are essentially small information models with "bindings" to clinical terminology. That is, for each element defined in a FHIR resource, the allowable type and range of values is explicitly defined. For those elements of the model that must contain a value from a specific set of concepts, this "binding" is specified. Figure 7.17 depicts part of the defining for the FHIR *condition* resource. One element of the resource is *clinical status*. This element is used to define the status of the condition, and the binding for this field limits allowable values to a predefined FHIR value set that includes 'active', 'recurrence', 'relapse', 'inactive', 'remission', and 'resolved' (Fig. 7.17a). Similarly, element *code* specifies that the value can come from any number of terminologies used to code conditions, problems or diagnoses, and lists SNOMED as an example of one such terminology (Fig. 7.17b).

7.5   Repositories of Standards

7.5.1   FAIRSharing

As standards have evolved, a number of repositories and websites have been developed to catalog these standards. One valuable resource in this space is the FAIRSharing website [38]. This resource has evolved over time. It began life as the MIBBI Project (Minimum Information for Biological and Biomedical Investigations), a website that cataloged minimum information checklists [39]. MIBBI evolved into to BioSharing.org, a curated website of data standards, databases, and data policies. BioSharing linked these artifacts together, indicating for example which data repositories use which data standards, and which journals or funders require use of which standards, or deposition of data into which repositories. More recently, with the formalization of FAIR guidelines for data sharing (see Chap. 15), BioSharing changed its name to FAIRSharing. Its creators describe it as "an informative and educational resource that describes and interlinks community-driven standards, databases, repositories and data policies… covering natural sciences (for example, *biomedical*, chemistry, astronomy, agriculture, earth sciences and life sciences), engineering, and humanities and social sciences" [38]. Importantly, FAIRSharing includes a status attribute, indicating whether a given standard is "ready", "in development", or "deprecated." It is not uncommon to find a standard documented online that is no longer maintained and/or has been replaced by a different standard. That status can be difficult to ascertain e.g., from a static publication describing that standard from 10 years ago (Fig. 7.18).

Browsing through FAIRSharing for other clinical and mental health related content standards yields several results, but it should be noted that there are some surprising annotations and inconsistent external documentation. As of October 2020, there are 176 "reporting guidelines", 50 of which are tagged with the subject of "Biomedical

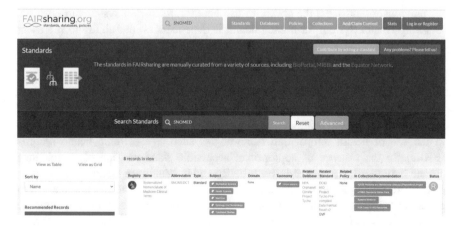

Fig. 7.18 FAIRSharing

Science" and eight with "Social and Behavioral Science." A guideline called MIfMRI is cataloged in FAIRSharing as a reporting checklist for Minimum Information about an fMRI Study. The FAIRSharing record points to the website for the Organization for Human Brain Mapping, but a search for "MIfMRI" on that site yields no hits. Searches for this standard in PubMed and Google Scholar yield similarly disappointing results. A standard known as MINI- Minimum Information about a Neuroscience Investigation- was described by Gibson et al. [40] and is cataloged in FAIRSharing, but the website provided in the record appears to be no longer active. These cautionary tales are not meant to discourage the reader from using standards, but rather to encourage you to perform due diligence in identifying the right standard to use. Also, whenever possible, try hard to find an existing, maintained standard that meets your needs, or comes close, and work with the owners of that standard to modify it as needed. This is far preferable to creating your own, only for that standard to end up in the dustbin of forgotten standards with broken links and no users. (Again, see Fig. 7.10).

7.5.2 Interoperability Standards Advisory (ISA)

One of the most useful resources for up-to-date information about clinical interoperability standards is the Interoperability Standards Advisory, or ISA (https://www.healthit.gov/isa/). This resource provides information regarding identification, assessment, and determination of "recognized" interoperability standards by the US Office of the National Coordinator for Health IT.

7.6 Addressing Gaps in Standards to Accommodate Mental Health

As previously described, the ability to use health information systems to enable a Learning Health System for mental health is dependent on our ability to represent clinical information accurately and unambiguously in a way that computerized systems understand. Unfortunately, while much progress has been made over the past decades in enhancing standards to enable technical and semantic interoperability in the biomedical domain, there remain substantial gaps in such systems of representation relative to mental health and the behavioral sciences [41]. Moreover, as described in Chap. 16, the mental health sector is currently undergoing an exponential increase in the use of health information technologies such as electronic health records (EHRs). In the absence of appropriate, accessible standards and clear guidance around how to use the standards, each EHR vendor, healthcare system, and practice creates proprietary information models using idiosyncratic value sets not mapped to coded terminology. The large number of distinct EHR products, combined with the multitude of small-scale implementations, each housing data for a relatively small number of people seeking mental health services, makes standardizing mental health information essential. Without standards, we cannot facilitate meaningful and reliable collection, exchange, pooling and aggregation of data required to generate the actionable knowledge required to improve mental healthcare.

In this section we provide an overview of gaps in standards and outline opportunities to improve systems for concept and knowledge representation relative to mental health. We summarize some of the specific challenges in modeling concepts for this domain and make recommendations for approaching terminology enhancement in this space. Finally, we outline a preliminary foundation from which the systematic enhancement of systems for the computational representation of clinical mental health information can occur.

7.6.1 Standards for Concept and Knowledge Representation in Mental Health

Table 7.9 enumerates several standards for concept and knowledge representation relevant to mental health. Two of the most important controlled vocabularies are

Table 7.9 Systems for concept and knowledge representation in mental health

System	Description
Controlled Vocabularies	
Thesaurus of Psychological Index Terms	Controlled vocabulary used for indexing publications in the PsycINFO database
Terminologies	
CPT	Classification and coding system used for health-related procedures performed in outpatient settings in the United States
LOINC	Terminology covering health measurement and assessment such as lab tests, radiology studies, and psychosocial surveys, questionnaires, and assessment instruments
MeSH	Terminology used for indexing publications in the MEDLINE database
ICD-10-PCS	Procedure classification and coding system used for coding health-related procedures performed in inpatient settings in the United States
Ontologies	
SNOMED-CT	Ontology covering the entire domain of healthcare including clinical findings, functions, diseases, procedures, and other health related information
Nosologies	
DSM-5	Classification (Nosology) of mental health disorders and related problems
ICD-10 ICD-10-CM	Classification (Nosology) of injuries, diseases, and health-related problems. ICD-10 is used internationally, ICD-10-CM is the modified US version.
ICD-11	Classification (Nosology) of injuries, diseases, and health-related problems

MeSH, or Medical Subject Headings and the Thesaurus of Psychological Index Terms [11]. MeSH is used to index biomedical publications in the MEDLINE (Medical Literature Analysis and Retrieval System Online) database. MEDLINE is a major publication database covering the life sciences and biomedical information, containing more than 26 million references journal articles. The Thesaurus of Psychological Index Terms is used to index publications in the PsycINFO® [42] database. PsycINFO® is the official publication indexing database of the American Psychological Association (APA) and is the most extensive and widely used publication indexing database in mental health and the behavioral sciences [43]. It indexes publications from more than 25,000 journals, including articles from more than 50 countries in 29 languages [44].

7.6.2 Minimum Clinical Data Sets

Over the past two decades, several authors have articulated the need to develop both condition-specific and intervention-specific minimal clinical data sets in mental health [45]. These authors have argued that condition-specific data sets will need to include information related not only to history, exposures, signs, and symptoms, but also methods for assessing and monitoring the course of illness. They have argued that intervention-specific minimum clinical data sets will need to include data elements related to pertinent details of the intervention, presumed mechanisms of action, and response to interventions, including adverse events.

7.6.3 Quality of Terminologies Relative to Mental Health

In assessing systems for concept and knowledge representation relative to utility in a specific domain of health, there are several factors to consider. The first factor is how well the system covers the domain of interest, in this case, MH. The second factor is the extent to which the system is capable of fully representing the domain (i.e., whether the system is "adequate"). Finally, there is the question of fully defining the concepts of interest. Moreover, to be useful in LHS and informatics paradigms, the terminology must be computable. It is worth noting that those products with content having the best coverage of mental health are often not developed using informatics-informed methods, and those products suitable for use in informatics methods do not contain significant mental health content (Table 7.10).

Table 7.10 Characteristics of technologies for data and knowledge representation relative to mental health

System	Content	MH content coverage	Enables computation	Adequacy for MH
MeSH	Indexing Publications	POOR	STRONG	STRONG
Psychological Index Terms	Indexing Publications	STRONG	POOR	STRONG
PsycINFO T&M Field	Tests	STRONG	POOR	STRONG
PsycTESTS	Indexing Publications	STRONG	POOR	STRONG
CEM/CIMI	Clinical (All)	POOR	STRONG	STRONG
SNOMED-CT	Clinical (All)	FAIR	STRONG	FAIR
ICD-10-PCS	Interventions, Procedures	POOR	STRONG	STRONG
CPT	Interventions, Procedures	POOR	STRONG	STRONG
LOINC	Measures, Assessments	FAIR	STRONG	STRONG
DSM-5	Problems	STRONG	POOR	STRONG
ICD-10-CM, ICD-11-CM	Problems	FAIR	STRONG	STRONG

Reused with permission from Ranallo et al. (2016) and updated

7.7 Conclusions and Recommendations

Standards are important for enabling storage, exchange, interpretation, and analysis of data. While content and syntactic standards in the mental health space largely share the same challenges as those in other areas of medicine, semantic standards introduce hurdles that are unique to mental health due to its interdisciplinary nature, epistemological challenges, and the lack of objectively observed *things* to describe. To overcome these challenges will require engaging both informaticians and behavioral scientists in the important work of terminology development. Arguably the first hurdle is simply recognizing that systems for concept representation carry with them specific epistemological assumptions (assumptions about what can be known, by whom, and how- see Chap. 6), and the epistemological assumptions of one discipline may or may not be shared by another. Differences in these assumptions between the biological and behavioral sciences have implications for concept modeling, and therefore must be explicitly addressed. Making explicit the differences in the epistemological assumptions of the biological sciences and those of the behavioral sciences is important to facilitate efficient concept modeling.

To overcome these challenges, informaticians will need deeper insight into the various disciplines that comprise the behavioral sciences. We will need clearer insight into the scope of knowledge, the variation in theoretical models, and the inherent differences in epistemological assumptions within this domain. We need to recognize the terminologies commonly used in healthcare today were developed specifically for general physical healthcare. The structural aspects of these terminologies were developed in tandem with the content they were designed to model, including the attributes of, and relationships between, primarily physical and biological entities (environmental entities that impact biological processes). Work involving concept representation for mental health will involve more than simple additions to content. It will require substantive changes to the concept models themselves, and indeed to the way we conceptualize mental health and illness. Behavioral scientists will need insight into the value of, and best practices for, developing high quality terminologies for more rapid acquisition of knowledge. We will need to work together to refine best practices for terminology development to successfully address the novel challenges of this domain.

References

1. Skovira RJ. Ontological grounding of a knowledge mapping methodology: defining data, information, and knowledge. Issues Inf Sci. 2007;VII(2):258–64.
2. Zins C. Conceptual approaches for defining data, information, and knowledge. J Am Soc Inf Sci Technol. 2007;58(4):479–93.
3. Sanders J Defining terms: data, information and knowledge. In: 2016 SAI computing conference (SAI). 2016. IEEE.
4. Dervos DA, Coleman AS. A common sense approach to defining data, information, and metadata. Würzburg: Ergon-Verlag; 2006.
5. Boisot M, Canals A. Data, information and knowledge: have we got it right? J Evol Econ. 2004;14(1):43–67.
6. Aamodt A, Nygård M. Different roles and mutual dependencies of data, information, and knowledge—an AI perspective on their integration. Data Knowl Eng. 1995;16(3):191–222.
7. Kanehisa M, et al. Data, information, knowledge and principle: back to metabolism in KEGG. Nucleic Acids Res. 2014;42(D1):D199–205.
8. Chute CG. Clinical classification and terminology: some history and current observations. J Am Med Inform Assoc. 2000;7(3):298–303.
9. States U Data standards. 2021. Available from https://resources.data.gov/standards/concepts/
10. Cimino JJ. Desiderata for controlled medical vocabularies in the twenty-first century. Methods Inf Med. 1998;37(4–5):394.
11. Tuleya LGE. Thesaurus of psychological index terms. Washington, DC: American Psychological Association; 2007.
12. Zhu X, et al. A review of auditing methods applied to the content of controlled biomedical terminologies. J Biomed Inform. 2009;42(3):413–25.
13. Gruber TR. A translation approach to portable ontology specifications. Knowl Acquis. 1993;5(2):199–220.
14. Ogden CK, Richards IA. The meaning of meaning. San Diego, CA: Harcourt, Brace; 1923.
15. Kim TY, Coenen A, Hardiker N. A quality improvement model for healthcare terminologies. J Biomed Inform. 2010;43(6):1036–43.
16. Elkin PL, et al. Guideline and quality indicators for development, purchase and use of controlled health vocabularies. Int J Med Inform. 2002;68(1–3):175–86.
17. Bales ME, et al. Qualitative assessment of the international classification of functioning, disability, and health with respect to the desiderata for controlled medical vocabularies. Int J Med Inform. 2006;75(5):384–95.
18. Association, A.P. Diagnostic and statistical manual of mental disorders (DSM-5®). Arlington, VA: American Psychiatric Pub; 2013.

19. IHTSDO, Standard nomenclature of medicine-clinical terms. International Release January 2011.
20. Lee, Y.T. Information modeling: from design to implementation. In: Proceedings of the second world manufacturing congress. 1999. Canada/Switzerland: International Computer Science Conventions.
21. Oniki TA, et al. Lessons learned in detailed clinical modeling at Intermountain Healthcare. J Am Med Inform Assoc. 2014;21(6):1076–81.
22. Martínez-Costa C, et al. Isosemantic rendering of clinical information using formal ontologies and RDF. Stud Health Technol Inform. 2013;192:1085.
23. Schulz S, Martínez-Costa C. How ontologies can improve semantic interoperability in health care. In: Process support and knowledge representation in health care. Cham: Springer; 2013. p. 1–10.
24. Tenenbaum JD, Sansone S-A, Haendel M. A sea of standards for omics data: sink or swim? J Am Med Inform Assoc. 2014;21(2):200–3.
25. Baker M. 1,500 scientists lift the lid on reproducibility. Nature. 2016;533:452–4.
26. Society F. Minimum Information about a high-throughput SEQuencing Experiment. 2012 10/4/2020]; Available from http://fged.org/projects/minseqe/
27. Ghitza UE, et al. Common data elements for substance use disorders in electronic health records: the NIDA clinical trials network experience. Addiction. 2013;108(1):3–8.
28. Saver JL, et al. Standardizing the structure of stroke clinical and epidemiologic research data: the National Institute of Neurological Disorders and Stroke (NINDS) stroke common data element (CDE) project. Stroke. 2012;43(4):967–73.
29. Health N.I.O NIH CDE repository. 2020 [cited 2020 10/09/2020].
30. Svensson-Ranallo PA, Adam TJ, Sainfort F. A framework and standardized methodology for developing minimum clinical datasets. AMIA Jt Summits Transl Sci Proc. 2011;2011:54.
31. Werley HH, Devine EC, Zorn CR. Nursing needs its own minimum data set. Am J Nurs. 1988;88(12):1651–3.
32. Glover G. Adult mental health care in England. Eur Arch Psychiat Clin Neurosci. 2007;257:71–82.
33. Morris R, et al. The Irish nursing minimum data set for mental health--a valid and reliable tool for the collection of standardised nursing data. J Clin Nurs. 2010;19(3–4):359–67.
34. Regenstrief Institute. Logical observation identifiers names and codes (LOINC®). Indiana, IN: Regenstrief Institute, Inc.; 2021.
35. Benson T, Grieve G. Hl7 version 2. In: Principles of health interoperability. Cham: Springer; 2016. p. 223–42.
36. Beeler GW. HL7 version 3—an object-oriented methodology for collaborative standards development. Int J Med Inform. 1998;48(1–3):151–61.
37. (HL7), H.L., HL7 CDA R2 IG: Consolidated CDA Templates for Clinical Note (US Realm), DSTU R2.1—Vol. 1: Intro. August 2015 with 2019 June errata.
38. Sansone SA, et al. FAIRsharing as a community approach to standards, repositories and policies. Nat Biotechnol. 2019;37(4):358–67.
39. Taylor CF, et al. Promoting coherent minimum reporting guidelines for biological and biomedical investigations: the MIBBI project. Nat Biotechnol. 2008;26(8):889–96.
40. Gibson F, et al. Minimum information about a neuroscience investigation (MINI): electrophysiology. Nat Prec. 2009:1–1. https://doi.org/10.1038/npre.2009.1720.2.
41. Ranallo PA, et al. Psychological assessment instruments: a coverage analysis using SNOMED CT, LOINC and QS terminology. AMIA Annu Symp Proc. 2013;2013:1333–40.
42. American Psychological Association. PsycINFO®. Washington, DC: APA EBSCO; 2012.
43. American Psychological Association. APA Databases. Washington, DC: APA EBSCO; 2012.
44. American Psychological Association. APA Databases: PsycINFO® Homepage. 2012 October [cited 2012 November 9]; Available from http://www.apa.org/pubs/databases/psycinfo/index.aspx
45. Institute of Medicine. Improving the quality of health care for mental and substance-use conditions. Quality chasm series, vol. xxiii. Washington, DC: National Academies Press; 2006. 504 p

Chapter 8
Use of Medical Imaging to Advance Mental Health Care: Contributions from Neuroimaging Informatics

Randy L. Gollub and Nicole Benson

Abstract Although medical imaging is not routinely deployed in the day-to-day structure of mental health care delivery, physicians and other healthcare providers are at a tipping point where such objective, quantitative physiological assessments are likely to become ever more important in the future. Such a development would generate new, actionable knowledge and information, at both an individual person and population public health levels. Mental health informatics could expand to encompass the acquisition of structured imaging data to augment other widely available data types.

In this chapter, pioneering examples that illustrate the clinical, catalytic potential of medical imaging within mental health informatics are presented and those aspects of biomedical imaging informatics that are pertinent for mental health are introduced. Efforts in translational medical imaging informatics are reviewed, highlighting ways in which incredible advances from the research side are starting to approach clinical utility. Equally important, medical imaging data collected during the delivery of routine clinical care is becoming increasingly available and can be used, together with the wealth of clinical data in the electronic health record, to play a critical role in advancing our understanding, prevention and treatment of mental health disorders.

Keywords Neuroimaging · MRI · Quantitative imaging metrics morphometry · DICOM · PACS · Brain imaging · Atlas

R. L. Gollub (✉) · N. Benson
Massachusetts General Hospital, Boston, MA, USA
e-mail: rgollub@partners.org; nbenson@mgh.harvard.edu

© Springer Nature Switzerland AG 2021
J. D. Tenenbaum, P. A. Ranallo (eds.), *Mental Health Informatics*, Health
Informatics, https://doi.org/10.1007/978-3-030-70558-9_8

8.1 Introduction

Biomedical imaging technologies continue to advance our ability to capture rich human data sets that can inform mental healthcare. Such technologies describe anatomy and physiology in ever greater detail and at increasing spatiotemporal resolutions. The use of these biomedical imaging technologies during the routine delivery of healthcare, and the electronic recording and storage of the resultant data in various archives and databases, some not yet linked to the electronic healthcare record (EHR), creates the opportunity to extract far more specific, objective and quantitative information than would otherwise be typically captured in the EHR. Historically, EHR anatomic and physiologic data have been limited to minimal extracts in the form of free text formats such as Radiology and Pathology reports, and a few vanguard structured fields of quantitative imaging metrics primarily in oncology [1, 2]. Properly instrumented for inclusion in the EHR and/or for facilitated extraction, this detailed anatomic and physiologic data has the potential to contribute to the ability of those working in the field of Mental Health Informatics to advance knowledge and improve patient care. It is important to note that medical imaging recordered as part of the work-up for mental health disorders is most commonly used to rule out other clinical conditions rather than as a way to diagnose mental health conditions or to monitor treatment. Thus, at this point in time, the potential value of these content-laden data has barely been tapped. However, exciting prospects are on the horizon as exemplified by some ground-breaking research studies.

One study that nicely illustrates this approach evaluated long-hypothesized [3] neuroprotective effects of prenatal folic acid exposure on postnatal brain development through late adolescence. Fully prospective studies of this question would take decades to operationalize, at a cost of many millions of dollars. Instead, Roffman and colleagues deployed human brain MRI scans acquired during the delivery of routine clinical care from an academic healthcare center [4], in concert with a "natural experiment" design, to address this question on an accelerated timetable and far more modest budget [5]. These researchers leveraged the fact that, in late 1996, and fully in effect by mid-1997, the United States government mandated that grain products be fortified with folic acid. The investigators used the mature informatics infrastructure at their institution [6, 7] to identify and to access the brain scans from a cohort of 315 youths, aged 8 to 18 years, born between January 1993 and December 2001 (inclusive of folic acid fortification rollout ±3.5 years) who had a clinically normal brain MRI scan done during that timeframe [4] (Fig. 8.1). The cohort was then divided into 3 age-matched groups based on birthdate and related level of prenatal folic acid fortification exposure (none, partial, or full). The brain scans were processed with software tools to extract quantitative metrics of brain structure. What they found was that cortical thickness in bilateral frontal and temporal regions increased with folate exposure and that age-associated thinning in temporal and parietal regions was delayed by folate exposure (Fig. 8.2). These changes in regional cortical thickness were replicated in two independent, observational, community-based cohorts, the Philadelphia Neurodevelopmental Cohort (PNC) [8] and the National Institutes of Health Magnetic Resonance Imaging Study of Normal Brain Development [9]. In the PNC cohort, decreased thinning in frontal, temporal, and parietal regions was associated with

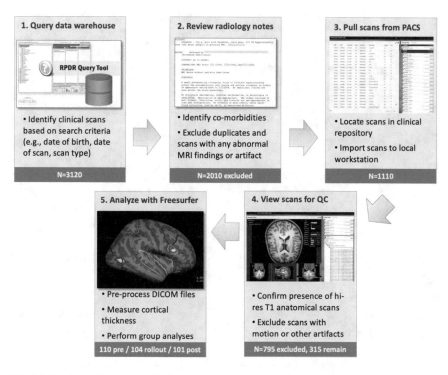

Fig. 8.1 To obtain the data needed to test the proposed association between the neuroprotective effects of prenatal folic acid and a reduced risk of schizophrenia, Roffman and colleagues [5]. (1) used their institutional informatics infrastructure, the Research Patient Data Registry (RPDR) at Partners Healthcare, to identify a cohort of youth, born between January 1993 and December 2001 (inclusive of folic acid fortification rollout ±3.5 years) who had a brain MRI scan done when they were between the ages of 8 to 18 years. They identified a potential cohort of 3120 youth who met those criteria. (2) The investigators then manually reviewed the radiology reports to exclude any youth with medical conditions that could potentially influence brain structure or with known imaging artifacts or other abnormalities, excluding 2012 on that basis. (3) The remaining 1110 scans were accessed and copied from the institutional Radiology archives (**Picture Archiving and Communication Systems (PACS)**) using a module of the RPDR, the Medical imaging Bench to Bedside (mi2b2) workbench [4]. (4) Each brain MRI scan was manually curated to identify those that met quality criteria (absence of image artifacts, sufficiently high spatial resolution and image contrast) yielding a final cohort of 315 youth who met all inclusion/exclusion criteria and could be used for the study. (5) The cohort was then divided into 3 age-matched groups based on birthdate and related level of prenatal folic acid fortification exposure (none, partial, or full) and the brain scans processed with the Freesurfer suite of software tools to extract quantitative metrics of brain structure

lower odds of psychosis spectrum symptoms. Future work will illuminate how these quantitative structural changes in cortical regions, as detected by MRI, are related to the pathophysiological processes underlying psychotic symptoms and potential targets for treatment. This landmark work demonstrates the exciting potential of existing EHR data, including clinically acquired brain MRI scans, and the Learning Health System (see Chap. 1) to yield information on par with clinical research studies that were conducted over decades at the cost of many millions of dollars.

Critical to the success of this pioneering neuropsychiatric work on folic acid exposure and schizophrenia outcomes was the availability of neuroimaging data in

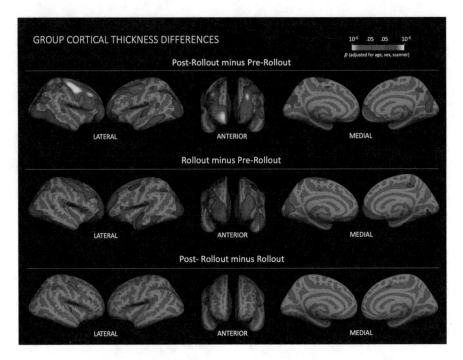

Fig. 8.2 Cortical thickness in bilateral frontal and temporal regions increased with folate exposure and age-associated thinning in temporal and parietal regions was delayed by folate exposure. Results are displayed as pseudo-colored statistical maps painted onto the inflated surfaces of the left and right cortex of a template (average) brain. In the top row, the contrast between cortical thickness in cohort with no exposure to folate (Pre-Rollout) and full exposure to folate (Post-Rollout) is displayed as pseudo-color statistical maps painted overlaying the inflated cortical surface. The hotter colors indicate thicker cortical surface in the children exposed to folate during gestation. In the middle row the contrast between the cohort with partial exposure to folate (Rollout) and no exposure to folate (Pre-Rollout) is displayed indicating that partial exposure appears to be protective. In the bottom row the contrast between the cohort with partial exposure to folate (Rollout) and full exposure to folate (Post-Rollout) is displayed indicating that the incremental change from partial to full exposure to gestational folate is less pronounced. See [5] for full details

the population of interest stored in EHR data repositories. There are significant stores of brain images in hospital imaging repositories that have been reported to be "normal" and/or "normative" in that any subtle anomalies or variations captured by the imaging were not detected by visual inspection, even when interpreted by an expertly trained radiologist. For example, there is evidence that brain imaging is ordered for patients who present with acute and chronic headaches at a rate that exceeds best practice clinical guidelines. This is true because it is rare that headaches, in the absence of other symptoms, result from a intracranial pathological condition that can be detected using routine radiological practices of image acquisition and analysis [10]. Thus, in current practice, brain imaging is performed to reveal information that reliably enables the clinician to rule out uncommon, but potentially serious, causes of headache (e.g. tumor). However, at present the image data are not otherwise used for further refining the differential diagnosis or for guiding treatment decisions.

In another example, clinically acquired diffusion-weighted MR images from neonates and children were used to build age-specific "normative" atlases that provide essential knowledge about early brain development and may guide the detection of abnormal patterns of maturation. In this work, a set of age-specific Apparent Diffusion Coefficient (ADC) atlases from 201 healthy full-term children, imaged between 0–6 years, with MRI acquired at a single large academic hospital from 2006–2013, were generated after using the informatics infrastructure [6, 7] to identify and to access the brain scans [11]. The atlases capture quantitative brain tissue metrics that contribute to knowledge of neurodevelopment as well as guiding clinical detection of

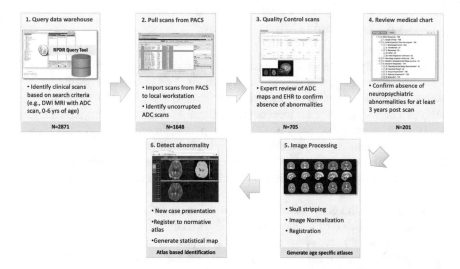

Fig. 8.3 Development of age specific "normative" atlases of Apparent Diffusion Coefficient (ADC) values extracted from brain Diffusion Weighted (DWI) MRI brain scans acquired during the provision of clinical care (1.). The investigators used their institutional informatics infrastructure, the RPDR at Partners Healthcare, to identify a cohort of 2871 infants and children who had a brain MRI scan done when they were between birth and 6 years old. (2.) The investigators then accessed those scans from institutional Radiology archives **(PACS)** using a module of the RPDR, the mi2b2 workbench, and identified 1648 cases where ADC maps had been generated from the DWI scans and were stored in the PACS. (3.). The expert imaging processing data scientist and neuroradiologist team members manually reviewed both the ADC maps and the EHR data for the identified cases, and confirmed the absence of abnormal findings at the time of the scan for 705 cases. (4.) The team neonatologist and pediatric neuroradiologist, with the help of clinical coordinator and collaborating pediatric residents reviewed the medical records of each case and confirmed the absence of signs and symptoms of neurodevelopmental and mental health conditions for at least 2 years post scan in 201 of the cases. (5.) These carefully curated ADC scans were binned by age, and the images processed through a workflow that included field of view correction, skull stripping, image intensity normalization, and registration to yield a set of age specific ADC atlases. (6.) The clinical application of the age specific atlases is to use them to support clinicians' interpretation of individual patient ADC maps by making statistical comparison to a "normative" reference thus increasing the visibility of subtle abnormalities and providing more quantitative, spatially interpretable information. Reference: Ou Y, Zollei L, Retzepi K, Castro V, Bates SV, Pieper S, et al. Using clinically acquired MRI to construct age-specific ADC atlases: Quantifying spatiotemporal ADC changes from birth to 6-year old. Hum Brain Mapp. 2017;38(6):3052–68

abnormalities (Fig. 8.3). Future work that advances our sensitivity to detect subtle anatomic variations through the use of machine learning algorithms trained on curated data such as these culled from the vast stores of clinical brain images might in fact begin to contribute to a deeper understanding of "normal" brain structure and function and how they are impacted by a person's mental health status [12]. In particular, for severe mental health conditions such as those characterized by violent or antisocial behavior, the ability to diagnose and predict the outcomes of a course of care could have signficant benefits for both the individual and society.

8.2   Capturing Meaningful Neuroscientific Anatomic and Physiologic Data

Clinical imaging ordered in the context of mental healthcare provision is most commonly used to rule out other clinical conditions. For example, when an elderly patient presents with an acute mental status change, imaging may be obtained to rule out a cerebrovascular accident or brain cancer. As clinical imaging technologies advance, the hope is that when an 18-year-old patient presents with an acute mental status change, imaging may be obtained to help differentiate between schizophrenia and bipolar disorder. Clinical tools combined with informatics techniques will shift the field towards a shared knowledge with the potential to yield interpretable, clinically actionable data.

As applied to the goal of advancing Mental Health Informatics (MHI), we focus on technologies that capture the static anatomy and dynamic physiology of the central and peripheral nervous systems. But it is important to acknowledge that brain-body connections are integral to many mental health concerns such as the profound relation between autism and gastrointestinal disorders [13] or the multiple systemic side-effects (e.g. megacolon/agranulocytosis/myocarditis) manifested by people with schizophrenia who are treated with medications such as clozapine [14]. Many thorough informatics resources are available that detail the relevant non-mental health aspects of anatomy and physiology of the immune, endocrine, sensory, musculoskeletal, and digestive systems [2]. In addition to clinical presentation data, there is also a tremendous potential for the integration of genomic data with a variety of imaging data to identify any relationships between known basic science genotypes and aspects of the disease imaging phenotype. This relationship is referred to as radiogenomics and looks at the associations between image features or phenotypes and molecular phenotypes or markers providing the capacity for enhanced association analyses [15]. This is a growing area of importance in medicine providing capacity to identify imaging features associated with genomic characteristics [16]. Here, we will focus on those aspects of static anatomy and dynamic physiology that are unique to clinical neuroscience and, in particular, to mental health.

While anatomic and physiologic information about the central and peripheral nervous systems exist in EHR data, the level of specificity of this information is often limited. Frequently, data generated by orders, scheduling processes, encounters, and billing claims provide evidence that imaging was performed, but the actual imaging data are not present in the data set. The limited formation is useful in guiding the informatician to what data does exist and where to find it. However, only when working with the actual MR image data and its derivatives is it possible to make use of all the available physiologic and anatomic information contained therein. Revolutions in the use of advanced imaging processing and Artificial Intelligence (AI) in medical imaging [17] are steadily driving forward progress in the medical imaging informatics field. Industry, healthcare systems and researchers are all working towards improved instrumentation of clinical systems to extract this meaningful anatomic and physiological data in the service of improved, efficient and specific patient care.

Clinical imaging systems generate multimodal imaging data sets such as electroencephalographic (EEG) recordings, computed tomography (CT) images, Positron Emission Tomography (PET) with metabolic and receptor binding, many types of Magnetic Resonance Imaging (MRI), and some digitized molecular pathology images that detail central and peripheral nervous systems structure and function. Access to a few of these valuable data stores is possible by some currently available clinical workflows, and a few advanced research technologies. But many of these valuable clinical resources are yet to be tapped by informaticians.

Inherently, medical images are an unstructured data type. Moving and storing medical image data is relatively straightforward; but extracting information and meaning from the images is not as easy. Quantitative feature extraction converts images into mineable data [18]. Image processing to derive features and create meaning from these features, such as identification of abnormalities, volumes of structures, velocity of flows, and other "phenotypic" characteristics, requires technically demanding and highly nuanced image processing steps as well as expensive resources in terms of both personnel and equipment to support the computational demands.

8.3   Radiology Workflow: From Order to Storage

Radiologists were early adopters of electronic medical records, and, working with modalities that are inherently digital, such as CT and MRI, worked to establish many best practices for the field of healthcare informatics. Over the last half-century, medical imaging has evolved from primarily analog to almost exclusively digital image construction transmitted through institutional electronic media. This digital radiological revolution was accompanied by the development of industry standards. There are now robust, standardized, and continually evolving methods for ordering, scheduling, protocoling (the specific details for how imaging study will be performed), acquiring, analyzing, reporting, storing, visualizing, and transmitting digital radiology images due to the coordinated efforts of multiple professional organizations and societies [1, 19]. This comprehensive corpus of standards, now known as the **Digital Imaging and Communications in Medicine (DICOM)** standard, was initially developed in 1983 by the National Electrical Manufacturers

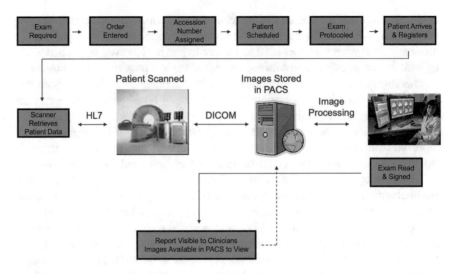

Fig. 8.4 Progression of patient imaging study through the Hospital Information System. There are many steps involved in the image acquisition, each generating fields of data in the EHR

Association in conjunction with the American College of Radiology to facilitate the sharing of information across manufacturers and equipment.

The electronic radiology workflow is depicted in Fig. 8.4. It begins with a clinician ordering an exam which generates a unique ID or **accession number** for the patient's study. This process is increasingly rule-based, with evidenced-based criteria that guide ordering providers to clinically justify the exam. Once the order is entered, the person is scheduled for the study. Prior to the study, the exam is protocoled, meaning that the details of the specific scan acquisition sequences needed to answer the clinical question being asked by the ordering provider is specified by the imaging experts. When the person arrives, the study is identified by the **accession number** which is used throughout the duration of the exam to track the progress of the study and interpretation.

During the examination, imaging data is acquired, transmitted to a system for optimal viewing and clinical interpretation (reading), and then archived. **Picture Archiving and Communication Systems (PACS)** is a medical imaging technology that facilitates access to images of multiple types (e.g., ultrasound, MRI, CT) and provides efficient storage with quick retrieval capabilities [1]. When digital images are acquired, they are transmitted electronically to the central PACS repository using the DICOM standard. The DICOM standard, when applied, facilitates image transmission and viewing across a variety of PACS platforms allowing for interoperability of distribution, viewing, and annotation of images from a variety of image acquisition devices. The DICOM standard can be applied to images, their annotations and associated imaging reports such that all can be stored under the same unique encounter identifier and linked for subsequent, coordinated viewing. Each radiologic study comprises multiple image data files, each of which is tagged with a unique identifier. Images may be tagged for post-processing steps so additional details can be transmitted and stored. With PACS, the compiled DICOM data can be viewed remotely and simultaneously on the same network, a key requirement for coordinating clinical care. There are some limitations in the (re)use of clinical images for research purposes (see later sections), that are due to vendor-specific use of proprietary DICOM fields for holding critical acquisition parameters and to technological advances in image acquisition and processing that happen faster than updates to the DICOM standard [20].

8.4   Data and Standards

Physician interpretation of medical images, known as reports, may be generated using structured templates, free text, or a combination of the two. When radiology reports are generated using structured data, their common data elements (CDE) allow for easy extraction for clinical and research purposes [21]. This information is supplemental to other portions of the encounter such as text within the history of present illness, neurological and mental status exams, and family history sections that are discussed elsewhere.

At present, the majority of clinical data stored in radiology reports are free text [22]. Natural language processing (NLP) has been used to extract information from these reports both for clinical care and research [23]. For example, NLP has been used to obtain information from reports to help practices meet quality metrics (e.g., information used to determine whether follow-up imaging is required for incidental findings) that are required for Merit-based Incentive Payment System scores and these algorithms have, in some cases, replaced human coders [24]. Recent work highlights the potential for NLP algorithms to enable automatic identification of abnormal findings in brain images from Radiology reports, not only those associated with disorders with known structural pathology such as stroke and tumors, but also cerebral atrophy, and small vessel disease that are more subtle findings associated with situations when mental healthcare services are obtained [25] (see Chap. 13 for more on NLP).

Similar to mental healthcare disciplines, the discipline of radiology is working to define common data elements for establishing quality metrics and/or benchmarking parameters. Multiple fields, including cardiology and pathology, are more actively developing structured reporting standards to facilitate quality assessment. Like mental health, radiology is working towards this effort by developing exam reporting templates across institutions that will improve extraction of meaningful metrics for understanding the clinical status of the patient (see for example, BI-RADS for breast imaging [26], and PI-RADS for prostate imaging [27]). As visionary leadership within radiology understands the critical importance of uniform report standards, the radiology field is moving steadily in this direction. For example, the American Society of Neuroradiology, the American College of Radiology, and the Radiological Society of North America collaborated to define a set of common data elements to be used to describe the essential concepts, features and observations found in radiology reporting to standardize this process [28–31]. The goal is to create report features that are simultaneously human and machine readable. The currently available common data elements with relevance for mental health pertain to localization and quantitation of brain lesions (e.g. due to stroke, multiple sclerosis), and to disruption in quantitative metrics from diffusion- and susceptibility-weighted MRI acquisitions, which reveal localized disturbances in brain tissue properties.

In addition to these generated reports, the images themselves can contain structured data (e.g., input by the radiologist or technician) to augment the content of the image in a graphical overlay (e.g., identifying an area of interest on an image with an arrow, demarcating the boundary of a lesion with a line, etc.). A robust, mature, open-sourced, research-based framework for this was developed under the leadership of Daniel Rubin's Annotation and Image Markup (AIM) project [32]. AIM provides a mechanism for standardizing the way image annotations are formatted and stored [33]. The AIM platform also incorporates quantitative metrics extracted from the medical images, such as the volume of a segmented anatomic feature within the image. Not surprisingly, since the project was closely aligned with the NIH National Cancer Institute's informatics efforts, the utility of AIM is best demonstrated in oncology where tumors are measured using Response Evaluation Criteria in Solid Tumors (RECIST) to follow the course of treatment, and marked on the images themselves [34]. Once images are annotated with RECIST measures, AIM allows for the tracking and storage of these measurements over the course of an individual's treatment.

There are few exemplars in mental health that have the RECIST level of functionality, incorporating both extracted quantitative information from the medical image, and incorporating the information directly into the image as an annotation. The closest mental health equivalent is the use of quantitative metrics of hippocampal and entorhinal cortical volumes in the assessment of mild cognitive impairment and dementias [35]. However, as capabilities for routine extraction of more quantitative features that yield interpretable metrics for human cognition, emotion and behavior advance, it is highly likely that such features will make essential contributions to automated phenotyping [36].

8.5 Image-Derived Features for Mental Health

As noted above, current medical practice does not include the systematic extraction and reporting of quantitative anatomic or physiologic metrics of brain health from medical images to the treating mental health clinician for direct patient care. However, rapid progress is being made in the broader domain (e.g [37]) and promising signals from the human neuroimaging research community suggest it will not be long before such data become part of routine clinical practice (see for example [38] and [39]). Critically, the clinical translational research community that works with human brain imaging data, is acutely aware of the importance of generating reliable, reproducible data; the cornerstone of any meaningful biomarkers. Professional societies promulgate best practices for the acquisition, analysis and reporting of quantitative brain-imaging-derived features at both the group and individual level (see for example [40–42]).

Rapid progress is being made across all domains of medical imaging, towards automated and/or semiautomated image processing, and artificial intelligence (AI) support for extraction of quantitative imaging metrics and assessing their predictive value. Image processing methods include algorithms that identify and locate various image characteristics (e.g. intensity boundaries, morphological texture features, and curves) and assign a label to every image voxel (volume element) such that voxels that have similar characteristics are assigned the same label. This work requires advances in automated brain image registration (alignment of the image of interest to a reference image such as previous time point of the same person or normative atlas), segmentation (delineation of features within an image), and labeling, as just a few examples. Adoption of this trend is increasing [17, 43, 44], with appropriate attention being paid to develop ethical guidelines to govern access and protect patients (see for example, [45]). Current state of the art research for medical imaging analytics is on the cusp of becoming the "norm" for clinical practice, as exemplified by work on retinopathy of prematurity [46], body composition metrics relevant for cardiometabolic, cardiovascular and cancer care [47] as well as myriad quantitative metrics useful for diagnosis and prognostication of cancers (e.g. tumor volume, blood vessel permeability, and perfusion) [48]. Although some of the most innovative and impactful advances in healthcare IT infrastructure, such as the Substitutable Medical Applications and Reusable Technologies (SMART) that builds on the openly licensed HL-7 draft standard called Fast Health Interoperability Resources (FHIR), have limitations in their initial versions that preclude use for working with medical imaging data [49, 50], there are examples of successful informatics infrastructures that enable robust workflows to repurpose clinically acquired neuroimaging data for meaningful secondary research [4, 51]. However, there is significant work to be done to harmonize clinical images in order to pool them for secondary research use (see Table 8.1).

Table 8.1 Clinical images and associated data are different when obtained for research or clinical purposes

	Research setting	Clinical setting
Acquisition	Standardized, typically with a research protocol	Varies based on patient needs, may be customized to the patient
Quality	High image resolution	Only as high resolution as needed to answer the clinical question
Subjects	Typically normal subjects	Rarely normal, often seeking images for a clinical reason
Data	Quantitative data, standardized	Qualitative, written reports

In the next section we briefly describe specific modalities where imaging metrics are beginning to contribute to the provision of mental health care by illuminating plausible mechanistic understanding of pathophysiological processes underlying presenting symptoms and/or have already been demonstrated to have the sensitivity to contribute to decision making for the clinical care of an individual. For a more complete description of the underlying physics, acquisition and image generation details for medical image modalities please see detailed reviews of this information [2].

8.5.1 Magnetic Resonance Imaging

Magnetic resonance imaging (MRI) is the most widely used imaging modality to assess brain structure and function. A standard, whole brain clinical imaging protocol typically includes several different scans, or acquisition sequences, each uniquely capturing meaningful information about brain tissue properties and function. The workhorse sequences are T1-weighted images, diffusion weighted images (DWI) and T2*-weighted sequences of various types used for functional magnetic resonance imaging (fMRI). A detailed explanation for the underlying magnetic resonance technology is beyond the scope of this chapter, but in short, the different techniques differ in the timing of their radiofrequency pulses, and consequently in the characteristics of the tissue they highlight. These sequences are routinely collected at 1.5 T or 3 T field strengths, depending on the locally available MR scanners. (In this context, T stands for Tesla, the unit of strength of the magnet used.) As field strength increases, so too does spatial resolution and signal strength. The standard 1.5 T and 3 T scanners in widespread clinical use are able to provide resolution of ~1 mm for structural scans and 3-5 mm for functional scans. This resolution is more than adequate for extracting and visualizing many clinically meaningful signals. However, ongoing frontier efforts are looking towards acquisitions at up to 20 T [52, 53], which may well be required to extract subtle findings most relevant for mental health practice. Because image acquisition parameters (e.g. manufacturer, field strength, gradient coil properties, spatial resolution, etc.) greatly impact extracted metrics, generating meaningful quantitative results requires harmonization of the images at the time of acquisition and/or during post processing (e.g., [54–56]).

Structural MR data, most often T1-weighted sequences, is currently used for most quantitative imaging work. From this 3D sequence, robust software tools and workflows enable systematic extraction and labeling of cortical surfaces (pial, gray and white matter), labeling of regionally specific cortical areas and subcortical structures, and other quantitative metrics such as cortical curvatures. There are several dominant software packages in current research use including FreeSurfer [57] (and see the wealth of clinical translational applications of this software at [58] and the Connectome Workbench [59]). The use of hippocampal volume as a vendor-provided, clinically meaningful metric as noted above [35] is based on a software package that has common roots with the FreeSurfer tool.

Excellent examples of the imminent clinical translation of this modality come from studies using the UK Biobank data [60]. One of the earliest, and most widely attempted, approaches to the use of quantitative brain imaging to generate a clinically meaningful signal was to estimate brain age from a large sample of "healthy" or "normative" whole brain MRI scans using various AI algorithms, then determine if the scan from a single individual deviated in some predictable way from the expected value [61]. Specifically, accelerated aging (positive change) and resilience (negative change) have been found to correlate with factors such as dementia and preservation of cognitive function, respectively. As another example, UK BioBank T1-weighted brain MR data, from more than 19,700 people, was used to generate hippocampal volume "nomograms", or predicted values for hippocampal volume as it changes over 45 to 75 years of age [62]. Of particular relevance for mental health care, preliminary investigation of the impact of lifestyle choices such as smoking status and sociocultural determinants such as education were demonstrated to have significant, predictable impact on hippocampal volume (e.g. smoking decreases it, greater education increases it). The sensitivity to detect these subtle effects in the UK BioBank data was the direct consequence of the rigorous study design whereby all data were collected with a single MR scan acquisition protocol, on a small set of calibrated MR scanners from the same manufacturer [60, 63], thus the variance introduced during acquisition of the images was greatly minimized compared to other published studies that relied on the aggregation of image data across multiple sites with a more heterogenous set of acquisition parameters.

Functional magnetic resonance imaging (fMRI), the most common example of which relies on the Blood Oxygen Level Dependent (BOLD) signal, is a $T2^{*}$-weighted acquisition that is the method most widely used by the human brain imaging research community. FMRI studies can be divided into two basic approaches: resting state and task based. Resting state fMRI measures exactly what the name suggests; the on-going function of the awake brain at "rest" or, more accurately, how the brain functions in the absence of having a specified task to perform. This technique can be used to map functional brain networks and network properties of healthy volunteers and/or to discern differences between cohorts. In contrast, task based studies use an experimental paradigm (as simple as flashing lights or as complex as resolving an ethical dilemma) to probe brain function. Current clinical use of fMRI is limited to pre-surgical motor, language and memory mapping in patients with epilepsy, brain tumors, arteriovenous malformations or other pathologies [64, 65].

The use of fMRI to inform the clinical practice of mental health is the promise of the future. Despite thousands of research studies, and tens of thousands of research scans investigating the entire gamut of mental health conditions, virtually none have yielded actionable biomarkers to support the care of people with depression, anxiety, or psychosis. That isn't to say that there aren't myriad positive findings in the neuroimaging literature that provide meaningful insights to pathophysiological mechanisms, or that the field lacks enthusiasm and resolve to move forward to that goal [66]. As just two examples, neuroimaging-based insights have provided support for the development of educational strategies to address learning differences in dyslexia [67]; and visualization of neural activity associated with placebo analgesia gave a potent "lift" to the realignment of medical education to embrace the importance of the therapeutic encounter as an element of the healing experience [68, 69]. There will be much more to say in this domain in the coming years.

Other MR imaging modalities, including magnetic resonance spectroscopy (MRS) and diffusion weighted imaging (DWI) are active research tools for investigating the pathophysiological mechanisms underlying mental health conditions. Diffusion imaging, a rapidly evolving technique for non-invasively mapping the "wiring" of the brain by quantifying the molecular movements of water molecules, is a key clinical tool for presurgical mapping, along with fMRI. MRS techniques focus on the spectral profiles of brain metabolites (e.g. choline, creatinine, lactate and others) and provide quantitative data on the neurochemical state of the brain. Specifically, the MRS signals can be tuned to measure the metabolic status of the brain and can be imaged with sufficient spatial resolution to study brain regions. One of the most commonly imaged metabolites is N-acetylaspartate (NAA), a marker of neuronal density and viability. In current clinical practice, MRS measures of NAA is of great use in the differential diagnosis and monitoring of therapeutic treatment responses in brain cancers. In research studies, MRS is used to investigate glutamatergic dysfunction and impairments in energy metabolism [70], and this method is being used to probe the impact of stress on human brain function [71].

8.5.2   Nuclear Medicine Imaging

Positron emission tomography (PET) and single-photon emission computed tomography (SPECT) are nuclear medicine imaging methods that measure various radioactively labeled, metabolic and/or pharmacologic probes that bind to, or are taken up by, specific tissues after being injected into a patient's peripheral circulation [72]. The information generated by these methods have both spatial information (where in the brain) and functional information (specified by the probe that is employed). Due to radiation safety considerations which limit agent administration, the signals are relatively subtle, which, in addition to features of the scanners such as photodetector design, limits spatial resolution and continues to spur technological advances in acquisition and analysis methods. There are multiple imaging probes in current clinical use that evaluate brain function; most commonly for patients who present with or are being followed for epilepsy, Parkinson's disease, mild cognitive impairment and more severe dementias especially Alzheimer's Disease, as well as for primary and metastatic brain tumors.

One research domain within nuclear medicine imaging that has intriguing neuropsychiatric clinical potential is the use of a class of imaging probes that bind to the

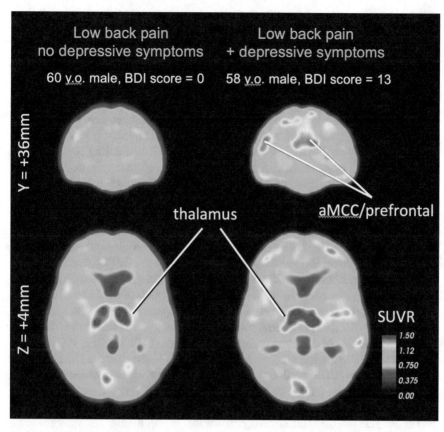

Fig. 8.5 Neuroinflammatory correlates of negative affect in people with chronic pain. Positron emission tomography (PET) imaging with the glial marker 18 kDa translocator protein (TSPO) ligand [^{11}C]PBR28 generated maps from two people with low back pain either without (left) or with (right) depressive symptoms. While both subjects demonstrate comparable PET signal in the thalamus, the participant with comorbid depressive symptoms displays additional signal elevation in aMCC, prefrontal and other regions. *aMCC* anterior middle cingulate cortex, *BDI* Beck Depression Index, *SUVR* Standardized uptake value ratio [74]

18 kDa translocator protein (TSPO), commonly referred to as a biomarker of 'neuroinflammation' or 'microglial activation' [73]. Altered TSPO binding or expression has been reported in a number of mental health conditions including depression, schizophrenia, autism spectrum disorders and bipolar disorder, as well as neurologic disorders including multiple chronic pain disorders, multiple sclerosis, stroke, traumatic brain injury, and many dementias. Regionally specific alterations in binding have even been associated with negative affect in people with chronic pain (Fig. 8.5) [74]. It is likely that these intriguing results will spur further research to tease apart complex cellular and molecular alterations relevant for mental health by identifying markers that can be used for diagnosis, prognostication and treatment targets.

8.5.3   Neurophysiology Workflows

Non-invasive electrical recordings of brain activity (electroencephalograms (EEG)) are an important diagnostic tool in clinical work-ups to assess the central nervous system and are commonly used to evaluate conditions including sleep disorders, seizures, and others. Recent research efforts have demonstrated the potential for quantitative EEG data to help predict neurocognitive outcomes after cardiac arrest [75]. Electrical recordings of brain activity also include evoked potentials associated with sensory testing and electrical recordings collected during some biofeedback treatments. For example, evoked potentials (EPs) reflect the electrophysiologic response of a specific region of the nervous system in response to a stimulus (e.g., light, sensory or motor inputs). EPs can be used to augment physical exam findings (e.g., the neurological exam), identify sensory abnormalities, or monitor changes in disease progression. Data generated through EP testing include amplitude and latency of response to the stimulus [76]. There is neurophysiological evidence from research studies using EEG and magnetoencephalography (MEG) that individuals with schizophrenia have a specific deficit in sleep spindles [77]. If shown to be true, therapies that preserve or enhance sleep oscillatory dynamics would be a promising therapeutic approach to improve cognition in schizophrenia [78].

The process for data collection, management, storage, and incorporation of key quantitative metrics of electrical brain activity into the EHR for these studies is not standardized. In current practice, time-course EEG data gathered may not be integrated with the EHR at all, or only portions of the study may be included (e.g., as an insert to the text finding included in the final report). Further, text reports from these studies are not yet standardized, yielding variation in reporting and practice. However, standardized terminology software is beginning to emerge (e.g., Standardized Computer-based Organized Reporting of EEG) [79, 80]. And the clinical translational research community is contributing to this effort through the NIH-funded National Sleep Research Resource (NSRR) [81], which supports a web-based data portal that aggregates, harmonizes, and organizes sleep and clinical data from thousands of individuals studied as part of cohort studies or clinical trials [82]. The NSRR provides a growing suite of open-source software tools to facilitate data exploration and data visualization [83]. Each deidentified study record minimally includes the summary results of an overnight sleep study, annotation files with scored events, the raw physiological signals from the sleep record, and available clinical and physiological data. NSRR is designed to be interoperable with other public data resources such as the Biologic Specimen and Data Repository Information Coordinating Center Demographics (BioLINCC) data [84] and analyzed with methods provided by the Research Resource for Complex Physiological Signals (PhysioNet) [85].

The PhysioNet project is yet another significant effort towards robust EHR data curation, mining and sharing coming from the research community [86]. PhysioNet provides the research infrastructure and knowledge to support the Medical Information Mart for Intensive Care (MIMIC) project. The MIMIC project makes available large-scale clinical databases of detailed health care data from intensive care units. The work of this team of clinical domain experts (physicians, nurses, pharmacists, respiratory therapists, and others) and data scientists has provided critical "how-to" methods to successfully overcome the challenges of using complex EHR derived data for research. MIMIC makes publicly accessible a database of over 40,000 individuals who were cared for on the critical care units of the Beth Israel Deaconess Medical Center between 2001 and 2012. This resource enables research scientists to analyze finely detailed time course physiology data obtained in the ICU in combination with more typically used EHR data elements to be used, for example, to generate a machine learning algorithm for an early warning score that predicts which patients will develop septic shock [87] .

The MIMIC effort has grown over decades with incremental improvements in the methods for primary data acquisition at the point of care in hospital intensive care units [88], through instrumentation of the data recording devices, their input to the EHR, extraction into rigorously curated, freely-accessible research databases, and development of a Code Repository for the research community to facilitate meaningful, reproducible studies [89]. The online, open-source Code Repository provides a framework for collaboration. The resources available promote greater understanding of the shared datasets, and tools that can improve the consistency and validity of users' work. The MIMIC Code Repository, built using best practices for scientific computing [90], includes code as standardized scripts in languages including Structured Query Language (SQL), Python, and R, that allow users to extract key concepts from the datasets (e.g. identification of the specific cohort of individuals used in a published manuscript or method for quantifying administration of a particular medication). The Code Repository also includes resources to support the community of users, including public discussion forums and bug trackers. While not yet wrapped around electroencephalographic (EEG) and other modalities of brain imaging, this might be in the future as the detrimental mental and behavioral sequela of the severe medical illnesses treated in ICUs are well known [91]. The negative consequences of severe medical illness on mental health has been brought to keen public attention by the COVID 19 pandemic [92, 93].

8.5.4   Neuroimaging Informatics

Robust image data management software and practices are as critical as advances in image acquisition and analytics for the development of clinically meaningful quantitative metrics derived from brain imaging [94]. While not yet incorporated into the clinical practice domain, much work has been done by the neuroimaging research community. One of the earliest efforts in this domain is the Biomedical Informatics Research Network (BIRN), a collaboratory funded by the NIH to begin to build infrastructure between technological advances in computer science and the biomedical technologies- using neuroimaging as the driving application [95]. The foundational work done by BIRN investigators included development of neuroimaging ontologies [96], and cross site calibration method development for structural [97–99] and functional MR scans [100, 101]. The NIH-funded Neuroimaging Informatics Tools and Resources Clearinghouse (NITRC—[102]) is widely used by the neuroimaging community to find and share information, tools and data. NITRC support includes a resources registry for data, tools and expertise, a brain image repository and a cloud computing environment integrated with the image repository [103].

To address the need for large enough cohorts to derive clinically meaningful knowledge from expensive brain images, substantial investments have been and continue to be made in the aggregation of large scale neuroimaging data repositories ([104] and also see the individual articles referenced therein). Simply stated, it is necessary to aggregate very large numbers of healthy ("normative") individuals, especially to follow them longitudinally, as only a small proportion will develop any particular mental health condition. Visionary leadership in this effort has come from the United Kingdom through the inclusion of systematic collection of high quality, multi-modal brain imaging in 100,000 predominately healthy participants as part of their national Biobank project [60].

In the US, the NIH has initiated, and continues to support, the collection of large scale, harmonized and richly phenotyped brain image data sets, each of which target specific clinical translational goals. The Alzheimer's Disease Neuroimaging Initiative (ADNI [105]), a longitudinal, multi-center study designed to develop clinical, imaging, genetic and biochemical biomarkers for the early detection and tracking of Alzheimer's Disease was funded jointly by the NIH and pharmaceutical industry partners. The ADNI project built upon lessons learned for harmonization of MR image acquisition parameters, calibration of fMRI activation, and data management from the early BIRN project and ongoing efforts at the participating sites. The NIH Mental Health Data Archive (NDA, [106]) integrates several neuroimaging data repositories harmonized into one database for querying and retrieval. Repositories currently supported by the NDA include the NIMH Data Archive, the Adolescent Brain Cognitive Development Study (ABCD, [107]), the Connectome Coordination Facility (CCF), the Osteoarthritis Initiative (OAI), and the NIAAA Data Archive (NIAAADA). The NDA grew out of the infrastructure supporting the National Database for Autism Research containing neuroimaging data from over 25,000 participants [108]. The Connectome Coordination Facility manages the neuroimaging data from all of the Human Connectome Projects (HCP, [59]). HCP projects include lifespan and multiple disease specific studies that aim to map the human brain at the highest possible spatial and temporal resolution in the service of connecting brain structure to function and behavior. The HEALthy Brain and Child Development (HBCD) study [109] one component of the Helping to End Addiction Long-term (HEAL) Initiative [110], is currently in the planning stages. The HBCD Study will recruit and follow a large cohort of pregnant women and their children from regions of the country significantly affected by the opioid crisis. Findings from this cohort, including, comprehensive neuroimaging assessments, will help researchers understand normative childhood brain development as well as the long-term impact of prenatal and postnatal opioid and other drug and environmental exposures.

Community commitment to practices of Free and Open Source Software (FOSS), data sharing and collaboration are essential to speed identification of clinically meaningful and actionable quantitative brain imaging metrics [111]. This is especially true in the area of functional neuroimaging where there is a dizzying array of variation in how the richly detailed data is acquired, analyzed and interpreted (see for example [112]). Comprehensive, machine readable and actionable provenance describing all elements of an imaging study: input data, processing steps, computational environment, statistical assessment, and complete results are all required in order for brain imaging data to be Findable, Accessible, Interoperable and Reusable (i.e., FAIR; [113]). The International Neuroinformatics Coordinating Facility (ICNF), a standards organization that is comprised of researchers, infrastructure providers, industry partners, and publishers from 18 countries with more than 120 affiliated institutions has been active in this domain for decades [114]. The ICNF supports numerous active Working Groups devoted to the development of key standards such as those focused on Neuroimaging Quality Control and Special Interest taskforces working on multiple fronts towards improving reproducibility in neuroimaging [115]. Another international effort devoted to this work is supported by the Organization for Human Brain Mapping (OHBM [40, 116]). Substantial support comes from the NIH funded Brain Research through Advancing Innovative Neurotechnologies (BRAIN) Initiative [117], which is making investments not only in novel methods for brain imaging data acquisition, but also in the development of informatics infrastructure specifically for analysis of human brain imaging data. And while not specifically devoted to brain imaging, the National Alliance for Medical Image Computing (NA-MIC; [118]) has a substantial focus in neuroimaging applications and has helped create and lead this culture through community-based open-access hackathons [119].

The Center for Reproducible Neuroimaging Computation (CRNC) supports the development and dissemination of a comprehensive set of brain image data management, analysis and utilization frameworks for both basic research and clinical activities. Also known as ReproNim, this center provides a community based organizational framework that encompasses the efforts of multiple related open source projects. The CRNC promulgates fundamental principles such as the consistent use of brain image data standards (e.g. DICOM [19], NIfTI [120], and the Brain Imaging Data Structure (BIDS), a standard for organizing and describing MRI datasets [121] and platforms for the sharing of code and data management (e.g. Git, GitHub, DataLad [122], as well as workflow systems (e.g. the Laboratory for NeuroImaging (LONI) pipeline [123] and Nipype (Neuroimaging in Python: Pipelines and Interfaces; [124]), the use of robust software package and execution management systems (NeuroDebian [125]), Docker [126], NeuroDocker [127], Singularity [128], NITRC-CE [102], and broad dissemination of results (NeuroVault [129]), NeuroSynth [130], [131]). A standard data model for the description of all these research elements, the Neuroimaging Data Model (NIDM, [132, 133]), is also in place to facilitate and distribute semantically annotated and unambiguous representations of the complete experimental cycle.

8.6 Challenges and Opportunities

Despite the fact that neuroimaging is not in common practice during the routine delivery of mental health services, there is good reason to believe that the future holds immense promise for high impact contributions from this source of biological data [134]. There are unquestionably a myriad of remaining technological and logistical hurdles to the incorporation of clinically useful metrics derived from imaging data into the provision of mental healthcare. However, the increasing availability of neuroimaging data collected during the delivery of routine clinical care that can be used together with the wealth of clinical data in the EHR will play a critical role in the advancement of our understanding of mental health disorders [12].

References

1. Erickson B, Greenes RA. Imaging Systems in Radiology. In: Shortliffe EH, Cimino JJ, editors. Biomedical informatics: computer applications in health care and biomedicine. London: Springer; 2014. p. 593–611.
2. Shortliffe EH, Cimino JJ. Biomedical informatics: computer applications in health care and biomedicine. London: Springer; 2013.
3. Roffman JL. Neuroprotective effects of prenatal folic acid supplementation: why timing matters. JAMA Psychiat. 2018;75(7):747–8.
4. Murphy SN, Herrick C, Wang Y, Wang TD, Sack D, Andriole KP, et al. High throughput tools to access images from clinical archives for research. J Digit Imaging. 2015;28(2):194–204.
5. Eryilmaz H, Dowling KF, Huntington FC, Rodriguez-Thompson A, Soare TW, Beard LM, et al. Association of prenatal exposure to population-wide folic acid fortification with altered cerebral cortex maturation in youths. JAMA Psychiat. 2018;75(9):918–28.
6. Murphy SN, Gainer V, Chueh HC. A visual interface designed for novice users to find research patient cohorts in a large biomedical database. AMIA Annu Symp Proc. 2003:489–93.
7. Kohane IS, Churchill SE, Murphy SN. A translational engine at the national scale: informatics for integrating biology and the bedside. J Am Med Inform Assoc. 2012;19(2):181–5.
8. Satterthwaite TD, Elliott MA, Ruparel K, Loughead J, Prabhakaran K, Calkins ME, et al. Neuroimaging of the Philadelphia neurodevelopmental cohort. NeuroImage. 2014;86:544–53.
9. Evans AC. Brain development cooperative G. The NIH MRI study of normal brain development. NeuroImage. 2006;30(1):184–202.
10. Callaghan BC, Kerber KA, Pace RJ, Skolarus LE, Burke JF. Headaches and neuroimaging: high utilization and costs despite guidelines. JAMA Intern Med. 2014;174(5):819–21.
11. Ou Y, Zollei L, Retzepi K, Castro V, Bates SV, Pieper S, et al. Using clinically acquired MRI to construct age-specific ADC atlases: quantifying spatiotemporal ADC changes from birth to 6-year old. Hum Brain Mapp. 2017;38(6):3052–68.
12. Sotardi S, Gollub RL, Bates SV, Weiss R, Murphy SN, Grant PE, Ou Y. Voxelwise and regional brain apparent diffusion coefficient changes on MRI from birth to 6 years of age. Radiology. 2021;298(2):415–24.
13. Benson NM, Kadzielski S. Gastroenterology. In: Hazen EP, McDougle CJ, editors. Massachusetts general hospital textbook of medical care in autism spectrum disorder. New York City: Humana Press Springer International Publishing; 2018.
14. De Berardis D, Rapini G, Olivieri L, Di Nicola D, Tomasetti C, Valchera A, et al. Safety of antipsychotics for the treatment of schizophrenia: a focus on the adverse effects of clozapine. Ther Adv Drug Saf. 2018;9(5):237–56.

15. Kuo MD, Jamshidi N. Behind the numbers: decoding molecular phenotypes with radiogenom-ics–guiding principles and technical considerations. Radiology. 2014;270(2):320–5.
16. Mazurowski MA. Radiogenomics: what it is and why it is important. J Am Coll Radiol. 2015;12(8):862–6.
17. Gajawelli N, Tsao S, Kromnick M, Nelson M, Lepore N. Image postprocessing adoption trends in clinical medical imaging. J Am Coll Radiol. 2019;16(7):945–51.
18. Gillies RJ, Kinahan PE, Hricak H. Radiomics: images are more than pictures, they are data. Radiology. 2016;278(2):563–77.
19. DICOM Standards committee. Digital imaging and communications in medicine. Available from: https://www.dicomstandard.org.
20. Fedorov A, Beichel R, Kalpathy-Cramer J, Clunie D, Onken M, Riesmeier J, et al. Quantitative imaging informatics for cancer research. JCO Clin Cancer Inform. 2020;4:444–53.
21. Rubin DL, Kahn CE Jr. Common data elements in radiology. Radiology. 2017;283(3):837–44.
22. Pons E, Braun LM, Hunink MG, Kors JA. Natural language processing in radiology: a systematic review. Radiology. 2016;279(2):329–43.
23. Silveira PC, Ip IK, Goldhaber SZ, Piazza G, Benson CB, Khorasani R. Performance of wells score for deep vein thrombosis in the inpatient setting. JAMA Intern Med. 2015;175(7):1112–7.
24. Siwicki B. Radiology practices using AI and NLP to boost MIPS paymentsMay 31, 2020. Available from: https://www.healthcareitnews.com/news/radiology-practices-using-ai-and-nlp-boost-mips-payments.
25. Wheater E, Mair G, Sudlow C, Alex B, Grover C, Whiteley W. A validated natural language processing algorithm for brain imaging phenotypes from radiology reports in UK electronic health records. BMC Med Inform Decis Mak. 2019;19(1):184.
26. D'Orsi CJ, Sickles EA, Mendelson EB, Morris EA, et al. ACR BI-RADS® Atlas, breast imaging reporting and data system. Reston, VA: American College of Radiology; 2013.
27. Turkbey B, Rosenkrantz AB, Haider MA, Padhani AR, Villeirs G, Macura KJ, et al. Prostate imaging reporting and data system version 2.1: 2019 update of prostate imaging reporting and data system version 2. Eur Urol. 2019;76(3):340–51.
28. Alkasab TK, Bizzo BC, Berland LL, Nair S, Pandharipande PV, Harvey HB. Creation of an open framework for point-of-care computer-assisted reporting and decision support tools for radiologists. J Am Coll Radiol. 2017;14(9):1184–9.
29. Flanders AE, Jordan JE. The ASNR-ACR-RSNA common data elements project: what will it do for the house of neuroradiology? AJNR Am J Neuroradiol. 2019;40(1):14–8.
30. American Society of Neuroradiology. ASNR Neuroradiology CDE distribution supporting documentation. Available from: https://www.asnr.org/resources/cde/
31. Radiological society of North America. Common DATA Elements (CDEs) for radiology. Available from: https://www.radelement.org/about
32. National Cancer Institute. Annotation and Image Markup–AIM. Available from: https://wiki.nci.nih.gov/display/AIM/Annotation+and+Image+Markup+-+AIM
33. Channin DS, Mongkolwat P, Kleper V, Sepukar K, Rubin DL. The caBIG annotation and image Markup project. J Digit Imaging. 2010;23(2):217–25.
34. Schwartz LH, Litiere S, de Vries E, Ford R, Gwyther S, Mandrekar S, et al. RECIST 1.1-Update and clarification: from the RECIST committee. Eur J Cancer. 2016;62:132–7.
35. Louis S, Morita-Sherman M, Jones S, Vegh D, Bingaman W, Blumcke I, et al. Hippocampal sclerosis detection with neuroquant compared with neuroradiologists. AJNR Am J Neuroradiol. 2020;41(4):591–7.
36. Yu S, Ma Y, Gronsbell J, Cai T, Ananthakrishnan AN, Gainer VS, et al. Enabling phenotypic big data with PheNorm. J Am Med Inform Assoc. 2018;25(1):54–60.
37. Zwanenburg A, Vallieres M, Abdalah MA, Aerts H, Andrearczyk V, Apte A, et al. The image biomarker standardization initiative: standardized quantitative radiomics for high-throughput image-based phenotyping. Radiology. 2020;295(2):328–38.
38. Raichlen DA, Klimentidis YC, Bharadwaj PK, Alexander GE. Differential associations of engagement in physical activity and estimated cardiorespiratory fitness with brain volume in middle-aged to older adults. Brain Imaging Behav. 2020;14:1994–2003.

39. Mateos-Perez JM, Dadar M, Lacalle-Aurioles M, Iturria-Medina Y, Zeighami Y, Evans AC. Structural neuroimaging as clinical predictor: a review of machine learning applications. Neuroimage Clin. 2018;20:506–22.
40. Nichols TE, Das S, Eickhoff SB, Evans AC, Glatard T, Hanke M, et al. Best practices in data analysis and sharing in neuroimaging using MRI. Nat Neurosci. 2017;20(3):299–303.
41. Alsop DC, Detre JA, Golay X, Gunther M, Hendrikse J, Hernandez-Garcia L, et al. Recommended implementation of arterial spin-labeled perfusion MRI for clinical applications: a consensus of the ISMRM perfusion study group and the European consortium for ASL in dementia. Magn Reson Med. 2015;73(1):102–16.
42. Gilmore CD, Comeau CR, Alessi AM, Blaine M, El Fakhri GN, Hunt JK, et al. PET/MR imaging consensus paper: a joint paper by the society of nuclear medicine and molecular imaging technologist section and the section for magnetic resonance technologists. J Nucl Med Technol. 2013;41(2):108–13.
43. Allen B, Agarwal S, Kalpathy-Cramer J, Dreyer K. Democratizing AI. J Am Coll Radiol. 2019;16(7):961–3.
44. Wang KC, Kohli M, Carrino JA. Technology standards in imaging: a practical overview. J Am Coll Radiol. 2014;11(12 Pt B):1251–9.
45. Larson DB, Magnus DC, Lungren MP, Shah NH, Langlotz CP. Ethics of using and sharing clinical imaging data for artificial intelligence: a proposed framework. Radiology. 2020;295(3):675–82.
46. Bellsmith KN, Brown J, Kim SJ, Goldstein IH, Coyner A, Ostmo S, et al. Aggressive posterior retinopathy of prematurity: clinical and quantitative imaging features in a large North American cohort. Ophthalmology. 2020;127(8):1105–12
47. Bridge CP, Rosenthal M, Wright B, Kotecha G, Fintelmann F, Troschel F, et al. Fully-Automated analysis of body composition from CT in cancer patients using convolutional neural networks. In: Stoyanov D, Taylor Z, Sarikaya D, et al, eds. OR 2.0 Context-aware operating theaters, computer assisted robotic endoscopy, Clinical image-based procedures, and Skin image analysis. CARE 2018, CLIP 2018, OR 2.0 2018, ISIC 2018. Lecture Notes in Computer Science, vol 11041. Cham, Switzerland: Springer, 2018;204–13.
48. Yankeelov TE, Mankoff DA, Schwartz LH, Lieberman FS, Buatti JM, Mountz JM, et al. Quantitative imaging in cancer clinical trials. Clin Cancer Res. 2016;22(2):284–90.
49. Mandel JC, Kreda DA, Mandl KD, Kohane IS, Ramoni RB. SMART on FHIR: a standards-based, interoperable apps platform for electronic health records. J Am Med Inform Assoc. 2016;23(5):899–908.
50. Wagholikar KB, Mandel JC, Klann JG, Wattanasin N, Mendis M, Chute CG, et al. SMART-on-FHIR implemented over i2b2. J Am Med Inform Assoc. 2017;24(2):398–402.
51. Milchenko M, Snyder AZ, LaMontagne P, Shimony JS, Benzinger TL, Fouke SJ, et al. Heterogeneous optimization framework: reproducible preprocessing of multi-spectral clinical MRI for neuro-oncology imaging research. Neuroinformatics. 2016;14(3):305–17.
52. Polimeni JR, Wald LL. Magnetic resonance imaging technology-bridging the gap between noninvasive human imaging and optical microscopy. Curr Opin Neurobiol. 2018;50:250–60.
53. Budinger TF, Bird MD. MRI and MRS of the human brain at magnetic fields of 14T to 20T: Technical feasibility, safety, and neuroscience horizons. NeuroImage. 2018;168:509–31.
54. Fennema-Notestine C, Gamst AC, Quinn BT, Pacheco J, Jernigan TL, Thal L, et al. Feasibility of multi-site clinical structural neuroimaging studies of aging using legacy data. Neuroinformatics. 2007;5(4):235–45.
55. Ou Y, Gollub RL, Retzepi K, Reynolds N, Pienaar R, Pieper S, et al. Brain extraction in pediatric ADC maps, toward characterizing neuro-development in multi-platform and multi-institution clinical images. NeuroImage. 2015;122:246–61.
56. Weiss RJ, Bates SV, Song Y, Zhang Y, Herzberg EM, Chen YC, et al. Mining multi-site clinical data to develop machine learning MRI biomarkers: application to neonatal hypoxic ischemic encephalopathy. J Transl Med. 2019;17(1):385.
57. FreeSurfer. FreeSurfer. Available from: https://surfer.nmr.mgh.harvard.edu
58. FreeSurfer. Zotero. Available from: https://www.zotero.org/freesurfer/collections/5KQCZFRB

59. NIH Blueprint for Neuroscience Research. Connectome coordination facility. Available from: https://www.humanconnectome.org
60. Miller KL, Alfaro-Almagro F, Bangerter NK, Thomas DL, Yacoub E, Xu J, et al. Multimodal population brain imaging in the UK Biobank prospective epidemiological study. Nat Neurosci. 2016;19(11):1523–36.
61. Smith SM, Vidaurre D, Alfaro-Almagro F, Nichols TE, Miller KL. Estimation of brain age delta from brain imaging. NeuroImage. 2019;200:528–39.
62. Nobis L, Manohar SG, Smith SM, Alfaro-Almagro F, Jenkinson M, Mackay CE, et al. Hippocampal volume across age: nomograms derived from over 19,700 people in UK Biobank. Neuroimage Clin. 2019;101904:23.
63. Littlejohns TJ, Holliday J, Gibson LM, Garratt S, Oesingmann N, Alfaro-Almagro F, et al. The UK Biobank imaging enhancement of 100,000 participants: rationale, data collection, management and future directions. Nat Commun. 2624;11(1):2020.
64. Buchbinder BR. Functional magnetic resonance imaging. Handb Clin Neurol. 2016;135:61–92.
65. Black DF, Little JT, Johnson DR. Neuroanatomical considerations in preoperative functional brain mapping. Top Magn Reson Imaging. 2019;28(4):213–24.
66. Gabrieli John DE, Ghosh Satrajit S, Whitfield-Gabrieli S. Prediction as a humanitarian and pragmatic contribution from human cognitive neuroscience. Neuron. 2015;85(1):11–26.
67. Zuk J, Dunstan J, Norton E, Yu X, Ozernov-Palchik O, Wang Y, et al. Multifactorial pathways facilitate resilience among kindergarteners at risk for dyslexia: a longitudinal behavioral and neuroimaging study. Dev Sci. 2020:e12983.
68. Finniss DG, Kaptchuk TJ, Miller F, Benedetti F. Biological, clinical, and ethical advances of placebo effects. Lancet. 2010;375(9715):686–95.
69. Harvard Health Publishing. The power of the placebo effect. Available from: https://www.health.harvard.edu/mental-health/the-power-of-the-placebo-effect
70. Duarte JMN, Xin L. Magnetic resonance spectroscopy in schizophrenia: evidence for glutamatergic dysfunction and impaired energy metabolism. Neurochem Res. 2019;44(1):102–16.
71. Houtepen LC, Schur RR, Wijnen JP, Boer VO, Boks MP, Kahn RS, et al. Acute stress effects on GABA and glutamate levels in the prefrontal cortex: a 7T (1)H magnetic resonance spectroscopy study. Neuroimage Clin. 2017;14:195–200.
72. Mettler Jr FA, Guiberteau ML. Essentials of nuclear medicine and molecular imaging. 7th ed: Elsevier; 2018.
73. Notter T, Coughlin JM, Sawa A, Meyer U. Reconceptualization of translocator protein as a biomarker of neuroinflammation in psychiatry. Mol Psychiatry. 2018;23(1):36–47.
74. Albrecht DS, Kim M, Akeju O, Torrado-Carvajal A, Edwards RR, Zhang Y, et al. The neuroinflammatory component of negative affect in patients with chronic pain. Mol Psychiatry. 2021;26(3):864–74
75. Amorim E, van der Stoel M, Nagaraj SB, Ghassemi MM, Jing J, O'Reilly UM, et al. Quantitative EEG reactivity and machine learning for prognostication in hypoxic-ischemic brain injury. Clin Neurophysiol. 2019;130(10):1908–16.
76. Walsh P, Kane N, Butler S. The clinical role of evoked potentials. J Neurol Neurosurgery & Psychiatry. 2005;76(suppl 2):ii16–22.
77. Purcell SM, Manoach DS, Demanuele C, Cade BE, Mariani S, Cox R, et al. Characterizing sleep spindles in 11,630 individuals from the National Sleep Research Resource. Nat Commun. 2017;8:15930.
78. Manoach DS, Mylonas D, Baxter B. Targeting sleep oscillations to improve memory in schizophrenia. Schizophr Res. 2020;221:63–70
79. Beniczky S, Aurlien H, Brogger JC, Hirsch LJ, Schomer DL, Trinka E, et al. Standardized computer-based organized reporting of EEG: SCORE - Second version. Clin Neurophysiol. 2017;128(11):2334–46.
80. McCarthy LH, Longhurst CA, Hahn JS. Special requirements for electronic medical records in neurology. Neurol Clin Pract. 2015;5(1):67–73.
81. NHLBI. National Sleep Research Resource. updated 2020. Available from: https://sleepdata.org

82. Dean DA, Goldberger AL, Mueller R, Kim M, Rueschman M, Mobley D, et al. Scaling up scientific discovery in sleep medicine: the national sleep research resource. Sleep. 2016;39(5):1151–64.

83. MkDocs. Luna: software for the analysis of sleep signal data. Available from: http://zzz.bwh.harvard.edu/luna/

84. NHLBI. BioLINCC. Available from: https://biolincc.nhlbi.nih.gov/home/

85. MIT Laboratory for Computational Physiology. PhysioNet. Available from: https://physionet.org

86. Goldberger AL, Amaral LA, Glass L, Hausdorff JM, Ivanov PC, Mark RG, et al. PhysioBank, PhysioToolkit, and PhysioNet: components of a new research resource for complex physiologic signals. Circulation. 2000;101(23):E215–20.

87. Henry KE, Hager DN, Pronovost PJ, Saria S. A targeted real-time early warning score (TREWScore) for septic shock. Sci Transl Med. 2015;7(299):299ra122.

88. Johnson AEW, Pollard TJ, Shen L, Lehman WH, Feng M, Ghassemi M, et al. MIMIC-III, a freely accessible critical care database. Scientific Data. 2016;3(1):160035.

89. Johnson AEW, Stone DJ, Celi LA, Pollard TJ. The MIMIC code repository: enabling reproducibility in critical care research. J Am Med Inform Assoc. 2017;25(1):32–9.

90. Wilson G, Aruliah DA, Brown CT, Chue Hong NP, Davis M, Guy RT, et al. Best practices for scientific computing. PLoS Biol. 2014;12(1):e1001745.

91. LaBuzetta JN, Rosand J, Vranceanu AM. Review: post-intensive care syndrome: unique challenges in the neurointensive care unit. Neurocrit Care. 2019;31(3):534–45.

92. Holmes EA, O'Connor RC, Perry VH, Tracey I, Wessely S, Arseneault L, et al. Multidisciplinary research priorities for the COVID-19 pandemic: a call for action for mental health science. Lancet Psychiatry. 2020;7(6):547–60.

93. Benson NM, Ongur D, Hsu J. COVID-19 testing and patients in mental health facilities. Lancet Psychiatry. 2020;7(6):476–7.

94. Marcus DS, Erickson BJ, Pan T, Group CIIW. Imaging infrastructure for research. Part 2. Data management practices. J Digit Imaging. 2012;25(5):566–9.

95. Helmer KG, Ambite JL, Ames J, Ananthakrishnan R, Burns G, Chervenak AL, et al. Enabling collaborative research using the Biomedical Informatics Research Network (BIRN). J Am Med Inform Assoc. 2011;18(4):416–22.

96. Bug WJ, Ascoli GA, Grethe JS, Gupta A, Fennema-Notestine C, Laird AR, et al. The NIFSTD and BIRNLex vocabularies: building comprehensive ontologies for neuroscience. Neuroinformatics. 2008;6(3):175–94.

97. Jovicich J, Czanner S, Greve D, Haley E, van der Kouwe A, Gollub R, et al. Reliability in multi-site structural MRI studies: effects of gradient non-linearity correction on phantom and human data. NeuroImage. 2006;30(2):436–43.

98. Han X, Jovicich J, Salat D, van der Kouwe A, Quinn B, Czanner S, et al. Reliability of MRI-derived measurements of human cerebral cortical thickness: the effects of field strength, scanner upgrade and manufacturer. NeuroImage. 2006;32(1):180–94.

99. Jovicich J, Czanner S, Han X, Salat D, van der Kouwe A, Quinn B, et al. MRI-derived measurements of human subcortical, ventricular and intracranial brain volumes: Reliability effects of scan sessions, acquisition sequences, data analyses, scanner upgrade, scanner vendors and field strengths. NeuroImage. 2009;46(1):177–92.

100. Keator DB, van Erp TGM, Turner JA, Glover GH, Mueller BA, Liu TT, et al. The function biomedical informatics research network data repository. NeuroImage. 2016;124(Pt B):1074–9.

101. Yendiki A, Greve DN, Wallace S, Vangel M, Bockholt J, Mueller BA, et al. Multi-site characterization of an fMRI working memory paradigm: reliability of activation indices. NeuroImage. 2010;53(1):119–31.

102. NeuroImaging Tools & Resources Collaboratory. NITRC. Available from: https://www.nitrc.org

103. Kennedy DN, Haselgrove C, Riehl J, Preuss N, Buccigrossi R. The NITRC image repository. NeuroImage. 2016;124(Pt B):1069–73.
104. Eickhoff S, Nichols TE, Van Horn JD, Turner JA. Sharing the wealth: neuroimaging data repositories. NeuroImage. 2016;124(Pt B):1065–8.
105. Alzheimer's Disease Neuroimaging Initiative. Alzheimer's disease neuroimaging initiative. Available from: http://adni.loni.usc.edu
106. National Institutes of Health. NIMH Data Archive. Available from: https://nda.nih.gov
107. US Department of Health and Human Services. Adolescent brain cognitive development. Available from: https://abcdstudy.org.
108. Hall D, Huerta MF, McAuliffe MJ, Farber GK. Sharing heterogeneous data: the national database for autism research. Neuroinformatics. 2012;10(4):331–9.
109. National Institutes of Health. HEALthy brain and child development study. Available from: https://heal.nih.gov/research/infants-and-children/healthy-brain
110. Collins FS, Koroshetz WJ, Volkow ND. Helping to end addiction over the long-term: the research plan for the NIH HEAL initiative. JAMA. 2018;320(2):129–30.
111. Halchenko YO, Hanke M. Open is Not Enough. Let's Take the Next Step: An Integrated, Community-Driven Computing Platform for Neuroscience. Front Neuroinform. 2012;6:22.
112. Carp J. On the plurality of (methodological) worlds: estimating the analytic flexibility of FMRI experiments. Front Neurosci. 2012;6:149.
113. Wilkinson MD, Dumontier M, Aalbersberg IJ, Appleton G, Axton M, Baak A, et al. The FAIR guiding principles for scientific data management and stewardship. Sci Data. 2016;3:160018.
114. International Neuroinformatics Coordinating Facility. A standards organization for open and FAIR neuroscience. Available from: https://www.incf.org
115. International Neuroinformatics Coordinating Facility. INCF special interest groups. Available from: https://www.incf.org/activities/special-interest-groups
116. Nichols T, Das S, Eickhoff SB, Evans AC, Glatard T, Hanke M. et al. Best practices in data analysis and sharing in neuroimaging using MRI. Nat Neurosci. 2017;20:299–303.
117. National Institutes of Health. The BRAIN Initiative. Available from: https://braininitiative.nih.gov
118. National Alliance for Medical Image Computing. National Alliance for Medical Image Computing (NA-MIC). Available from: https://www.na-mic.org
119. Kapur T, Pieper S, Fedorov A, Fillion-Robin JC, Halle M, O'Donnell L, et al. Increasing the impact of medical image computing using community-based open-access hackathons: The NA-MIC and 3D Slicer experience. Med Image Anal. 2016;33:176–80.
120. ReproNim. NIfTI-1 data format. Available from: https://nifti.nimh.nih.gov/nifti-1/
121. Gorgolewski KJ, Auer T, Calhoun VD, Craddock RC, Das S, Duff EP, et al. The brain imaging data structure, a format for organizing and describing outputs of neuroimaging experiments. Sci Data. 2016;3:160044.
122. Gorgolewski K, Burns CD, Madison C, Clark D, Halchenko YO, Waskom ML, et al. Nipype: a flexible, lightweight and extensible neuroimaging data processing framework in python. Front Neuroinform. 2011;5:13.
123. Rex DE, Ma JQ, Toga AW. The LONI pipeline processing environment. NeuroImage. 2003;19(3):1033–48.
124. Neuroimaging in Python. Nipype: neuroimaging in python pipelines and interfaces. Available from: https://nipype.readthedocs.io/en/latest/
125. NeuroDebian Team. The ultimate neuroscience software platform. Available from: http://neuro.debian.net
126. Docker Inc. Docker. Available from: https://www.docker.com
127. NeuroDocker. NeuroDocker. Available from: https://github.com/ReproNim/neurodocker
128. Sylabs. Singularity Examples. Available from: https://sylabs.io/docs/
129. NeuroVault. NeuroVault. Available from: https://neurovault.org
130. Neurosynth. Neurosynth. Available from: https://neurovault.org

131. Kennedy DN, Abraham SA, Bates JF, Crowley A, Ghosh S, Gillespie T, et al. Everything matters: the Repronim perspective on reproducible neuroimaging. Front Neuroinform. 2019;13(1)

132. NIDM Working Group. NIDM 2018. Available from: http://nidm.nidash.org

133. Keator DB, Helmer K, Steffener J, Turner JA, Van Erp TG, Gadde S, et al. Towards structured sharing of raw and derived neuroimaging data across existing resources. NeuroImage. 2013;82:647–61.

134. Shen L, Thompson PM. Brain imaging genomics: integrated analysis and machine learning. Proc IEEE. 2020;108(1):125–62.

Chapter 9
Informatics Technologies for the Acquisition of Psychological, Behavioral, Interpersonal, Social and Environmental Data

Elena Tenenbaum, Piper A. Ranallo, and Janna Hastings

Abstract The collection, capture, storage, sharing, and interpretation of data are essential to all research and practice in mental health. A wide range of informatics technologies and tools have been developed to facilitate data use across the full knowledge acquisition lifecycle. In this chapter, we focus on data acquisition. We introduce the field of psychometrics—the science of measurement in psychology. We discuss the unique challenges of data acquisition in mental health by exploring the nature of psychological, behavioral, interpersonal, social, and environmental data in the context of mental health. Finally, we discuss some current challenges in the use of informatics technologies for data in these domains and how those challenges might be addressed in the future.

Keywords Psychometrics · Reliability · Validity · Measurement · Social, Behavioural, Interpersonal and Environmental data · Data Acquisition

9.1 Introduction

Mental healthcare is focused on optimizing the mental, emotional, behavioral, and social functioning of individuals, families, and communities. High quality mental healthcare prevents, detects, and treats mental health problems. As in physical

E. Tenenbaum (✉)
Duke University, Durham, NC, USA
e-mail: elena.tenenbaum@duke.edu

P. A. Ranallo
Six Aims for Behavioral Health, Minneapolis, MN, USA
e-mail: pranallo@sixaims.org; sven0018@umn.edu

J. Hastings
Clinical, Educational and Health Psychology, University College London, London, UK
e-mail: j.hastings@ucl.ac.uk

© Springer Nature Switzerland AG 2021
J. D. Tenenbaum, P. A. Ranallo (eds.), *Mental Health Informatics*, Health Informatics, https://doi.org/10.1007/978-3-030-70558-9_9

healthcare, our ability to deliver high quality and safe clinical care depends on effectively and consistently acquiring and applying new and improved knowledge. This knowledge acquisition process includes basic research on the etiology of disease and the mechanism underlying normative and pathological development; clinical research about the most effective targeted interventions; and both health services and implementation science research about how to effectively translate what we have learned from basic and clinical research into practice.

Knowledge discovery in mental health, as in any healthcare domain, depends on our ability to identify, name, and empirically measure relevant phenomena. In mental health, this is no easy task! In physical healthcare, the entities and processes of interest are often more tangible—they describe physical phenomena. Increasingly sophisticated and reliable technologies that allow researchers and clinicians to see, measure, and quantify biological entities and processes have been developed and widely disseminated. The challenge in mental health lies largely in how we objectively define and reproducibly quantify the relevant entities and processes: the behaviors, internal experiences, and interpersonal and social interactions relevant to mental health and illness. Compared to physiologic phenomena, such as temperature, blood pressure, or weight, "psychological" phenomena such as level of introversion, depth of sadness, ability to detect social cues, and cognitive capacities are much more challenging to quantify. Interpersonal phenomena, such as quality of attachment, manifestations of racial contempt, or level of interpersonal respect between members of a family, team, or community are equally difficult to measure. Still, in order to improve a person's social, emotional, interpersonal, and cognitive functioning, we need objective ways to measure such phenomena.

In short, the kinds of things we most need to measure in mental healthcare are fundamentally different from the kinds of things we measure in physical healthcare. As a result, the tools we use for measurement in mental health are fundamentally different from those used in physical health. But as in physical health, they are developed using robust scientific methods that have been empirically demonstrated to produce high quality representations of the phenomena they seek to measure. Just as medical measurement technologies are grounded in the best and most current knowledge from the physical and biological sciences, so too are social and behavioral measurement technologies grounded in the best and most current knowledge from the behavioral and social sciences. With that said, mental health data do present unique challenges in assessing the distinction between the real-world thing being measured (e.g., the emotional state of sadness), the observable manifestation of that thing as a "signal" (e.g., tears, facial expression, body language, social behaviors), and the representation of the signal as "data" in a research repository or clinical record (e.g., "affect is sad"). This is important in mental health because the relationship between the underlying state and the signal used to detect it is less certain than it is in the biological sciences. For example, a person experiencing a profound depression may smile and say they feel content, but an anemic person will have a hard time faking a normal red blood cell count.

In this chapter, we start with an introduction to psychometrics - the science concerned with the measurement of psychological phenomena. We give an overview of the types of clinical phenomena (emotions, thoughts, personal relationships, and one's role in the larger community) relevant in mental health research and practice. We introduce technologies that allow us to detect and objectively measure these phenomena. We conclude with limitations and outstanding challenges, in particular relating to the heterogeneity of datasets needed for mental health informatics.

9.2 Psychometrics: A Brief Primer

Psychomerics is the field of study concerned with the theory and technique of psychological measurement. The origins of the belief that we can measure the psychological features (i.e. mental processes and characteristics) of a person are often traced back to 1859 when Darwin published *The Origin of Species* and drew attention to the notion of individual differences. Sir Francis Galton, a relative of Darwin's, later applied Darwin's conceptualization to the study of humans. Galton, often referred to as "the father of psychometrics" began his investigation of individual differences with measures of concrete abilities including reaction time and visual perception, arguing that those with superior performance on these measures would be most likely to thrive [1]. These early studies of psychological phenomena were largely restricted to *psychophysics*, or the relationship between physical stimuli and perception. In psychophysics, one can draw a direct parallel between physical units and the brain's ability to process those stimuli in the physical world. In this way, psychological functions were assessed as if they were concrete entities with concrete values, as in the weight or length of a specimen in biology. When attempting to measure introversion, apathy, or pleasure, such a direct line becomes much less practical. *Psychometric theory* allows for the scientific and statistically driven measurement of these unobservable abilities, attitudes, and traits.

Unlike psychophysics, modern psychometrics relies on the assumption that an underlying trait or state such as depression or IQ, often called a *latent trait*, exists and can be estimated (with some level of error) by asking multiple questions or observing multiple behaviors that one would expect to be associated with that trait. This approach to measurement development in psychology was formalized by a taskforce assembled by the American Psychological Association (APA) in the 1950s in an effort to establish the criteria necessary for publishing a psychological test.

Because we cannot determine a direct connection between the underlying traits and the mental capacities that can be observed, rigorous statistical analysis must be performed to assess a measure before it is considered "psychometrically valid". A test must be both *reliable* and *valid* to be of scientific use. Reliability can be assessed in a number of ways. *Test-retest reliability* refers to the tendency for the same person given the same test to receive the same score at two time points. *Internal consistency* is another type of reliability which assesses the extent to which different items on the same measure are related to each other. This can be assessed with *a split-half correlation analysis* which, as the name would suggest, explores the correlation between two halves of the same measure. *Inter-rater reliability* describes the consistency with which two raters administering the same test to the same individuals would score responses and interpret results in the same way. Inter-rater reliability is particularly relevant for assessments that involve behavioral observations.

Validity is the other critical piece of psychometric validation. Validity refers to the extent to which the instrument measures what it claims to measure. In its weakest form, this can be described with *face validity* which refers to the extent to which questions on, or observations from, the measure are likely to be related to the underlying trait under investigation. This is often assessed informally by asking "experts in the field" how consistent the measure is with their experience of the feature being measured. *Content validity* addresses the completeness with which the measure assesses a given construct. For example, asking whether a person is having difficulty sleeping might be one indication of anxiety, but that item alone would not be sufficient for content validity in assessing anxiety. *Discriminant validity* measures the lack of correlation between two measures that you would not expect to be related. This is particularly important when you are attempting to develop a measure of one specific feature or ability (*i.e.*, social skills) and need to demonstrate that your measure is not attributable to more general measures (e.g., IQ).

Criterion validity, also called *convergent validity* assesses the extent to which the result of a measure is consistent with other measures or behaviors we would expect to be related. For example, although the two US standardized academic tests—SATs and ACTs—have convergent validity (i.e., scores on the two measures are highly correlated and likely represent similar abilities), their criterion validity as reasonable predictors of how one will perform in college has been called into question [2].

One of the most famous outcomes of the APAs 1950 taskforce was an article by Cronbach and Meehl [3], in which they coined the terms *construct validity* and *nomological network*. According to Cronbach and Meehl, in order for a construct to be "scientifically admissible," it must be meaningfully related to other theoretical constructs or observable behaviors (i.e., it must have construct validity). Put simply, if you want to claim that your measure of a given construct is meaningful, it should be related to other behaviors or constructs one would expect to find in a network of related behaviors, inferred latent traits, and constructs.

Cronbach and Meehl defined a nomological network as "the interlocking system of laws which constitute a theory." In order to provide evidence that your measure has construct validity, Cronbach and Meehl argued, you had to develop a nomological network for your measure. Nomological networks may therefore be used to assess the empirical support for psychological theories (see Fig. 9.1).

In one recent example of the utility of the nomological network for empirical analysis, Hyatt et al. [5] used it to test the theory that narcissism is related to self-esteem. If true, tests that are purported to measure these traits ought to correlate. In fact, using a combination of self-report measures, behavioral observations, and clinical interviews to measure narcissism and self-esteem, the authors demonstrated that while both constructs are related to assertive interpersonal styles, self-esteem is adaptive

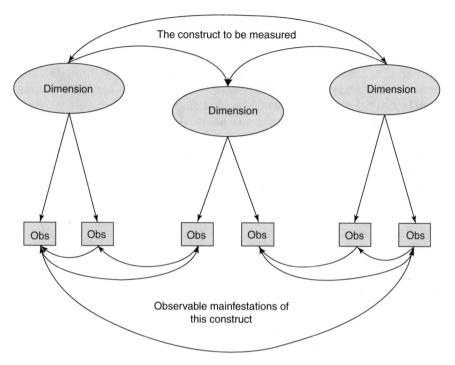

Fig. 9.1 The nomological network. A nomological network "includes a theoretical framework for what is being measured, specifying linkages between different hypothetical constructs, between different observable attributes, and between hypothetical constructs and observable attributes. Qualitatively different measurement operations may be said to measure the same attributes if their locations in the nomological network link them to the same hypothetical construct variable" [4]

and negatively associated with psychopathology while narcissism was uniquely related to callousness, grandiosity, entitlement, and demeaning attitudes towards others.

As the field of psychometrics was emerging, so too were high speed supercomputers [6]. This allowed psychometricians to run *factor analyses* more efficiently, which they used to determine empirically what latent factors (or theorized underlying traits) were driving responses to their tests and measures. Factor analysis, while a powerful tool, leaves open the largely subjective question of how many latent factors one ought to include in a model. (See Chap. 12 for more detail.)

With increasingly accessible statistical packages for running these types of psychometric analyses, a vast number of psychological instruments have been developed [7]. Some estimates suggest that nearly 20,000 psychological measures are created each year [8]. Unfortunately, most of these measures are proprietary and overlap, at least to some extent, with existing measures. This leaves measure selection to the researcher or clinician who bases that decision on the merits of a given measure for their specific clinical practice or research question, thereby creating a nightmare for data standardization. Comparability of research findings and one's capacity to integrate data from multiple studies for meta-analyses is significantly hampered by these disparate measures.

9.3 Types of Data Relevant for Mental Health

Measurement in mental health is used to synthesize across different symptomatic, behavioral, social and psychological elements in order to support the diagnosis of, or assign a quantitative metric to, the risk or severity of a given syndrome or condition. Mental health conditions and associated diagnoses are of course a prominent type of data of core relevance for mental health. However, the focus of this chapter is not only such conditions and diagnoses, but also the types of the elementary units of data that are included as questions in these questionnaires and metrics, the distinguishable individual elements that in total give evidence for the syndromes and conditions that are inferred on their basis. To this end, we distinguish several broad groupings of types of data relevant for mental health (Fig. 9.2) relating to different categories of phenomena in the world: psychological, behavioral, interpersonal, social, and environmental.

9.3.1 Psychological Data

With its roots in philosophical discussions of the distinction between mind and body (Descartes, 1596–1650), the mind as a blank slate or *tabula rasa* (Locke, 1632–1704), and the misguided efforts of phrenology to make sense of the mind from the shape of the head (Franz Joseph Gall, 1758–1828), it has been said that "Psychology has a long past but a short history," (Hermann Ebbinghaus, 1850–1909). When the American philosopher and psychologist William James published *The Principles of Psychology* in 1890, he defined psychology as "the science of mental life." This science has evolved significantly in the last two centuries, to encompass theories of behavior, cognition, personality, intelligence and most recently, social psychology. The psychological data that have been used to test these theories present some of the most challenging areas for standardized data acquisition as they involve subjective entities to which observational access is typically indirect.

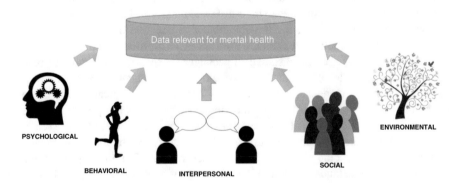

Fig. 9.2 Types of data relevant for mental health

9.3.1.1 What Is Measured

A broad range of psychological phenomena are relevant for mental health. One of the most widely studied is intelligence. Some of the earliest efforts at objective measurement of intelligence are attributed to Alfred Binet who was tasked with determining which French children should be removed from typical education classes for lack of ability. Binet went on to develop the first intelligence test, which, following many iterations, is still used today. Around the same time, Spearman put forth the notion that human ability across domains was based on a unidimensional factor he described as general ability, or "g." This notion of a single intelligence was quite popular at the start of the twentieth century, but has largely been replaced by models that include multiple forms of intelligence. Intelligence and ability testing gained much attention during the first and second world wars when the American military adopted this type of testing to optimize placement of soldiers. Today, intelligence is assessed with any number of validated measures, each of which includes different domains and subscales which are then combined to yield one cumulative intelligence quotient (IQ) (see Fig. 9.3). IQ is the ratio between the estimate of a person's "mental age" based on their performance on a measure of intelligence and their actual chronological age. The broad range of subscales included and abilities tested in determining intelligence presents one of many challenges for data standardization [1].

Another phenomenon of interest is personality. Personality refers to stable, long-lasting patterns of dispositions and tendencies that characterize a person's behavior, responses and preferences. One popular model of personality attributes is the 'five-factor' model of personality [13] which holds that personality consists of variability in five main dimensions: Extraversion, Agreeableness, Conscientiousness, Neuroticism, and Openness to Experience (Fig. 9.4). People have attributes along each of these dimensions that vary on a pole of oppositions. For example, in the Extraversion dimension people can vary from quiet and reserved to assertive and

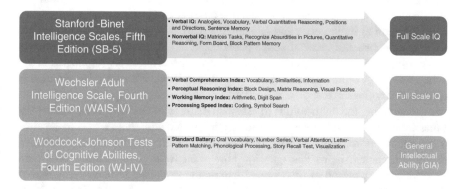

Fig. 9.3 Subscales and domain scores that factor into IQ on three widely used measures of intelligence. Notes: The WAIS-IV can also be used to calculate a General Ability Index (GAI) based on the Verbal Comprehension and Perceptual Reasoning Index scores only [9–12]

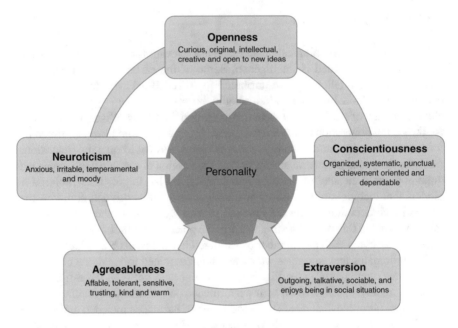

Fig. 9.4 Illustration of the Big Five personality dimensions

sociable, while on the Neuroticism dimension people vary from emotionally stable to highly reactive. Assessment instruments are widely available for evaluating where individuals are placed on those dimensions [14], including for use in clinical mental health contexts [15].

As with IQ, there are multiple options for assessing personality including the Myers-Briggs Type Indicator [16], the Personality Assessment Inventory [17], and the California Psychological Inventory (CPI) [18]. One of the most widely used and well validated measures of personality is the Minnesota Multiphasic Personality Inventory (MMPI), a self-report measure of personality that consists of true/false statements and assesses personality features on 52 scales [19].

In addition to intelligence and personality, there is a ubiquitous need to collect data on emotions and other affective phenomena in clinical and research contexts involving mental health. This is because affective disturbances are implicated in the symptomatology of many mental health conditions. While it is normal to experience a range of emotions in response to different situations, of key importance in evaluating and studying mental health is to establish patterns of emotional responses over time, consider the overall severity and relation to the stimulus as well as level of impairment. For example, many commonly used inventories for the evaluation of depression contain items that question how often feelings of sadness have been experienced in a period of time—persistent and unexplained sadness being one of the key symptoms of depression. Another emotion that may be relevant is irritability. Table 9.1 provides examples of some of the diverse measures used to assess for the most common mental health conditions.

Table 9.1 A select set of common measures used to assess presence and severity of the most common mental health disorders

	Assessment	Reference	Proprietary	Format
Depression	Beck Depression Inventory (BDI)	[20]	Yes	21-Item self-report measure
	Hamilton Depression Rating Scale (HAM-D)	[21]	No	21-Item clinician-administered scale
	Center for Epidemiologic Studies Depression Scale (CES-D)	[22]	No	20-Item self-report measure
	Patient Health Questionnaire-9 (PHQ-9)	[23]	No	9-Item self-report measure
Anxiety	Beck Anxiety Inventory (BAI)	[20]	Yes	21-Item self-report measure
	State Trait Anxiety Inventory	[24]	Yes	20-Item self-report measure
	Hamilton Anxiety Rating Scale	[25]	No	14-Item clinician-administered scale
	Anxiety disorders interview schedule-revised (ADIS-R)	[26]	Yes	Clinician-administered structured interview
	Generalized Anxiety Disorder 7 (GAD-7)	[27]	No	7-Item self-report measure

Apart from the presence or absence and degree of a specific emotion, something that is linked prominently to many mental health conditions is emotion *regulation*, which is the extent to which emotions are able to be amplified or reduced as needed in order to function optimally in a given context [28].

Other psychological data pertains to cognitive processes. Examples include patterns of thought such as rumination and reflection. Factors that affect psychological functioning, such as stress, can also be risk factors in mental health conditions [29–31]. Of course, there are interrelationships between all of these different aspects of psychological data. For example, emotion regulation and patterns of emotions are related to personality and to the patterns of functioning involved in specific mental health conditions [32]. Cognitive factors influence emotions and can mediate against the worsening of mental health conditions under triggering conditions—thus, one of the objectives of cognitive therapy (one of the most widely used treatments in mental health) is to increase resilience through improved cognitive processes [33].

9.3.1.2 Measurement Approaches

Measures used in mental health take a number of forms. Self-report measures, like the MMPI ask individuals to respond to a series of true-false or Likert scale type questions (e.g., strongly disagree to strongly agree). These measures often include scales that allow the examiners to assess for problematic response patterns including positive or negative-biased responses (i.e., someone who consistently answers in a positive or negative manner regardless of question content) or inconsistent responses (i.e., different answers to multiple questions regarding the same content but with varied phrasing).

Clinical interviews are another approach used regularly in mental health. These can be structured or semi-structured. In a structured clinical interview, the examiner asks specific questions verbatim and moves between test items based on the individual's responses. The most widely used structured interview for diagnostic assessments is the Structured Clinical Interview for DSM-5 (SCID-5) [34] which allows for assessment of multiple disorders at the same time [35, 36]. This uses broad questions to determine whether an individual is endorsing symptoms of a given disorder, and if so, moves into more detailed questions about the severity and duration of those symptoms to determine whether the individual meets criteria for that particular DSM-5 diagnosis. Another structured interview that allows for assessment of multiple disorders is the Diagnostic Interview for Anxiety, Mood, OCD and Related Neuropsychiatric Disorders (DIAMOND) [37].

In contrast with structured interviews, semi-structured interviews rely on less specific questions but give general guidelines and leave the evaluator more freedom to pursue specific items or delve further into a given topic. The Autism Diagnostic Observation Schedule 2nd Edition (ADOS-2) [38] is one example of a semi-structured interview in which some items include specific questions (which do not need to be read verbatim) and others offer general guidelines for interacting with the individual for the purpose of eliciting specific opportunities for behavioral observation.

9.3.2 Behavioral Data

To understand how behavioral data are collected today, it is helpful to revisit the history of behaviorism. In an effort to circumvent the challenges of psychological traits being unobservable, early modern psychology focused on behaviorism. Ivan Pavlov (1849–1936), John Watson (1878–1958) and later B.F. Skinner (1904–1990) are credited with their efforts to drill down the study of the human mind into the behaviors that can be observed directly and objectively. Behaviorism is often described with Pavlov's work on conditioned reflexes. Pavlov demonstrated that repeated presentation of a bell paired with food can cause dogs to salivate at the sound of a bell even in the absence of food. Watson later demonstrated how an emotional response such as fear can also be conditioned. Watson and his graduate student (and later wife) Rosalie Rayner are most well known for their attempts to condition a fear response in an infant called "Little Albert" by pairing a previously non-frightening stimulus (a white rat) with a startling loud bang, thereby conditioning Little Albert to demonstrate fear when presented with the rat, even in the absence of the loud bang.

Today, we continue to study observable behavior as a means for understanding the workings of the mind. In research, great effort is taken to painstakingly record or "code" the behavior of study participants for observation of such acts as smiling, turn-taking, initiating or responding to joint attention, presence or absence of stereotypies (repetitive movements often observed in individuals with autism spectrum disorder), body posturing, and reaching behavior (as in the famous Marshmallow study [39]). Behavioral measures are often used in the study and treatment of children, who may not have the insight or the language to allow self-reporting of mental states. Behavioral data can also be particularly informative when studying unconscious behaviors (e.g. tic disorders). Due to the laborious nature of this type of coding, this approach is far more common in research than in clinical realms where the offline coding required to meaningfully assess change would not be feasible. Advances in automation, e.g. computer vision analysis, may soon yield more clinical utility for the observation and analysis of "observable" (as in recognizable using automated computer vision) behaviors.

Of note, it is important to distinguish between traditional behaviorism and the modern use of the term in the context of behavioral medicine, which refers to the intersection between behavior, psychology, and biomedical science and has become a dominant approach to improving both mental and physical wellbeing. Behavioral medicine, or behavioral health, targets a range of lifestyle changes (e.g., physical activity, smoking cessation) and also includes biofeedback, an approach that involves training bodily processes such as muscle tension to reduce blood pressure, heart rate and pain.

Behavioral data may also appear in measures of other types, e.g. self-report measures. For example, Beck's Depression Inventory contains several items that refer to behavior: it includes questions regarding sleep, crying, and decision-making. Similarly, other composite measures that are used in mental health research and practice include questions relating to behavior. In addition, prominent examples of behaviors relevant to mental health include substance use. In research involving adolescents and young people, aggression and compliance with instructions may be the dimensions of behavior that are most relevant.

9.3.3 Social and Interpersonal Data

Humans are social organisms. Social and interpersonal data relates to interactions and relationships, both at the microcosm of an individual family or couple relationship, and at the larger scale of being embedded in a particular community or within a given culture. A breakdown in interpersonal and social relations is often one of the key early stage symptoms of mental health conditions, and in severe cases there may be great difficulties in establishing a satisfying level of embeddedness. In addition, social and interpersonal data is of particular importance in longitudinal studies of mental health. Early life stressors including emotional, physical, verbal or sexual abuse, neglect, severe conflicts, parental divorce, substance abuse, and poverty have also been shown to predict mental health status [40].

As described above, the quality of early childhood relationships are key predictors of mental health status later in life, and not surprisingly the quality of the relationship with caregivers and treatment providers can be predictive of the rate of recovery or response to treatment. Psychological measures and behavioral data have both been used to study the role of early childhood relationships and later mental health. Attachment theory [41, 42], which posits that early relationships between infants and their caregivers predict the way an individual will form relationships with others throughout their life, has long been assessed in a behavioral task called the "strange situation" [43]. In this approach, a 1-year-old child is brought into a novel space with their caregiver. The child is then presented with a series of scenarios including presence and absence of the caregiver and a stranger. The child's behavior in each situation is observed to determine both how the child responds to the novel presence of a stranger and the absence of their caregiver and how the child acts when reuniting with the caregiver. In contrast with this approach to assessing attachment in infants, for adults we can simply ask the individual about their relationships with others using a clinical interview such as the Adult Attachment Interview [44].

Alongside the nature of social relationships, socioeconomic factors such as level of financial resources are important for mental health. Low socioeconomic status is known to strongly mediate both rates of illness and outcomes, not only due to the environmental factors described below, but also in part through social stress experienced by people living under those conditions.

9.3.4 Environmental Data

The nature of the environment is also important to accurate research and treatment in mental health contexts. For example, related to socioeconomic status is quality of housing, and concomitantly quality of the neighboring environment. Environmental data of relevance for research and practice in mental health includes amount of green space, pollution levels including of course air pollution but also noise and light pollution that may interfere with sleep [45]. The setting for the provision of health care encounters is also very relevant, along with ease of access to health care.

9.4 Informatics Technologies for Data Acquisition

Data acquisition is an area where informatics technologies are having a large-scale and transformative impact on mental health research and practice. The transition from paper records to electronic records in health contexts enables sophisticated downstream applications. Data acquisition for the electronic health record (EHR) can be structured and standardized in a way that is more difficult to implement in paper-based systems, with input templates and drop-down menus from controlled vocabularies and ontologies. (See Chap. 16). This "digitization" of data enables data from different healthcare settings to be integrated, compared, and mined for downstream research [46]. Although still not trivial, this was much more difficult before EHR systems became widely adopted.

One way in which informatics technologies are being leveraged for the acquisition of data relating to mental, behavioral, and psychological phenomena is through computer-based psychometric assessment. This technology, variously referred to as *computer based assessment* (CBA), *computer mediated assessment* (CMA), *computre based testing* (CBT) involves the use fo computerized systems to administer tests and record test responses, scores, or both. A wide variety of instruments are being developed specifically for computer-based administration. That is, they are natively designed to be delivered via computer rather than paper. Online versions of many commonly used screening measures for mental health are also being developed and validated [47]. However, as computerized metrics are novel, they have not yet been standardized and validated to the same extent as existing paper-based metrics and instruments have been, and therefore the uptake of these *computerized psychometrics* within the clinic directly has been slow.

One relatively novel and prominent informatics-driven source for the acquisition for social and interpersonal data of relevance for mental health is social media. Social media usage patterns on platforms such as Facebook and Twitter provide information about the social contacts, friendships over time, communication patterns and behavior of individuals within social contexts. Users often express their emotions and thoughts, and these expressions are a valuable source of data for research in mental health which has increasingly been harnessed accordingly [48]. For example, social media usage has been used to investigate population patterns of mental health responses during crisis periods [49], and to investigate suicidal ideation in at-risk groups [50]. In order to interpret the information that is available on the social media platforms, it is often necessary to use sophisticated text and data mining algorithms [51].

Another modern source of data of significant importance for mental health, and discussed in detail in Chap. 17, is smartphones and wearable devices such as fitness monitors. In developed countries, these devices have become ubiquitously a part of most people's lives and, as they are embedded with multiple sensors which continuously create data such as tracking usage, location and movement, they are a rich resource for pattern and data mining for research and management [52]. For example, data from passive sensors can be used to predict mood [53]. Sensors can also be used in combination with smartphones in order to report environmental variables for which specific sensors may be available, for example, air pollution and radiation levels. Activity profiles are a highly relevant type of data for mental health contexts, not only for predicting psychological variables: physical activity is known to be protective against mental health conditions and may be used in self-management programs for mild conditions [54]. Moreover, location information tracked also provides one of the only systematic ways to track environmental influences on mental health. For example, location information may indicate access to public green spaces, which in turn are known to have a positive impact on mental health [55]. Smartphones and wearables also lend themselves to more frequent sampling, in techniques which strive for *ecological momentary assessment* [56], the objective of measuring psychological and behavioral states in the moment with high *ecological validity*—that is, validity for real-world settings rather than just research contexts—rather than reporting them retroactively, which has to be mediated by memory.

9.5   Challenges, Limitations and Future Directions

Data acquisition and capture are at the heart of research, and mental health is no exception. Informatics technologies are changing the landscape of data acquisition and capture on multiple fronts, and this "digital revolution" should be welcomed [45]. However, like other areas of informatics in mental health, it is not without challenges.

As mentioned above, one major challenge in mental health is the lack of standardization across labs and clinics in which measures, or clinical assessments, are used to measure various phenomena. When each lab and clinical setting uses a different measure of the same phenomena (such as empathy or emotion regulation), it is difficult to pool and aggregate the data across data sets. In addition to the massive number of measures available in mental health, a number of other challenges inherent to psychological research must be kept in mind when considering measurement in mental health. This includes the Hawthorne Effect [57], which refers to the finding that observation itself can alter responses. This concept emerged from studies of working conditions in factories in which it was shown that simply asking questions and showing interest in the workers improved productivity before any changes were actually implemented.

Another challenge is related to the accuracy of reporting, given what is referred to as *social desirability*. Because clinical interviews are inherently social, and because people tend to want to please others and demonstrate their social acceptability, it is difficult to obtain true answers to difficult and socially undesirable questions. Further, the phrasing of the questions themselves can have significant effects on how individuals respond (e.g., Do you engage in X behavior? vs. How often do you do X?). With so many measures in existence, this becomes an incredibly challenging factor for studying combinations of groups that have not been assessed with precisely the same measure. Of more significant concern is evidence that some measures are fraught with inherent bias, meaning that certain groups perform systematically differently than other groups irrespective of the trait being measured. This has been a particularly contentious matter for IQ tests [58].

Measurement and other forms of data capture are potential sources of researcher degrees of freedom which can—knowingly or unknowingly—allow for studies that report essentially false positives, or unreproducible results. This can occur, for example, if the measure or data capture technique is chosen from a wide range of possibilities in a way that best suits the given problem, rather than the underlying theoretical framework that structures the research as a whole [7]. The same effect may apply if multiple possibilities are available for standardizing and structuring data, allowing researchers the freedom to arbitrarily choose the measure that gives the best results on their study, potentially artificially improving the results. Working towards community-wide shared theoretical frameworks [59], as well as community-wide standards of best practice, is essential alongside other measures to achieve robust and cumulative science in practice [60, 61]. When there are a range of different perspectives on an underlying research question, which is often the case in mental health, it may be particularly difficult to arrive at standardized theoretical frameworks and data capture and description tools that work equally well for all the different perspectives, since standards development is usually driven within communities of practice within a given field rather than across several different disciplines and communities of practice [62]. For mental health, an inherently interdisciplinary problem space, improving the informatics support for translations and comparisons that cut across these disciplinary boundaries will be an important driver for accelerating progress [60, 63].

As discussed in Chap. 18, issues around ethics and privacy are highly relevant in all contexts in which data are shared or made publicly available [64]. It is essential that individual privacy be maintained, for example by de-identification of data, and consent needs to be given for data sharing, possibly even on a case by case basis depending on how the data will be used.

Dense large-scale datasets, such as those generated by novel wearable technologies, digital media, and even electronic healthcare systems, can be subject to large-scale noise and systematic biases which need to be corrected for. And such challenges in data quality may be obscured by advanced informatics analysis pipelines such as popular "deep learning" approaches, which may act as "black boxes" hindering the interpretability of the findings; interpretability is of paramount importance to achieve trust in newly emerging informatics-based systems [65].

Nevertheless, the promise of informatics-based systems to revolutionize mental health research and practice is clear; this revolution will in turn lead to improvements in our general understanding of mental health, and also our ability to create novel and individualized treatments [66].

References

1. Kaplan RM, Saccuzzo DP. Psychological testing: principles, applications, and issues. 5th and 9th ed. Cengage Learning. 2017. https://doi.org/10.1017/CBO9781107415324.004
2. Aguinis H, Culpepper SA, Pierce CA. Differential prediction generalization in college admissions testing. J Educ Psychol. 2016; https://doi.org/10.1037/edu0000104.
3. Cronbach LJ, Meehl PE. Construct validity in psychological tests. Psychol Bull. 1955; https://doi.org/10.1037/h0040957.
4. Colman. A.M. A dictionary of psychology: Oxford University Press; 2009.
5. Hyatt CS, Sleep CE, Lamkin J, Maples-Keller JL, Sedikides C, Campbell WK, Miller JD. Narcissism and self-esteem: a nomological network analysis. PLoS One. 2018; https://doi.org/10.1371/journal.pone.0201088.
6. Nunnally JC. Psychometric theory. 25 years ago and now. Educ Researcher. 1975; https://doi.org/10.2307/1175619.

7. Flake JK, Fried EI. Measurement schmeasurement: questionable measurement practices and how to avoid them. PsyArXiv (Preprint). 2019. https://doi.org/10.31234/osf.io/hs7wm.

8. Hand DJ. Measurement: A very short introduction. Oxford University Press; 2016.

9. Dumont R, Willis JO, Veizel K, Zibulsky J. Wechsler adult intelligence scale. In: Encyclopedia of Special Education. 4th ed; 2014. https://doi.org/10.1002/9781118660584.ese2520.

10. Roid GH, Pomplun M. The Stanford-Binet intelligence scales: The Guilford Press; 2012.

11. Woodcock, K. S., Schrank, R. W., Mather, F. A., & McGrew, N. (2014). Woodock Johnson IV – Tests of cognitive ability, oral language, and achievement.

12. Zibulsky J, Veizel K. Wechsler memory scale. In: Encyclopedia of Special Education. 4th ed; 2014. https://doi.org/10.1002/9781118660584.ese2524.

13. McCrae RR, John OP. An introduction to the five-factor model and its applications. J Pers. 1992; https://doi.org/10.1111/j.1467-6494.1992.tb00970.x.

14. Widiger TA, Trull TJ. Assessment of the five-factor model of personality. J Pers Assess. 1997; https://doi.org/10.1207/s15327752jpa6802_2.

15. Widiger TA, Presnall JR. Clinical application of the five-factor model. J Pers. 2013; https://doi.org/10.1111/jopy.12004.

16. Myers IB. The Myers-Briggs type indicator: manual (1962); 2014. https://doi.org/10.1037/14404-000.

17. Morey LC. The personality assessment inventory. In: Personality assessment. 2nd ed; 2014. https://doi.org/10.4324/9780203119143.

18. Gough HG. The California psychological inventory. In: Testing and assessment in counseling practice. 2nd ed; 2012. https://doi.org/10.4324/9781410604323-9.

19. Butcher JN, Williams CL. Essentials of MMPI-2 and MMPI-A interpretation: University of Minnesota Press; 1992.

20. Beck AT, Ward CH, Mendelson M, Mock J, Erbaugh J. An inventory for measuring depression. Arch Gen Psychiatry. 1961; https://doi.org/10.1001/archpsyc.1961.01710120031004.

21. Hamilton M. A rating scale for depression. J Neurol Neurosurg Psychiatry. 1960;23:56–62. https://doi.org/10.1136/jnnp.23.1.56.

22. Radloff LS. The CES-D scale: a self-report depression scale for research in the general population. Appl Psychol Measurement. 1977; https://doi.org/10.1177/014662167700100306.

23. Kroenke K, Spitzer RL, Williams JBW. The PHQ-9: validity of a brief depression severity measure. J Gen Intern Med. 2001; https://doi.org/10.1046/j.1525-1497.2001.016009606.x.

24. Spielberger CD, Gorsuch RL, Lushene R, Vagg PR, Jacobs GA. Manual for the state-trait anxiety inventory. Palo Alto, CA: Consulting Psychologists Press; 1983.

25. Hamilton M. The assessment of anxiety states by rating. Br J Med Psychol. 1959;32:50–5. https://doi.org/10.1111/j.2044-8341.1959.tb00467.x.

26. Di Nardo PA, Barlow DH. Anxiety disorders interview schedule-revised (ADIS-R). New York: Phobia and Anxiety Disorders Clinic, Center for Stress and Anxiety Disorders, State University of New York at Albany; 1988.

27. Spitzer RL, Kroenke K, Williams JBW, Löwe B. A brief measure for assessing generalized anxiety disorder: the GAD-7. Arch Intern Med. 2006; https://doi.org/10.1001/archinte.166.10.1092.

28. McRae K, Gross JJ. Emotion regulation. Washington, DC: Emotion; 2020. https://doi.org/10.1037/emo0000703.

29. Chu DA, Williams LM, Harris AWF, Bryant RA, Gatt JM. Early life trauma predicts self-reported levels of depressive and anxiety symptoms in nonclinical community adults: relative contributions of early life stressor types and adult trauma exposure. J Psychiatr Res. 2013; https://doi.org/10.1016/j.jpsychires.2012.08.006.

30. Clark C, Caldwell T, Power C, Stansfeld SA. Does the influence of childhood adversity on psychopathology persist across the lifecourse? A 45-year prospective epidemiologic study. Ann Epidemiol. 2010; https://doi.org/10.1016/j.annepidem.2010.02.008.

31. Marin MF, Lord C, Andrews J, Juster RP, Sindi S, Arsenault-Lapierre G, et al. Chronic stress, cognitive functioning and mental health. Neurobiol Learn Mem. 2011; https://doi.org/10.1016/j.nlm.2011.02.016.

32. Sloan E, Hall K, Moulding R, Bryce S, Mildred H, Staiger PK. Emotion regulation as a trans-diagnostic treatment construct across anxiety, depression, substance, eating and borderline personality disorders: a systematic review. Clin Psychol Rev. 2017; https://doi.org/10.1016/j.cpr.2017.09.002.

33. Kingdon D, Mander H. Cognitive behavioral therapy. In: International encyclopedia of the social & behavioral sciences. 2nd ed; 2015. https://doi.org/10.1016/B978-0-08-097086-8.27011-6.

34. American Psychiatric Association. DSM-5 Diagnostic Classification. Diagn Statist Manual Mental Disorders. 2013; https://doi.org/10.1176/appi.books.9780890425596.x00diagnosticclassification.

35. First MB. Structured clinical interview for the DSM (SCID). In: The encyclopedia of clinical psychology; 2015. https://doi.org/10.1002/9781118625392.wbecp351.

36. First MB, Williams JBW, Karg RS, Spitzer RL. Structured clinical interview for DSM-5 research version. Washington DC: American Psychiatric Association; 2015.

37. Tolin DF, Gilliam C, Wootton BM, Bowe W, Bragdon LB, Davis E, et al. Psychometric properties of a structured diagnostic interview for DSM-5 anxiety, mood, and obsessive-compulsive and related disorders. Assessment. 2018; https://doi.org/10.1177/1073191116638410.

38. Lord C, Rutter M, DiLavore P, Risi S, Gotham K, Bishop S. Autism diagnostic observation schedule – Second edition (ADOS-2). Los Angeles, CA: Western Psychological Corporation; 2012.

39. Mischel W, Ebbesen EB. Attention in delay of gratification. J Pers Soc Psychol. 1970; https://doi.org/10.1037/h0029815.

40. Cohen RA, Hitsman BL, Paul RH, McCaffery J, Stroud L, Sweet L, et al. Early life stress and adult emotional experience: an international perspective. Int J Psychiatry Med. 2006; https://doi.org/10.2190/5R62-9PQY-0NEL-TLPA.

41. Ainsworth MS. Infant–mother attachment. Am Psychol. 1979;34(10):932.

42. Bowlby J. Attachment and loss, Vol. I: Attachment. New York: Basic Books; 1969.

43. Ainsworth MDS, Bell SM. Attachment, exploration, and separation: Illustrated by the behavior of one-yearolds in a strange situation. Child development. 1970;49–67.

44. George C, Kaplan N, Main M. Adult Attachment Interview; 1985.

45. Shilo S, Rossman H, Segal E. Axes of a revolution: challenges and promises of big data in healthcare. Nat Med. 2020; https://doi.org/10.1038/s41591-019-0727-5.

46. Velupillai S, Suominen H, Liakata M, Roberts A, Shah AD, Morley K, et al. Using clinical Natural Language Processing for health outcomes research: overview and actionable suggestions for future advances. J Biomed Inform. 2018; https://doi.org/10.1016/j.jbi.2018.10.005.

47. van Ballegooijen W, Riper H, Cuijpers P, van Oppen P, Smit JH. Validation of online psychometric instruments for common mental health disorders: a systematic review. BMC Psychiatry. 2016; https://doi.org/10.1186/s12888-016-0735-7.

48. Wongkoblap A, Vadillo MA, Curcin V. Researching mental health disorders in the era of social media: systematic review. J Med Internet Res. 2017; https://doi.org/10.2196/jmir.7215.

49. Karmegam D, Ramamoorthy T, Mappillairajan B. A systematic review of techniques employed for determining mental health using social media in psychological surveillance during disasters. Disaster Med Public Health Preparedness. 2019; https://doi.org/10.1017/dmp.2019.40.

50. De Choudhury M, Kiciman E, Dredze M, Coppersmith G, Kumar M. Discovering shifts to suicidal ideation from mental health content in social media. In: Conference on Human Factors in Computing Systems – Proceedings; 2016. https://doi.org/10.1145/2858036.2858207.

51. Tsakalidis A, Liakata M, Damoulas T, Cristea AI. Can we assess mental health through social media and smart devices? Addressing bias in methodology and evaluation. In: Lecture Notes in Computer Science (including subseries Lecture Notes in Artificial Intelligence and Lecture Notes in Bioinformatics); 2019. https://doi.org/10.1007/978-3-030-10997-4_25.

52. Mohr DC, Zhang M, Schueller SM. Personal sensing: understanding mental health using ubiquitous sensors and machine learning. Annu Rev Clin Psychol. 2017; https://doi.org/10.1146/annurev-clinpsy-032816-044949.

53. Morshed MB, Saha K, Li R, D'Mello SK, De Choudhury M, Abowd GD, Plötz T. Prediction of mood instability with passive sensing. Proceedings of the ACM on Interactive, Mobile, Wearable and Ubiquitous Technologies. 2019; https://doi.org/10.1145/3351233.
54. Morgan WP. Physical activity and mental health. 2013; https://doi.org/10.4324/9780203782361.
55. Nutsford D, Pearson AL, Kingham S. An ecological study investigating the association between access to urban green space and mental health. Public Health. 2013; https://doi.org/10.1016/j.puhe.2013.08.016.
56. Shiffman S, Stone AA, Hufford MR. Ecological momentary assessment. Annu Rev Clin Psychol. 2008; https://doi.org/10.1146/annurev.clinpsy.3.022806.091415.
57. Adair JG. The Hawthorne effect: a reconsideration of the methodological artifact. J Appl Psychol. 1984; https://doi.org/10.1037/0021-9010.69.2.334.
58. Reynolds CR, Suzuki LA. Bias in psychological assessment: an empirical review and recommendations. In: Handbook of psychology, Vol. 10: Assessment psychology. 2nd ed; 2013.
59. Robinaugh DJ, Haslbeck JMB, Ryan O, Fried EI, Waldorp LJ. Invisible hands and fine calipers: a call to use formal theory as a toolkit for theory construction. Perspect Psychol Sci. 2020;
60. Hastings J. Mental health ontologies: how we talk about mental health, and why it matters in the digital age: University of Exeter Press; 2020.
61. Hastings J, Michie S, Johnston M. Theory and ontology in behavioural science. Nat Hum Behav. 2020; https://doi.org/10.1038/s41562-020-0826-9.
62. Hastings J, Frishkoff GA, Smith B, Jensen M, Poldrack RA, Lomax J, et al. Interdisciplinary perspectives on the development, integration, and application of cognitive ontologies. Front Neuroinf. 2014; https://doi.org/10.3389/fninf.2014.00062.
63. Larsen RR, Hastings J. From affective science to psychiatric disorder: ontology as a semantic bridge. Front Psychiatry. 2018; https://doi.org/10.3389/fpsyt.2018.00487.
64. Martone ME, Garcia-Castro A, VandenBos GR. Data sharing in psychology. Am Psychol. 2018; https://doi.org/10.1037/amp0000242.
65. Vellido A. The importance of interpretability and visualization in machine learning for applications in medicine and health care. Neural Comput Applic. 2019; https://doi.org/10.1007/s00521-019-04051-w.
66. Harvey A, Brand A, Holgate ST, Kristiansen LV, Lehrach H, Palotie A, Prainsack B. The future of technologies for personalised medicine. New Biotechnol. 2012; https://doi.org/10.1016/j.nbt.2012.03.009.

Chapter 10
Data to Information: Computational Models and Analytic Methods

Shyam Visweswaran and Mohammadamin Tajgardoon

Abstract Computational models and analytic methods are increasingly important in the modeling and analyses of mental health and illness. The increased availability of data, the development of a wide range of analytic methods, and powerful and ubiquitous computing capability provide an unprecedented opportunity to develop computational models. Broadly speaking, two types of computational models are used in the context of mental health. Theory-based approaches generate explanatory models that describe the mechanisms of neural or psychological processes. Data-driven approaches typically extract predictive relations between variables and relevant outcomes or uncover patterns such as disease subtypes in data. Machine learning methods are increasingly used to develop models, especially data-driven models. This chapter will describe key methods and application examples, the workflow in machine learning, data preprocessing, feature selection methods, and the main categories of machine learning algorithms including supervised learning, unsupervised learning, semi-supervised learning, and deep learning. In addition, this chapter will briefly describe standards for reporting models and ethical and safety issues related to the development and use of computational models.

Keywords Computational model · Explanatory model · Predictive model Machine learning · Dimensionality reduction · Supervised learning Unsupervised learning

S. Visweswaran (✉) · M. Tajgardoon
University of Pittsburgh, Pittsburgh, USA
e-mail: shv3@pitt.edu; mot16@pitt.edu

© Springer Nature Switzerland AG 2021   235
J. D. Tenenbaum, P. A. Ranallo (eds.), *Mental Health Informatics*, Health
Informatics, https://doi.org/10.1007/978-3-030-70558-9_10

10.1   Introduction

A computational model, broadly speaking, is a set of mathematical expressions that represents a process or predicts a state [1]. Such a mathematical model can be a simple equation or a complex series of mathematical expressions. Typically, the development and evaluation of such a model are sufficiently intensive that they require a computer and hence it is termed a computational model. In mental health, computational models are useful to understand the social, environmental, behavioral, mental, and biological basis of mental function and dysfunction, to uncover the etiology and evolution of mental disorders, to reveal the effects of drugs and interventions, and to predict response to therapy [2]. Further, computational models can perform predictions, discover patterns, and provide explanations in mental health. That is, they can be used to characterize, predict, and explain the complex interactions between phenomena studied within—and at the interface of—the biological, behavioral, and social sciences.

Biological processes relevant to mental function and dysfunction span many levels of biological scale from the genetic, molecular and cellular to neural circuits, the nervous system and behavior [3]. Deciphering mental function and dysfunction in mental illness often requires comprehension and integration of phenomena at multiple levels. Schizophrenia due to a genetic mutation provides an example of a mental health disorder whose mechanism spans multiple levels [3]. At the genetic level, the deletion of a small part of chromosome 22 (22q11.2 deletion) is associated with greatly increased risk of developing schizophrenia. At the molecular level, the genetic defect results in a decrease in the production of an enzyme that, at the cellular level, results in insufficient axonal growth and branching [4]. At the neural circuit level, transmission is decreased between the hippocampus and the prefrontal cortex, and at the behavioral level, this manifests as deficits in working memory. A computational model has the potential to integrate phenomena at one or more levels in a mathematically rigorous way.

Recent advances in data availability, the development of a wide range of analytic methods, and powerful and ubiquitous computing capability provide an unprecedented opportunity to develop computational models. First, data sets related to normal and abnormal mental, behavioral, and biological function are increasingly available and include a broad range of types of data. Experimental data sets that are typically collected in research studies include types of data such as clinical, psychological, behavioral, social, genetic, environmental, metabolomic, epidemiological, and neuroimaging data. Observational data sets are becoming available from sources such as electronic health records (EHRs), social media, passive sensing, monitoring of communication through mobile smartphones, and wearable technologies with sensors that measure behavior such as physical activity, sleep quality, and blood pressure [5]. Several large efforts are collecting multiple types of data on a large scale. The Alzheimer's Disease Neuroimaging Initiative (ADNI) has generated a wide range of data types to research Alzheimer's disease [6]. The All of Us Research Program is enrolling a diverse group of at least 1 million people in the U.S. and is collecting a range of data including EHRs and genomic data [7]. The NIH Human Biomolecular Atlas Program is generating multi-omic data at the single-cell level across a range of human tissue types [8].

Second, a broad range of analytic methods has been developed and is readily available for application. Third, access to faster and ever more powerful computers is becoming inexpensive and ubiquitous. The convergence of readily available data, analytic methods, and powerful computing has led to the development of a wide range of explanatory and correlational computational models. These models have great potential to facilitate understanding the social, behavioral, psychological, and biological correlates of normal mental phenomena, uncover the pathogenesis of mental illnesses, enable more precise diagnoses, better predict prognosis, comprehend the mechanisms of drugs, and optimally allocate healthcare resources in mental illnesses.

10.2 Analytic Approaches to Computational Modeling

Broadly speaking, computational models are used in two ways related to mental health and illness (and in biomedicine more generally). The first way is to express descriptive theories of mental function and dysfunction in a precise and quantitative way. For example, a model may represent a cognitive process such as learning or a dysfunctional psychological process that underlies panic disorder [1] or denote an abnormal neural circuit that gives rise to perceptual difficulties in autism [9]. The second way is to represent the result of computer-based analyses of data. For example, a model may represent patterns or natural divisions, such as subtypes of psychosis. A model may also represent the risk of developing an illness, or the likely benefit of a therapy in an individual. Corresponding to these two types of models, the analytic methods used in developing the first type are called theory-based and those used in developing the second type are called data-driven [10, 11]. Models developed using theory-based methods often seek to uncover causal relationships in data, while those developed using data-driven methods predominantly seek to identify correlations in data.

Theory-based approaches aim to develop computational models of causation or explanation (see Box 10.1) and describe the mechanisms of neural, psychological or behavioral processes [12]. Theory-based approaches often use mathematical equations that represent neural or psychological mechanisms. For example, a causal model may describe quantitatively the effect that a change in the concentration of a given neurotransmitter has on the behavior of a neural circuit [13]. In causal or explanatory models, the variables (see Box 10.1) correspond to neural or psychological processes, and the parameters (see Box 10.1) corresponding to the variables are calculated from data using statistical methods.

Data-driven approaches, in contrast, seek to develop computational models for classification, prediction, or pattern mining (see Box 10.1). Such models might be used to classify whether an individual has psychosis or not, to predict the risk of an individual developing psychosis in the future, or to uncover patterns of psychosis that have distinct cognitive patterns. Typically such models do not provide causal knowledge or explanations of underlying biological mechanisms. Statistical and machine learning methods are used to develop data-driven models. For example, a machine learning model may predict antidepressant medication response from several variables including demographics, neuroimaging biomarkers, and genetic variants [14]. Though the model is able to predict which individuals are likely to respond to antidepressant medication, no knowledge can be inferred regarding the causal mechanisms of antidepressant response because the model does not represent underlying neural or psychological processes.

Theory-based approaches typically uncover causal relations or provide insight into underlying mechanisms of neural or psychological processes [15]. Data-driven approaches typically extract predictive relations between variables and relevant outcomes or uncover patterns such as disease subtypes in data. The two approaches, thus, provide complementary knowledge [11].

10.3   Theory-Based Approaches

Theory-based approaches seek to represent descriptive theories of mental function and dysfunction in a computable way. This allows for simulating or predicting behaviors by solving the equations in the model that represent neural or psychological processes. A key goal is to represent in a precise and quantitative way neural or psychological mechanisms of normal and abnormal mental processes such as thinking, reasoning, planning, emotion, and behavioral strategy. Theory-based approaches include constructing *dynamical systems* and *causal networks*.

10.3.1   Dynamical Systems

Dynamical systems are models that describe the evolution of neural and psychological states over time using equations [3]. Simpler examples of such models include those that describe the swinging of a clock pendulum and the movement of the Earth around the sun. Many biophysical, connectionist, and reinforcement-learning models are dynamical systems.

One approach to developing such a model is to translate a descriptive theory into a mathematical model. Typically, the model is described in two parts; the structural component is a pictorial representation of relations among relevant variables in the domain, and the quantitative component consists of differential equations with parameters [16]. Figure 10.1 shows part of a model that was developed for panic disorder [17]. Panel (a) shows the structure of the model; a circle denotes a variable and an arrow from one circle to another indicates the influence of the first variable on the other. The three variables that are shown include arousal, perceived threat,

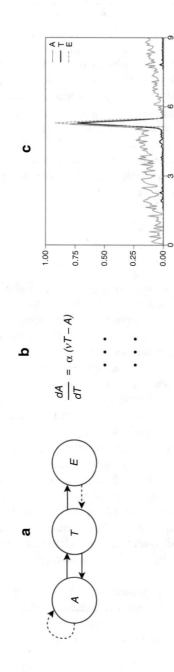

Fig. 10.1 Theory-based model for panic disorder. Panel (**a**) shows the structure of the model; the circles indicate the concepts arousal (A), perceived threat (T), and escape (E), and the arrows indicate causal relationships. Panel (**b**) shows one of the differential equations specified in the model. Panel (**c**) depicts the simulated behavior defined by the equations. (Adapted from [16])

and escape, which are key concepts in a theory used to describe panic disorder [18]. The theory posits that perception of threat leads to arousal that in turn results in bodily sensations of fear and anxiety. However, the precise form and strength of this effect are unspecified in the theory. In the computational model, this relation is specified by a differential equation as shown in panel (b). A differential equation states how a rate of change in one variable is related to another variable. In this example, the equation relates the rate of arousal A to the level of perceived threat T. After the model structure and the differential equations have been specified, the model can simulate how a panic attack occurs. Panel (c) depicts the simulated behavior for a period of time with plots of the levels of arousal, perceived threat, and escape. When the effect of perceived threat on arousal is sufficiently strong, there is positive feedback that produces a surge in the levels of arousal, perceived threat, and escape behavior that constitutes the panic attack. Details of methods for developing dynamical systems are provided in reference (16).

10.3.2 Causal Networks

Causal networks are models that represent cause-effect relations. The structure of the model is represented by a directed acyclic graph (DAG) and the quantitative component of the model consists of probability distributions. A graph consists of nodes (shown as ovals) that denote variables and arcs (lines) that link pairs of nodes. In a directed graph the arcs have direction. A directed arc that links two nodes denotes that the variable at the tail of the arc is the cause and the variable at the head of the arc is its effect. As an example, the variable worry in the causal network shown in Fig. 10.2 is connected by a directed arc to the variable sleep problems implying that worry causes sleep problems [19]. Further, the node denoting worry is called the parent node, and the node denoting sleep problems the child node. A directed pathway such as the one from the variable bullying to the variable sleep problems also implies a causal relationship between the two, albeit one that is effected through the intermediate variable worry on the path. A directed acyclic graph has no cycles, which means that it is not possible to begin at a node, traverse the graph following the directed arcs, and loop back to the starting node. Thus, a DAG represents direct causes and chains of causal relations. The causal strength is quantified by a probability distribution that is associated with a node; a probability distribution consists of the probability of each possible value of a node based on the values of its parent node(s).

One approach to developing a causal network is to specify the graphical structure from knowledge in the domain. A second approach is to derive the structure from data. In both approaches, the parameters are typically derived from data. Details of methods for developing causal networks from data are provided in references [20, 21].

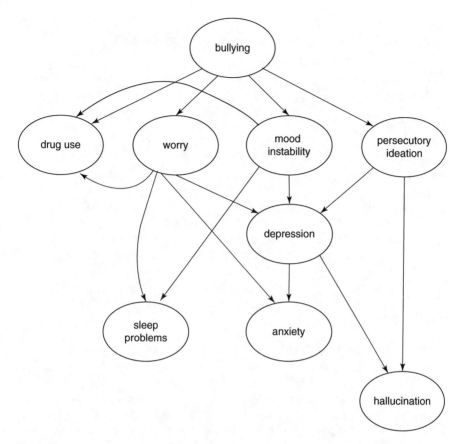

Fig. 10.2 Causal network of relationships between variables related to bullying. (Adapted from [19])

10.4   Data-Driven Approaches

Data-driven approaches use statistical, and increasingly, machine learning (ML) methods to develop models for classification of disease, prediction of clinical outcomes, or defining disease subtypes. A data-driven model captures patterns or relations in the data, often in the form of an equation, and contains parameters that specify the equation. The process of model construction is called training, during which relations and parameters are calculated from the data. This is followed by model evaluation when the performance of the model is assessed. A list of commonly used terms in ML with brief descriptions is given in Box 10.1.

Box 10.1 Glossary of Terms Associated with Machine Learning

Model: A model captures patterns or relations, often in the form of an equation, and it consists of a structure and parameters (see Structure and Parameter). A model may be developed using a theory-driven or a data-driven computational method.

Algorithm: A computational method to achieve a specific goal, especially by a computer. A model is produced by the application of an algorithm, often to a data set.

Explanatory (causal) model: A model that quantitatively describes neural and psychological mechanisms that produce mental illnesses.

Predictive model: A model that quantitatively predicts a clinical outcome such as the risk of development of psychosis in the future. Often, a classification model is called a predictive model (see Classification model).

Classification model: A model that identifies or classifies an existing clinical state such as the presence or absence of psychosis.

Pattern mining: Process of identifying clusters or rules that describe specific patterns in the data such as identifying subtypes of psychosis with distinct cognitive patterns.

Variable: A variable is any characteristic that is measured in a data set. Broadly speaking, a variable can be categorical or continuous. An example of a categorical variable is presence or absence of psychosis and an example of a continuous variable is body weight.

Structure: The structure is part of the specification of a model that describes the variables that are included in the model and the relationships among them. Examples of structures are the variables in a logistic regression model and the graph in a causal network model.

Parameter: A parameter is part of the specification of the model that quantifies variables and the relationships among them. Examples of parameters are the coefficients of the regression equation in a logistic regression model and the probability distributions that are associated with the nodes of the graph in a causal network model.

Feature: A feature is a variable that has been processed so that it is usable for modeling or analysis. An example of a feature is rescaled body weight where the values in a data set have been converted to fractions that lie between 0 and 1.

Target: A target is a variable that a model will predict. A target is also called a class or label. For example, in a model that predicts the future risk of psychosis, the target is the presence or absence of psychosis in the future.

Preprocessing: The process of converting the original data into a format that is suitable for model construction. Converting variables to features is a key preprocessing step.

Training: The process of computing parameters of a model from data. Sometimes, the structure of a model is also computed from data.

Training data set: The data set that is used to train a model.
Evaluation: The process of assessing a model's performance or accuracy, for example its sensitivity and specificity.
Validation data set: The data set that is used to evaluate a model.
Overfitting: Overfitting is the scenario where a model performs very well on the training data set and performs poorly on the validation data set.

10.4.1   The Workflow in Machine Learning

While there are many types of models and an even larger number of algorithms, most applications of ML use the same basic workflow. As shown in Fig. 10.3, the main steps are data collection, data preprocessing, selection of algorithm, application of an algorithm to construct the model, and evaluation of the model.

Data collection may be laborious, or data may be readily available because it was previously collected. Broadly speaking, data come from two main sources: either they are generated from experiments (e.g., data from a randomized controlled trial) or they are produced as a byproduct of some activity (e.g., EHR data that are collected during clinical care). As data sets become freely available beyond the entity that generated them, they may be reused extensively for ML. The steps of data preprocessing, selection of appropriate algorithm, and model construction are typically iterative, and these three steps may be repeated several times. Data preprocessing converts the original data into a format that is suitable for ML and is described in more detail below in the Preprocessing section.

The rapid rise of ML has generated so many algorithms that it can feel overwhelming to choose the appropriate one. Broadly speaking, there are three main categories of ML algorithms: supervised learning, unsupervised learning, and semi-supervised learning. These are described in detail in the Machine Learning Algorithms section below. The type of variables and the nature of the task guide the selection of a suitable algorithm. Variables can be broadly classified as categorical or continuous. Categorical variables contain a finite number of categories, such as psychosis (present, absent) and race (Caucasian, African American, Asian, etc.). Continuous variables are numeric, such as body weight and blood pressure. Broadly speaking, tasks may be categorized as *classification*, *regression*, *prediction*, and

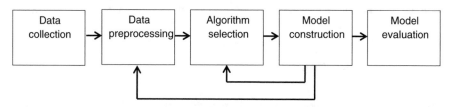

Fig. 10.3 Typical workflow in machine learning. The arrows at the bottom indicate that the steps in the middle are often iterative

pattern mining. An example of a classification task is identifying the clinical state when the target variable is categorical (e.g., has psychosis or not) and an example of a regression task is estimating the value of a physiological parameter when the target variable is continuous (e.g., current blood pressure value). Prediction typically refers to forecasting an outcome in the future, and examples of prediction tasks include assessing the risk of developing an illness when the target variable is categorical (e.g., develop psychosis or not in the future) and forecasting the value of a physiological parameter when the target variable is continuous (e.g., the blood pressure value after starting the antipsychotic medication clozapine). Examples of pattern mining tasks include uncovering subtypes of schizophrenia from symptom profile, cognitive profile, genetic signature, or brain-based assessments [22].

For classification and prediction tasks, supervised ML algorithms are appropriate. More specifically, if the outcome is categorical (e.g., identifying whether an individual has psychosis or not from structural magnetic resonance imaging [23], or predicting whether an individual will develop psychosis in the future or not from linguistic and behavioral information [24]), then classification algorithms like classification trees or support vector machines are suitable. On the other hand, if the outcome is continuous (e.g., the current blood pressure in an individual, or the blood pressure if an individual were to be prescribed clozapine [25]), then regression algorithms like linear regression or support vector regression are suitable.

Pattern mining tasks are often focused on discovering subtypes from data and unsupervised ML algorithms are appropriate for these tasks. For example, for discovering cognitive subtypes in schizophrenia from neuropsychological measures, verbal comprehension, perceptual organization, cognitive flexibility, auditory learning, and memory, a clustering algorithm that groups the data is suitable [26]. Details of clustering algorithms and other algorithms that are applicable for more complex tasks are described in detail in the Machine Learning Algorithms section below.

After the algorithm appropriate to the task and variables is selected, it is applied to a *training data set*, a data set that is used to construct a model. Typically, the workflow is iterative, and the middle three steps may be repeated several times with the construction of interim models (see Fig. 10.3). After the model is finalized it is evaluated on a *validation data set* that is distinct from the training data set. When an evaluation is performed, it is good practice that only the final model, and not the interim models, is assessed on the validation data set to provide a fair assessment of the expected performance on future data to which the model will be applied [27, 28]. More extensive validation may be needed to assess the applicability of the model to data that is obtained from different time periods or geographical locations, or to data that differ in prevalence or severity of the disease under study [27, 28].

10.5   Preprocessing

Preprocessing involves converting raw data to data that is ready for model construction. Preprocessing involves a range of activities such as *data cleaning, data integration, imputation of missing data* if appropriate, and *dimensionality reduction*.

Data cleaning focuses on identifying and removing discrepancies and correcting errors. Data from multiple sources may have to be combined into a single data set; this must be done carefully to avoid redundancies and inconsistencies. Imputation of missing data involves filling in values for data that is missing with a suitable value since some ML algorithms cannot handle missing data. Dimensionality reduction is the process of reducing the number of variables under consideration and is described in more detail below in the Dimensionality Reduction section. The original values in a data set are called *variables*, and after preprocessing of the values, the variables are referred to as *features*. For example, the variable body weight is referred to as the feature body weight when the original body weight values are converted to fractions that lie between 0 and 1.

10.5.1   Dimensionality Reduction

Increasingly, biomedical data sets contain a large number of variables, numbering in the tens of thousands or more, and sometimes the number of variables is greater than the number of observations. In data sets with a large number of variables, many of the variables are either redundant or irrelevant for model construction. Such variables, when included in modeling, can result in models that perform poorly due to the inclusion of the irrelevant variables. Dimensionality reduction is used to reduce the number of variables and the resulting features, so that better models are developed. In addition to developing better models, dimensionality reduction may speed up model construction by reducing the computational cost and may provide simpler and more easily interpretable models [29].

Two main approaches to dimensionality reduction are *feature selection* and *feature extraction*. Feature selection is the process of selecting a subset of the original set of features to obtain fewer features that are relevant for model construction [30]. Feature extraction, in contrast, is the process of creating fewer new features from the original set of features by combining them in various ways. Thus, feature selection picks some of the original features while feature extraction creates new features from the original features. Compared to feature extraction, an advantage of feature selection is that it preserves the original semantics of the features that is useful for interpreting the model.

10.5.2   Feature Selection Methods

Feature selection methods can be grouped into four categories that include *knowledge-based selection*, *filter methods*, *wrapper methods*, and *embedded methods* (Table 10.1) [31]. Knowledge-based selection uses expert knowledge from a human expert or obtained from the scientific literature. This method offers features with high interpretability; however, it is laborious and time-consuming [32, 33].

Table 10.1 Feature selection methods with brief descriptions and examples

Method	Advantages	Disadvantages	Examples
Knowledge-based	Features are likely to be highly interpretable	Laborious and time-consuming	Selection of genomic variables curated from a gene-disease association database [33]
Filter	Fast; can handle large numbers of features; feature selection is independent of which ML algorithm is used	Selected features may be worse than wrapper and embedded methods; univariate filter methods cannot capture interactions among features	Univariate filter methods include chi-square test and t-test; multivariate filter methods include forward selection and backward elimination [34]
Wrapper	Captures interactions among features; selected features often better than filter methods	Slow; feature selection is dependent on which ML algorithm is used	Stepwise regression [36], forward and backward feature selection algorithms [35]
Embedded	Captures interactions among features; faster than wrapper methods	Feature selection is dependent on which ML algorithm is used	ML algorithms such as classification and regression trees, random forests, and regularized regression

Filter methods evaluate the relevance of features by assessing the intrinsic characteristics of the data without considering the properties of the subsequent ML algorithm. Univariate filter methods evaluate a single feature at a time, while multivariate filter methods evaluate subsets of features at a time [34]. In univariate filter methods, individual features are ranked according to a specific criterion, and the top ranked n features are selected. Examples of ranking criteria are the *chi-square statistic, mutual information,* and *variance* of the feature. A major drawback of univariate filter methods is that they may select redundant features because the relationships among features are not considered. Multivariate filter methods, on the other hand, are capable of eliminating redundant features by assessing relationships among features. In contrast to univariate methods that apply a criterion to single features, multivariate filter methods apply the criterion, such as mutual information, to subsets of features. Multivariate filter methods typically search over subsets of features and evaluate each subset with the ranking criterion. Two common approaches for searching are *forward selection* and *backward elimination* [35]. In forward selection, the method begins with an empty feature set and adds one feature at a time that best improves the criterion and ends when the addition of a feature does not improve the criterion. In backward elimination, the algorithm begins with all features and removes one feature at a time that best improves the criterion and ends when the removal of a feature does not improve the criterion. Filter methods are fast and scale well to high-dimensional data with large numbers of features. However, the features selected by filter methods may be worse than those selected by the wrapper and embedded methods that are described next.

Wrapper methods assess the suitability of features by evaluating their performance in the ML algorithm that is chosen to construct the model. For example, with supervised ML algorithms (e.g., logistic regression), a wrapper may evaluate subsets of features based on the accuracy of the model. As another example, with unsupervised ML algorithms (e.g., k-means clustering), a wrapper may evaluate subsets based on the goodness of the clusters. The wrapper methods search over subsets of features in the same way as multivariate filter methods. The features selected by wrapper methods are typically better than those selected by filter methods because the feature subsets are evaluated using the ML algorithm that will be subsequently used for model construction. However, wrapper methods are slow and may not scale well to high-dimensional data or if the ML algorithm itself is slow.

Embedded methods integrate feature selection in the ML algorithm; thus, as the ML algorithm constructs a model, it also performs feature selection. Commonly used ML algorithms that are integrated with embedded feature selection methods include classification and regression trees, random forests, and regularized regression. Embedded methods are faster than wrapper methods and scale better to high-dimensional data and slower ML algorithms.

10.5.3   Feature Extraction Methods

In contrast to feature selection methods that do not alter the original features, feature extraction methods construct new features that are more relevant in model construction. Examples of common feature extraction methods include linear discriminant analysis (LDA) and principal component analysis (PCA). These methods produce fewer features by combining the original features.

For example, Fig. 10.4 shows a data set with two features, F1 and F2, that are represented by the x- and y-axes and two classes represented by red and black colors. LDA is applied to this data set to produce a single feature that will be most relevant to distinguish between the two classes. With feature selection, the only options are to use F1 or F2 that correspond to projecting the data onto the x-axis or y-axis, respectively, and neither one is useful in separating the two classes (Panel b in Fig. 10.4 shows the projection on F1). With LDA, new features are created by projecting the data onto new axes and then selecting the one that produces the best separation. In Fig. 10.4, two new features, F3 and F4, are shown as new axes onto which the data is projected. As can be seen, of the features F1, F3, and F4, F3 separates the two classes perfectly. Thus, F3 is a better new feature than F4.

While LDA creates new features that maximize the separation of the classes, PCA creates new features that maximize the variance in the data. More complex feature extraction methods include kernel learning and neural networks that project the data in complex ways.

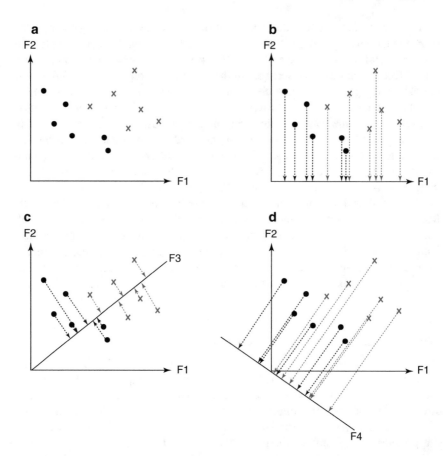

Fig. 10.4 Linear discriminant analysis (LDA). Panel a shows data from two classes (red and black). Panel b shows the projection of the data onto the x-axis that represents feature F1. Each of panels c and d show a new axis that represents a new feature. Projections of the data on the various axes show that feature F3 produces the best separation of the two classes

10.6 Machine Learning Algorithms

The goal of ML is to infer patterns from data and use them to make predictions or provide insights into relations in the data. Rapid progress in ML in the past few decades has led to the development of a wide range of ML algorithms, including those that can be applied to big data sets. ML algorithms can be categorized broadly into *supervised learning, unsupervised learning,* and *semi-supervised learning.* Lately, a subfield of ML called *deep learning* has developed that is concerned with algorithms that are inspired by artificial neural networks.

10.6.1   Supervised Learning

In supervised learning the training data set contains a special variable called the target (also called class or label), and is referred to as labeled. The goal of supervised learning is to classify or predict the target (or the class or label). For example, in a model predicting the risk of psychosis, the target is the presence or absence of psychosis in the future. The goal of supervised learning is to learn a pattern that relates the features to the target such that when the pattern is applied to new data, it classifies or predicts the target accurately. When the target is binary (i.e., it has only two possible values, for example, presence or absence of psychosis) the supervised learning is called classification (see Fig. 10.5). Logistic regression, classification trees, naive Bayes, support vector machines, and random forests are commonly used classification methods. When the target is a continuous variable (e.g., body weight) the supervised learning is called regression. Linear regression, regression trees, support vector regression, and random forests are commonly used regression methods. In linear regression, the model is an equation that describes a line that is closest to all data points (see Fig. 10.5). The line can then be used to predict the value of the target for a new data point. Some methods like classification and regression trees and random forests can be used for both classification and regression. Although logistic regression (not to be confused with linear regression) is called regression, it is typically used for classification when the target is binary because it predicts the probability that a data point belongs to one of two classes.

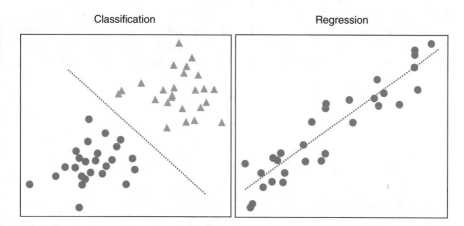

Fig. 10.5 Supervised learning. On the left, the classification model is a line (red dotted) that separates the triangular data from the circular data. On the right, the regression model is a line that is close to all of the data

10.6.2   Unsupervised Learning

In contrast to supervised learning, in unsupervised learning the training data set does not contain a target, and is referred to as unlabeled. The goal of unsupervised learning is to uncover patterns or natural divisions, such as subtypes of psychosis. Clustering and dimensionality reduction (that is used for preprocessing) are commonly used for unsupervised learning.

Clustering partitions the data into groups that are meaningful and useful. (Though it is worth noting that "meaningful and useful" can sometimes be challenging to ascertain.) An example of an application of clustering is identifying subtypes of schizophrenia based on features such as symptoms, neuropsychological measures, cognitive measures, and brain imaging [23]. The goal of clustering data points into groups (clusters) is to achieve both good cohesion and separation. Cohesion refers to making each cluster compact, which means that the data points in a cluster are very similar or close to one another. Separation refers to making each cluster distinct or isolated from other clusters, which means that the data points in a cluster are very different or far away from the data points in other clusters. Clustering methods include (1) hierarchical methods that find successive clusters using previously established clusters, (2) partitional methods that determine all clusters at once, and (3) Bayesian clustering methods that provide a probability distribution over the collection of all ways to partition the data. A commonly used method is k-means, a partitional method that partitions the data into k clusters where k is specified by the user and each cluster minimizes the distance of the members of the cluster from the cluster center (see Fig. 10.6). The value of k may be specified by the user based on knowledge of the domain. Often, such knowledge is lacking, and in such situations, the k-means algorithm is applied to the data with different values of k to generate different numbers of clusters and the optimal number of clusters is chosen to have both good cohesion and separation. The section

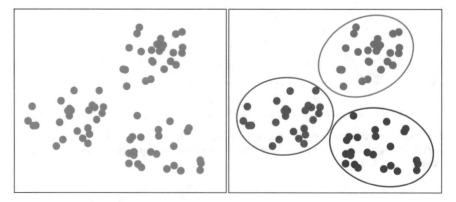

Fig. 10.6 Before clustering (left panel) and after clustering with k-means that reveals three clusters (right panel)

Evaluation of Model Performance below provides details on measuring cluster cohesion and separation.

Dimensionality reduction refers to reducing the number of features in the data and is described in more detail above in the Dimensionality Reduction section. Dimensionality reduction is typically useful to apply to data with a large number of features such as brain image or genomic data.

10.6.3   Semi-Supervised Learning

Traditionally, learning has consisted of either supervised learning, where all data is labeled, or unsupervised learning, where all data is unlabeled. Semi-supervised learning is concerned with learning from a combination of labeled and unlabeled data for tasks such as classification and clustering. Semi-supervised learning is applicable in many applications where there is limited labeled data but a large amount of unlabeled data.

Semi-supervised learning is based on the assumption that data points that are closer to each other are more likely to have the same label. The simplest semi-supervised learning method for classification is self-training. In self-training, a classification model like logistic regression is constructed from the labeled data and is applied to the unlabeled data. Unlabeled data that has been classified with high probability is added to the training data set and the model is retrained on the larger data set, and this process is repeated several times. Self-learning has the advantages that it is simple and can be used with any classification method; however, it has the disadvantage that mistakes in the labeling of the unlabeled data may be reinforced, leading to a poor model. Another semi-supervised learning method for classification is co-training. Co-training uses two different views of the data, where each view may arise from distinct data types, to construct a pair of models. For example, in schizophrenia classification, one model is constructed from brain imaging and another from neuropsychological measures. In a fashion similar to self-training, the models are applied to unlabeled data, and data that are labeled with high probability by either model are added to the training data set that is used to retrain the models. The intuition is that the two models are likely to make different mistakes and mistakes in labeling are fewer than with self-training [37].

Semi-supervised learning can also be used for clustering, in which the knowledge of labels in the small amount of labeled data is leveraged by the algorithm. One example of a semi-supervised learning method for clustering is constrained k-means clustering, which is an extension of standard k-means clustering. The algorithm first identifies a set of *seed clusters* using only the labeled data such that data of the same class are assigned to the same cluster. Next, the algorithm applies standard k-means clustering to the unlabeled data using the centers of the seed clusters for initialization rather than using random values for cluster centers as is done in standard k-means [38].

10.6.4   Deep Learning

The methods described so far depend heavily on the representation of the data that is provided to the algorithm. For example, when logistic regression is used to predict the risk of psychosis, the model does not use the raw data directly. Rather, specific features are provided to the model. However, in many applications, it is difficult to know what features should be used. For example, when predicting the risk of psychosis from individual pixels in a magnetic resonance imaging scan, it is challenging to define relevant features for a logistic regression model.

Deep learning solves this challenge by automatically defining features from raw data, and enables the construction of complex features from simpler ones. For example, to recognize the image of a cat in a picture, deep learning extracts simple features consisting of edges from pixels, combines edges to form complex features like corners and contours, and further combines these to construct more complex features like parts of a cat's face. The archetypal example of a deep learning model is the multilayer neural network (see Fig. 10.7). A multilayer neural network uses the first layer to translate input features to simple mathematical functions and uses additional layers to successively combine simpler functions into complex functions. Figure 10.7 shows an illustrative example of a multilayer neural network that was developed to classify individuals as autistic or not from magnetic resonance images of the brain [39].

10.7   Evaluation of Model Performance

Evaluation of supervised ML models is well developed compared to the evaluation of unsupervised ML models. We will focus on the evaluation of supervised models and only briefly discuss unsupervised models.

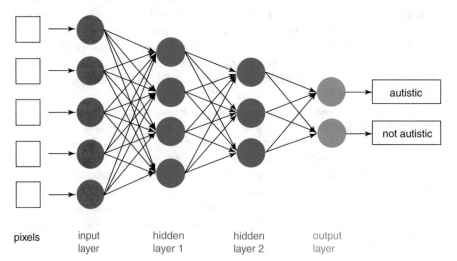

Fig. 10.7 An illustrative multilayer neural network that takes pixels from magnetic resonance images as input and produces as output whether an individual is autistic or not. It has two intermediate layers (hidden layers) that transform the input to the output

10.7.1   Supervised Models

The correctness of a supervised model such as a logistic regression model is measured by the degree to which the classification (e.g., has psychosis) or prediction (e.g., will develop psychosis) matches the current state or future outcome. A common application is one where the target has only two classes (e.g., has psychosis or does not have psychosis) and the classifications or predictions are stated numerically (e.g., a number between 0 and 1 from a logistic regression model where the number denotes the probability of having psychosis). The numerical value from a model is converted into a class by using a threshold such that if the value is above the threshold one class (e.g., has psychosis) is assigned, and if below the threshold the other class is assigned (e.g., does not have psychosis). A model that produces numerical classifications or predictions is evaluated on various measures of performance that include *discrimination* and *calibration*.

Discrimination measures the ability of the model to separate one class from the other (e.g., those who have psychosis from those who do not). It is assessed with the Receiver Operating Characteristic (ROC) curve that is based on the concepts of sensitivity and specificity, which are computed after a model's output is converted into classes by applying a threshold. Sensitivity is the ability of the model to correctly identify individuals with psychosis or who will develop psychosis (e.g., the percentage of individuals with psychosis and are correctly identified), whereas specificity is the ability of the model to correctly identify individuals without psychosis or who will not develop psychosis (e.g., the percentage of individuals who do not have psychosis and are correctly identified). The ROC curve graphically displays the trade-off between sensitivity and specificity as the threshold for categorization is varied from the lowest value to the highest (e.g., from 0 to 1 for a logistic regression model). As shown in Fig. 10.8, a ROC curve goes from the bottom left corner to the top right corner. Points on the curve in the lower left are thresholds at which the

Fig. 10.8 Receiver Operating Characteristic (ROC) curves. ROC curves for three hypothetical models are shown. Curve A represents a model with perfect discrimination. Curve B represents discrimination of a realistic model that is potentially useful. Curve C shows a model that performs no better than chance

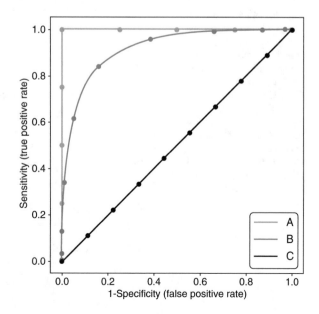

model's classification ability has high specificity and low sensitivity. In contrast, points in the upper right are thresholds at which the model has high sensitivity but low specificity. Thus moving along the curve from the bottom left to the top right represents the trade-off between sensitivity (increasing) and specificity (decreasing).

The area under the ROC curve (AUC) is a number between 0.5 to 1 that provides a single number summary of discrimination [40]. An AUC of 1 represents perfect discrimination that would be achieved by a perfect model, for example, a logistic regression model that correctly assigns a probability of 1 to every individual who has psychosis and a probability of 0 to every individual without psychosis. An AUC of 0.5 indicates discrimination that is no better than chance and denotes a useless model, for example, one that has no ability at all to distinguish between individuals with or without psychosis (see Fig. 10.8).

Calibration measures the extent of agreement between the numerical classifications or predictions and the actual current state or future outcome in groups of individuals with similar numerical values [41]. For example, if a logistic regression model assigns a probability of 0.2 (i.e., predicts a 20% risk) of developing psychosis to an individual, then the fraction of individuals who have been assigned similar probabilities of developing psychosis should be approximately 0.2 (i.e., approximately 20 out of 100 individuals with similar probabilities should develop psychosis). A calibration curve provides a graphical assessment of calibration and consists of predictions on the x-axis and the outcome on the y-axis. A perfectly calibrated model will have a calibration line that is identical to the diagonal line (see Fig. 10.9).

A perfect calibration curve is achieved by a perfectly calibrated model, for example, a logistic regression model that correctly assigns a probability of 0.2 to one group of individuals where the fraction 0.2 of the group will later develop psychosis, assigns a probability of 0.4 to the second group of individuals where the fraction 0.4 of the group will later develop psychosis, assigns a probability of 0.7 to the third group of individuals where the fraction 0.7 of the group will later develop psychosis, and so on (see Fig. 10.9).

Fig. 10.9 Calibration curves. Calibration curves for three hypothetical models are shown. Curve A represents a model with perfect calibration. Curves B and C represent calibrations of realistic models that are potentially useful. Curve B denotes better calibration than Curve C because it is closer to the diagonal line that represents perfect calibration

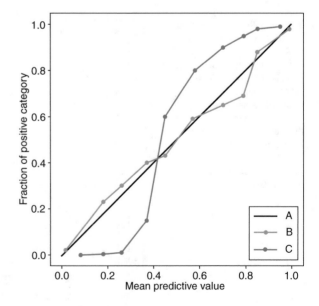

A model with excellent discrimination (AUC close to 1) may be poorly calibrated. For example, a naive Bayes model that assigns a probability of 0.9 to every
individual who will develop psychosis and a probability of 0.8 to every individual
who will not has perfect discrimination but will have poor calibration because it is
assigning probabilities that are too high to the group of individuals who will not
develop psychosis (i.e., it is unlikely that the fraction 0.8 of this group will develop
psychosis). Some ML algorithms like naive Bayes and classification and regression
trees may produce models with poor calibration. ML algorithms are often sensitive
to the incidence of the condition in the training data set. When a model is developed
from a data set with high incidence, it may be miscalibrated for a setting where the
incidence is lower and generate systematically overestimated risk probabilities [42].

10.7.2 Unsupervised Models

No standard approach exists for the validation of cluster models because, contrary
to supervised learning where we have the ground truth in the data to evaluate the
model's performance, in unsupervised learning typically no ground truth is available. However, some evaluation measures are available that are useful to evaluate
clusters without reference to ground truth [43].

The goal of clustering is to create clusters that have good cohesion and separation. Cohesion or compactness of clusters can be assessed by the variation of the
distances of data points to the cluster center. For a single data point, the measure that
is used is the square of the distance of the data point from its cluster center. The
average squared distance over all points serves as an overall measure of how compact the clusters are. The number of clusters at which there is an elbow in the plot
of the average squared distance versus number of clusters is considered to be an
optimal number of clusters on this measure (see Fig. 10.10).

Fig. 10.10 The averaged
squared distance decreases
as the number of clusters
increase. The elbow of the
curve occurs when the
number of clusters is 3

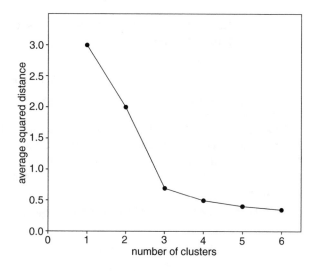

Fig. 10.11 The average silhouette coefficient increases and then decreases as the number of clusters increase. The peak of the curve occurs when the number of clusters is 3

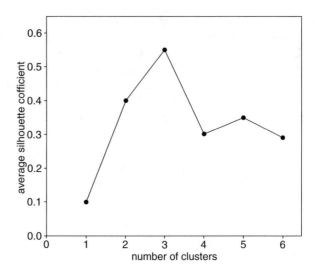

Separation or cluster isolation can be assessed by the silhouette coefficient. For a single data point, the silhouette coefficient is calculated as the difference between the mean nearest-cluster distance (i.e., mean distance between the data point and all other points of the nearest cluster that the data point is not a part of) and the mean intra-cluster distance (i.e., mean distance between the data point and all other points in the same cluster) that is normalized by the maximum value. A high silhouette coefficient indicates that the data point is well-matched to its own cluster and poorly matched to neighboring clusters. The average silhouette coefficient over all points serves as an overall measure of how well the clusters are separated. The number of clusters at which the average silhouette coefficient peaks is considered to be an optimal number of clusters for this measure (see Fig. 10.11).

10.8 Applications of Computational Models in Mental Health

One way of categorizing computational models is by the level(s) of biological scale at which they are applicable from a lower level of molecular process to a higher level of behavioral expression.

Biophysical models, used at the lower biological levels, are constrained by the biological details and physiological properties of ion channels (e.g., temporal and voltage-dependent behavior of the flow of ions), neuronal cell membranes (e.g., temporal evolution of the membrane electrical potential), synapses (e.g., long increase or decrease in signal transmission), and neural circuits (e.g., feed-forward and feedback propagation of signals). Biophysical models are typically used at the molecular, cellular, or circuit levels. At the cellular level, a biophysical model may represent the electrical properties of neurons with the component cell bodies, axons, and dendrites in minute detail. At the next higher level, a biophysical model may represent the electrical features of a population of neurons as a set of compartments (e.g., one compartment for cell bodies of neurons and another for dendrites). For example, Purkinje cell models have been developed that incorporate the electrical properties of 15 types of ion channels, and such models can be used to study the effects of genetic mutations of ion channel genes on Purkinje cell function [44].

Connectionist models use neural networks and are based on the idea that the knowledge underlying neural or psychological activity is stored in the connections among neurons. Adjustments to the strengths of connections lead to changes in behavior. Connectionist models can provide a link between mechanistically based neural networks and expression of behavior and are applicable at the circuit and system levels. Examples of connectionist models include models of hallucinations and delusional thoughts in schizophrenia and perceptual difficulties in autism [9].

Reinforcement-learning models represent systems that learn to gain rewards and avoid punishments in complicated environments [45]. Further, they can be used to represent and reason about how information obtained at one point in time affects beliefs and behavior at another [3]. These models are applicable at the system and behavior levels and tend not to be biophysically detailed. An example of a reinforcement-learning model is one that models how dopamine and cortico-basal ganglia-thalamocortical (CBGTC) circuits stimulate behavior to acquire rewards and avoid punishments [13].

Classification models categorize data such as individuals into several classes. Such models are typically learned from data and can be used, for example, in identifying whether an individual has a disease or not, and differentiating among several mental illnesses with similar symptomatology. For example, a classification model can distinguish individuals with and without bipolar disorder using clinical, neuroimaging, neurocognitive, and biomarker data [46, 47].

Regression models estimate a continuous value such as blood pressure or the score on a mental health instrument. For example, a regression model can estimate the score on the Positive Mental Health instrument from demographic characteristics such as age and gender and clinical characteristics such as duration of illness, anxiety and depression [48]. Classification and regression models as well as predictive models and cluster models, which follow, apply to any level of biological scale from a lower level of molecular process to a higher level of behavioral expression.

Predictive models typically forecast an outcome or a future event. Prediction is critical to many clinical activities related to mental health disorders as in other areas of medicine and includes risk assessment (assessing the risk of developing a disease in the future), prognosis (forecasting the likely course of a disease), and therapeutics (predicting treatment response) [48]. Beyond the care of individuals, prediction plays a critical role in public health and research. Predictive models are typically derived from data and can help guide decision-making related to mental health disorders and public health. Risk assessment models are useful in clinical management and research. For example, similar to the benefits of early detection of breast cancer, prediction of a high risk of psychosis by early detection of prodromal phase can lead to early intervention and improvement of outcomes [49]. Furthermore, risk prediction can increase the efficiency of research studies by evaluating interventions on at-risk individuals [50].

Better prediction of the most likely diagnosis allows timely initiation of therapy, which minimizes suffering and increases adherence. For example, the ability to distinguish major depression from bipolar disorder earlier can enable earlier and appropriate interventions [51]. Predicting prognosis is also clinically valuable. For example, accurate prediction models for social and occupational disability in individuals with prodromal symptoms of psychosis or with recent-onset depression can guide personalized prevention of functional impairment [32, 52].

The prediction of response to treatment enables the selection of optimized interventions. For example, clinical information and genetic variants can predict outcomes in psychotherapy and drug therapies [53, 54]. Individualized and more precise treatment increases adherence and decreases undesired side effects. Additionally, better prediction of poor responders to treatment advances research by focusing on the evaluation of new drugs and treatments in treatment-resistant individuals [50].

Cluster models group data such as individuals in such a way that individuals in the same group or cluster are more similar to each other than to those in other clusters. Cluster models have been extensively used to subtype or stratify a range of mental illnesses. For example, schizophrenia and depression have been subtyped using symptoms, neuropsychological measures, cognitive measures, and brain imaging [55].

With the rapid growth of analytic methods to develop computational models, increasingly such algorithms are being applied to understand neural and psychological processes and across several mental health disorder domains. Table 10.2 lists some domains with illustrative applications of computational modeling. Applications in elucidating the mechanisms of psychological or neural processes focus on modeling normal and abnormal neuronal activity at the level of ion channels, cells, and circuits, as well as mental and psychological phenomena such as perception, planning, and emotion. Detection and diagnosis applications emphasize the risk of developing mental health disorders and their diagnosis. Prognosis, treatment, and support applications concentrate on the progression, treatment, or support opportunities for mental illnesses. Applications in public health focus on estimating prevalence and monitoring mental health disorders. Finally, applications in research and clinical administration are aimed at improving mental health research and in improving processes in clinical workflows [56].

Table 10.2 Application domains in mental health and illness and illustrative applications of computational models. (Adapted from [24])

Domain	Applications
Mechanisms of psychological or neural processes	• Characterization and quantification of the electrical properties of neurons • Modeling normal perception and perceptual dysfunction in schizophrenia and autism • Modeling behavior to acquire rewards and avoid punishments
Detection and diagnosis	• Developing risk models to identify an individual's predisposition for, or risk of, progressing to a mental health disorder • Classifying a new individual as diseased or not • Differentiating among mental health disorders with similar symptomatology
Prognosis, treatment, and support	• Predicting long-term clinical outcomes • Detecting changes in behavior indicative of a mental health disorder from mobile and sensor data • Providing personalized and timely treatment or interventions • Analysis of online support groups for mental health communities
Public health applications	• Assessing mental illnesses in both specific and broader populations • Monitoring mental health following an event or disaster • Creating models of risk to improve health system delivery
Research and clinical administration	• Improving resource allocation • Improving research methodologies (e.g., data sharing, participant selection, and analysis) • Extracting mental health symptoms from existing sources (e.g., research publications, clinical notes, and databases)

10.9   Standards for Reporting Models

Computational models are poorly reported in the literature [57]. Missing details in the title, abstract, model-building procedures, description of the final model, and report of model performance make it difficult for the scientific and healthcare community to judge the validity and applicability of computational models.

One initiative to standardize reporting of the key details of studies that develop models for clinical application is the Transparent Reporting of a multivariable predictive model for Individual Prognosis Or Diagnosis (TRIPOD) Statement [58]. TRIPOD includes a 22-item checklist that focuses on reporting how a model that provides a diagnosis or prognosis was conducted, analyzed, and interpreted. This checklist guides the details that should be included in the title, abstract, descriptions of the data, predictors, and outcomes, and descriptions of model specification, development, and performance of the model. For example, the checklist specifies that in the introduction of the study description, the clinical context (including whether it is diagnostic or prognostic) and rationale for developing or validating the predictive model should be described. As another example, the objectives of the study should be specified clearly, including whether the study describes the development or validation of the model, or both.

The TRIPOD checklist is available at www.tripod-statement.org. Adherence to this checklist by researchers, peer reviewers, and editors will lead to more complete reporting of details of computational models [59].

10.10   Policy, Ethical, and Safety Issues

The increasing availability of data and the growing application of analytic methods have led to the development of a wide range of computational models both for biomedical discovery and clinical use. When these models are deployed, especially in a clinical context to provide targeted care, to improve outcomes, and to lower healthcare costs, policy, ethical, and legal challenges arise [60, 61]. (See Chapter 18.) A comprehensive consideration of such issues is presented in a recent publication [60], a few key issues are summarized in the next paragraph, and some examples of ethical and safety issues are given in Table 10.3 [62].

A primary consideration is whether or not the data used in model development is representative of the whole population. Historically, members of certain racial and ethnic groups, people with disabilities, individuals in prison, and members of other vulnerable groups have been underrepresented in research studies. Such inequitable representation can lead to models that are not valid for parts of the population [63, 64]. A second consideration is that models need to be evaluated in real-world settings before deployment [60]. A third consideration is a liability. Makers as well as users of computational models in clinical care may face liability if there are errors in the model or if the model malfunctions. Increasingly, regulators of medical devices and software will regulate the application and deployment of computational models in clinical care. The U.S. Food and Drug Administration (FDA) is ensuring the safety, efficacy, and security of computational models for clinical use by regulating such models as Software as a Medical Device (SaMD) [65]. One of the first computational models that received marketing authorization in the U.S. in 2018

Table 10.3 Examples of safety issues in the clinical use of computational models of mental health and illnesses

Issue	Description
Model drift	A mismatch between the data on which the model was trained and that used in operation, due to changes over time or use of the model at a different location, may result in erroneous predictions.
Automation complacency	Human users come to unduly rely on the model's predictions because they perceive the model to be infallible, which may result in accepting erroneous predictions.
Adversarial hacking	Model weaknesses allow a small, carefully designed change to inputs to completely alter the model's output, causing it to confidently arrive at erroneous predictions.

detects diabetic retinopathy from retinal images [66, 67]. However, the regulation of computational models is a challenge because they differ from existing medical technologies: they can continuously adapt, they have the potential to be widely used in clinical interactions, and the way they reach their recommendations is often opaque to physicians [68]. A fourth consideration is safety related to the clinical use of these models (see Table 10.3). Examples of safety issues include model drift [69, 70], automation complacency [71], and adversarial hacking [72], as described in Table 10.3. A fifth consideration with the widespread use of predictive models is the availability of explanations that describe the basis of predictions [73]. Predictive explanation provides reasoning for the prediction that is made by a model for an individual. For example, the insight that an explanation provides about why an individual is assigned a high probability of developing psychosis, may lead a physician to gain trust in that prediction. Good explanations are parsimonious so that they are readily and rapidly understood by the user [74].

10.11   Conclusion

The complexity of mental function and dysfunction and their underlying neural and psychological mechanisms pose a unique challenge. Because of the increased availability of data, analytic methods, and computing capability, investigators have an unprecedented opportunity to develop computational models [11, 75]. Modern theory-based and data-driven methods have the potential to elucidate neural and psychological mechanisms of mental function, more precisely classify mental health disorders, better predict the risk of developing mental health disorders, and discover new molecular mechanisms that can be targeted by new interventions.

References

1. Stoddard J, Jones M. Computational modeling in pediatric mental health. J Am Acad Child Adolesc Psychiatry. 2019;58(5):471.
2. Stephan KE, Bach DR, Fletcher PC, Flint J, Frank MJ, Friston KJ, et al. Charting the landscape of priority problems in psychiatry, part 1: classification and diagnosis. Lancet Psychiatry. 2016;3(1):77–83.
3. Kurth-Nelson Z, O'Doherty J, Barch D, Deneve S, Durstewitz D, Frank M, et al. Computational approaches for studying mechanisms of psychiatric disorders. Computational psychiatry: New perspectives on mental illness. 2016:77–99.
4. Mukai J, Tamura M, Fénelon K, Rosen AM, Spellman TJ, Kang R, et al. Molecular substrates of altered axonal growth and brain connectivity in a mouse model of schizophrenia. Neuron. 2015;86(3):680–95.
5. Trull TJ, Ebner-Priemer U. Ambulatory assessment. Annu Rev Clin Psychol. 2013;9:151–76.
6. Weiner MW, Veitch DP, Aisen PS, Beckett LA, Cairns NJ, Cedarbaum J, et al. Impact of the Alzheimer's disease neuroimaging initiative, 2004 to 2014. Alzheimers Dement. 2015;11(7):865–84.
7. Investigators AoURP. The "All of Us" research program. N Engl J Med. 2019;381(7):668–76.

8. Consortium H. The human body at cellular resolution: the NIH Human Biomolecular Atlas Program. Nature. 2019;574(7777):187.
9. Lanillos P, Oliva D, Philippsen A, Yamashita Y, Nagai Y, Cheng G. A review on neural network models of schizophrenia and autism spectrum disorder. Neural Netw. 2020;122:338–63.
10. Bennett D, Silverstein SM, Niv Y. The two cultures of computational psychiatry. JAMA Psychiat. 2019;76(6):563–4.
11. Huys QJ, Maia TV, Frank MJ. Computational psychiatry as a bridge from neuroscience to clinical applications. Nat Neurosci. 2016;19(3):404.
12. Maia TV, Huys QJ, Frank MJ. Theory-based computational psychiatry. Biol Psychiatry. 2017;82(6):382–4.
13. Maia TV, Frank MJ. From reinforcement learning models to psychiatric and neurological disorders. Nat Neurosci. 2011;14(2):154.
14. Chang B, Choi Y, Jeon M, Lee J, Han K-M, Kim A, et al. ARPNet: antidepressant response prediction network for major depressive disorder. Genes. 2019;10(11):907.
15. Huys QJ. Advancing clinical improvements for patients using the theory-driven and data-driven branches of computational psychiatry. JAMA Psychiat. 2018;75(3):225–6.
16. Haslbeck J, Ryan O, Robinaugh D, Waldorp L, Borsboom D. Modeling psychopathology: from data models to formal theories. 2019.
17. Robinaugh D, Haslbeck J, Waldorp L, Kossakowski J, Fried EI, Millner A, et al. Advancing the network theory of mental disorders: a computational model of panic disorder. 2019.
18. Steimer T. The biology of fear-and anxiety-related behaviors. Dialogues Clin Neurosci. 2002;4(3):231.
19. Moffa G, Catone G, Kuipers J, Kuipers E, Freeman D, Marwaha S, et al. Using directed acyclic graphs in epidemiological research in psychosis: an analysis of the role of bullying in psychosis. Schizophr Bull. 2017;43(6):1273–9.
20. Glymour C, Zhang K, Spirtes P. Review of causal discovery methods based on graphical models. Front Genet. 2019;10:524.
21. Glymour CN, Cooper GF. Computation, Causation, and Discovery. AAAI Press; 1999.
22. Green MJ, Girshkin L, Kremerskothen K, Watkeys O, Quidé Y. A systematic review of studies reporting data-driven cognitive subtypes across the psychosis spectrum. Neuropsychol Rev. 2019:1–15.
23. Salvador R, Radua J, Canales-Rodríguez EJ, Solanes A, Sarró S, Goikolea JM, et al. Evaluation of machine learning algorithms and structural features for optimal MRI-based diagnostic prediction in psychosis. PLoS One. 2017;12(4):e0175683.
24. Rezaii N, Walker E, Wolff P. A machine learning approach to predicting psychosis using semantic density and latent content analysis. NPJ Schizophr. 2019;5(1):1–12.
25. Gonsai N, Amin V, Mendpara C, Speth R, Hale G. Effects of dopamine receptor antagonist antipsychotic therapy on blood pressure. J Clin Pharm Ther. 2018;43(1):1–7.
26. Dawes SE, Jeste DV, Palmer BW. Cognitive profiles in persons with chronic schizophrenia. J Clin Exp Neuropsychol. 2011;33(8):929–36.
27. Labarère J, Bertrand R, Fine MJ. How to derive and validate clinical prediction models for use in intensive care medicine. Intensive Care Med. 2014;40(4):513–27.
28. Hendriksen JM, Geersing G-J, Moons KG, de Groot JA. Diagnostic and prognostic prediction models. J Thromb Haemost. 2013;11:129–41.
29. Guyon I, Elisseeff A. An introduction to variable and feature selection. J Mach Learn Res. 2003;3(Mar):1157–82.
30. Kohavi R, Sommerfield D. Feature subset selection using the wrapper method: overfitting and dynamic search space topology. KDD; 1995.
31. Tay D, Poh CL, Goh C, Kitney RI. A biological continuum based approach for efficient clinical classification. J Biomed Inform. 2014;47:28–38.
32. Koutsouleris N, Kambeitz-Ilankovic L, Ruhrmann S, Rosen M, Ruef A, Dwyer DB, et al. Prediction models of functional outcomes for individuals in the clinical high-risk state for psychosis or with recent-onset depression: a multimodal, multisite machine learning analysis. JAMA Psychiat. 2018;75(11):1156–72.

33. Raghu VK, Ge X, Chrysanthis PK, Benos PV, editors. Integrated theory-and data-driven feature selection in gene expression data analysis. 2017 IEEE 33rd International Conference on Data Engineering (ICDE); 2017: IEEE.
34. Bolón-Canedo V, Sánchez-Maroño N, Alonso-Betanzos A. A review of feature selection methods on synthetic data. Knowl Inf Syst. 2013;34(3):483–519.
35. Devijver PA, Kittler J. Pattern Recognition Theory and Applications. Springer Science & Business Media; 2012.
36. Miller A. Subset Selection in Regression. CRC Press; 2002.
37. Chapelle O, Schölkopf B, Zien A. Introduction to semi-supervised learning. Semi-Supervised Learning. 2017:1–12.
38. Bair E. Semi-supervised clustering methods. Wiley Interdisciplinary Reviews: Computational Statistics. 2013;5(5):349–61.
39. Kong Y, Gao J, Xu Y, Pan Y, Wang J, Liu J. Classification of autism spectrum disorder by combining brain connectivity and deep neural network classifier. Neurocomputing. 2019;324:63–8.
40. Alba AC, Agoritsas T, Walsh M, Hanna S, Iorio A, Devereaux P, et al. Discrimination and calibration of clinical prediction models: users' guides to the medical literature. JAMA. 2017;318(14):1377–84.
41. Steyerberg EW, Vickers AJ, Cook NR, Gerds T, Gonen M, Obuchowski N, et al. Assessing the performance of prediction models: a framework for some traditional and novel measures. Epidemiology (Cambridge, Mass). 2010;21(1):128.
42. Van Calster B, McLernon DJ, Van Smeden M, Wynants L, Steyerberg EW. Calibration: the Achilles heel of predictive analytics. BMC Med. 2019;17(1):1–7.
43. Steinbach M, Kumar V, Tan P. Cluster Analysis: Basic concepts and algorithms. Introduction to Data Mining. Pearson Addison Wesley. 2005.
44. Mäki-Marttunen T, Kaufmann T, Elvsåshagen T, Devor A, Djurovic S, Westlye LT, et al. Biophysical psychiatry—how computational neuroscience can help to understand the complex mechanisms of mental disorders. Front Psych. 2019;10
45. Montague PR, Dolan RJ, Friston KJ, Dayan P. Computational psychiatry. Trends Cogn Sci. 2012;16(1):72–80.
46. Wu M-J, Mwangi B, Bauer IE, Passos IC, Sanches M, Zunta-Soares GB, et al. Identification and individualized prediction of clinical phenotypes in bipolar disorders using neurocognitive data, neuroimaging scans and machine learning. NeuroImage. 2017;145:254–64.
47. Pinto JV, Passos IC, Gomes F, Reckziegel R, Kapczinski F, Mwangi B, et al. Peripheral biomarker signatures of bipolar disorder and schizophrenia: a machine learning approach. Schizophr Res. 2017;188:182.
48. Visweswaran S, Cooper GF. Risk stratification and prognosis using predictive modelling and big data approaches. Personalized and Precision Medicine Informatics: Springer; 2020. p. 87–105.
49. Strobl EV, Eack SM, Swaminathan V, Visweswaran S. Predicting the risk of psychosis onset: advances and prospects. Early Interv Psychiatry. 2012;6(4):368–79.
50. Hahn T, Nierenberg A, Whitfield-Gabrieli S. Predictive analytics in mental health: applications, guidelines, challenges and perspectives. Mol Psychiatry. 2017;22(1):37.
51. Fung G, Deng Y, Zhao Q, Li Z, Qu M, Li K, et al. Distinguishing bipolar and major depressive disorders by brain structural morphometry: a pilot study. BMC Psychiatry. 2015;15(1):298.
52. Voineskos AN. Predicting functional outcomes in early-stage mental illness: prognostic precision medicine realized? JAMA Psychiat. 2018;75(11):1105–6.
53. Eley TC, Hudson JL, Creswell C, Tropeano M, Lester KJ, Cooper P, et al. Therapygenetics: the 5HTTLPR and response to psychological therapy. Mol Psychiatry. 2012;17(3):236.
54. Hou L, Heilbronner U, Degenhardt F, Adli M, Akiyama K, Akula N, et al. Genetic variants associated with response to lithium treatment in bipolar disorder: a genome-wide association study. Lancet. 2016;387(10023):1085–93.
55. Marquand AF, Wolfers T, Mennes M, Buitelaar J, Beckmann CF. Beyond lumping and splitting: a review of computational approaches for stratifying psychiatric disorders. Biological psychiatry: cognitive neuroscience and neuroimaging. 2016;1(5):433–47.

56. Shatte AB, Hutchinson DM, Teague SJ. Machine learning in mental health: a scoping review of methods and applications. Psychol Med. 2019;49(9):1426–48.
57. Heus P, Damen JA, Pajouheshnia R, Scholten RJ, Reitsma JB, Collins GS, et al. Poor reporting of multivariable prediction model studies: towards a targeted implementation strategy of the TRIPOD statement. BMC Med. 2018;16(1):1–12.
58. Collins GS, Reitsma JB, Altman DG, Moons KG. Transparent reporting of a multivariable prediction model for individual prognosis or diagnosis (TRIPOD). Ann Intern Med. 2015;162(10):735–6.
59. Heus P, Damen JA, Pajouheshnia R, Scholten RJ, Reitsma JB, Collins GS, et al. Uniformity in measuring adherence to reporting guidelines: the example of TRIPOD for assessing completeness of reporting of prediction model studies. BMJ Open. 2019;9(4):e025611.
60. Cohen IG, Amarasingham R, Shah A, Xie B, Lo B. The legal and ethical concerns that arise from using complex predictive analytics in health care. Health Aff. 2014;33(7):1139–47.
61. Kelly CJ, Karthikesalingam A, Suleyman M, Corrado G, King D. Key challenges for delivering clinical impact with artificial intelligence. BMC Med. 2019;17(1):195.
62. Char DS, Shah NH, Magnus D. Implementing machine learning in health care—addressing ethical challenges. N Engl J Med. 2018;378(11):981.
63. Obermeyer Z, Powers B, Vogeli C, Mullainathan S. Dissecting racial bias in an algorithm used to manage the health of populations. Science. 2019;366(6464):447–53.
64. McCradden MD, Joshi S, Mazwi M, Anderson JA. Ethical limitations of algorithmic fairness solutions in health care machine learning. The Lancet Digital Health. 2020;2(5):e221–e3.
65. Allen B. The role of the FDA in ensuring the safety and efficacy of artificial intelligence software and devices. J Am Coll Radiol. 2019;16(2):208–10.
66. FDA. FDA permits marketing of artificial intelligence-based device to detect certain diabetes-related eye problems. 2019. Available from: http://www.fda.gov/news-events/press-announcements/fda-permits-marketing-artificial-intelligence-based-device-detect-certain-diabetes-related-eye.
67. Gulshan V, Peng L, Coram M, Stumpe MC, Wu D, Narayanaswamy A, et al. Development and validation of a deep learning algorithm for detection of diabetic retinopathy in retinal fundus photographs. JAMA. 2016;316(22):2402–10.
68. Gerke S, Babic B, Evgeniou T, Cohen IG. The need for a system view to regulate artificial intelligence/machine learning-based software as medical device. NPJ Digital Medicine. 2020;3(1):1–4.
69. Challen R, Denny J, Pitt M, Gompels L, Edwards T, Tsaneva-Atanasova K. Artificial intelligence, bias and clinical safety. BMJ Qual Saf. 2019;28(3):231–7.
70. Nestor B, McDermott M, Boag W, Berner G, Naumann T, Hughes MC, et al. Feature robustness in non-stationary health records: caveats to deployable model performance in common clinical machine learning tasks. arXiv preprint arXiv:190800690. 2019.
71. Goddard K, Roudsari A, Wyatt JC. Automation bias: a systematic review of frequency, effect mediators, and mitigators. J Am Med Inform Assoc. 2011;19(1):121–7.
72. Finlayson SG, Bowers JD, Ito J, Zittrain JL, Beam AL, Kohane IS. Adversarial attacks on medical machine learning. Science. 2019;363(6433):1287–9.
73. Suermondt HJ, Cooper GF. An evaluation of explanations of probabilistic inference. Comput Biomed Res. 1993;26(3):242–54.
74. Caruana R, Lou Y, Gehrke J, Koch P, Sturm M, Elhadad N, editors. Intelligible models for healthcare: Predicting pneumonia risk and hospital 30-day readmission. Proceedings of the 21th ACM SIGKDD International Conference on Knowledge Discovery and Data Mining; 2015: ACM.
75. Adams RA, Huys QJ, Roiser JP. Computational psychiatry: towards a mathematically informed understanding of mental illness. J Neurol Neurosurg Psychiatry. 2016;87(1):53–63.

Chapter 11
Bioinformatics in Mental Health: Deriving Knowledge from Molecular and Cellular Data

Krithika Bhuvaneshwar and Yuriy Gusev

Abstract Translational bioinformatics plays a crucial role in biomarker discovery as it helps to bridge the gap between bench research and bedside clinical applications. Thanks to newer and faster molecular profiling technologies and decreasing costs, there are many opportunities for researchers to explore the molecular and physiological mechanisms of diseases. Biomarker discovery, or the identification of observable indicators of underlying biological state, enables researchers to characterize patients better, predict treatment responses and monitor disease outcomes. In addition, biomarker tests specialized for a disease can enable early detection and intervention or prevention.

Due to increasing prevalence and rising treatment costs, mental health disorders have become an important area for biomarker discovery and for improved patient treatment and care. Exploration of underlying biological mechanisms is key to the understanding of pathogenesis and pathophysiology of mental disorders.

In this chapter, we cover various data types commonly used in bioinformatics, file formats, and common methods for acquisition of such data. We also address the strengths and limitations of the different types of data used in biomarker discovery. We cover data and knowledge related to molecular and cellular phenomena, and their relationships to other phenomena in mental health. Finally, we address methods to transform molecular and cellular data into meaningful information about higher level human function.

Keywords Bioinformatics · Biomarker · Genomics · Proteomics · Metabolomics Epigenetics · Microbiome · microRNA · Translational bioinformatics · Precision medicine

K. Bhuvaneshwar (✉) · Y. Gusev
Innovation Center for Biomedical Informatics (Georgetown-ICBI), Georgetown University, Washington, DC, USA
e-mail: kb472@georgetown.edu; yg63@georgetown.edu

© Springer Nature Switzerland AG 2021
J. D. Tenenbaum, P. A. Ranallo (eds.), *Mental Health Informatics*, Health Informatics, https://doi.org/10.1007/978-3-030-70558-9_11

11.1 Introduction

11.1.1 Translational Bioinformatics and Biomarker Discovery

Bioinformatics is the science of storing, retrieving, analyzing and interpretating large amounts of biological information [1]. It includes computational methods that can be applied to biomedical data to gain new insights about disease etiology, progression and outcomes. Often referred to as "big data", these large data collections include genetic sequences, cell populations, gene expression profiles, etc. The goal of bioinformatics is to analyze and interpret this large-scale biological data to make new predictions or discover new biology [2]. Though the scope of bioinformatics extends beyond genomic data into proteomics, metabolomics, and more, genomic data is a major focus of the field, and where a significant portion of activity has concentrated. As shown in Table 11.1, there is an order of magnitude differences between the number of PubMed hits for the respective terms above. Thus bioinformatics is arguably a superset of other, more genome-focused subfields such as *computational genomics* or *genomic data science* [3].

Bioinformatics scientists often start their research by trying to understand the biology or the molecular basis for disease. There are various molecular scale biological data types that are studied. Referred to as *molecular features*, these data types generate voluminous amounts of molecular and clinical data which are studied under the emerging field of translational bioinformatics. The aim of translational bioinformatics is to provide a better understanding of the molecular basis of disease, which can help guide clinical practice and ultimately improve human health (see Chap. 2).

When studying the molecular basis of disease, researchers look for a short list of molecular features that can separate two groups of individuals. Referred to as *biomarkers*, these are important because they can be used for better diagnostics, and

Table 11.1 PubMed searches for genomics, proteomics, and metabolomics respectively return result counts that differ by an order of magnitude between each term

Query Term	Search Details	Results
Genomics	"Genome"[MeSH terms] OR "genome"[all fields] OR "genomes"[all fields] OR "genome s"[all fields] OR "genomically"[all fields] OR "genomics"[MeSH terms] OR "genomics"[all fields] OR "genomic"[all fields]	1,535,287
Proteomics	"Proteom"[all fields] OR "proteome"[MeSH terms] OR "proteome"[all fields] OR "proteomes"[all fields] OR "proteomical"[all fields] OR "proteomically"[all fields] OR "proteomics"[MeSH terms] OR "proteomics"[all fields] OR "proteomic"[all fields]	135,578
Metabolomics	"Metabolome"[MeSH terms] OR "metabolome"[all fields] OR "metabolomes"[all fields] OR "metabolomics"[MeSH terms] OR "metabolomics"[all fields] OR "metabolomic"[all fields]	42,529

prediction of outcome in research and clinical practice [4]. The discovery of these biomarkers in translational bioinformatics research is called *biomarker discovery*. There are many different types of biomarkers, including those that indicate the presence of a disease (diagnostic biomarkers), those that indicate the likely course of a disease (prognostic biomarkers) and those that can predict how an individual is likely to respond to a certain treatment (theranostic biomarkers) [5]. These biomarkers described are more predictive in nature. There are other biomarkers that help understand the pathophysiological processes of the underlying disease, referred to as *mechanistic biomarkers*. These biomarkers also enable better classification of a phenotype [6].

11.1.2 How Bioinformatics and Data Science Contribute to Biomarker Discovery in Mental Health

Thanks to the digitization of healthcare data, larger than ever amounts of data are being generated and collected from electronic health record (EHR) systems, medical imaging, laboratory and genomics tests, mobile health and wearable technology [7]. This explosion of healthcare data exemplifies what is commonly referred to as Big Data. It is in the exabyte scale now, and was projected to grow to close to 2 zettabytes (10^{21} bytes!) in 2020 [8]. With advances in artificial intelligence methodologies, scientists are able to apply machine learning and deep learning techniques to structured and unstructured data in ways previously unimaginable. Despite the complexity, scalable computational power and the interdisciplinary nature of bioinformatics has enabled scientists and researchers to explore the mechanisms of complex diseases [9, 10].

In this Big Data revolution, bioinformatics and data science play a crucial role as they enable scientists to extract and integrate biological information from a molecular and cellular level. At the molecular level, the different components include the DNA, mRNA, protein, microRNA and metabolites. Bioinformatics also enables researchers to understand diseases at a cellular level by looking at the pathways and networks associated with each disease. Empowered by initiatives like the Precision Medicine Initiative [11], now referred to as the All of Us Program (https://allofus. nih.gov/), bioinformatics enables the practice of precision medicine in the clinic by offering clinicians a comprehensive view of the patient, unique as they are, so that the doctors can treat the person as a whole, often described by the Latin phrase 'cura personalis' i.e. cure of the entire person.

Biomarkers are measurable indicators of a biological state or condition that can enable outcome prediction [12]. The Big Data revolution and cloud computing has allowed for complex investigation of biomedical data and enabled discovery of new biomarkers [13]. A good biomarker must be reliable, reproducible, and independently confirmed by more than one study. It should have high sensitivity and specificity, as well as positive predictive value. Chapter 10 of this book offers detailed explanation of these concepts. It is also advantageous for the diagnostic technology

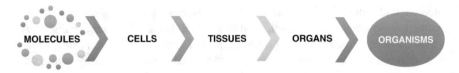

Fig. 11.1 Hierarchy of physiological functions

to be affordable and covered by patient insurance, in addition to using simple experimental methodology for analysis [14, 15]. Biomarkers can also enable identification of various disease sub-types, better prediction of disease progression, and better monitoring of treatment response [15]. Biomarkers can be identified at any level of physiological function, be it in a cell or at an organism level (Fig. 11.1).

In recent years, mental health disorders have become an important target for biomarker discovery and an area of great need for improved patient outcomes due to increasing prevalence and rising treatment costs [5]. Exploration of underlying biological mechanisms is key to the pathogenesis and pathophysiology of mental disorders [16].

Translational bioinformatics plays a vital role in biomarker discovery as it bridges the gap from the bench to the bedside. In the MH realm, a good MH biomarker needs to be scalable, must conform to social and systemic interaction, respect privacy, and avoid bias [17]. At present, very few or no biomarker tests have been approved for use in the clinic for MH, making this research even more important [18].

Newer molecular profiling and diagnostic technologies and lower costs have enabled researchers to explore the molecular and physiological mechanisms of diseases like never before and mental health is no exception [5]. In this chapter, we review the types of data used in biomarker discovery. We will also see how the data and information are related to various molecular and cellular phenomena in mental health, and how this can be transformed into meaningful knowledge about higher level human function.

11.2 Types of Data in Biomarker Discovery

In this Big Data revolution, bioinformatics and data science play a crucial role as they enable scientists to extract and integrate biological information from a molecular and cellular level. At the molecular level, the different components include the DNA, mRNA, protein, microRNA, metabolites, and others (Fig. 11.2). Each data type has a name that ends with the word "omics", that describes the field of study, such as, *genomics* (study of the DNA or RNA), *transcriptomics* (study of the RNA), *proteomics* (study of proteins), *metabolomics* (study of metabolites), *glycomics* (study of glycans) etc. Together they are often referred to as "*multi-omics*" or

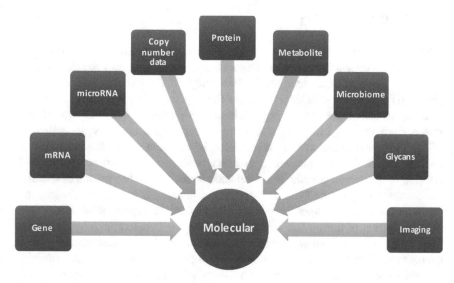

Fig. 11.2 Molecular scale biological data types

"omics" data. In this chapter we will review commonly used analysis workflows for each molecular data type, and their applications.

11.2.1 Genomics: The Study of the DNA

Cells are the building blocks of life and contain *chromosomes* which hold *DNA (deoxy-ribonucleic acid)*. The *DNA* in a cell exists as a double helix structure and can be thought of as a sequence of genetic 'letters' known as *nucleotides*—As, Cs, Gs, and Ts. These stand for adenine, cytosine, guanine, and thymine respectively. The human genome is made up of over 3 billion of these genetic letters [19]. The function of chromosomes is to store information, which is passed on to the progeny. The *genome* of a person includes a full set of the complete DNA sequence. The study of the whole genome, including analysis of its structure and function and its interpretation, is called *genomics*. It can help researchers understand how some diseases develop and can help to identify the most effective treatments [20] for those diseases.

Genome sequencing or whole genome sequencing (WGS or DNA-seq) technology determines the order of the DNA nucleotides in a genome. The sequencing of the first human, known as the *Human Genome Project* started in 1990 and was completed in 2003 at a cost of $2.7 billion [21] and using a method known as Sanger sequencing. Today, "next-generation sequencing" (NGS) technology is faster and more efficient, and a person's full genome can be sequenced in a matter of days, or even hours, for less than $1000 [21, 22]. Another variation on WGS is whole exome sequencing (WES), in which sequencing is only performed on the relatively small portion of the genome that codes for proteins.

11.2.1.1 Data Processing

DNA is extracted from a blood or tissue sample, cut into smaller fragments, and loaded into a *sequencing machine*. This machine determines short sequences of the 4 "letters" (4 types of nucleotides) in these fragments, referred to as *reads*. These reads are typically 75–150 letters long and the sequence of nucleotides of each fragment come out of the sequencing machine in a random order. This workflow is summarized in Fig. 11.3. About 600 million reads are typically generated for WGS. This data, essentially a list of letters, is represented in a file format called *FASTQ*. Due to their random order, these reads are difficult to interpret since their position in the human genome is not yet known. Only once the position of a read in the human genome is known, can we check if the read is located in a region that forms a gene or a protein, or a regulatory region, and determine its function.

The position of these reads in the human genome is determined by comparing them with a *reference genome,* which is a complete set of sequences from the human genome used internationally as a reference. This process is performed using computational algorithms and is referred to as *mapping or alignment*. At the end of this workflow, the position of each read in the human genome is known. This information is represented in a file format known as *Binary Alignment Mapping (BAM)*.

Once the BAM file is obtained, another computational algorithm is applied that extracts a large amount of information including changes in the normal sequence, referred to as a *mutation; insertions and deletions* in the normal sequence; detecting any changes in the number of copies of a DNA segment (*copy number variations); chromosomal aberrations* in the normal sequence, and more. The mutations, insertions and deletions are represented in a file format known as *Variant Call File* (VCF)

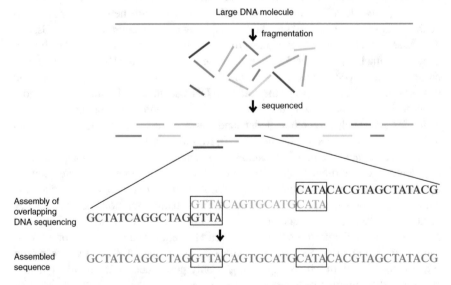

Fig. 11.3 DNA sequencing (*Image Courtesy of National Human Genome Research Institute* https://www.genome.gov/)

format, which enables the inclusion of additional information about the mutation including name of the gene, its function, and more.

It must be noted that in every step of this workflow, the file formats used (FASTQ, BAM and VCF, reference genome) are industry standards created to enable reproducibility. This genomic annotation and information in these standard file formats allows researchers to look deeper into the biology and function to better understand how a patient's genome could affect the outcome and disease.

11.2.1.2 Strengths and Limitations

- The cost of sequencing assays has been decreasing steadily over the past 10 years. The falling costs of genome sequencing has enabled researchers to pursue whole genome sequencing for their research projects. In addition, more consumers are able to get their entire genome sequenced through direct to consumer testing companies.
- Genome sequencing analysis is increasingly being integrated into clinical practice in recent years. Reports derived from genome sequencing analysis and other diagnostic tests (referred to as *molecular diagnostic reports*) can offer clinicians a prioritized list of gene mutations and therapies for every patient. Such reports allow a doctor to choose an off-label therapy or suggest a clinical trial based on a particular mutation. These molecular diagnostic reports are currently used typically in cancer and newborn screening. Such reports would also allow the physician to look at the genes involved in drug metabolism when deciding dosage. Many of these tests are increasingly being covered by insurance and the hope is that these diagnostic and theranostic tests will be applicable in more diseases in the future. This is the beginning of personalized or precision medicine, and allows for many such directions in the future.
- This type of sequencing generates massive amounts of data which can make the processing and analysis of data complex. The data, storage and analysis of this kind of data needs the cloud or a high-performance computing (HPC) environment which can be expensive. Due to the large volume of data, the identification of top features and biomarkers can be a challenge for many scientists without additional support from bioinformatics scientists.

11.2.1.3 Examples in Mental Health

NGS and genome wide association studies (GWAS) have shed light on several mutations that increase the risk of many psychiatric disorders. These results could be used as potential targets for developing new treatments [23–26]. Studies based on data from a large consortium found several genes that had a common molecular neuropathology to be implicated in several psychiatric disorders including Autism Spectrum Disorder (ASD), schizophrenia (SCZ), bipolar disorder (BD), depression and alcoholism (AAD) [27].

Pantazatos et al. used RNA sequencing (RNA-seq) to study gene expression in patients with depression, and a number of genes with altered expression levels including humanin-like-8 (MTRNRL8), interleukin-8 (IL8), serpin peptidase inhibitor, clade H (SERPINH1) and chemokine ligand 4 (CCL4) [28]. Molecular analysis has shown that the biological processes associated with MDD include immune response, innate immune response, immune system process, and immune system development.

11.2.2   Transcriptomics: The Study of the RNA

The flow of information from DNA to RNA to proteins is one of the fundamental principles of molecular biology, referred to as the Central Dogma of biology. DNA uncoils its double helix structure allowing the sides to separate and for one strand to serve as a template to create a matching sequence of *ribonucleic acid (RNA)* called a *messenger RNA (mRNA) transcript,* or simply a *transcript* (Fig. 11.4). This process is called *transcription*, and the study of RNA *transcriptomics*. It is an important part of the puzzle because its gives researchers a window into what happens dynamically in cells at the RNA level, not just at the relatively static level of DNA.

A *gene* is the functional unit of heredity [29]. It is a region of DNA that has a certain function, and encodes the information needed to create either a protein via processes of transcription and translation or a non-coding RNA molecule [30]. Findings from the Human Genome Project suggest that there are about 20,000 genes in the human genome that encode for proteins. *Gene expression* is the process by which the instructions in our DNA are converted into a functional product, such as a protein [29].

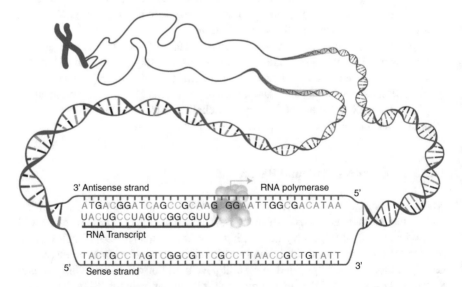

Fig. 11.4 The process of transcription. It shows how the RNA transcript is formed from the uncoiled DNA segment representing a gene. Image courtesy: National Human Genome Research Institute (https://www.genome.gov)

In a given cell, only a fraction of the genes are "turned on" or activated, and the rest are turned off. This process is known as *gene regulation* and is affected both by the DNA sequence itself and by changes in the environment. This regulation controls the transcription and translation, and not only whether the proteins are produced by a gene but also the amount of protein being made [31].

In this field of *transcriptomics*, one of the main aspects of research study is the measurement of the expression of the genes in an organism. There are two popular methods of measuring gene expression data—one is by using a technology called a *microarray chip*; and another newer method by simply sequencing the RNA known as *RNA-sequencing (RNA-seq)*.

Affymetrix is a company that offers different types of microarray chips for data capture. Illumina is another company that offers not only microarray chip platforms, but also sequencing machines for DNA and RNA sequencing, and more.

11.2.2.1 Data Processing

In brief, a blood or tissue sample is taken from a patient, from which *total RNA* is extracted. Microarrays chips are glass slides with thousands or even millions of tiny spots printed on them in defined positions, with each spot containing fragments of DNA with a known sequence of nucleotides. The sample being analyzed is labeled with fluorescent markers that attach to individual RNA molecules. That sample is then washed over the spotted microarray, and those labeled RNA molecules bind to the specific spots on the array that contain the complementary sequence. The amount of RNA in the sample being analyzed can then be quantified by detecting the level of fluorescence at each spot. This process is summarized in Fig. 11.5. Once the level

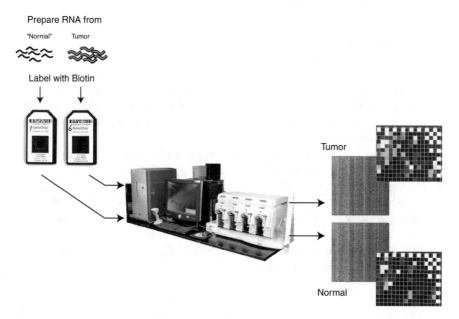

Fig. 11.5 DNA microarray technology (*Image Courtesy of National Human Genome Research Institute* https://www.genome.gov/)

of RNA from the samples is measured using such a microarray, the *raw gene expression data* are generated for each sample analyzed, and a series of data wrangling steps are applied to obtain gene expression data in a *normalized data matrix format* ready for the next steps of analysis, e.g. with genes as rows and samples as columns.

For RNA-sequencing, the total RNA extracted from blood or tissue sample, is cut into smaller fragments, converted into complimentary DNA fragments and loaded into a *sequencing machine*. Similar to the WGS process described above, the sequencing machine determines the sequence of letters in these fragments, and the data is represented in a *FASTQ* file. About 20–40 million reads are typically generated by RNA-seq technology for a single sample. The reads are then compared to the *reference genome* using *alignment* algorithms to determine the location of each read. Once the BAM file is obtained, a specialized *quantification algorithm* is run that estimates a relative abundance of the reads aligned to a transcript. The output of RNA-seq is also a matrix and is equivalent to the gene expression values obtained using microarrays, although the data representation (units of data) are different between the two.

Once the gene expression data matrix is obtained, one can compare the gene expression values across two or more groups of patients stratified by some clinical attribute and determine the genes that differ most between the two groups. These genes are referred to as *differentially expressed genes, or DEGs*. Common comparisons include patients with and without disease, mild vs. severe disease, patients that responded to treatment vs. those that did not, etc. Once these DEGs are obtained, it allows for further studies on the function of the differentially expressed genes, sometimes referred to as *downstream analysis*.

There are other applications of RNA-seq data including fusions that are out of scope for this chapter.

11.2.2.2 Strengths and Limitations

- The study of RNA offers a window into the regulation events that happen after transcription. These events, known as *post-transcriptional regulation events,* can alter gene expression. By studying the RNA, we can understand the dynamic state of the cell and the biological processes affected during post transcriptional regulation events.
- The analysis is relatively straightforward and many bench scientists are comfortable using software that can perform this kind of analysis.
- The volume of data is significantly smaller than for whole genome sequencing, making the data extraction, data storage, and analysis relatively affordable.
- While the study of RNA-seq data does provide information about gene expression, fusions and novel transcripts; scientists still need to sequence the DNA to get information about mutations at the DNA level, insertions and deletions, as well copy number alternations.

11.2.2.3 Examples in Mental Health

Researchers have studied differently expressed genes (DEGs) comparing samples from people with and without diagnoses of Autism and SCZ. Once the DEGs are identified, researchers can look at other genes expressed with the DEGs (referred to as *co-expressed genes*), and the networks involved to understand the underlying molecular foundations [32]. Analysis of RNA-seq data of brains with bipolar disorder showed downregulation of cell adhesion, neurodevelopment, and synaptic pathways; and upregulation of immune signaling genes [33]. Genes known for increased risk of SCZ include ZNF804A [34, 35]. Xiao et al. studied the methylome and transcriptome in SCZ and BD. The mRNA levels of RELN were affected in SCZ and BD patients [36]. Kohen et al. applied RNA-seq to patients with MH disorders including SCZ, MDD and BD, and found miR-182 levels changed in these disorders. miR-182 was found activated in patients with BD and healthy controls, while it was found downregulated in MDD and SCZ [37]. Wang et al. reviewed RNA-seq based studies in SCZ, and found GABA function, glutamate function, myelin- and oligodendrocyte-related processes affected. Other biological processes related to immune and inflammatory pathways including genes IL6 and SERPINA3 were also affected [38].

11.2.3 Proteomics: The Study of Proteins

As mentioned above, the human genome is made up of over 3 billion of the genetic 'letters'—As, Cs, Gs, and Ts. However only approximately 1% of it is occupied by sequences of the genes that encode for proteins (referred to as *coding regions*) [39]. Proteins are important as they are the building blocks of the cells and also determine the function and regulation of the tissues and organs in the human body [40]. *Proteomics* is the field of science concerned with applying the modern techniques of molecular biology, biochemistry, and genetics to analyzing the structure, function, and interactions of proteins on a large scale.

Proteomics technologies also enable measurement of the abundance or level of expression of the proteins that determine the cell type (as a result of cell differentiation) and the biological state of the cell. Measurement of proteins in different tissues and under different conditions offers researchers a critical understanding of the underlying biological mechanisms and how they could be disrupted in a disease [19].

11.2.3.1 Data Processing

A popular data capture technique used in proteomics and metabolomics is *mass spectrometry* (MS). It involves the separation, ionization, and detection of molecules that make up a protein. The protein molecule can be quantified relative to the known concentration of another labeled molecule [19]. Another method of data capture is called *Reverse-phased protein microarrays (RPPA)*. It allows monitoring of the fluctuating state of the protein regions among different cell populations. This is especially useful to trace the state of cellular signaling molecules in a set of samples that has both case and control samples, for instance, diseased and normal cells in the same tissue section. This high-throughput technology is very sensitive and can detect proteins from low abundance inputs [41].

The study of the *protein structure* is another important area of research. It offers more information about how a drug binds to a receptor in a cell and enables the development of more effective and personalized drug treatment options. It can also help understand how a virus or foreign body binds to the receptors in the human body and causes disease.

11.2.3.2   Strengths and Limitations

• Structure and function of proteins are more complex than of DNA or RNA, and hence quantification of protein observations is also complex [19].
• RPPAs are dependent on appropriate antibodies for the detection of proteins, so this method may be not be applicable for all proteins [41].

11.2.3.3   Examples in Mental Health

Bot et al. studied 171 serum proteins in 1589 patients from the Netherlands Study of Depression and Anxiety. They found serum analytes associated with current MDD linked to diverse cell communication, signal transduction processes, immune response, and protein metabolism [42]. Advances in proteomics have allowed the development of new biomarker discovery methods for early detection and diagnosis of AD [43, 44]. Liao et al. studied the proteomic characterization of amyloid plaques and discovered more than 400 different proteins associated with it [45]. Other proteomics studies also found oxidative damage, major disturbances in protein homeostasis and energy production in AD.

11.2.4   Metabolomics: The Study of Metabolites

Humans consume food which is converted into energy for various biochemical reactions. This energy allows the cells in the body to grow and run various cellular processes [46]. During these biochemical reactions, proteins are broken down (i.e. metabolized) into small molecules knowns as metabolites, which are eventually eliminated from the cell. The study of these small molecules on a large scale is known as *metabolomics*. These small molecules include sugars, lipids, amino acids, fatty acids, phenolic compounds, and alkaloids, among others [47].

The metabolites in an organism are easily affected by changes in the environment and/or disease, making them ideal candidate for biomarkers. They can also help us better understand diseases and drug interactions, toxicities, and mechanisms of action [46].

11.2.4.1 Data Processing

Like proteomics, metabolomics data can also be captured through mass spectrometry (MS). Samples are prepared using standard protocols and input into the mass spectrometer, which produces a unique spectrum for each molecule. The molecule size and its charge are captured by the spectrometer. These numerical measurements are in the form of abundances for each molecule, with each molecule represented by its molecular weight. This technique is referred to as *untargeted metabolomics* since any measurable small molecule is captured. It is typically performed using a combination of liquid chromatography and mass spectrometry (LCMS) technique [48]. Another common data capture technique for metabolomics is Nuclear magnetic resonance (NMR) spectroscopy. In this analytical technique, the individual analytes in a sample are separated by their magnetic resonance shift, and a unique spectrum is produced for each analyte [49]. NMR involves minimal sample preparation and is highly reproducible, but less sensitive in comparison to mass spectrometry [50].

The data are then represented in the form of a data matrix and can be compared between two or more groups of interest to find features (metabolites) with significantly changed abundance between the groups. These features can also be compared with standard reference databases to identify the *putative small molecules* based on molecular weight [19]. Researchers can then perform an independent validation to verify the presence and the amount of the putative molecule in the sample. This is done using a technique called *targeted metabolomics*—where the experiment is focused on a small set of small molecules of interest, to obtain accurate absolute quantification. It uses standardized controls, and is typically performed using a combination of two mass analyzers in one mass spectrometry instrument (referred to as MS/MS or tandem mass spectrometry) which allows for increased sensitivity and higher precision [48, 51].

11.2.4.2 Strengths and Limitations

- Metabolites are influenced by genes, proteins, and the environment. They in turn affect various biochemical pathways in the human body. This relationship can help researchers in biomarker discovery and to better understand the underlying mechanisms of action.
- Metabolites can be found in blood (serum or plasma) and other biofluids, enabling this type of analysis using non-invasive and inexpensive analysis techniques.

- Metabolomics is often used along with other omics data types including genomics to get an additional insights and fuller understanding of human health and disease [46].

11.2.4.3   Examples in Mental Health

Mapstone et al. identified a set of 10 lipids from the peripheral blood of people who went on to develop AD 2–3 years later with 90% accuracy [52]. Studies have shown that the metabolic pathways for ATP production are dysfunctional in MDD [53, 54]. Studies have also investigated psychiatric medications including antipsychotics, and antidepressants, in animals. A metabolite related to the glutamate/GABA–glutamine cycle pathway was found dysregulated in depressed animal models. Additionally, mitochondrial dysregulation through alterations in amino acid and energy metabolism was found [55].

11.2.5   Epigenetics/Epigenomics

Scientists have learned that the permanent changes to the DNA sequence (mutations) is only one of the ways the human genome affects gene expression. There are other ways the transcriptome can be affected, for instance, by the presence of a chemical compound such as a methyl group (referred to as *DNA methylation*), or a histone group (referred to as *histone modification*). Known as *epigenetic* changes, these modifications can also regulate the activity of a gene (gene expression) and affect the function of a protein. Environmental changes including pollution and a person's diet can also affect the epigenome. The study of the epigenome on a large scale is referred to as *epigenetics* [56]. More specifically, epigenetics is the study of heritable changes in gene expression that do not involve changes to the underlying DNA sequence, i.e. changes in phenotype without the changes in genotype. Epigenetics is often performed in conjunction with other omics data modalities including gene expression and WGS. It allows researchers to detect the genomic regions that bind to a protein of interest [57].

11.2.5.1   Data Processing

Popular techniques used to study epigenetic data includes a process called *ChIP-sequencing (ChIP-seq)*. It combines the experimental technique of *chromatin immunoprecipitation (ChIP)* with high throughput parallel DNA sequencing to identify the sites where protein interacts with the DNA (referred to as *DNA binding sites*) [58].

By capturing how proteins interact with DNA to regulate gene expression, researchers are able to understand in more detail the disease states and related biological processes [58]. This technique also allows for identification of *transcription factors* which are proteins involved in the process of transcribing DNA into RNA [59, 60].

11.2.5.2 Strengths and Limitations

- ChIP-Seq offers higher resolution, better coverage, and less noise compared to its array-based predecessor technique known as *ChIP-chip* [61].
- Epigenetics performed in conjunction with other omics technologies, referred to as *multi-omics analysis*, could help to put the pieces of the puzzle together and reveal more about the underlying mechanisms in mental health disorders.
- Similar to other NGS high throughput sequencing methods, ChIP-Seq technique generates a lot of data, and has the same strengths and limitations as other NGS methods. This includes higher cost than traditional array data capture methods [61]. However the cost of sequencing assays has been decreasing steadily over past 10 years.
- One of the challenges with ChIP-seq is that the DNA binding sites tend to be more common in certain genomic regions. These regions have a higher concentrations of the Guanine (G) and Cytosine (C) nucleotides. Referred to as *GC-content,* these could potentially bias the ChIP-seq signal. In newer algorithms, this bias is accounted for within the quantification algorithms [57].

11.2.5.3 Examples in Mental Health

Various epigenetics changes have been found in many mental health studies. Epigenetic changes in the gene BDNF or receptor TRKB were found in multiple psychiatric disorders including MDD, BD, SCZ, and borderline personality disorder (BPD) [62]. Epigenetic changes in serotonin transporter SLC6A4 have also been implicated as well in MDD, BD, PTSD, SCZ, and ADHD [62, 63]. Epigenetic changes were found in gene HDAC4 in the blood of patients with PTSD [64].

According to Kumsta et al., DNA methylation levels of two genes related to stress regulation (NR3C1 and FKBP5) may be used as a predictive marker for therapy. DNA methylation of the serotonin transporter gene (SLC6A4) was found to be significantly different between responders and non-responders to psychotherapy treatment. Studies found that changes in the DNA methylation over the course of therapy were linked to treatment outcome. There is hence potential for epigenetic markers to be used in the prediction of treatment outcome [65].

11.2.6   microRNA

We know that only ~1% of the human genome is occupied by sequences of genes that encode for proteins. The remaining 99% does not code for proteins and is called the *non-coding regions*. Some of these regions encode a type of RNA referred to as non-protein coding RNA or simply non-coding RNA. They include many different types of RNA, and the most widely known and studied amongst them is called *microRNA (miRNA)*.

A miRNA is a small non-coding RNA molecule about 22 nucleotides long, found in plants, animals and some viruses. The main function of the miRNA is to regulate gene expression via inhibition of translation initiation or RNA degradation. miRNA provides a mechanism of fine-tuned regulation of protein production in the cells. mirBase (http://www.mirbase.org/) is a biological database that is an archive of microRNA information such as IDs, annotations and sequences.

11.2.6.1 Data Processing

miRNA data is typically captured by three popular techniques. One is a technology called *Real-time quantitative PCR (RT-qPCR)*. Similar to gene expression data capture, expression of miRNAs can be quantified using microarray chips, or by using next generation sequencing technique called *microRNA-sequencing (or miRNA-seq)*. In all three techniques, the abundance of the miRNA is captured in numerical format and represented as data matrices. These numerical matrices can be used to compare various case and control groups in order to identify differentially expressed microRNAs. Further analysis of microRNA results in potential genes targeted by the microRNAs, which are typically experimentally validated through RT-qPCR [66].

These can then be explored by further downstream analysis to identify those miRNA that show strong association with the phenotypes and also to extrapolate connections with disease outcome. Figure 11.6 shows an example of the network of interactions between 4 microRNAs and their experimentally validated targets.

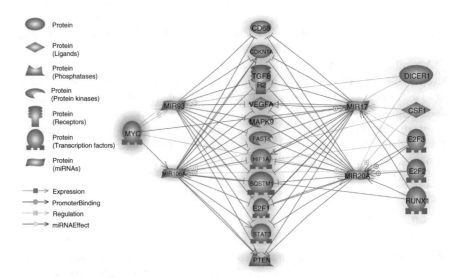

Fig. 11.6 An example of the network of interactions between four microRNAs and their experimentally validated targets. *Experimentally validated targets (blue highlights) and regulators (yellow and red highlights) are shown connected to their corresponding microRNAs (green highlights). The four microRNAs shown are from miR-17/92 cluster and play important roles in health and disease.* The image was created using the Elsevier Pathway Studio software [67].

11.2.6.2 Strengths and Limitations

- MicroRNAs are extremely important and known for their role in biogenesis and human diseases.
- It is predicted that microRNAs regulate more than 10,000 protein coding genes, and hence can easily affect many cellular processes [68].
- miRNAs can be detected in whole blood, plasma, and serum as well as in other biofluids [68]. These miRNAs are called circulating miRNAs and are released by many types of cells in various tissues and organs.

11.2.6.3 Examples in Mental Health

miRNAs are best known for their regulation of behavior, cognition, and emotion in psychiatric disorders. miRNAs have been most studied in subjects with Major Depressive Disorders (MDD). They have been implicated in increased vulnerability to early life stress, and its related depression [69, 70].

Circulating miRNAs in body fluids have shown to be promising biomarkers for the diagnosis of Parkinson's disease (PD), and other psychiatric and neurodegenerative disorders [71, 72]. miRNA hsa-miR409-3p targets gene FAM117B and other genes, and is known to be linked with SCZ [73–75]. miR-182 was found activated in patients with Bipolar Disorder (BD) and healthy controls, while it was found downregulated in MDD and SCZ [37].

11.2.7 DNA Copy Number

Normal human cells contain two copies of each gene, one copy inherited from each parent. From the Human Genome Project, it was discovered that the human genome can experience gains and losses of some genomic regions i.e. copy number of the genes can either be increased (more than 2 copies) or decreased (fewer than 2 copies).

These DNA copy number alterations also known as copy number changes or copy number variations are actually structural abnormalities in the chromosome that could be one of many types, including duplications, deletions, or translocations. These abnormalities typically occur when there is an error in cell division resulting in cells with too few or too many copies of the entire chromosome or a fragment of chromosome.

Known risk factors that increase the risk of such abnormalities include disease (for example cancer), environmental factors such as exposure to radiation or UV light, certain drugs, maternal age, etc.

11.2.7.1 Data Processing

DNA copy number data is typically captured using various technologies—including microarray-based comparative genome hybridization (arrayCGH), genotyping arrays, and, more recently, high-resolution NGS. These days, researchers are able to extract DNA copy number alterations by using specialized computational algorithms from high-resolution NGS data [76].

The DNA copy number alterations are mathematically summarized in the form of *segments*. Each segment reflects a genomic region that has a similar genomic alteration profile. It has a numeric value that reflects the genomic instability in that region and is unique to each patient. Specialized algorithms, referred to as segmentation algorithms are used to perform this quantification [76].

11.2.7.2 Strengths and Limitations

- The study of copy number variation can identify the genomic regions of instability. With this information, the genes located in the unstable regions can be identified and studied in more detail. It allows researchers to explore the function of the genes, and the pathways affected and how they are linked to clinical outcome.
- Bioinformaticians also correlate copy number data with other available genomic data including gene expression, or microRNA expression. Studying these correlation patterns can reveal a great deal about underlying biological mechanisms of a disease.
- Many such *DNA copy number alterations* are common in cancer. This area has not been studied much in mental health and has a great potential for biomarker discovery.

11.2.7.3 Examples in Mental Health

There are a few studies that have identified genomic regions of variation. Cuccaro et al. studied copy number variation (CNV) in AD and found variations in several genomic regions including 1p36, 1q21,1q32, 2p23, and 2q14 [77]. Genomic regions 1q32 and 22q11.22 were identified as "hot spots" i.e. regions of large copy number variation for SCZ and Bipolar Disorder (BD) [78, 79]. Genes in these regions were found to be methylated in both disorders [36].

11.2.8 Neuro-Imaging

Medical imaging is a technique wherein a visual representation of the body interior is taken. It is different from other molecular data types because is unstructured. Molecular imaging techniques can be used to visualize biological processes taking place in the cells of organisms, and is used to detect early stage disease and identify abnormalities.

11.2.8.1 Data Processing

Imaging informatics is a diverse area that includes understanding of the major types of imaging data, methods for processing imaging information and analysis tools, and integration with other types of health data. Biomedical imaging informatics involves various steps including image acquisition, image content representation, management/storage of images, image processing, image analysis and image interpretation/computer reasoning. These are covered in detail in Chap. 8.

Once the images are acquired and processed, they are analyzed to extract meaningful information with the help of machine learning or deep learning models to compare groups of patients, identify abnormalities, etc. Then the results from analyses are presented to the imaging professional to make clinical or research decisions [80, 81].

The end to end workflow for image analysis is quite complex and many open source and commercial software and toolkits exist for this purpose. Some examples include Cancer Imaging Phenomics Toolkit (CaPTk) [82] and The Medical Imaging Interaction Toolkit (MITK) [83].

11.2.8.2 Strengths and Limitations

- Since the data are in the form of image pixels, the analysis workflows are quite complex and often requires specialized imaging professionals as well as bioinformatics expertise.
- Medical imaging technologies produce large amounts of data at the terabyte scale so the storage, analysis and results of analysis is not trivial, and often needs cloud based resources or super computers.
- Due to the size and nature of the data generated, deep learning based algorithms have recently been applied to this data type to enhance performance and analyses [84].

11.2.8.3 Examples in Mental Health

Genetics and brain images have been used to diagnose schizophrenia [85]. Brain imaging has been used to predict treatment outcome for social anxiety disorder [86]. According to Okano et al., real-time fMRI neurofeedback could reduce auditory hallucinations [87].

11.2.9   Emerging Data Types: Microbiome

The gastrointestinal (GI) tract contains a hundred trillion microorganisms such as bacteria and viruses that play a crucial role in digestion, regulation of the immune system, and managing stress response. These microorganisms, referred to as the gut microbiome, have also been found, somewhat surprisingly, to affect human behavior and brain function. The Gut-Brain-Axis (GBA) describes the bidirectional connection between the gut and the brain via different systems including the immune system, the nervous system and the endocrine system [88].

11.2.9.1   Data Processing

Most recently, next generation sequencing techniques have been used to capture microbiome data. Referred to as *metagenomic sequencing*, the technique allows the thousands of microbes including bacteria, archaea and viruses to be identified with relative ease. The technique also captures abundance of major types of microbes, and then compared with standard databases to not only identify, but to chart the phylogenetic relationships between these microbes in a diagram known as phylogenetic trees. Once researchers understand the etiology and type of microbes in the sample, it allows for further understanding of disease mechanisms and treatment.

11.2.9.2   Strengths and Limitations

- The microbiome offers the potential to not only help researchers with understanding mental health disorders, but also to be used in treatment [89]. In conjunction with psychotherapy, psychiatrists are now considering complementary treatments including treatment with probiotics, herbal remedies, and vitamins that can improve GI symptoms via microbiome [88, 90, 91].
- 'Psychobiotics' is a term has been given to a set of drugs that contain beneficial microbes that can reduce both inflammation and anxiety [88, 90, 91]. These new drugs could be administered in addition to standard therapy to improve treatment response in mental health disorders.
- Fecal transplants are currently being tested in mouse models for their efficacy to improve mental health outcomes [88, 90, 91].

11.2.9.3   Examples in Mental Health

The alterations of gut microbiota have been associated with neurodegenerative diseases as well as mood disturbance and depression. In a mentally and physically healthy person, the pro-inflammatory cytokines are in equilibrium with the anti-inflammatory cytokines. But when the human body has as a bacterial infection, the immune system in the body is activated and that can increase the activity of the pro-inflammatory cytokines such as interleukins, which in turn lowers the metabolism of neurotransmitters and causes depressive symptoms. Hence through the function of the immune system, the brain converts chronic inflammation into depression and anxiety symptoms [88, 90].

Many studies suggest that when a person is under a lot of stress, it activates the stress response in the human body. This can cause potentially permanent changes in the way the neurons activate and deplete the microbiome. Due to the GBA, this action causes an immune response in the body and causes depressive symptoms. Studies also show that stress induces neuroendocrine hormones which affects bacterial growth, which in turn can influence behavior, metabolism, appetite and immune response [88, 90, 92]. Depression is known to be closely related to elevations in C-reactive proteins, inflammatory cytokines, and oxidative stress, which are connected through the immune system.

The inflammasome, a multiprotein complex responsible for the activation of inflammatory response, has been associated with MDD [93] through a mechanism linked with the gut microbiota. Wong *el al.* discovered caspase-1 affects brain function and causes depression-like symptoms through the gut-inflammasome-brain axis [94].

11.3 Cellular Attributes in Biomarker Discovery

The cellular attributes used in biomarker discovery include molecular function, cellular component, and biological processes (Fig. 11.7).

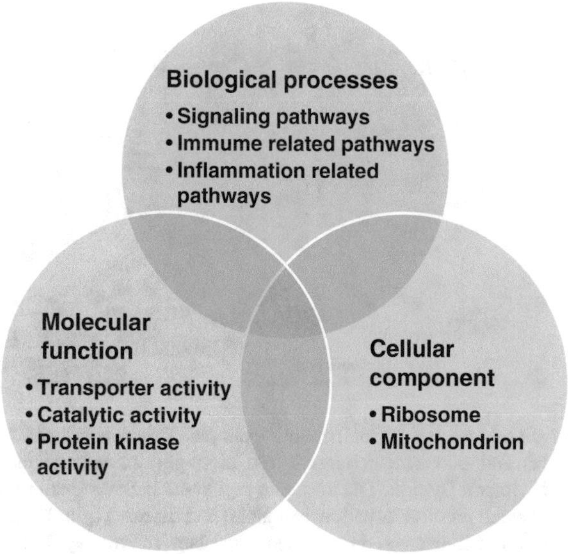

Fig. 11.7 Cellular attributes used in biomarker discovery. These attributes represent the three component vocabularies of the Gene Ontology [95] and also shows example terms in each category

Biological processes
- Signaling pathways
- Immune related pathways
- Inflammation related pathways

Molecular function
- Transporter activity
- Catalytic activity
- Protein kinase activity

Cellular component
- Ribosome
- Mitochondrion

Once a short list of genes and/or molecular features of interest are obtained from analysis of molecular data, the next step is to add functional annotation—to see which biological processes or molecular functions these features are associated with [96]. There are several ways of achieving this.

Gene ontology (GO) http://www.geneontology.org is a standard annotation of genes and gene products across many species. It's essentially a set of three controlled vocabularies that catalog the molecular function of a gene product, the biological process in which the gene product participates, and the cellular component where the gene product can be found [97]. It allows researchers to perform *gene ontology enrichment analysis* wherein the list of genes of interest are compared against the GO database to derive the biological processes, molecular functions and cellular locations that are statistically over-represented in the input gene list.

Similar to GO, annotated biological pathways can capture interactions between genes and other molecules that have the same or similar function. These pathways include signaling pathways, immune or inflammation related pathways, and more. Popular pathway databases include KEGG (https://www.genome.jp/kegg/), Reactome (https://reactome.org/), and Wikipathways (https://www.wikipathways.org/index.php/WikiPathways. Analogous to GO enrichment, *pathway enrichment analysis* is performed wherein the list of genes of interest are compared against the pathway databases to identify the most important pathways related to the input gene list.

Biological interaction networks can be built using specialized software to expand on the input gene or protein list with molecules and other features that directly interact with the inputs through a physical interaction or through microRNA targets or regulators. Such tools allow researchers to better understand the underlying biological mechanisms causing disease. Examples of such interaction networks are shown in Figs. 11.6 and 11.8.

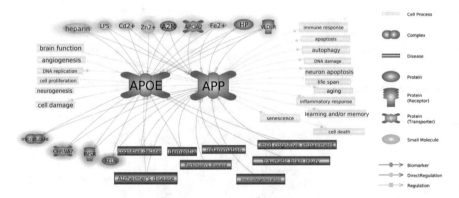

Fig. 11.8 An interaction network example. This network shows upstream regulators (blue highlight) and downstream targets (red highlight) of two genes of interest, APOE and APP, in Alzheimer's Disease. The upstream regulators include small molecules and other proteins. It also shows cell processes (yellow rectangle) and diseases (purple rectangle) associated with these two genes. The image was created using the Elsevier Pathway Studio software [67]

11.4   Systems Biology in Mental Health

Biological systems are dynamic and complex, so it's not easy to predict their behavior by studying individual components and properties. By integrating both theories and methods from biology, computer science, engineering, bioinformatics, and physics, researchers can begin to understand how these complex systems change over time, and to develop solutions to the most important health related questions [98–100].

Systems biology is an interdisciplinary approach to understanding the big picture of molecules, cells, organisms or species by integrating the experimental and computational aspects of research across the molecules, cells, tissues and organs in the biological systems [101]. This integrative approach applies various types of models including pathway analysis, molecular and cellular network models, and knowledge bases to multi-omics data to enable new discoveries. These discoveries could be in the fields of biomarkers, toxicology, diagnostics, drug targets and drug discovery, disease stage and clinical trials [102] (Fig. 11.9).

Mental disorders are complex not only due to the complexity of the hard to access brain areas, but also because of their inherent heterogeneity [103]. Applications of systems biology methods could shed new light on mental disorders from a systems medicine perspective.

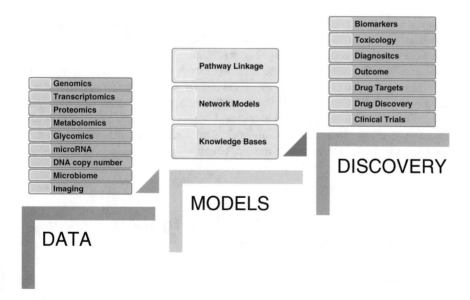

Fig. 11.9 Integrative bioinformatics through Systems Biology

11.5   Mental Health Vs. Medical Conditions

Bioinformatics methods can be applied to biomedical data to get new insights about disease ethology, progression and outcomes in any disease area, be it for a medical condition or mental health. It can be used to compare groups of patients, for example patients with and without disease, early vs. late disease, pre- vs post-treatment, responders vs. non-responders etc. Models can also be built using the data to understand the relationships between different molecular data types, or other variables.

Before the era of genomics in clinics, all brain cancer patients were given the same drug, but only a few responded. According to the National Brain Tumor Society (NBTS), there are more than 120 types of tumor of the brain and central nervous system (CNS) [104]. The World Health Organization (WHO) had originally grouped brain cancers based on histological tumor grade into four groups namely grades I, II, III and IV. But this classification was not very helpful in the prediction of clinical outcome [105]. In 2010, a landmark paper used The Cancer Genome Atlas (TCGA) multi omics data collection to identify four distinct molecular sub-types in brain cancers [106]. The four molecular sub-types included IDH mutation status, ATRX loss, H3K27M mutation, TP53 mutation, and 1p/19q co-deletion [105, 107, 108]. This discovery of brain cancer molecular sub-types was enabled by bioinformatics, and consequently WHO upgraded their classification to include these molecular sub-types [108]. The identification of the IDH mutation sub-type triggered new research and clinical trials in brain cancers [109]. Patients who fall under certain subtypes are known to have better prognosis. Similar examples exist for sub-types of other cancers as well. And such an approach could be extended to MH disorders as well to better understand various disease states.

Mental Health disorders are similar in many ways to medical conditions including diabetes, cancer, heart disease etc. Each mental health disorder is different and unique and must be studied in detail to better understand its molecular underpinnings. For each molecular data type, standard outcome measures exist in most MH disorders to allow studies to correlate biological variables (biomarkers) with psychological variables (measures of mental, cognitive, emotional, social, and behavioral phenomena).

11.5.1   Bioinformatics Knowledge Discovery and Application: An Example in Mental Health

In this example, we demonstrate a typical bioinformatics research workflow setting using Alzheimer's disease (AD) as an example. AD is a progressive neurodegenerative disorder that is estimated to affect one in nine senior adults. Its risk factors include age, family history and surrounding environment [110]. Many studies have been conducted to understand the underlying molecular mechanisms but no cure has been found so far [111].

Early onset Alzheimer's disease (EOAD) affects people before the age of 65 and was observed in the family history of affected families across several generations. It is quite rare and accounts for less than 10% of all patients with AD [112]. Genes associated with this sub-type of AD include amyloid precursor protein (APP), presenilin 1 (PSEN1) and presenilin 2 (PSEN2). Hundreds of mutations were found in these genes that could increase the risk of acquiring AD. These mutations were found to be associated with increased accumulation of the Amyloid-β (Aβ)1–42 peptide. Amyloid-β is the main component of amyloid plaques found in the brains of AD patients [113].

In contrast, late onset Alzheimer's disease (LOAD) affects people older than 65 and is about 80% due to genetic variation. The most widely known genetic risk factor for LOAD is the apolipoprotein E (APOE) gene [113]. People who inherit one copy of this allele have an increased chance of AD and those with two copies have an even greater risk [112]. In AD patients, abnormal changes to Tau leads to blocks in the transportation and communication system in neurons [114].

Pathway studies of AD brain tissue and blood revealed different types of pathways affected. Systems biology analysis allows researchers to combine the knowledge gleaned from molecular and cellular attributes by focusing on the higher level biological phenomena including synapse structure or function, cell lifespan, etc. Results obtained from these analyses could be used to improve treatment outcome and to correct or minimize effects of disrupted function. New studies could also employ the new ways of detection including microbiome, metabolomics and imaging.

In recent years, several potential biomarkers for AD have been discovered in the cerebrospinal fluid (CSF) of the human body and have shown promise for clinical applications. Imaging biomarkers including functional and structural magnetic resonance imaging (MRI) were used to indicate the changes in CSF flow that happen in AD patients [115]. Many AD patients have amyloid-β (Aβ) plaques present in their brains long before they develop the disease, and researchers took advantage of this for screening purposes. As a result, a PET tracer was developed that could specifically detect these Aβ plaques.

11.6   Conclusion

Neuroscience, the scientific study of the nervous system, has made tremendous progress in understanding the processes that govern the system. But not much progress has been made in translating this research into the clinic to treat psychiatric disorders. Biomarkers can bridge this gap which is why it is crucial to extract knowledge from molecular and cellular research using a broad array of bioinformatics methods, tools and resources [116].

The Genomics Workgroup of the National Advisory Mental Health Council (NAMHC) in 2018 developed three main recommendations to move forward in genomic neuropsychiatry. These include creating unbiased, well-powered studies; applying rigorous, and novel approaches; and using common resources based on universal data sharing concepts [117].

In the long run, a range of biomarker types ranging from genetic variation, DNA copy number changes, DNA methylation patterns, and gene and microRNA expression, in conjunction with clinical information, could help to guide treatment options and help us move towards more personalized medicine approaches in treatment of mental health disorders [65]. As we strive to integrate MH disorders into mainstream medical care and health information technology systems, the power of translational bioinformatics and systems medicine will enable us to overcome the stigma associated with these disorders, and accelerate new funding, research studies, and in-silico and lab analyses and findings.

References

1. EMBL-EBI. What is bioinformatics ? May 21 2020; Available from: https://www.ebi.ac.uk/training/online/course/bioinformatics-terrified/what-bioinformatics-0.
2. TowardsDataScience. What is bioinformatics. 2017; Available from: https://towardsdatascience.com/what-is-bioinformatics-703170763999
3. Biospace. Careers in bioinformatics: hot and getting hotter. 2019. May 21 2020; Available from: https://www.biospace.com/article/careers-in-bioinformatics-hot-and-getting-hotter.
4. Strimbu K, Tavel JA. What are biomarkers? Curr Opin HIV AIDS. 2010;5(6):463–6.
5. Tenenbaum JD, et al. Translational bioinformatics in mental health: open access data sources and computational biomarker discovery. Brief Bioinform. 2019;20(3):842–56.
6. Rush AJ, Ibrahim HM. A Clinician's perspective on biomarkers. Focus (Am Psychiatr Publ). 2018;16(2):124–34.
7. evariant.com. What is healthcare big data? 2019. Dec 23 2019; Available from: https://www.evariant.com/faq/what-is-healthcare-big-data.
8. PRNewswire. $11.45 bn big data in healthcare market, 2025. 2018 Dec 23 2019; Available from: https://www.prnewswire.com/news-releases/1145-bn-big-data-in-healthcare-market-2025-300623544.html.
9. Channels IE. How data analytics helps mental health issues. Dec 23 2019; Available from: https://channels.theinnovationenterprise.com/articles/how-social-media-analysis-can-improve-mental-health.
10. Wikipedia. Bioinformatics. Dec 23 2019; Available from: https://en.wikipedia.org/wiki/Bioinformatics.
11. NLM. What is the precision medicine initiative? Dec 24 2019; Available from: https://ghr.nlm.nih.gov/primer/precisionmedicine/initiative.
12. Wikipedia. Biomarker. Dec 24 2019; Available from: https://en.wikipedia.org/wiki/Biomarker.
13. Lin Y, et al. Computer-aided biomarker discovery for precision medicine: data resources, models and applications. Brief Bioinform. 2019;20(3):952–75.
14. Cook I. Biomarkers in psychiatry: potentials, pitfalls, and pragmatics. Primary Psychiatry. 2008;15(3):54–9.
15. Sokolowska I, et al. The potential of biomarkers in psychiatry: focus on proteomics. J Neural Transm (Vienna). 2015;122(Suppl 1):S9–18.
16. Herron JW, Nerurkar L, Cavanagh J. Neuroimmune Biomarkers in Mental Illness. Curr Top Behav Neurosci. 2018;40:45–78.
17. Harris KM, Schorpp KM. Integrating biomarkers in social stratification and Health Research. Annu Rev Sociol. 2018;44:361–86.
18. Biologically-inspired biomarkers for mental disorders. EBioMedicine. 2017;17:1–2.
19. Payne PRO, Embi, PJ, Translational informatics: realizing the promise of knowledge-driven healthcare. 2014.

20. NHGRI. Genomics and medicine. 2019. April 27, 2020; Available from: https://www.genome.gov/health/Genomics-and-Medicine.
21. NHGRI. The cost of sequencing a human genome. Feb 7 2020; Available from: https://www.genome.gov/about-genomics/fact-sheets/Sequencing-Human-Genome-cost.
22. Wikipedia. $1,000 genome. Sep 14 2020; Available from: https://en.wikipedia.org/wiki/$1,000_genome.
23. Alexander Arguello P, et al. From genetics to biology: advancing mental health research in the genomics ERA. Mol Psychiatry. 2019;24(11):1576–82.
24. ScienceDaily. Largest study of its kind reveals that many psychiatric disorders arise from common genes. 2019. May 21 2020; Available from: https://www.sciencedaily.com/releases/2019/12/191212142634.htm.
25. Cross-Disorder Group of the Psychiatric Genomics Consortium. Electronic address, p.m.h.e. and C. Cross-disorder Group of the Psychiatric Genomics. Genomic relationships, novel loci, and pleiotropic mechanisms across eight psychiatric disorders. Cell. 2019;179(7):1469–82. e11
26. Sabatello M. Psychiatric genomics and public mental health in the young mind. Am J Bioeth. 2017;17(4):27–9.
27. Gandal MJ, et al. Shared molecular neuropathology across major psychiatric disorders parallels polygenic overlap. Science. 2018;359(6376):693–7.
28. Pantazatos SP, et al. Whole-transcriptome brain expression and exon-usage profiling in major depression and suicide: evidence for altered glial, endothelial and ATPase activity. Mol Psychiatry. 2017;22(5):760–73.
29. NLM. Gene. April 27, 2020; Available from: https://ghr.nlm.nih.gov/primer/basics/gene.
30. Wikipedia. Gene. April 27 2020; Available from: https://en.wikipedia.org/wiki/Gene.
31. NLM. Can genes be turned on and off in cells? April 27 2020; Available from: https://ghr.nlm.nih.gov/primer/howgeneswork/geneonoff.
32. Wang W, Wang GZ. Understanding molecular mechanisms of the brain through transcriptomics. Front Physiol. 2019;10:214.
33. Kathuria A, et al. Transcriptome analysis and functional characterization of cerebral organoids in bipolar disorder. Genome Med. 2020;12(1):34.
34. Zhou Y, et al. Interactome analysis reveals ZNF804A, a schizophrenia risk gene, as a novel component of protein translational machinery critical for embryonic neurodevelopment. Mol Psychiatry. 2018;23(4):952–62.
35. Park DI, Turck CW. Interactome studies of psychiatric disorders. Adv Exp Med Biol. 2019;1118:163–73.
36. Xiao Y, et al. The DNA methylome and transcriptome of different brain regions in schizophrenia and bipolar disorder. PLoS One. 2014;9(4):e95875.
37. Kohen R, et al. Transcriptome profiling of human hippocampus dentate gyrus granule cells in mental illness. Transl Psychiatry. 2014;4:e366.
38. Wang X, Cairns MJ. Understanding complex transcriptome dynamics in schizophrenia and other neurological diseases using RNA sequencing. Int Rev Neurobiol. 2014;116:127–52.
39. ENCODE. ENCODE: Deciphering function in the human genome. Sep 16 2020; Available from: https://www.genome.gov/27551473/genome-advance-of-the-month-encode-deciphering-function-in-the-human-genome#.
40. NLM. Protein. April 27 2020; Available from: https://ghr.nlm.nih.gov/primer/howgeneswork/protein.
41. Wikipedia. Reverse phase protein lysate microarray. April 27 2020; Available from: https://en.wikipedia.org/wiki/Reverse_phase_protein_lysate_microarray.
42. Bot M, et al. Serum proteomic profiling of major depressive disorder. Transl Psychiatry. 2015;5:e599.
43. Lista S, et al. Evolving relevance of Neuroproteomics in Alzheimer's disease. Methods Mol Biol. 2017;1598:101–15.
44. Brinkmalm A, et al. Explorative and targeted neuroproteomics in Alzheimer's disease. Biochim Biophys Acta. 2015;1854(7):769–78.
45. Liao L, et al. Proteomic characterization of postmortem amyloid plaques isolated by laser capture microdissection. J Biol Chem. 2004;279(35):37061–8.

46. Metabolon. About metabolomics. April 27 2020; Available from: https://www.metabolon.com/what-we-do/about-metabolomics.
47. EMBL-EBI. Small molecules. Jan 8 2020; Available from: https://www.ebi.ac.uk/training/online/course/introduction-metabolomics/what-metabolomics/no-glossary-small-molecules-no-glossary.
48. Roberts LD, et al., Targeted metabolomics. Curr Protoc Mol Biol, 2012. Chapter 30: Unitas 30.2.1–24.
49. Shah SH, Kraus WE, Newgard CB. Metabolomic profiling for the identification of novel biomarkers and mechanisms related to common cardiovascular diseases: form and function. Circulation. 2012;126(9):1110–20.
50. Emwas AH, et al. NMR spectroscopy for metabolomics research. Metabolites. 2019;9(7):123.
51. MayoClinic. Targeted metabolomics. 2020. Aug 18 2020; Available from: https://www.mayo.edu/research/core-resources/metabolomics-core/services/targeted-metabolomics.
52. Mapstone M, et al. Plasma phospholipids identify antecedent memory impairment in older adults. Nat Med. 2014;20(4):415–8.
53. Martins-de-Souza D, et al. Identification of proteomic signatures associated with depression and psychotic depression in post-mortem brains from major depression patients. Transl Psychiatry. 2012;2:e87.
54. Kahl KG, Stapel B, Frieling H. Link between depression and cardiovascular diseases due to epigenomics and proteomics: focus on energy metabolism. Prog Neuro-Psychopharmacol Biol Psychiatry. 2019;89:146–57.
55. Humer E, Probst T, Pieh C. Metabolomics in psychiatric disorders: What we learn from animal models. Meta. 2020;10(2):72.
56. NLM. Epigenome. April 27 2020; Available from: https://ghr.nlm.nih.gov/primer/howgeneswork/epigenome.
57. Teng M, Irizarry RA. Accounting for GC-content bias reduces systematic errors and batch effects in ChIP-seq data. Genome Res. 2017;27(11):1930–8.
58. Wikipedia. ChIP sequencing. 2020. May 21 2020; Available from: https://en.wikipedia.org/wiki/ChIP_sequencing.
59. ScienceDirect. ChIP-sequencing. 2013. May 21, 2020; Available from: https://www.sciencedirect.com/topics/neuroscience/chip-sequencing.
60. Nature. Transcription factor. 2014. May 21 2020; Available from: https://www.nature.com/scitable/definition/transcription-factor-167/.
61. Park PJ. ChIP-seq: advantages and challenges of a maturing technology. Nat Rev Genet. 2009;10(10):669–80.
62. Kular L, Kular S. Epigenetics applied to psychiatry: clinical opportunities and future challenges. Psychiatry Clin Neurosci. 2018;72(4):195–211.
63. Palma-Gudiel H, Fananas L. An integrative review of methylation at the serotonin transporter gene and its dialogue with environmental risk factors, psychopathology and 5-HTTLPR. Neurosci Biobehav Rev. 2017;72:190–209.
64. Nievergelt CM, et al. Genomic approaches to posttraumatic stress disorder: the psychiatric genomic consortium initiative. Biol Psychiatry. 2018;83(10):831–9.
65. Kumsta R. The role of epigenetics for understanding mental health difficulties and its implications for psychotherapy research. Psychol Psychother. 2019;92(2):190–207.
66. Augustin R, et al. Computational identification and experimental validation of microRNAs binding to the Alzheimer-related gene ADAM10. BMC Med Genet. 2012;13:35.
67. Elsivier. Pathway studio. Sep 16 2020; Available from: https://www.elsevier.com/solutions/pathway-studio-biological-research.
68. Issler O, Chen A. Determining the role of microRNAs in psychiatric disorders. Nat Rev Neurosci. 2015;16(4):201–12.
69. Narahari A, Hussain M, Sreeram V. MicroRNAs as biomarkers for psychiatric conditions: a review of current research. Innov Clin Neurosci. 2017;14(1–2):53–5.
70. Allen L, Dwivedi Y. MicroRNA mediators of early life stress vulnerability to depression and suicidal behavior. Mol Psychiatry. 2020;25(2):308–20.

71. van den Berg MMJ, et al. Circulating microRNAs as potential biomarkers for psychiatric and neurodegenerative disorders. Prog Neurobiol. 2020;185:101732.
72. Roser AE, et al. Circulating miRNAs as diagnostic biomarkers for Parkinson's disease. Front Neurosci. 2018;12:625.
73. Wang X, Gardiner EJ, Cairns MJ. Optimal consistency in microRNA expression analysis using reference-gene-based normalization. Mol BioSyst. 2015;11(5):1235–40.
74. Beveridge NJ, Cairns MJ. MicroRNA dysregulation in schizophrenia. Neurobiol Dis. 2012;46(2):263–71.
75. Wang J, et al. microRNAs as novel biomarkers of schizophrenia (review). Exp Ther Med. 2014;8(6):1671–6.
76. Song L, et al. CINdex: a Bioconductor package for analysis of chromosome instability in DNA copy number data. Cancer Inform. 2017;16:1176935117746637.
77. Cuccaro D, et al. Copy number variants in Alzheimer's disease. J Alzheimers Dis. 2017;55(1):37–52.
78. Nothen MM, et al. New findings in the genetics of major psychoses. Dialogues Clin Neurosci. 2010;12(1):85–93.
79. Malhotra D, Sebat J. CNVs: harbingers of a rare variant revolution in psychiatric genetics. Cell. 2012;148(6):1223–41.
80. Wikipedia. Image segmentation. 2020. May 21 2020; Available from: https://en.wikipedia.org/wiki/Image_segmentation.
81. Wikipedia. Medical imaging. 2020. May 21 2020; Available from: https://en.wikipedia.org/wiki/Medical_imaging.
82. Davatzikos C, et al. Cancer imaging phenomics toolkit: quantitative imaging analytics for precision diagnostics and predictive modeling of clinical outcome. J Med Imaging (Bellingham). 2018;5(1):011018.
83. Wolf I, et al. The medical imaging interaction toolkit. Med Image Anal. 2005;9(6):594–604.
84. Shen D, Wu G, Suk HI. Deep learning in medical image analysis. Annu Rev Biomed Eng. 2017;19:221–48.
85. Jiang W, King TZ, Turner JA. Imaging genetics towards a refined diagnosis of schizophrenia. Front Psych. 2019;10:494.
86. Whitfield-Gabrieli S, et al. Brain connectomics predict response to treatment in social anxiety disorder. Mol Psychiatry. 2016;21(5):680–5.
87. Okano K, et al. Real-time fMRI feedback impacts brain activation, results in auditory hallucinations reduction: part 1: superior temporal gyrus -preliminary evidence. Psychiatry Res. 2020;286:112862.
88. Wikiversity. Microbiome and mental health. Jan 14 2020; Available from: https://en.wikiversity.org/wiki/Microbiome_and_Mental_Health.
89. Bastiaanssen TFS, et al. Gutted! Unraveling the role of the microbiome in major depressive disorder. Harv Rev Psychiatry. 2020;28(1):26–39.
90. Skonieczna-Zydecka K, et al. Microbiome-the missing link in the gut-brain axis: Focus on its role in gastrointestinal and mental health. J Clin Med. 2018;7(12):521.
91. Rottig S, Rujescu D. Microbiome in psychiatry: where will we go? Eur Arch Psychiatry Clin Neurosci. 2018;268(1):1–2.
92. Cryan JF. Stress and the microbiota-gut-brain Axis: an evolving concept in psychiatry. Can J Psychiatr. 2016;61(4):201–3.
93. Licinio J, Wong ML. The role of inflammatory mediators in the biology of major depression: central nervous system cytokines modulate the biological substrate of depressive symptoms, regulate stress-responsive systems, and contribute to neurotoxicity and neuroprotection. Mol Psychiatry. 1999;4(4):317–27.
94. Wong ML, et al. Inflammasome signaling affects anxiety- and depressive-like behavior and gut microbiome composition. Mol Psychiatry. 2016;21(6):797–805.
95. Ashburner M, et al. Gene ontology: tool for the unification of biology. Nat Genet. 2000;25(1):25–9.

96. EBI. Gene set enrichment analysis and pathway analysis. 2020 May 21 2020; Available from: https://www.ebi.ac.uk/training/online/course/functional-genomics-ii-common-technologies-and-data-analysis-methods/gene-set-enrichment.

97. EBI. Gene ontology. 2020 May 21 2020; Available from: https://www.ebi.ac.uk/training/online/glossary/gene-ontology.

98. NIH. Systems biology as defined by NIH. April 27 2020; Available from: https://irp.nih.gov/catalyst/v19i6/systems-biology-as-defined-by-nih.

99. ISB. What is systems biology? April 27, 2020; Available from: https://isbscience.org/about/what-is-systems-biology/.

100. Harvard. Welcome to the department of systems biology. April 27 2020; Available from: https://sysbio.med.harvard.edu/.

101. Kitano H. Systems biology: a brief overview. Science. 2002;295(5560):1662–4.

102. Wikipedia. Systems biology. April 27 2020; Available from: https://en.wikipedia.org/wiki/Systems_biology.

103. Gutierrez Najera NA, Resendis-Antonio O, Nicolini H. "Gestaltomics": Systems biology schemes for the study of neuropsychiatric diseases. Front Physiol. 2017;8:286.

104. NBTS. Tumor types: Understanding brain tumors. Sep 16 2020; Available from: https://braintumor.org/brain-tumor-information/understanding-brain-tumors/tumor-types/.

105. Behnan J, Finocchiaro G, Hanna G. The landscape of the mesenchymal signature in brain tumours. Brain. 2019;142(4):847–66.

106. Verhaak RG, et al. Integrated genomic analysis identifies clinically relevant subtypes of glioblastoma characterized by abnormalities in PDGFRA, IDH1, EGFR, and NF1. Cancer Cell. 2010;17(1):98–110.

107. van den Bent MJ. Interobserver variation of the histopathological diagnosis in clinical trials on glioma: a clinician's perspective. Acta Neuropathol. 2010;120(3):297–304.

108. Louis DN, et al. The 2016 World Health Organization classification of tumors of the central nervous system: a summary. Acta Neuropathol. 2016;131(6):803–20.

109. DeWeerdt S. The genomics of brain cancer. Nature. 2018;561(7724):S54–5.

110. APA. What is Alzheimer's disease? Dec 28 2019]; Available from: https://www.psychiatry.org/patients-families/alzheimers/what-is-alzheimers-disease.

111. Di Resta C, Ferrari M. New molecular approaches to Alzheimer's disease. Clin Biochem. 2019;72:81–6.

112. NIA. Alzheimer's disease genetics fact sheet. Dec 31 2019; Available from: https://www.nia.nih.gov/health/alzheimers-disease-genetics-fact-sheet.

113. Verheijen J, Sleegers K. Understanding Alzheimer disease at the Interface between genetics and transcriptomics. Trends Genet. 2018;34(6):434–47.

114. NIA. What happens to the brain in Alzheimer's disease? Aug 18, 2020; Available from: https://www.nia.nih.gov/health/what-happens-brain-alzheimers-disease.

115. Huang CC, et al. The combination of functional and structural MRI is a potential screening tool in Alzheimer's disease. Front Aging Neurosci. 2018;10:251.

116. Jones KA, Menniti FS, Sivarao DV. Translational psychiatry--light at the end of the tunnel. Ann N Y Acad Sci. 2015;1344:1–11.

117. NIMH. Towards a genomic psychiatry: Recommendations of the genomics workgroup of the NAMHC. 2018. May 21 2020. Available from: https://www.nimh.nih.gov/about/director/messages/2018/towards-a-genomic-psychiatry-recommendations-of-the-genomics-workgroup-of-the-namhc.shtml.

Chapter 12
Integrative Paradigms for Knowledge Discovery in Mental Health: Overcoming the Fragmentation of Knowledge Inherent in Disparate Theoretical Paradigms

Janna Hastings and Rasmus Rosenberg Larsen

Abstract The domain of mental health is inherently complex, spanning across multiple disciplines, data types, descriptive levels, and approaches. This complexity has brought considerable challenges in terms of how to facilitate efficient knowledge discovery and integration across disciplines in the domain. The vocabulary and semantic frameworks in use across these different descriptive levels are fragmented and contested, and it is difficult to gain an overview of what is known across all the relevant bodies of knowledge and practice. In this chapter, we review progress that has recently been made towards integrative semantic and computational frameworks for structuring and advancing mental health research. This includes the paradigm shift incubated in the NIMH's RDoC effort, which offers a roadmap for studying the nature of the complex interactions within and between human systems: biological (body, brain), mental (mind), behavioral, social, and environmental. We also review computational approaches to infer and model relationships between entities that explicitly cross levels of explanation and disciplinary boundaries. We describe the quantitative methods that are used to integrate and analyze across heterogeneous datasets, and the epistemological challenges that face the field when attempting to determine mechanistic explanations that move the global understanding of mental health forward.

Keywords Semantic Frameworks · Diagnostic and Statistical Manual (DSM) · Research Domain Criteria (DSM) · Factor Analysis · Network Analysis · Epistemology

J. Hastings (✉)
Clinical, Educational and Health Psychology, University College London, London, UK
e-mail: j.hastings@ucl.ac.uk

R. R. Larsen
Department of Philosophy, University of Toronto Mississauga, Toronto, ON, Canada
e-mail: rosenberg.larsen@utoronto.ca

© Springer Nature Switzerland AG 2021
J. D. Tenenbaum, P. A. Ranallo (eds.), *Mental Health Informatics*, Health
Informatics, https://doi.org/10.1007/978-3-030-70558-9_12

12.1 Introduction

Research and discovery in any scientific discipline depends on a plethora of processes for acquiring and transforming evidence, in the form of data, into conclusions, in the form of assertions. Discovery processes depend on complex disciplinary theoretical commitments and practical constraints, in ways that differ from discipline to discipline. Theoretical commitments in this context encompass basic assumptions about the world and what can be or should be investigated by research, while practical constraints include the methods that make such investigations possible. Various aggregates of theories and practices in each discipline constitute different 'epistemic cultures', that is, ways of knowing about the world [1].

Over the last hundred years, segregation of research efforts into distinct academic disciplines or fields has become the norm, beginning early in educational trajectories. Each field develops its own vocabulary, methods, and tools. This disciplinary fragmentation and specialization have increased to the extent where some have proposed that from a certain perspective, it could be said that knowledge is no longer shared, but individualized [2]. And this fragmentation affects not only bodies of knowledge and research practices, it affects education and ways of thinking and reasoning. Those who study medicine receive different foundational information than those who study psychology, biology, statistics and so on. Some courses emphasize and train quantitative skills and reasoning, while others focus more on descriptive interpretation and memorizing a large body of factual knowledge.

Disciplinary specialization is not necessarily problematic in and of itself, as long as the subject matter and research questions of different disciplines are sufficiently distinguishable. However, in interdisciplinary fields such as mental health, in which the subject matter is shared between multiple disciplines, these disciplinary specializations and separate vocabularies can provide barriers to successful cumulative progress. Examples of different broad disciplinary areas that are relevant for mental health include psychiatry, psychology, neuroscience, biology, and epidemiology. Each of these disciplinary groupings is further sub-divided into a myriad of different specialties and sub-disciplines. Complex standardized discovery protocols have evolved and grown during the history of each discipline. Different protocols are used in each discipline both for the measurement of phenomena in standardized ways, and for interpretation of the results of such measurements. The differences extend also to which entities are believed to exist, or be the most relevant, in which contexts.

In mental health, there are significant theoretical and practical obstacles to conducting research that addresses questions spanning across historically separate domains [2–5]. These are partly due to the wide range of factors that affect mental health and the complexity of the conditions themselves. No single researcher can be an expert in all the different aspects of these phenomena from each of the different disciplinary perspectives, and cross-disciplinary collaboration can pose challenges [6, 7]. As a result, studies investigating the relationships between different discipline-specific phenomena (for example, the relation between emotion dysregulation and endocrine dysfunction) are significantly outnumbered by studies dealing with individual discipline-specific categories in isolation (e.g. psychometric models of specific disorders) [8]. However, there is a growing community-wide recognition that the standard practices of research in isolated disciplines and single-entity categories have not led to sufficient progress in mental health treatment innovation, and thus that enabling interdisciplinary knowledge integration is becoming a more urgent objective [9, 10].

The previous chapters in this textbook have covered a broad scope and provided detailed discussions of many of the specific techniques, methods, vocabularies, and tools that are used in the various (but inter-related) disciplinary perspectives within mental health. Now, in this chapter, we look at frameworks and techniques that aim to achieve integrative and interdisciplinary research. We explore recent approaches, paradigms and frameworks that have been proposed to address the problem of fragmentation, and to support integrative research and practice in mental health.

In the next section, we explore the challenge of fragmented vocabularies and the need for semantic integration. In the subsequent section, we explore computational methods that support integrative empirical analyses. Thereafter, we conclude with a discussion about epistemic considerations, reproducibility, and the inherent limitations in current integrative research paradigms.

12.2 Integrative Semantic Frameworks and the RDoC Initiative

Almost all empirical research aims to investigate regularities and repeatable phenomena in nature, in search of commonalities and truths that are generalizable beyond a single, limited, experimental setting. Research is thus directed at types of entities rather than specific entities, and samples are selected that are believed to exemplify such commonalities and types sufficiently so as to support generalizable conclusions. For that reason, a system of classification, or semantic framework, that specifies type of entity, is needed.

Psychiatric research and practice for the past several decades has largely been structured according to the diagnostic categories formalized in the various editions of the *Diagnostic and Statistical Manual of Mental Disorders* (DSM; most recent edition DSM-5 published in 2013 [11]) and the largely aligned *International Classification of Disorders and Related Health Problems* (ICD; most recent edition ICD-10 [12]). These classifications specify types of mental health disorder corresponding to syndromes of interrelated symptoms and patterns of behavior. The disorders that are specified in the latest version of the DSM[1] are listed in Table 12.1

---

[1] Note that the DSM is also discussed in some detail in Chap. 5.

Table 12.1 Classification of psychiatric entities in the DSM-5

DSM Chapter (classification grouping)	Examples of classified disorders (where applicable, not comprehensive)
Neurodevelopmental disorders	Autism spectrum disorder, specific learning disorders, intellectual developmental disorder
Schizophrenia spectrum and other psychotic disorders	Schizophrenia, schizoaffective disorder, brief psychotic disorder
Bipolar and related disorders	Bipolar I disorder, bipolar II disorder, cyclothymic disorder
Depressive disorders	Disruptive mood dysregulation disorder, major depressive disorder, persistent depressive disorder (dysthymia), premenstrual dysphoric disorder
Anxiety disorders	Separation anxiety disorder, selective mutism, specific phobia, social anxiety disorder (social phobia), panic disorder, agoraphobia, generalized anxiety disorder
Obsessive-compulsive and related disorders	Obsessive-compulsive disorder (OCD), body dysmorphic disorder (BDD), hoarding disorder, trichotillomania (hair-pulling disorder), and excoriation (skin-picking) disorder
Trauma- and stressor-related disorders	Acute stress disorder (ASD) and posttraumatic stress disorder (PTSD).
Dissociative disorders	Dissociative identity disorder, dissociative amnesia, depersonalization/derealization disorder
Somatic symptom and related disorders	Somatic symptom disorder, illness anxiety disorder, conversion disorder, factitious disorder
Feeding and eating disorders	Anorexia nervosa, bulimia nervosa, binge eating disorder
Elimination disorders	Enuresis (wetting), encopresis (soiling)
Sleep-wake disorders	Insomnia disorder, hypersomnolence disorder, narcolepsy, nightmare disorder
Sexual dysfunctions	Delayed ejaculation, erectile disorder, genito-pelvic pain/penetration disorder
Gender dysphoria	
Disruptive, impulse-control, and conduct disorders	Intermittent explosive disorder, pyromania, kleptomania
Substance-related and addictive disorders	
Neurocognitive disorders	Delirium, mild neurocognitive disorder, and major neurocognitive disorder
Personality disorders	Paranoid, schizoid, schizotypal, antisocial, borderline, histrionic, narcissistic, avoidant, dependent and obsessive-compulsive personality disorder
Paraphilic disorders	Voyeuristic, exhibitionistic, frotteuristic, sexual masochism, sexual sadism, pedophilic paraphilic disorder

along with their grouping categories [13]. For example, 'major depressive disorder' belongs to the class of depressive disorders, and is described as being characterized by a cluster of symptoms including persistent depressed mood, loss of interest in activities, fatigue and loss of energy, and slowing down of thoughts [14].

The development of the DSM was motivated by the need to address heterogeneity in clinical treatment and interpretation of mental health conditions. Before the introduction of the DSM, it was common for different clinicians to arrive at different diagnoses for the same clinical presentation [15, 16]. It was thus difficult to perform empirical studies that relied on studying the same phenomenon in a cohort of persons with the same or similar conditions, since samples tended to be heterogeneous. By creating a standard set of categories for describing psychiatric phenomena along with assessment tools and guidance for performing diagnoses, reliability in clinical diagnoses was improved, and it became possible to perform large-scale population studies with increased homogeneity across samples. However, the definitions of disorders, and the general approach to classification that is manifested within the DSM, have been criticized in various different ways [9, 17].

Firstly, there is widespread concern about the use of arbitrary thresholds in the described symptomatology. For example, since the last revision of the DSM, major depression can be diagnosed as early as two weeks after a major bereavement, but there is no substantial evidence base to support why two weeks is the most appropriate timeframe to distinguish between depression and the normal responses associated with grief [18]. It is understandable that many of the thresholds used in the DSM have been subject to wide debate. In general, there is a difficult balance when defining thresholds such as these between the need to offer appropriate medical care in cases of clinical necessity and urgency, and the imperative to avoid medicalizing normal experiences [19]. This is exacerbated in situations where medical care or reimbursement is conditional on the receipt of a definite diagnosis.

Secondly, a problem of diagnostic overlap or co-morbidity exists between most of the major categories, in that individuals with severe mental health conditions tend to meet the criteria for multiple disorders, which suggests that the categories are not as distinct in reality as they appear in the classification hierarchy. There is also evidence from genetic studies that many of the disorder categories share their genetic risk factors [20], again suggesting that the underlying biological reality does not divide neatly into distinct categories.

Thirdly, research being structured rigidly into diagnostic categories has hindered research on mental health phenomena that cut across categories or are present in members of the population that do not meet the criteria for any specific condition. This has been particularly obvious in countries where a specific categorization system has been institutionalized to the extent that research funding depends on targeting a specific disorder as it is defined in that categorization [15], which was the case until recently in the US with the DSM.

However, it is no longer the case. In response to the longstanding problems with the DSM, the US's National Institute of Mental Health proposed the Research Domain Criteria (RDoC) framework as a new way to structure research, envisioned as 'breaking out of the confines' of diagnostic categories [21–24]. In contrast to the categorical approach followed by the DSM, the RDoC is built from the bottom up as a multifaceted classification addressing various *dimensions* of mental health phenomena. Thus, rather than proposing rigid groupings to which people are assigned as belonging by a concrete diagnosis, RDoC proposes a series of variables within a multi-dimensional space, into which people may be heterogeneously placed according to their signs and symptoms. RDoC is explicitly multi-domain and integrative in its design, providing a structure in which research is classified into a matrix of high-level traits and cross-cutting constructs. One of the incentives behind the

Table 12.2 The RDoC domains and constructs

RDoC domain	Examples of constructs (not comprehensive)
Negative valence systems	Acute threat ("fear"), potential threat ("anxiety"), sustained threat, loss, frustrative nonreward
Positive valence systems	Reward responsiveness, reward learning, reward valuation
Cognitive systems	Attention, perception, declarative memory, language, cognitive control, working memory
Social processes	Social communication, perception and understanding of the self, perception and understanding of others
Arousal and regulatory systems	Arousal, circadian rhythms, sleep-wakefulness
Sensorimotor systems	Motor actions, agency and ownership, habit, innate motor patterns

development of the RDoC was the hope that re-directing research efforts into a shared framework of high-level dimensional traits might facilitate a more efficient integration of knowledge across different sciences [25–27].

The RDoC matrix is divided into six major domains. Within each domain, different phenomena, called 'constructs', are classified, each of which may vary dimensionally from normal to abnormal. The domains and examples of constructs are listed in Table 12.2. It should be apparent that there are some clear mappings between constructs as envisioned in the RDoC and corresponding disorder categories in the DSM. For example, there is a clear relationship between the construct 'potential threat' in the RDoC's 'negative valence systems', and the DSM classification of anxiety disorders. However, not all DSM categories have obvious mappings, and indeed such direct mappings were not intended by the design of the RDoC. The RDoC is not intended for use in clinical contexts yet, rather focusing solely on research contexts. This is reflected also in the fact that the RDoC is explicitly put forward as a proposal subject to change in the future, rather than a finalized new classification system to replace existing classification systems.

The RDoC also has an explicit representation of the different ways that constructs can be measured. These measurements are called 'units of analysis', which can include molecular, cellular, neurological and behavioral assessments. The RDoC framework is thus typically represented as a matrix, or table, in which the rows are constructs and the columns are units of analysis (for example, 'cells' and 'circuits'). The RDoC knowledgebase available online[2] is populated with links to elements of the relevant type (for example, types of cell), that have been implicated in some way in the relevant construct, for each element of the table. Thus, the RDoC project brings together or *integrates* fundamentally different types of knowledge, arising from fundamentally different perspectives—biological, behavioral, etc.—insofar as they bear on the same construct. In other words, RDoC is explicitly *integrative by design*. It has already been hailed in the US as enabling mental health to transcend the boundaries of individual diagnostic categories and disciplinary categories [28]. However, it has also been criticized for being semantically vague, that is, lacking clear definitions for the entities to which it refers [9, 29–31]. Moreover, the distinction between 'constructs' and 'units of analysis' is not always clear. For example, many of the

---

[2] https://www.nimh.nih.gov/research/research-funded-by-nimh/rdoc/constructs/rdoc-matrix.shtml

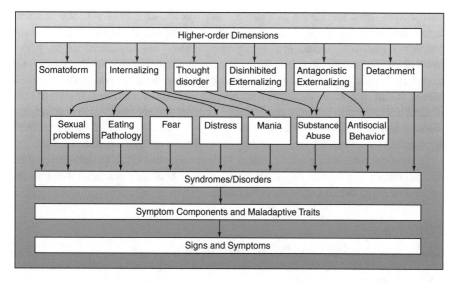

Fig. 12.1 A schematic illustration of the HiTOP hierarchical structure, adapted from that shown in [32]. The illustrated levels are "super-spectra", "spectra", "subfactors", "syndromes/disorders", "components" and "symptoms"

constructs are behavioral in nature, while there is also a unit of analysis of type 'behavior'. To address these gaps, approaches that assign more explicit semantics, such as ontologies, might be applied to flesh out and define the semantics of the RDoC matrix [5].

The RDoC is not the only initiative that aims to re-think the classification of entities of relevance for mental health. One alternative proposal is the hierarchical taxonomy of psychopathology (HiTOP), which posits a hierarchical structure amongst psychopathological conditions rooted in a measure of generalized psychopathology [32]. HiTOP has been developed quantitatively, using methods such as factor analysis (described further below) to determine a dimensional structure directly from observed clinical data. As illustrated in Fig. 12.1, the top level of the HiTOP consists of what are called 'spectra', broad groupings of or dimensions of symptomatology in psychopathological conditions. These are 'somatoform', 'internalising', 'thought disorder', 'externalising-disinhibited', 'externalising-antagonistic', and 'detachment'. Spectra are then further divided into sub-factors, for example, 'sexual problems', 'eating problems', 'fear', 'distress', 'mania' and 'antisocial behavior'. Beneath the sub-factors, syndromes and disorders are at the next hierarchical level, thereafter signs, symptoms, components, and traits are included at the lowest level of the hierarchy. Symptoms are transient, while traits are stable.

Although hierarchical approaches such as HiTOP are not explicitly integrative across disciplinary perspectives—their domain is restricted to 'classical' psychopathology, as is that of the DSM—they offer an interestingly empirical approach whereby the hierarchy and the groupings at each hierarchical level are based on and informed by large-scale empirical studies, using for example factor analysis as an approach to identify dimensions of variability in the data. As will be detailed in the next section, what this means is that the groupings included in HiTOP are deduced based on empirically observed covariation of symptoms, and the hierarchical structure proposes higher-order dimensions by deriving "factors" that explain variability in the lower dimensions [33]. It thus represents an important shift, alongside the RDoC, towards evaluating and interpreting the full body of knowledge and evidence about mental health *as a whole* rather than compartmentalized into different bodies of evidence associated with different categories of disorder that are assumed to be relatively distinct. It also reflects a shift further towards a data-driven and computational approach to advancing the understanding of conditions in mental health.

In the next section, we take a deeper look at some examples of data-driven and computational approaches for research in mental health informatics that can be applied in a way that is explicitly integrative.

12.3   Integrative Computational Methods

12.3.1   Factor Analysis

The empirical approaches that have been used to define hierarchical semantic frameworks for mental health have used *factor analysis* to determine general or shared factors behind observations of different symptoms. In a dataset with multiple observations across multiple variables, each variable is a *dimension*. Factor analysis is a statistical method commonly used in psychology and psychometrics that aims to reduce the number of dimensions, i.e. the *dimensionality,* of a large-scale dataset, by identifying jointly shared *latent* (or hidden) variables that are able to explain some of the variability in the whole dataset more succinctly [34, 35].

For example, a study might have several measurements of variables relating to the bodies of a number of people, e.g. their height, leg length, hand size, head circumference, waist circumference, and weight, each of which is mutually correlated (see Fig. 12.2). If we were to apply factor analysis on this dataset, we may detect a hidden variable that explains a portion of the overall variance across the other variables, which in this case might be called 'body size' (illustrated by the box labelled '?' in Fig. 12.2c). Hidden variables are not themselves measured, thus, they are called *latent,* that is, they are suggested by the data. The overall aim of factor analysis is to identify this type of latent variable, or explanatory factor. The observed variables can then be represented as a sum of the variation in the hidden variables, together with a portion of variance that is unique to each specific variable, simplifying interpretation of the overall dataset.

There are many subtleties to performing a factor analysis that may affect the results, such as deciding on the optimal number of factors and associated parameters in the analysis. Note that in the example given earlier, if the dataset had been from a group of children, the hidden factor might be better identified as 'age'—highlighting that factor analysis can give evidence that there is a hidden explanatory

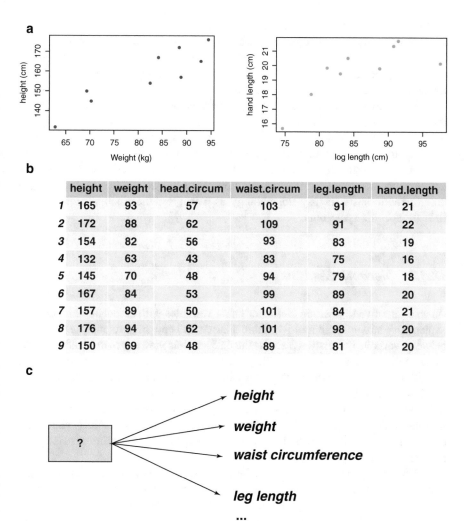

Fig. 12.2 Factor analysis. An example dataset (**b**) illustrating measurements, for nine individual persons, of several mutually correlated variables (e.g. **a** shows plots of height vs weight and leg length vs. hand length) that may have a hidden or latent factor that explains a significant proportion of the variance (**c**)

variable, but not necessarily tell you what that variable *is* (so to speak). Factor analysis is often used as an exploratory form of analysis, in which the statistical methods aim to discover the presence of latent variables. It can also be used in confirmatory analyses, in which a specific hypothesis about latent variables is tested. Interpretation of the results of a factor analysis is quite often far from straightforward, and it has been noted that statistics alone cannot arbitrate between different possible underlying structures [36].

Although it was not explicitly developed to be integrative, factor analysis can be applied to multi-level datasets of variables and thereby serve as an integrative approach. For example, in [37] connections are found between symptoms such as distress and underlying risk factors such as information processing bias and autonomic dysregulation, indicating a multi-level conceptual model of psychopathology. In another example ([38]), factor analysis is used to explore cross-level relationships between genetic risks and observed psychopathologies, finding that multi-gene genetic risk factors were good predictors of latent general factors of psychopathological symptomatology (especially in the negative dimension), but once these latent factors had been taken into account, the genetic risk factors were not specific predictors for individual symptoms such as psychosis, suggesting a broad genetic basis for psychopathology as a whole rather than specific genetic risks for specific symptoms.

12.3.2   Network Analysis

As an alternative to positing factors or latent variables with associated hierarchical explanatory structures in multi-variable datasets, it is possible to analyse the direct between-variable correlations[3] across the dataset, thus viewing each variable on the same footing as each other variable. The correlational structure between distinct variables (i.e. the ways in which the variables change similarly) can be viewed as a *network* of between-variable interactions, where nodes correspond to variables (e.g. individual symptoms), and edges correspond to correlations above some threshold in strength and significance. Networks are inferred based on variability, which can be dynamic variability across time, or a static snapshot of variability across symptoms at a particular moment [39].

Networks of this form may even be considered to be a representation of the *nature* of the relevant conditions. In other words, conditions can be viewed as syndromes involving networks of interacting symptoms rather than as distinct individual or categorical entities with common or higher-level causes [40, 41]. For example, from a network perspective depression can be viewed not as a single categorical entity with diverse manifestations, but as a heterogeneous cluster of causally interacting symptoms in which, for example, insomnia may lead to fatigue, which in turn may lead to concentration problems and psychomotor problems [42].

Network approaches are becoming increasingly popular in mental health research [43, 44]. An example of a network analysis for a fictitious dataset is shown in Fig. 12.3. In this example, six anonymous individuals have given scores on a symptom scale for eight distinct symptoms: sadness, anhedonia, suicidal thoughts, insomnia, low self-esteem, worry, obsessions, and distress.

---

[3] Note that 'correlation' is used broadly here, to cover several different statistical measures in practice: various different correlation measures or other co-variance metrics may be used.

a

	sadness	anhedonia	suicidal	insomnia	selfesteem	worry	rumination	distress
1	10	12	4	8	9	13	13	18
2	12	18	5	18	10	14	15	19
3	14	13	6	17	9	13	14	20
4	10	15	4	12	8	14	15	20
5	8	10	5	10	7	11	10	19
6	15	13	4	17	8	13	12	18

b

	rowname	worry	anhedonia	rumination	selfesteem	insomnia	sadness	distress
1	worry							
2	anhedonia	.87						
3	rumination	.94	.85					
4	selfesteem	.70	.73	.74				
5	insomnia	.43	.60	.40	.45			
6	sadness	.41	.32	.29	.39	.82		
7	distress	.20	.24	.46	.00	.21	-.08	
8	suicidal	-.22	.00	.04	.28	.42	.18	.55

c

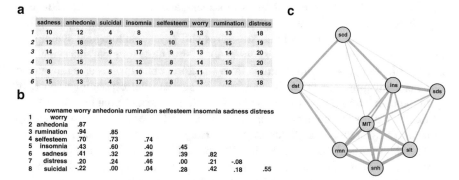

Fig. 12.3 Network analysis of fictitious data gives a network of interacting symptoms in depression. Fictitious data for six anonymous individuals, and eight symptoms. The fictitious scores for the different symptoms (**a**) result in between-symptom correlations (**b**) that are illustrated in the network plot (**c**; node labels abbreviated). Correlations are shown as lines between nodes, with green colour for positive correlation and red colour for negative correlation. Strength of correlation is indicated by line thickness. This example is based on that presented in the tutorial at [45] and makes use of the qgraph package in R [46]

The symptoms that are represented in these types of networks are not specific to one condition, although some symptoms may feature more prominently in the network related to one condition rather than another, and some symptoms such as insomnia tend to act as bridges between different conditions, which may help to explain patterns of comorbidity [47]. The network approach allows for feedback cycles and mutual influences between symptoms, which are not typically allowed by hierarchical or latent variable approaches that try to map out shared or common causes and attribute the remainder of the variability to aspects that are assumed to be independent. However, some have argued that the differences between latent variable approaches and network approaches are not as dramatic as they might appear [39].

In common with other empirically based data-driven methods, network approaches can be used to integrate across different levels and paradigms when used in conjunction with data that spans different levels and paradigms. For example, a network structure was computed to infer causal pathways between childhood trauma and psychopathological symptoms [48]. In this study, individual symptoms from a commonly used psychosis rating scale were used together with those of a childhood trauma rating scale in a sample of over 500 persons as input to an integrative network analysis. It was determined that childhood trauma as a whole was not specifically correlated with any distinct psychotic symptoms but rather with the general psychopathological severity as a whole. However, specific types of childhood trauma were strongly correlated with specific symptoms: physical abuse was associated with the symptoms "somatic concern" and "poor impulse control"; emotional abuse was associated with anxiety; sexual abuse was associated with item guilt, and physical neglect was associated with motor retardation. In the overall network that was inferred from the data, "unusual thought content" was the symptom with the highest betweenness, closeness, and strength measures, suggesting this as an important symptom within causal chains. The network approach has also been used to link across brain structures and psychopathological symptoms. For example, [49] correlated responses to a structured clinical interview for DSM-IV in 455 persons with features from structural brain images using magnetic resonance imaging. The DSM-IV questionnaire subscale corresponding to positive symptoms was found to correlate inversely with gray matter volume (GMV) and cortical thickness in frontal and temporal regions, while the subscale corresponding to negative symptoms was found to be inversely correlated with the measure of right frontal cortical surface area. In [50] the links between specific depression symptoms and neuroanatomical regions were explored in a network study comparing item responses from the Beck Depression Inventory scale (see Chap. 9) and an anatomical segmentation of whole-brain images obtained using functional magnetic resonance imaging (fMRI).

12.3.3 Computational Psychiatry

The network approach offers a systematic way to integrate across data involving variables which would otherwise have been treated separately, enabling integrative analyses. However, it is possible to go even further, by explicitly representing and evaluating mechanistic cross-level connections as detailed mathematical models. A family of approaches that aims to develop such models is commonly referred to as *computational psychiatry* [51].

Computational psychiatry grew out of advances in computational neuroscience applied to psychiatry [51]. It posits that the working of the brain, broadly understood, can be represented as if the brain were a processor of information (i.e. as if the brain were itself performing computations) of which it makes sense to ask (a) what are the mathematical properties and algorithms followed when processing the information, as well as (b) how those algorithms are realized by activity in neurons and brain circuits. Focusing on the algorithmic and mathematical levels of description allows the development of complex mechanistic models that can be systematically compared with empirical observations. Computational psychiatry makes use of *generative* models rather than just *descriptive* models. That is, the models not only aim to fit the observations, but also enable mechanistic predictions of *how* high-level causes actually generate low-level observations. A generative model operates as a 'forward model' from parameters to observed data, allowing sampling of the parameter space to make predictions for novel outcomes ([52]). This allows different simulations to be run computationally to determine which amongst several possible mechanisms may best account for observed behavior, and to assess the evidence for competing theories formally, e.g. by using Bayesian model comparison [53, 54].

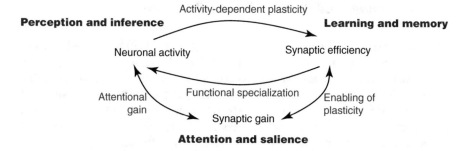

Fig. 12.4 A schematic example of a computational model of learning, taken from [56]. In the model, not shown here, each of the nodes in this network is associated with a mathematical expression, such that the model overall forms a system of equations that can be solved under different conditions

Consider, for instance, that a computational approach may describe 'learning' using a model with several parameters, which might include motivation, value representation, learning rate, confidence, exploratory behavior, prediction error, and meta-learning [55]. The model that is developed includes explicit representation of mathematical and algorithmic steps that link lower level entities through these posited parameters to the broader behavioral phenotypes that are observed, and enables different possible weightings of parameters or sub-processes to be explicitly modelled and tested. Figure 12.4 shows a simplified example of the multi-level computational model of learning represented in [56]. The schematic shown in Fig. 12.4 illustrates the broad connections between different entities (e.g. neuronal activity, synaptic efficiency) and the way that these entities are changed by activities (e.g. functional specialization). The schematic also illustrates the way in which these lower-level parameters are related to higher-level entities such as learning, perception and attention. However, the schematic leaves out the actual mathematical details that are presented in the original [56], as these are complex and there is not enough space in this chapter to sufficiently explain them here.

Similar to the RDoC, computational psychiatry is explicitly an integrative approach, yet it goes further than the RDoC in that it includes several mechanistic layers that are not accounted for in RDoC, related to intermediary processes between the RDoC levels 'circuits' and 'behavior'. Moreover, computational psychiatry explicitly represents mechanistic information for *how* each of the different RDoC levels (e.g. genes, cells, circuits, and cognitive and social processes) is associated and enacted through the other levels [51], using, for example, systems of differential equations. Different types of mathematical model can be used in computational approaches to psychiatry, e.g. by harnessing probabilistic or Bayesian statistics, or machine learning. Many of these computational models are initially developed from neuroimaging data as a key empirical foundation for selecting and estimating the value of parameters. These approaches can be used to make predictive models for disease mechanisms and progression, both within single subjects and across multiple subjects [57].

12.3.4 Within- and Between-Person Reasoning

There is a distinction between *within-person* (intraindividual) mechanistic reasoning, and *between-person* (interindividual) mechanistic reasoning. This distinction applies in network-based approaches and in other computational approaches. In factor analysis, factors may not represent *trait* differences between individuals, but rather *state* differences within individuals over time. For example, in the case of psychopathology, this distinction translates into differences in illness *trajectories* between individuals (i.e. state differences), rather than differences between *types of illness* (i.e. trait differences) [58]. In network-based approaches, within-person variability has been used to construct networks for a single participant over time, allowing insights at the personal level [59], as well as for insights into the structure of a condition by looking at multiple cases across a population. Individual level networks may differ from individual to individual despite their sharing a common diagnosis, meaning that the network-based approach may be more powerful than an approach based merely on discrete diagnoses [42]. This insight was harnessed, for example, to develop a program of individualized feedback based on determination of individual patterns of affect in the case of depression [60]. In this study, by means of digital technology, real-time experience sampling was used to determine current affective state of participants in a trial and enable individualised feedback to be provided. Feedback included, for example, information about activities or time frames that had been associated with greater overall positive affect. Participants receiving this type of feedback scored lower in depression ratings by the end of the study duration than did those participants who only received the normal standard of care.

Many computational and statistical approaches calculate either within- or between-person inferences separately. However, one approach that is able to simultaneously resolve both of these is multilevel structural equation modelling, a form of multi-level regression modelling that adjusts an overall linear regression model to accommodate nested data arising from within-person effects [61]. Multilevel structural equation modelling is used together with intensive longitudinal data which exhibits both a between-person structure reflecting the trait structure of patterns of behavior, and a within-person structure reflecting dynamic structures of the covariance of behaviors at a momentary level [58]. For example, a multi-level dynamic structural equation modelling approach was used to interpret affective differences within and between persons in the COGITO study which sampled two groups of 100 persons each (an older group and a younger group) for 100 days using a variety of cognitive and affective tests [62]. It was possible to attribute temporal variability in affective responsiveness to stressful events within persons, and associate that with between-person differences in traits (e.g. diagnoses), to confirm predictions such as that individuals who have been diagnosed with major depression dynamically respond more negatively to stressors than their non-depressed counterparts, and that individuals with a more negative patterns of affect were more at risk of becoming depressed. This study also highlighted that as composite variability in a longitudinal dataset would be due to both between- and within-individual variability, it was therefore necessary to pay attention to theoretical considerations, such as questions about which time scales are important for relevant features to appear, when designing studies and when choosing appropriate models for analysis.

12.4   Discussion: Epistemology and the Limitations of Integrative Paradigms

The subject matter of mental health does not easily split into separate disciplines. There are fundamental differences in epistemological frameworks and evaluation schemes between the different relevant disciplines. Epistemology, discussed in more detail in Chap. 6, refers to ways of knowing, or how we know what we know. For research in particular, it addresses how we derive new knowledge from scientific investigation. There are also superficial differences in methods of communicating findings and in associated vocabularies, which taken together may lead to contradictory results that are difficult to reconcile [3].

Approaches that aim to investigate the complex relationships within and between different types of entity in mental health research must necessarily commit themselves to a view of which entities exist (such as cells, circuits, diseases, etc.), which possible relationships may obtain between them (e.g. causal or constitutional), and how those entities and relationships can be operationally investigated. In other words, each approach therefore operates with certain implicit or explicit *ontological commitments*, that is, certain assumptions about the nature of the underlying reality that is being investigated. This is not only true of mental health research, but of all scientific disciplines. However, in some disciplines, ontological commitments are made explicitly clear through agreed standards for the domain (e.g. the standard model in physics), while in other domains ontological commitments remain implicit or are contested, hindering scientific transparency [63]. As the discussion of the DSM and the proposed alternatives such as the RDoC illustrates, there is currently no stable within- or between-discipline consensus about the fundamental ontological commitments in mental health research and practice. That is, there is no consensus as to which entities exist and which relations hold between them [3, 64]. There are significant theoretical and practical challenges accommodating the complexities and interrelationships of each domain and each discipline across the full range of biological and human sciences in order to cover the full scope of relevance to mental health [5].

Speaking to these theoretical and practical challenges, the philosopher Jacqueline Sullivan recently highlighted a problem facing mental health research across disciplines, which she called *uncoordinated conceptual pluralism* [65]. Sullivan highlights that a proliferation of conceptual entities to describe and subdivide mental functions, together with an accompanying proliferation of operational methods (paradigms or operationalizations) to isolate such mental functions for the purpose of research, has resulted in a pluralistic body of evidence that is difficult to integrate.

A related criticism is that the operationalizations used in individual studies may be too specific and detailed to provide adequate support for the broader and more general conclusions that are frequently drawn in the literature [66]. We have little insight in terms of the extent to which results arising from different paradigms are conflicting or disparate, since results from different studies may be described in different terms with respect to different entities, or described as though they are about the same entity when in fact they are not (due to differences in operationalisation). While an entity may be represented with the same *label* across different studies, that does not ensure that the entity *means* the same thing in different contexts. For example, a recent article on neuroscientific research in the legal domain noticed that the term 'lying,' was defined and operationalized in widely differing ways in neuroscientific investigations relative to the ways 'lying' was defined by the courts [67]. A 2015 journal article listed 50 words and phrases which it suggests are inaccurately or ambiguously used across mental health literature [68], including 'a gene for', 'lie detector', and 'neural signature'. Another recent article highlights the heterogeneity and diversity of things that are measured by different instruments across ten different mental health conditions [69], finding that similarity scores across different instruments ostensibly for the same condition ranged from 30% to at most 60%.

The problem of uncoordinated conceptual pluralism, as evidenced by label ambiguity and measurement heterogeneity, is exacerbated by an accompanying problem of *construct instability*, that is, adjustments to the meanings of terms, which continuously takes place in each discipline in which the semantic framework is undergoing active evolution. For a well-known example of construct instability in the wider medical context, the term 'diabetes' was updated after new discoveries were made to reflect the fact that it encompassed two distinct conditions, which are now called 'type 1 diabetes' and 'type 2 diabetes'. In the mental health context, similar examples of evolving constructs can be found in, for example, the incorporation in the DSM in 1994, and then removal again in 2013, of the condition 'Asperger's syndrome' [70]. Categories such as these are evolving across a multitude of different classification systems across a range of different relevant disciplines, posing significant challenges for integrative research.

There are further inherent challenges with ensuring that the methods used to standardize and operationalize mental health research map adequately onto the subject matter that is being investigated (i.e. that they are *valid*—see Chap. 8). Operationalization works differently in each discipline, and thus, constructs may be operationally limited in different ways in different disciplines. It may be helpful to consider some examples. In basic biological research, inferences may be extrapolated from the behavior and attributes of animal 'model organisms' or cells and tissues grown in the laboratory, with mutations in their genetic makeup, to the activity and causal role of different genes in different mental health conditions. For example, rodent models of depression are selected based on behavior that appears similar to human depression, similar types of molecular pathologies to what is known about the molecular pathology associated with depression, and similar responses to treatment as humans are known to have [71]. However, extrapolating from such animal-based research to humans has known limitations. In psychology and the behavioral sciences, theoretical nuances might be hidden behind different operationalizations designed to render a complex question tractable in a laboratory environment, and results may be idiosyncratically dependent on the posited constructs or specific measures. Generalizing from one specific operationalized construct to others, and to the situations that occur in wider everyday life, can be challenging. In medical research, the gold standard of evidence is the randomized controlled trial, in which participants are randomized into different groups and thereby a control is compared to an active treatment. However, such studies are expensive, not all types of intervention lend themselves to being blinded or controlled in a relevant fashion as would be needed to perform such studies [72], and for mental health related studies it can be difficult to recruit sufficient participants [73].

For example, in the restrictive experimental setups afforded to cognitive neuroscientific studies of emotion, perceptual pictures of emotional facial expressions are often used as a proxy for the study of the brain regions involved in emotional states. However, the neural state of viewing a picture of an angry person's face may not in fact have much in common with the neural state of being angry, and alternative paradigms include instructions for mental imagery, reading vignettes, and autobiographical recall [74]. In biological contexts, for example using rodent models, emotion research involves behavioural stimuli designed to elicit specific emotional states, while in clinical conditions the data may include clinical observational reports and self-reports. Comparing the results of these various different types of data is extremely challenging, and it should be evident that not all of these scenarios will be dealing with the same, or even a relevantly comparable, construct.

Thus, taken together, it follows that different forms of evidence about a single entity may have different epistemological limitations attached (limitations about what can be inferred from the study given its design and constraints), depending on the discipline and research paradigm from which it arises. What this means is that studies investigating, for example, 'depression' in one discipline, may be investigating a quite different phenomena as compared to studies investigating 'depression' in a different discipline, even to the extent that they agree on the existence of an entity with that name corresponding to a distinct category of disorder with a common cause or phenotype. And even then, within each discipline, the factors and variables that are determined to be related to each entity of this type will be different and not necessarily comparable.

Results arising from across disciplines are therefore difficult to tie together into coherent, structured, theoretically unified wholes. This is partly due to the lack of a perspective on how the different available theories and frameworks fit together and relate to the evidence at hand, and rendered even more intractable by the exponential increase in volumes of research outputs across all disciplines.

12.5   Conclusions

Mental health research and practice face significant, large-scale challenges both within and between disciplines. In a recent opinion article in the Proceedings of the National Academy of Sciences (PNAS) journal [75], the authors argue that philosophy is essential in scientific research, both for the purpose of conceptually clarifying the nature of the entities that are being investigated, and for the increasingly important work of facilitating inter-disciplinary conversations in subjects that cut across historical disciplinary boundaries, exactly as does mental health. As the authors write:

> Modern science without philosophy will run up against a wall: the deluge of data within each field will make interpretation more and more difficult, neglect of breadth and history will further splinter and separate scientific subdisciplines, and the emphasis on methods and empirical results will drive shallower and shallower training of students [75].

In the light of the above discussion on integrative paradigms in mental health and their limitations, this caution seems immediately relevant. But it is not only philosophy that will be needed to advance and integrate across disciplines for mental health: the systematic and large-scale application of *mental health informatics* will also be essential. In order for a meaningful vision of integrative knowledge discovery in mental health to become a reality, a coordinated effort involving funding, consensus building, and a widespread commitment to collaboration across disciplines will be needed.

In particular, over and above the computational approaches to analysis and interpretation that have been reviewed in this chapter, there is a need for systems that are able to store and integrate theory, data and knowledge [76] across all the different relevant entities from each discipline, and for *ontologies* [3, 5] that are able to support and enable the process of semantic integration into a cross-disciplinary, unified, consensus knowledge base.

References

1. Cetina KK, Reichmann W. Epistemic cultures. In: International encyclopedia of the social & behavioral sciences. 2nd ed. Oxford: Elsevier; 2015. https://doi.org/10.1016/B978-0-08-097086-8.10454-4.
2. Lybeck E. Reconstructing the academic profession, On Education. 2018;3(1). https://doi.org/10.17899/on_ed.2018.3.5.
2. Fung LK, Reiss AL. Moving toward integrative, multidimensional research in modern psychiatry: lessons learned from fragile X syndrome. Biological Psychiatry. 2016; https://doi.org/10.1016/j.biopsych.2015.12.015.
3. Hastings J. Mental health ontologies: how we talk about mental health, and why it matters in the digital age. Exeter: University of Exeter Press; 2020.
4. Kapur S, Phillips AG, Insel TR. Why has it taken so long for biological psychiatry to develop clinical tests and what to do about it. Mol Psychiatry. 2012; https://doi.org/10.1038/mp.2012.105.
5. Larsen RR, Hastings J. From affective science to psychiatric disorder: ontology as a semantic bridge. Front Psych. 2018; https://doi.org/10.3389/fpsyt.2018.00487.

6. Callard F, Fitzgerald D. Rethinking interdisciplinarity across the social sciences and neurosciences. Basingstoke: Palgrave Macmillan; 2015. https://doi.org/10.1057/9781137407962.
7. Callard F, Fitzgerald D, Woods A. Interdisciplinary collaboration in action: tracking the signal, tracing the noise. Palgrave Commun. 2015; https://doi.org/10.1057/palcomms.2015.19.
8. Kendler KS. The structure of psychiatric science. Am J Psychiatr. 2014; https://doi.org/10.1176/appi.ajp.2014.13111539.
9. Lilienfeld SO. DSM-5: centripetal scientific and centrifugal antiscientific forces. Clin Psychol Sci Pract. 2014; https://doi.org/10.1111/cpsp.12075.
10. Patel V, Saxena S, Lund C, Thornicroft G, Baingana F, Bolton P, et al. The lancet commission on global mental health and sustainable development. Lancet. 2018; https://doi.org/10.1016/S0140-6736(18)31612-X.
11. American Psychiatric Association. DSM-5 Diagnostic Classification. Diagnostic and Statistical Manual of Mental Disorders. 2013; https://doi.org/10.1176/appi.books.9780890425596.x00diagnosticclassification.
12. World Health Organization (1993) The ICD-10 classification of mental and behavioural disorders: Diagnostic criteria for research. The ICD-10 classification of mental and behavioural disorders: diagnostic criteria for research.
13. Regier DA, Kuhl EA, Kupfer DJ. The DSM-5: classification and criteria changes. World Psychiatry. 2013; https://doi.org/10.1002/wps.20050.
14. Uher R, Payne JL, Pavlova B, Perlis RH. Major depressive disorder in DSM-5: implications for clinical practice and research of changes from DSM-IV. Depress Anxiety. 2014; https://doi.org/10.1002/da.22217.
15. Clark LA, Cuthbert B, Lewis-Fernández R, Narrow WE, Reed GM. Three approaches to understanding and classifying mental disorder: ICD-11, DSM-5, and the National Institute of Mental Health's research domain criteria (RDoC). Psychol Sci Public Interest. 2017; https://doi.org/10.1177/1529100617727266.
16. Surís A, Holliday R, North CS. The evolution of the classification of psychiatric disorders. Behavioral Sciences. 2016; https://doi.org/10.3390/bs6010005.
17. Lilienfeld SO, Smith SF, Watts AL. Diagnosis and classification. In: Encyclopedia of mental health. 2nd ed; 2016. https://doi.org/10.1016/B978-0-12-397045-9.00085-9.
18. Iglewicz A, Seay K, Zetumer SD, Zisook S. The removal of the bereavement exclusion in the DSM-5: exploring the evidence. Curr Psychiatry Rep. 2013; https://doi.org/10.1007/s11920-013-0413-0.
19. Bolton D. Overdiagnosis problems in the DSM-IV and the new DSM-5: can they be resolved by the distress-impairment criterion? Can J Psychiatr. 2013; https://doi.org/10.1177/070674371305801106.
20. Martin J, Taylor MJ, Lichtenstein P. Assessing the evidence for shared genetic risks across psychiatric disorders and traits. Psychol Med. 2018; https://doi.org/10.1017/S0033291717003440.
21. Cuthbert BN, Insel TR. Toward the future of psychiatric diagnosis: the seven pillars of RDoC. BMC Med. 2013; https://doi.org/10.1186/1741-7015-11-126.
22. Insel TR. The nimh research domain criteria (rdoc) project: precision medicine for psychiatry. Am J Psychiatr. 2014; https://doi.org/10.1176/appi.ajp.2014.14020138.
23. Insel TR, Cuthbert B, Garvey M, Heinssen R, Pine D, Quinn K, et al. Research domain criteria (RDoC): toward a. American Journal of Psychiatry Online. 2010; https://doi.org/10.1176/appi.ajp.2010.09091379.
24. Insel TR, Cuthbert BN. Brain disorders? Precisely Science. 2015; https://doi.org/10.1126/science.aab2358.
25. Coghill D, Sonuga-Barke EJS. Annual research review: categories versus dimensions in the classification and conceptualisation of child and adolescent mental disorders – implications of recent empirical study. J Child Psychol Psychiatry Allied Discip. 2012; https://doi.org/10.1111/j.1469-7610.2011.02511.x.
26. Haslam N, Holland E, Kuppens P. Categories versus dimensions in personality and psychopathology: a quantitative review of taxometric research. Psychol Med. 2012; https://doi.org/10.1017/S0033291711001966.

27. Hengartner MP, Lehmann SN. Why psychiatric research must abandon traditional diagnostic classification and adopt a fully dimensional scope: two solutions to a persistent problem. Front Psych. 2017; https://doi.org/10.3389/fpsyt.2017.00101.
28. Carcone D, Ruocco AC. Six years of research on the national institute of mental health's research domain criteria (RDoC) initiative: a systematic review. Front Cell Neurosci. 2017; https://doi.org/10.3389/fncel.2017.00046.
29. Ceusters W, Jensen M, Diehl AD. Ontological realism for the research domain criteria for mental disorders. Stud Health Technol Inform. 2017; https://doi.org/10.3233/978-1-61499-753-5-431.
30. Weinberger DR, Glick ID, Klein DF. Whither research domain criteria (RDoC)? The good, the bad, and the ugly. JAMA Psychiat. 2015; https://doi.org/10.1001/jamapsychiatry.2015.1743.
31. Zoellner LA, Foa EB. Applying research domain criteria (RDoC) to the study of fear and anxiety: a critical comment. Psychophysiology. 2016; https://doi.org/10.1111/psyp.12588.
32. Kotov R, Waszczuk MA, Krueger RF, Forbes MK, Watson D, Clark LA, et al. The hierarchical taxonomy of psychopathology (HiTOP): a dimensional alternative to traditional nosologies. J Abnorm Psychol. 2017; https://doi.org/10.1037/abn0000258.
33. Kotov R, Krueger RF, Watson D. A paradigm shift in psychiatric classification: the hierarchical taxonomy of psychopathology (HiTOP). World Psychiatry. 2018; https://doi.org/10.1002/wps.20478.
34. Meehl PE. Bootstraps taxometrics: solving the classification problem in psychopathology. Am Psychol. 1995; https://doi.org/10.1037/0003-066X.50.4.266.
35. Yong AG, Pearce S. A Beginner's guide to factor analysis: focusing on exploratory factor analysis. Tutor Quant Methods Psychol. 2013; https://doi.org/10.20982/tqmp.09.2.p079.
36. Fried EI. Lack of theory building and testing impedes Progress in the factor and network literature. PsyArXiv (Preprint). 2020; https://doi.org/10.31234/osf.io/zg84s.
37. Hankin BL, Snyder HR, Gulley LD, Schweizer TH, Bijttebier P, Nelis S, et al. Understanding comorbidity among internalizing problems: integrating latent structural models of psychopathology and risk mechanisms. Dev Psychopathol. 2016; https://doi.org/10.1017/S0954579416000663.
38. Jones HJ, Heron J, Hammerton G, Stochl J, Jones PB, Cannon M, et al. Investigating the genetic architecture of general and specific psychopathology in adolescence. Transl Psychiatry. 2018a; https://doi.org/10.1038/s41398-018-0204-9.
39. Bringmann LF, Eronen MI. Don't blame the model: reconsidering the network approach to psychopathology. Psychol Rev. 2018; https://doi.org/10.1037/rev0000108.
40. Borsboom D. A network theory of mental disorders. World Psychiatry. 2017; https://doi.org/10.1002/wps.20375.
41. Goekoop R, Goekoop JG. A network view on psychiatric disorders:network clusters of symptoms as elementary syndromes ofpsychopathology. PLoS One. 2014; https://doi.org/10.1371/journal.pone.0112734.
42. Fried EI. Problematic assumptions have slowed down depression research: why symptoms, not syndromes are the way forward. Front Psychol. 2015; https://doi.org/10.3389/fpsyg.2015.00309.
43. Fried EI, van Borkulo CD, Cramer AOJ, Boschloo L, Schoevers RA, Borsboom D. Mental disorders as networks of problems: a review of recent insights. Soc Psychiatry Psychiatr Epidemiol. 2017; https://doi.org/10.1007/s00127-016-1319-z.
44. van Bork R, van Borkulo CD, Waldorp LJ, Cramer AOJ, Borsboom D. Network models for clinical psychology. In: Stevens' handbook of experimental psychology and cognitive neuroscience. Hoboken, NJ: John Wiley & Sons; 2018. https://doi.org/10.1002/9781119170174.epcn518.
45. Jones PJ, Mair P, McNally RJ. Visualizing psychological networks: a tutorial in R. Front Psychol. 2018b; https://doi.org/10.3389/fpsyg.2018.01742.
46. Epskamp S, Cramer AOJ, Waldorp LJ, Schmittmann VD, Borsboom D. Qgraph: network visualizations of relationships in psychometric data. J Stat Softw. 2012; https://doi.org/10.18637/jss.v048.i04.

47. Cramer AOJ, Waldorp LJ, Van Der Maas HLJ, Borsboom D. Comorbidity: a network perspective. Behav Brain Sci. 2010; https://doi.org/10.1017/S0140525X09991567.
48. Isvoranu AM, Van Borkulo CD, Boyette LL, Wigman JTW, Vinkers CH, Borsboom D, et al. A network approach to psychosis: pathways between childhood trauma and psychotic symptoms. Schizophr Bull. 2017; https://doi.org/10.1093/schbul/sbw055.
49. Padmanabhan JL, Tandon N, Haller CS, Mathew IT, Eack SM, Clementz BA, et al. Correlations between brain structure and symptom dimensions of psychosis in schizophrenia, schizoaffective, and psychotic bipolar i disorders. Schizophr Bull. 2015; https://doi.org/10.1093/schbul/sbu075.
50. Hilland E, Landrø NI, Kraft B, Tamnes CK, Fried EI, Maglanoc LA, Jonassen R. Exploring the links between specific depression symptoms and brain structure: a network study. Psychiatry Clin Neurosci. 2020; https://doi.org/10.1111/pcn.12969.
51. Adams RA, Huys QJM, Roiser JP. Computational psychiatry: towards a mathematically informed understanding of mental illness. J Neurol Neurosurg Psychiatry. 2016; https://doi.org/10.1136/jnnp-2015-310737.
52. Stephan KE, Mathys C. Computational approaches to psychiatry. Curr Opin Neurobiol. 2014; https://doi.org/10.1016/j.conb.2013.12.007.
53. Brodersen KH, Deserno L, Schlagenhauf F, Lin Z, Penny WD, Buhmann JM, Stephan KE. Dissecting psychiatric spectrum disorders by generative embedding. NeuroImage Clinical. 2014; https://doi.org/10.1016/j.nicl.2013.11.002.
54. Brodersen KH, Schofield TM, Leff AP, Ong CS, Lomakina EI, Buhmann JM, Stephan KE. Generative embedding for model-based classification of FMRI data. PLoS Comput Biol. 2011; https://doi.org/10.1371/journal.pcbi.1002079.
55. Corlett PR, Fletcher PC. Computational psychiatry: a Rosetta stone linking the brain to mental illness. Lancet Psychiatry. 2014; https://doi.org/10.1016/S2215-0366(14)70298-6.
56. Friston K. The free-energy principle: a rough guide to the brain? Trends Cogn Sci. 2009; https://doi.org/10.1016/j.tics.2009.04.005.
57. Stephan KE, Schlagenhauf F, Huys QJM, Raman S, Aponte EA, Brodersen KH, et al. Computational neuroimaging strategies for single patient predictions. NeuroImage. 2017; https://doi.org/10.1016/j.neuroimage.2016.06.038.
58. Wright AGC. The current state and future of factor analysis in personality disorder research. Pers Disord: Theory Res Treat. 2017; https://doi.org/10.1037/per0000216.
59. Bringmann LF, Vissers N, Wichers M, Geschwind N, Kuppens P, Peeters F, et al. A network approach to psychopathology: new insights into clinical longitudinal data. PLoS ONE. 2013; https://doi.org/10.1371/journal.pone.0060188.
60. Kramer I, Simons CJP, Hartmann JA, Menne-Lothmann C, Viechtbauer W, Peeters F, et al. A therapeutic application of the experience sampling method in the treatment of depression: a randomized controlled trial. World Psychiatry. 2014; https://doi.org/10.1002/wps.20090.
61. Muthén BO. Multilevel covariance structure analysis. Sociol Methods Res. 1994; https://doi.org/10.1177/0049124194022003006.
62. Hamaker EL, Asparouhov T, Brose A, Schmiedek F, Muthén B. At the frontiers of modeling intensive longitudinal data: dynamic structural equation models for the affective measurements from the COGITO study. Multivariate Behav Res. 2018; https://doi.org/10.1080/00273171.2018.1446819.
63. Smith B, Ceusters W. Ontological realism: a methodology for coordinated evolution of scientific ontologies. Appl Ontol. 2010; https://doi.org/10.3233/AO-2010-0079.
64. Bluhm R. The need for new ontologies in psychiatry. Philos Explor. 2017; https://doi.org/10.1080/13869795.2017.1312498.
65. Sullivan JA. Coordinated pluralism as a means to facilitate integrative taxonomies of cognition. Philos Explor. 2017; https://doi.org/10.1080/13869795.2017.1312497.
66. Yarkoni T. The generalizability crisis. PsyArXiv (Preprint). 2019; https://doi.org/10.31234/osf.io/jqw35.

67. Francken JC, Slors M. Neuroscience and everyday life: facing the translation problem. Brain Cogn. 2018; https://doi.org/10.1016/j.bandc.2017.09.004.
68. Lilienfeld SO, Sauvigné KC, Lynn SJ, Cautin RL, Latzman RD, Waldman ID. Fifty psychological and psychiatric terms to avoid: a list of inaccurate, misleading, misused, ambiguous, and logically confused words and phrases. Front Psychol. 2015; https://doi.org/10.3389/fpsyg.2015.01100.
69. Newson JJ, Hunter D, Thiagarajan TC. The heterogeneity of mental health assessment. Front Psych. 2020; https://doi.org/10.3389/fpsyt.2020.00076.
70. Barahona-Corrêa JB, Filipe CN. A concise history of asperger syndrome: the short reign of a troublesome diagnosis. Front Psychol. 2016; https://doi.org/10.3389/fpsyg.2015.02024.
71. Wang Q, Timberlake MA, Prall K, Dwivedi Y. The recent progress in animal models of depression. Prog Neuro-Psychopharmacol Biol Psychiatry. 2017; https://doi.org/10.1016/j.pnpbp.2017.04.008.
72. Guidi J, Brakemeier EL, Bockting CLH, Cosci F, Cuijpers P, Jarrett RB, et al. Methodological recommendations for trials of psychological interventions. Psychother Psychosom. 2018; https://doi.org/10.1159/000490574.
73. Liu Y, Pencheon E, Hunter RM, Moncrieff J, Freemantle N. Recruitment and retention strategies in mental health trials – a systematic review. PLoS One. 2018; https://doi.org/10.1371/journal.pone.0203127.
74. Siedlecka E, Denson TF. Experimental methods for inducing basic emotions: a qualitative review. Emotion Rev. 2019; https://doi.org/10.1177/1754073917749016.
75. Laplane L, Mantovani P, Adolphs R, Chang H, Mantovani A, McFall-Ngai M, et al. Why science needs philosophy. Proc Natl Acad Sci U S A. 2019; https://doi.org/10.1073/pnas.1900357116.
76. Hastings J, Michie S, Johnston M. Theory and ontology in behavioural science. Nat Hum Behav. 2020; https://doi.org/10.1038/s41562-020-0826-9.

Chapter 13
Natural Language Processing in Mental Health Research and Practice

Sam Henry, Meliha Yetisgen, and Ozlem Uzuner

Abstract Information relevant to mental health is commonly recorded as unstructured narrative text. This text may be part of a clinical record, a social media post, a diary, or a transcribed conversation between two or more people. Although the quantity and richness of this unstructured narrative text is vast, it is inaccessible to traditional computer systems which rely on structured data. Natural language processing (NLP) is a technology that solves the problem of making this information accessible to computer systems. NLP is a technology for converting unstructured narrative texts into a format that is more easily accessible to computerized systems. NLP is also a scientific field—the field concerned with developing and applying methods for making unstructured narrative texts computable. NLP is a field in computer science that combines artificial intelligence, statistics, and linguistics to process unstructured text and make it more easily accessible by computerized systems. In this chapter, we provide an overview of NLP within the mental health domain. We discuss different data sources, including electronic health records and social media text, and describe how to collect, process, and analyze these texts for mental health research and practice. Finally, we provide an overview of applications, challenges, limitations, and ethical considerations.

S. Henry (✉)
Christopher Newport University, Newport News, VA, USA
e-mail: samuel.henry@cnu.edu

M. Yetisgen
University of Washington, Seattle, WA, USA
e-mail: melihay@uw.edu

O. Uzuner
George Mason University, Fairfax, VA, USA

Harvard Medical School, Boston, MA, USA

Massachusetts Institute of Technology, Cambridge, MA, USA
e-mail: ouzuner@gmu.edu

© Springer Nature Switzerland AG 2021
J. D. Tenenbaum, P. A. Ranallo (eds.), *Mental Health Informatics*, Health Informatics, https://doi.org/10.1007/978-3-030-70558-9_13

Keywords Natural language processing · Text mining · Mental health · Psychiatry Applications

13.1 Introduction

Mental health related information is commonly recorded as unstructured narrative text. This text may be part of clinical records, social media posts, or transcribed conversations between a person seeking mental healthcare and the healthcare professional. Although the quantity and richness of this unstructured narrative text is vast, it is inaccessible to traditional computer systems which rely on structured data. The goal of NLP is to allow secondary analysis of this unstructured text by converting it into a format that is accessible to computer systems. This is a difficult task, and as such NLP combines methods from computer science, artificial intelligence, statistics, and linguistics [1]. In this chapter, we provide an overview of NLP concepts and approaches with an emphasis on its application to mental health. For a literature review on NLP for mental health up to the year 2013, we refer the reader to Abbe et al. [1], and for a scoping review up to the year 2015 focused on mental health and non-clinical texts to Calvo et al. [2].

NLP aims to convert unstructured narrative texts into a format that is more easily accessible to computerized systems. As noted in previous chapters, mental health related information is commonly recorded as unstructured narrative text. This text may be part of clinical records, social media posts, or transcribed conversations between a caregiver and patient. Although the quantity and richness of this unstructured narrative text is vast, it is inaccessible to traditional computer systems which rely on structured data. The goal of NLP is to allow secondary analysis of this unstructured text by converting it into a format that is accessible to computer systems. This is a difficult task, and as such NLP combines methods from computer science, artificial intelligence, statistics, and linguistics [1].

A typical NLP workflow (see Fig. 13.1) starts with gathering the unstructured text of interest, and processes this text to create what is called a *corpus*. This corpus is then processed to generate a *data representation* for analysis. These representations vary, and often include modified versions of the original text and various tags within the context of the text. The resulting representations are then combined either with heuristic rules or machine learning methods to understand the context of the information and to create a structured representation that captures the "meaning" of text.

In this chapter, we provide an overview of methods for corpus generation and data processing, present example NLP applications, and discuss the limitations and ethical considerations of NLP for mental health.

NLP methods vary depending on the requirements of the application. Table 13.1 summarizes some common NLP tasks. These tasks are commonly "pipelined" into a single larger NLP application. Applications often have a workflow similar to that shown in Fig. 13.1. First unstructured text data is collected, de-identified (if necessary), and manually annotated. Annotation allows for performance to be evaluated,

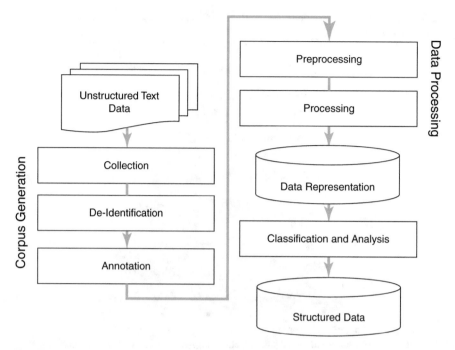

Fig. 13.1 Natural language processing converts unstructured text data into structured data which can be used by computer systems

Table 13.1 Common NLP Tasks

Information Retrieval	Collecting relevant documents or text snippets
Named entity recognition	Identifying entities of interest in text. E.g., *Patient Name, Symptom, Diagnosis*
De-identification	Identifying and disguising personally identifiable information
Relation extraction	Finding and labelling relations between entities in text. E.g., *<Drug > treats < Disease>*
Text classification	Adding a label to a document or text segment
Ontology construction	Analyzing language use to create a dictionary or hierarchy of terms
Natural language generation	Creating narrative text from structured information

and for supervised machine learning algorithms to be used. Next the data is cleansed in the preprocessing step and processed to generate representations for analysis. Processing may consist of one or more of the NLP tasks show in Table 13.1. This may include *named entity recognition* followed by *relation extraction* or *ontology construction*. The level of processing determines the granularity of the generated data representations.

These representations (shown in Table 13.2) capture information at increasing levels of understanding and may include sequences of letters or words, sentence

Table 13.2 Data Representations for NLP May Capture Information at Various Levels of Granularity, Including

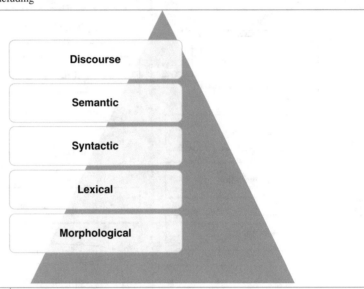

Morphological	Captures sub-word meaning, such as prefixes and suffixes
Lexical	Captures individual words (called *unigrams*), pairs of words (called *bi-grams*) or sequences of n words (referred to as *n-grams*)
Syntactic	Syntactic information captures how words are structured within a sentence or phrase, such as *part of speech (POS) tags* indicating whether a word is a noun, verb, adjective, etc.
Semantic	Captures the meaning of a word, such as whether it refers to a person's name, a location, a disease, etc.
Discourse	Captures information about how sentences, paragraphs, or documents are structured, such as document sections or document types

structure, word meaning or document structure. The granularity of the data representation is determined by the needs of the application and therefore the needs of the classification and analysis step. The generated data representations are combined and input into the classification and analysis step. This step uses heuristic rules, machine learning, or statistical analysis to create a structured representation that captures the "meaning" of text. This text meaning is converted into a structured form and constitutes the final output of the system.

13.2   Corpus Generation

The first step in the NLP process is to collect a corpus of documents. Different sources provide potentially different and complementary information. For mental health studies, there are two primary sources of narratives: Medical Records that

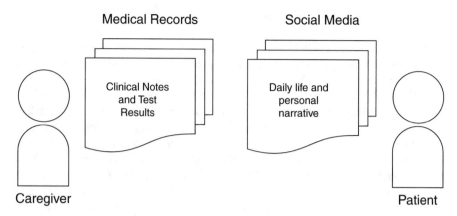

Fig. 13.2 Mental health contexts, users, and the information they capture. Medical records are relevant in terms of what others report about the patient. Social media content is relevant in terms of what the patient reveals about himself/herself

Table 13.3 Corpus Generation Tasks

Step	Tasks
Collection	Acquire a set of representative samples of narrative
De-identification	Remove all personally identifying information
Annotation	Manually generate a gold standard for desired outcome

capture the details of patient status and disease progress from the perspective of caregivers, and Social Media posts that captures the patient's perspective as a personal narrative which offers insights into the patient's daily life (Fig. 13.2). There are other data sources, but these are less commonly used. We highlight a few in the Other Data Sources section below.

No matter the data source, corpus generation requires the same three steps (Table 13.3). The implementation of these steps varies depending on the data sources, and in this section, we discuss these steps for medical records and social media content within the mental health domain.

13.2.1 Using Medical Records as a Corpus

Medical records are created as a result of interactions between a person and the health professionals from whom they seek care. They capture key observations about a person's health, summarize problems, interventions, goals, and care plans, and enable health professionals to make decisions based on a more complete information about health history. An estimated 80% of the information contained in a clinical record is stored as unstructured narrative text [4].

13.2.1.1 Collecting Medical Records

The first step of corpus generation is to draw a sample of records. Samples are often drawn from large hospital repositories. Examples include using diagnosis codes that may correlate with the health problem in focus [5–8]. Studies have shown, however, that diagnosis codes often fall short of representing the contents of the medical records [9], and only a small percentage of the health problems are actually coded. For example, Anderson et al. [9] reported that only 3% of cases with suicidal ideation mentions were coded for it. Therefore, when using diagnosis codes to draw data, the selected codes should capture a superset of the problem in focus, e.g., draw from a population that is known to be prone to the problem such as autism spectrum disorder diagnosis for studying suicidal ideation. Keywords are also commonly used to draw data, but similar care should be taken to avoid biased datasets. The section on Lexicon and Ontology Construction provides more information on how to develop an effective set of keywords. In some cases [10, 11] additional records are retrieved via *active learning,* an interactive machine learning technique (see Chap. 10) in which an annotated dataset is iteratively built via automatic identification of salient samples, additional human annotation, and model refinement. Table 13.4 summarizes some examples of medical record collection process.

13.2.1.2 De-Identification of Medical Records

After samples are collected, they must often be de-identified. Medical records are private information, protected by the Health Insurance Portability and Accountability Act (HIPAA) which dictates that their use for research requires either consent from

Table 13.4 A few characteristic examples and techniques for the medical record collection process

References	Data Repository	Retrieval Method	Notes
Gorrell et al. [10]	South London and Maudsley NHS trust (SLaM) [3]	Keyword matching	Retrieved additional samples via active learning
Jackson et al. [11]	Clinical record interactive search (CRIS) [12]	Keyword matching and manual review	Retrieved additional samples via active learning
Jackson et al. [13]	Clinical record interactive search (CRIS) [12]	ICD codes	–
Perlis et al. [14]	Partners HealthCare EHR data	ICD codes	Used i2b2 workbench software [15] for retrieval
Barak et al. [16]	Partners HealthCare EHR data	ICD codes of patients with 3+ visits	Data supplemented with death certificates
Rumshisky et al. [7]	Partners HealthCare EHR data	Patient diagnosis	–
Adekkanattu et al. [17]	Weill Cornell medicine EHR data	Prescription information	–

the patient or de-identification of the records through the removal of 18 categories of private health information [18]. De-identification can be manual [19], semi-automatic, or fully automatic [20]. The level of de-identification performance acceptable to different institutional review boards, and the intended recipient of the de-identified data (e.g., in-house use vs. distribution for research purposes) plays a role in decisions related to de-identification. For example, in-house use may require removal of all names, ID numbers, and locations. Whereas publicly released data may be stricter and may require the removal of both directly identifying information and indirectly identifying information (e.g., "the governor's wife").

13.2.1.3   Annotation of Medical Records

Following de-identification the corpora are annotated to create a gold standard [19]. This gold standard contains ground truth information necessary for creating, training, and evaluating for the desired task. The goal of the task defines what the gold standard annotations are. For example, a drug-name detection system will require all drug names in text to be manually annotated. An automatic diagnosis system will require document-level annotation of what the final diagnoses were, and possibly where in text the diagnosis is mentioned. Some studies use structured information such as diagnosis codes or information from the psychiatric review section [21] as gold standard annotations at the document level. However, document level annotations are not granular enough for all tasks, and health problems may be mentioned but not coded. Therefore, annotation of the narrative contents of a document is often necessary.

Annotating text often requires annotators with expertise in the problem under study [22–24]. Most studies use at least two annotators each of whom make independent passes over the data and a third annotator who serves as an arbitrator resolving disagreements. Quality of the annotated data and the reliability of the annotations are measured using metrics such as Cohen's Kappa [22, 23], which measures inter-annotator agreement, or F-measure [24] which quantifies an annotator's performance. See Figure 13.3 for an example of annotated text.

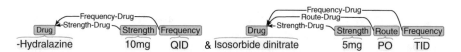

Fig. 13.3 Annotated text consists of the original or modified text and additional information. In this example, a medical record has been annotated with drug, strength, frequency, and route information

13.2.1.4 Publicly Available Medical Record Datasets

While all medical records are private, content related to mental health is considered extra-sensitive and is often treated with additional care [20]. As a result, to the best of our knowledge, the RDoC dataset [24] is the only publicly available dataset of clinical records for NLP mental health research. The RDoC dataset [24] was produced by the Centers of Excellence in Genomic Science (CEGS) Neuropsychiatric Genome-Scale and RDoC Individualized Domains (N-GRID) as part of the Research Domains Criteria (RDoC) project. It contains psychiatric intake records and interview-format yes/no questions and answers designed to evaluate the patient's mental health. These records have been de-identified and released to the research community with gold standard annotations for studies of de-identification and symptom severity prediction for positive valence disorders. The dataset was featured in the CEGS N-GRID shared tasks [5] resulting in many innovative solutions [21, 25–30].

13.2.2 Generating a Corpus from Social Media Data

Social media refers to web-enabled platforms that allow users to access and generate content and to form networks [31]. Individual instances of communications shared, i.e., posted, on social media are called *postings*. Postings that respond to each other are called *threads*. Example social media sites that have been used in mental health research include Reddit [32–39], Twitter [39–46], Facebook [39, 47], TrevorSpace [48], Tumblr [49], LiveJournal [50, 51], Weibo [52], and Mixi [53]. The content and networks captured in social media represent a wealth of health information voluntarily shared by users. This information is from the perspective of the users and provides a complementary perspective to information presented in medical records.

13.2.2.1 Collecting and Annotating Social Media Data

Collecting social media data requires identifying and downloading postings of interest. Most social media platforms provide an application programming interface (API) that allows efficient browsing and retrieval of the data they host[1,2,3] Postings of interest can be identified using surveys or through direct collection.

---

[1] https://developer.twitter.com

[2] http://www.reddit.com/dev/api

[3] https://www.tumblr.com › docs › api

Surveys created by the researcher identify a patient's mental health status (e.g., whether the patient is depressed or not) by directly asking them questions and requesting them to disclose their social media data to the researchers [39, 47, 54]. Surveys allows an assessment of specific constructs of the mental health status of the patients. However, these studies are typically limited in the amount of data used, and have several biases including selection and collection biases, and user's cognitive bias which may prevent participants from giving truthful responses to survey questions [45].

To overcome the limitation on data size, but not necessarily data bias, information may be directly collected from social media without surveys. Methods for direct collection often rely on self-reported diagnoses [45, 55–57] or via self-declared medication intake [44, 58]. These assertions can be found using rule-based or machine learning *classifiers* (an algorithm that assigns labels to data), or assuming that participation in mental health forums indicates a mental health problem. For example, Reddit organizes topics into subreddits that are specialized forums which may relate to mental health concerns such as suicide, addiction, and specific mental health conditions. These subreddits may be identified by keyword searches and manual classification [34]. Finally, where automatic retrieval with queries of social media text fall short, manually annotated text (individual posts, tweets, or text segments that are manually labeled as relevant to the study) can serve as examples of linguistic cues for the health problem. The manually annotated data can also serve as training data for a classifier that can automatically collect more samples [40, 59]. For example, Paul and Dredze [60] labeled 5128 tweets to train a classifier which then automatically collected more tweets by predicting if they were health related or not.

13.2.2.2   Privacy with Social Media Data

Expectations of privacy vary by social media platform. For example, Reddit is anonymous while Twitter is not. As a result, the information shared on the different social media platforms may vary both in its nature and in its detail. Some users may be more comfortable sharing mental health problems anonymously [61] while others feel comfortable volunteering their postings for research [54, 62] and even self-report their diagnoses [55–57]. As a result, data from social media has reduced privacy concerns relative to EHRs. However, it may still be appropriate to remove directly identifying information such as usernames. Ethical considerations are covered in more detail at the end of this chapter and in Chap. 18 of this text.

13.2.3   Other Data Sources

While EHRs and social media serve as the primary data sources for NLP in mental health, other data sources have been used. Althoff et al. [63] analyze text message conversations to discover the effectiveness of counseling strategies. Maenner et al.

[64] use the "The Autism and Developmental Disabilities Monitoring" network database, which contains children's developmental evaluations to classify autism spectrum disorder based on the language used in these assessments. Pestian et al. [65, 66] use a dataset of suicide notes to detect forgeries and identify word sentiment.

Finding novel data sources for NLP in mental health remains an open research direction. Some potential sources include, patient homework or diaries, legal records, patient emails, educational or social services records, therapy transcripts, and more. Additionally, combining multiple data sources and linking them to a single patient may be a promising research direction. For example, Thompson et al. [67] link Facebook posts to clinical records to predict suicide risk in veterans.

13.3   Data Processing

Once a corpus has been generated, the text in it can be processed and information can be extracted. This is the data processing step, and within it, tasks are accomplished by creating NLP pipelines. At a high level, a typical NLP pipeline includes preprocessing, featurization, analysis, and evaluation (see Table 13.5).

Figure 13.4 shows an example document classification pipeline in which raw text data is preprocessed, featurized, and classified to produce a yes or no decision. In the example preprocessing step, raw text is input into a series of steps that include: *stop word removal, lemmatization, part of speech (POS) tagging, dependency parsing*, and *negation detection*. The example featurization step includes creating a document embedding (e.g., the average of all *word embeddings*—vector representations of words—in the document), counting negated and non-negated keywords, and finding the average sentiment of all words in the document (e.g., to determine how positive or negative the tone of the document is). Lastly, this featurized document is input into a classifier (e.g., a support vector machine) which classifies the document with a yes or no decision

In this section, we describe each of these data processing steps in more detail. Since many NLP systems use similar components, it is common to use reusable NLP tools. These tools are often open-source and can be downloaded directly from the developers, or via code-sharing services such as GitHub.[4] Platforms such as

Table 13.5 Data processing steps of NLP pipeline

Step	Activities
Preprocessing	Cleaning, filtering, and normalizing data
Featurization	Transforming data into features which serve as an input representation for computational methods
Analysis	Identifying patterns in the data to draw conclusions; types of analysis include classification, regression, clustering, or statistical analysis
Evaluation	Quantifying the performance of a system for a specific task

---

[4] https://github.com/

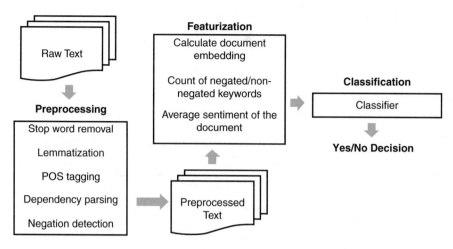

Fig. 13.4 An example document classification pipeline

Unstructured Information Management Architecture (UIMA) [68], or the Leo natural language processing platform [69] (which is based on UIMA) may be utilized to facilitate the integration of these re-usable components. These platforms provide a common framework to "plug-in" or re-use code and already-developed analysis components. As an example, Adekkanattu et al. [17] extend Leo for their system to extract PHQ-9 scores from clinical notes.

13.3.1 Preprocessing

Natural language is inherently noisy and difficult for machines to interpret. Preprocessing cleans, filters, and normalizes narratives to make downstream NLP tasks easier and more accurate. Common preprocessing tasks start with simple *lexical processing* tasks (i.e., processing of individual terms), followed by *syntactic processing* tasks (i.e., processing based on sentence structure), and end with more complex *semantic processing tasks* (i.e., meaning-based processing) (Table 13.6). Lexical processing typically begins with *stop word removal*—the removal of words that convey little information (e.g., "the", "a") or provide little information for a specific domain (e.g., "patient" in the context of mental health). Next, *stemming and lemmatization* map words to their root form (e.g., map "running" to "run"). Stemming is typically a heuristic-based method, where common affixes are removed (e.g., remove "-ing" from running). Lemmatization is a more complex and accurate normalization method, which is capable of normalizing more complex word forms. For example, stemming cannot normalize "*ran*" to its root form "*run*", but lemmatization can. Finally, multi-word terms are identified. Not all terms are expressed as a single word, but are instead multi-word terms (e.g., "borderline personality disorder" is a single term consisting of three words). *Multi-word term identification* is the

Table 13.6 Overview of the preprocessing tasks and tools discussed

Data representation	Overview of preprocessing	
	Task	Tool(s)
Lexical	Stop word removal	Natural language toolkit (NLTK)[a,b]
	Stemming, lemmatization	Natural language toolkit (NLTK)
	Multi-word term identification	word2vec::Interface package,[c] wordNet::Tools,[d] or Gensim[e]
Syntactic	POS tagging	Natural language toolkit (NLTK), Stanford CoreNLP processing toolkit [70, 71][f,g]
	Dependency parsing	Natural language toolkit (NLTK), Stanford CoreNLP processing toolkit [70, 72].[h]
	Negation detection	NegEx [73]
Semantic	Word sense disambiguation	–
	Concept mapping	Metamap [74]

[a]http://www.nltk.org/
[b]https://raw.githubusercontent.com/nltk/nltk_data/gh-pages/packages/corpora/stopwords.zip
[c]https://sourceforge.net/projects/word2vec-interface/
[d]https://metacpan.org/pod/WordNet::Tools
[e]https://radimrehurek.com/gensim/index.html
[f]https://stanfordnlp.github.io/CoreNLP/index.html
[g]https://nlp.stanford.edu/software/tagger.html
[h]https://nlp.stanford.edu/software/lex-parser.html

Table 13.7 Preprocessing tasks

Term	Description
Stop word removal	Removal of words that convey little information, e.g., "the", "a"
Stemming and lemmatization	Mapping words to their root form, e.g., "running" to "run"
Multi-word term identification	Identification of multi-word terms, e.g., "borderline personality disorder"
Part of speech (POS) tagging	Tagging words with their part of speech, i.e., noun, verb, adjective
Dependency parsing	Identifying the syntactic relationships between terms in a sentence (e.g., "compassionate" modifies the patient).
Negation detection	Identifying which terms or phrases are negated, e.g., "not feeling suicidal"
Word sense disambiguation (WSD)	Identifying the meaning of ambiguous terms, e.g., "patient" as a personality trait, not a person receiving treatment; and resolving acronyms, e.g., "serious mental illness" abbreviated as "SMI"

identification of multi-word terms. This is often performed by matching n-grams to terms in a dictionary, or by using statistical analysis to detect n-grams that occur much more frequently than would be expected by chance.

Syntactic processing tasks (Table 13.7) include *POS tagging, dependency parsing, and negation detection.* POS (part of speech) tagging is the task of

Preprocessing Example

1) The patient displayed symptoms of borderline personality disorder and was diagnosed with BPD

2) ~~The~~ patient displayed symptoms ~~of~~ borderline personality disorder ~~and was~~ diagnosed ~~with~~ BPD

3) ~~The patient~~ displayed symptoms ~~of~~ borderline personality disorder ~~and was~~ diagnosed ~~with~~ BPD

4) ~~The patient~~ displayed symptoms ~~of~~ borderline personality disorder ~~and was~~ diagnosed ~~with~~ BPD

5) ~~The patient~~ displayed symptoms ~~of~~ borderline personality disorder ~~and was~~ diagnosed ~~with~~ BPD

6) ~~The patient~~ displayed symptoms ~~of~~ borderline personality disorder ~~and was~~ diagnosed with BPD
                                 C0006012   C0006012

7)   display symptom C0006012 diagnos C0006012

Fig. 13.5 An example of how data is transformed in preprocessing. Line (1) shows the original sentence, (2) after stop word removal, (3) after domain specific stop words removal, (4) after stemming, (5) after multi-word terms identified, (6) after concept mapping, and (7) the final preprocessed text. This cleaner and simplified text may make downstream tasks more effective

tagging words with their part of speech. Knowing the part of speech (e.g., noun, verb, etc.) of terms is necessary for downstream tasks such as dependency parsing, negation detection, and word sense disambiguation, and also provides syntactic information used for featurization. Dependency parsing identifies the syntactic relationships between terms in a sentence (e.g., this noun is modified by that adjective). *Negation Detection* identities which terms or phrases are negated (e.g., "not depressed").

Semantic processing tasks include *word sense disambiguation* (WSD) and *concept mapping*, also referred to as *normalization*. Word sense disambiguation (WSD) identifies the meaning of ambiguous terms (e.g., "patient" as in "patience" versus "a person receiving medical treatment") or acronym resolution (e.g., "serious mental illness" abbreviated as "SMI"). Concept mapping, or normalization, maps synonymous terms to a single concept (e.g., "mental well-being" and "psychological health" to the same concept, "Mental Health") (Fig. 13.5).

13.3.2   Featurization

Featurization consists of converting text into a set of features. Features vary, and in the next sections we describe categories of features. Examples include *vector representations* of terms, *part of speech tag* counts, or the overall *sentiment* of language use. The process of developing a set of discriminative features is called *feature engineering*. It is a difficult, and often iterative task generally requiring domain expertise, and it is often the key to success or failure of the final application. Featurization may consist solely of creating *sentence or document vectors or embeddings*, but frequently, these vector representations are combined with other features.

13.3.2.1 Term Vectors

For many NLP applications, words and terms are represented as vectors. The simplest vector representation maps terms to *one-hot (binary) vectors*. These vectors consist of all zeros except for a single unique value of one, which indicates which term the vector represents. An example of this is shown in Fig. 13.6. In it, the vocabulary contains the terms "Cat", "Dog", "Fish", "Tree", "House", "Home", and so on. The vector of each word is shown as a row in the matrix. For one-hot vectors, the vectors are the size of the vocabulary, and contain a single value of one, at the index indicating the word. All other values are zero. One-hot vectors are very high dimensional (contain many elements) and create a sparse data-space (contains mostly zeros) which may not be ideal.

An alternative to one-hot vectors are *word embeddings*. Word embeddings are lower dimensional (contain few elements) vectors containing numeric values. Word embeddings are typically created by training a machine learning algorithm over a large corpus. These algorithms attempt to predict a word given its context (the surrounding words) or the context given a word. After training, the values in the internal layer of the neural network are used as word embeddings. Popular algorithms to generate word embeddings are *word2vec* [75] and *GLoVe* [76]. These algorithms exploit the observation that similar terms tend to have similar contexts, and their generated embeddings capture the meaning of terms. For example, in Fig. 13.6 the embeddings for terms "Cat", "Dog", "Fish", "Tree", "House", and "Home" are shown. Each embedding has a dimensionality of 5, meaning it contains 5 values. "Cat", "Dog", and "Fish" all have similar values in the first dimension, implying that the dimension is encoding information about how these are all animals. Similarly, House and Home contain similar values for dimension 5.

One-Hot Vectors

	Cat	Dog	Fish	Tree	...	House	Home
Cat	1	0	0	0	...	0	0
Dog	0	1	0	0	...	0	0
Fish	0	0	1	0	...	0	0
Tree	0	0	0	1	...	0	0
⋮	...	...	...	...	...	...	...
House	0	0	0	0	...	1	0
Home	0	0	0	0	...	0	1

Word Embeddings

	dim 1	dim 2	dim 3	dim 4	dim 5
Cat	0.5	0.4	0	0.1	0
Dog	0.6	0.3	0.1	0	0
Fish	0.4	0.1	0	0.5	0
Tree	0.2	0	0.7	0.1	0
⋮	...	...	...	...	...
House	0	0	0	0.2	0.8
Home	0.1	0	0.1	0.1	0.7

Fig. 13.6 Term vectorization methods

Because word embeddings are created by iterating over a large corpus, they are sensitive to the domain in which they are trained. In practice, this means that the encoded meaning of words will be different when trained on clinical text versus general English text. Pre-trained word embeddings generated from general English[5] and biomedical [77][6] domains are available, however word embeddings may also be easily created on data for a specific application. As examples, Tran et al. [21] used pre-trained word2vec vectors from PubMed,[7] Shen et al. [35] trained word2vec embeddings on Reddit data, and Jackson et al. [13] created word2vec vectors of unigrams and frequently occurring bigrams and trigrams of EHR data using Gensim.

More recently, *contextualized word embeddings*, such as those created by the algorithms *BERT* [78] and *ELMo* [79] have become popular. Rather than create static vector representations for all words in a corpus, contextualized word embeddings create vector representations for each instance of a word in text. Since word meaning can change based on its surrounding context, these algorithms incorporate both the meaning of the word and its surrounding context into the contextualized word embedding. Unlike word embeddings, pre-trained vector dictionaries are not possible for contextualized word embeddings. Instead, pre-trained models which generate embeddings on the fly are used. These models are most often trained on huge corpora and fine-tuned for application-specific data.

13.3.2.2 Sentence and Document Vectors

Just as terms may be represented as vectors, so can collections of terms such as sentences, social media posts, and documents. The simplest method of creating such vectors is to combine the individual term or component vectors. In the case of one-hot term representations, the term vectors may be combined using an OR operation to create a *binary vector* containing ones and zeros, where each value of one indicates the presence of the term specified by that index. Similarly, *bag of words* (BoW) vectors are commonly created by summing term vectors to create a vector of integer values, where each value indicates the count of terms specified by that index. Since some terms may occur frequently across all documents, they may be less informative, so instead of using the count of terms at each index, the *Term-Frequency Inverse Document Frequency (TF-IDF)* of each term may be calculated. *TF-IDF vectors* compute the value of a term's index as the number of times it occurs in that document divided by the number of times it occurs in all documents. When using word embeddings, sentence and document vectors are frequently built using either the sum or the average of the text's constituent term vectors.

---

[5] https://code.google.com/archive/p/word2vec/

[6] http://bio.nlplab.org/

[7] https://www.ncbi.nlm.nih.gov/pubmed/

13.3.2.3   Count-Based Features

Count-based features indicate the presence, absence, or frequency of some characteristic feature. This may be n-grams, keywords, POS tags, or even social media posts indicating a symptomatic outcome [44], the distribution of word usage [44], or the presence of definite articles and frequency of pronouns [34].

13.3.2.4   Rule-Based Features

Rule-based features incorporate human knowledge about the structure of language to elicit more detailed information. Examples are presence, absence, or exclusion rules within a context window [17], the presence of a verb before a noun [34], or if a term is negated or not [11]. Negation detection often uses rules; however, it can be more complex than checking for terms such as "no" or "not". Complex relations that negate words can cross sentence boundaries, and elements of language such as sarcasm can be hard to detect.

13.3.2.5   Sentiment and Psycholinguistic Features

Sentiment and psycholinguistic features can indicate the attitudes, opinions, and emotional or psychological state of the author. Examples include linguistic cues of social media posts [35, 44] and sentiment of a post [34]. These can be particularly important features for indicating the author's mental state. Sentiment features generally come from pre-existing sentiment dictionaries. These dictionaries typically contain a single sentiment value for each word, and do not take context, or the demographics of the writer into account. It is also possible to learn sentiment or fine-tune the sentiment of these dictionaries from annotated text. For example, Yazdavar et al. [46] include sentiment from users' profile description and linguistic clues from posts, integrated with information from posted images and profile pictures to indicate sentiment and predict depressed users. Mitchell et al. [56] develop linguistic markers of schizophrenia. Although not specifically focused on mental health, SemEval has hosted shared tasks focused on sentiment analysis of Twitter data for several years [80–82].

A variety of general English sentiment analysis tools exist, such as: Sentiwordnet [83] which contains the sentiment of words organized in a taxonomy; Affective Norm for English Words (ANEW) [84] vocabulary which holds a list of words and their sentiment tailored to micro-blogs; and, Linguistic Inquiry and Word Count Lexicon (LIWC) [85, 86][8] dictionary developed for psycholinguistic analysis of texts, which categorizes terms into one or more of several categories. LIWC has been widely used [42, 44, 46, 56, 87] for psycholinguistic analysis of language within the mental health domain.

---

[8] http://liwc.wpengine.com/

13.3.2.6   Sociability Features

Sociability features are used to estimate information about a user's online social life. Examples include the count of tweets, the number of followers, duration on the social media platform, frequency of posting [44], or user's ego-network and user engagement estimated by "@ replies" on Twitter [46].

13.3.2.7   Temporal Features

Temporal features are used to order sequential events. Temporal features are highly relevant for mental illness. As one example, "longer durations of untreated psychosis are associated with worse intervention outcomes" [88]. Additionally, mental health diagnoses often require monitoring the presence of symptoms over time [45]. There are relatively few examples using temporal features within the mental health domain. One notable example from Yazdavar et al. [45] monitors the presence of PHQ-9 symptoms of users' tweets over time. Another notable example from Saha et al. [44] monitors psychological states before and after drug treatments to estimate their effectiveness.

13.3.3   Analyzing Natural Language Data

Following featurization, data are analyzed to extract meaning. This step varies depending on the goals of the application, and it can involve either extraction of specific information from a narrative or the classification and grouping of narratives to support the end application. Analysis methods can be divided into the three broad groups: Rule-based systems, supervised machine learning systems, and unsupervised machine learning (Table 13.8).

Table 13.8 Methods for analyzing natural language data

Term	Description
Rule-based systems	Rule based systems consisting of a series of rules manually created by domain-experts
Supervised machine learning	Automatically learn from the data; learn to label data using manually annotated examples
Deep learning	A kind of supervised learning that uses multi-layer (deep) neural networks.
Unsupervised machine learning	Automatically learns patterns in data without annotation

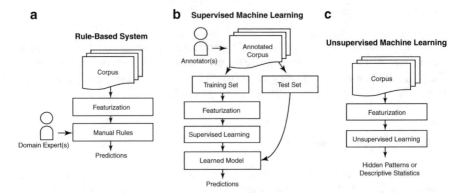

Fig. 13.7 Data analysis may consist of rule-based systems, supervised learning, or unsupervised learning

13.3.3.1 Rule-Based Systems

In rule-based systems (Fig. 13.7a), a domain expert creates a series of manually created rules. A corpus is featurized to accommodate these rules, the rules are applied, and predictions are made. Rule-based systems distinguish themselves from machine learning systems (supervised and unsupervised) because analysis is based purely on human-created rules, and patterns are not automatically found in the data. Rule-based systems tend to perform very well for a specific task, but since the rules are manually created, they are necessarily based on a limited number of observations in data. This means that rule-based systems may not generalize well. Regardless though, their simplicity, ability to perform well for specific tasks, and the interpretability of their output means they are commonly used, alone or as a part of larger systems.

13.3.3.2 Supervised Machine Learning Systems

Rather than manually creating rules, supervised machine learning systems automatically learn from the data (Fig. 13.7b). These systems require large volumes of manually annotated data. The annotated data is split between training and test sets. The *training set* is used to automatically learn a model from the annotated data. Predictions in the model may be categorical labels (classification), or real-valued numbers (regression). In either case, each sample in the training set is featurized, and those features are used to develop a model that minimizes the error between actual (annotated) labels, and the labels predicted by the model. Data is split between test and training because the learned model may "overfit" the data, meaning that while the model performs well for the samples in the training data, it may not generalize well to unseen samples. Since the samples in the test set were not used to generate the model, the model's prediction performance on them indicates how well the learned model will perform on new data.

As mentioned in the featurization section, the learned models are only as good as the predictive value of the features used to generate the model and identifying a concise set of highly descriptive features can be very challenging. As the saying goes, "garbage in, garbage out", and without successfully defining discriminative features, a machine learning algorithm will not perform well. Therefore, although domain experts are not required for supervised machine learning, they provide invaluable insight during the feature engineering process. Another key to machine learning success is accurate annotated data in large quantities. Annotating data often requires domain expertise and is a time-consuming process. However, with a good set of discriminative features and sufficient annotated data, supervised learning methods typically generalize better than rule-based systems.

The selection of the classification and regression algorithm is largely dependent on the application, and common algorithms such as *random forest classifiers* [34, 64], *support vector machines* [11, 33], *neural networks*, *logistic regression*, and *ensemble methods* [46] are used for NLP applications. Sequence learning algorithms, such as *conditional random fields* (CRFs) are, however a class of algorithms common to NLP, but uncommon elsewhere. CRFs classify based on a sequence of observations rather than just a single observation in isolation. Since language is represented as a sequence of words, these methods tend to perform well. Lastly, hybrid systems offer an alternative to purely machine learning based models. Hybrid systems combine supervised machine learning models with manually created rules, and offer a simple way to combine the precision of rule-based systems with the generalizability of supervised machine learning [10].

13.3.3.3 Deep Learning Systems

Deep learning systems are becoming increasingly common for NLP applications. Deep learning is a kind of supervised learning that uses multi-layer (deep) neural networks. A distinct advantage of deep learning systems is that they often forgo the difficult feature engineering process, and instead use only term vectors as input. This is possible, because deep learning methods theoretically learn features from data alone via the internal weights of the network. The thought is that features are learned at increasing levels of abstraction as the depth of the network increases. The drawback, however, is that deep learning systems typically require much larger amounts of training data than traditional supervised machine learning.

Figure 13.8 shows a deep learning system at a conceptual level. Vector representations of words in a sentence or phrase are input into a neural network with many layers. Theoretically, the first layers learn data representations which are input into a prediction layer which outputs a prediction. Deep learning systems therefore consist of two distinct components. A set of layers designed to learn a data representation, and a set of layers to make a prediction based on that representation. Commonly used architectures for generating data representations are *convolutional neural networks* (CNN) [89], *recurrent neural networks* (RNN), and their extension, *bidirectional long-short term memory* (BiLSTM). The prediction layer of these networks is most often a CRF (e.g., BiLSTM-CRF), where the CNN, RNN, or BiLSTM are used for feature generation and the CRF is used for prediction. *Attention mechanisms* [90] may also be included as an additional component to these networks. For example, Tran et al. [21] indicate that attention mechanisms allow for interpretability and therefore "quality control in a clinical setting."

Fig. 13.8 A conceptual view of a deep learning system. Word vectors of are input into a deep neural network which automatically learns a data representation and makes a prediction from it

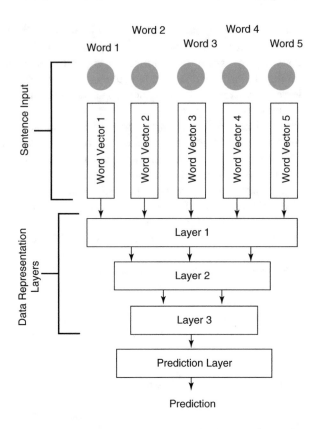

13.3.3.4 Unsupervised Machine Learning

Unsupervised machine learning methods do not require annotated data, but instead focus on characterizing or finding patterns in unannotated data (Fig. 13.7c). The most common unsupervised machine learning approaches for NLP are *topic modeling* and *clustering*.

Topic Modeling uses statistical methods to discover "topics" in documents. The most common topic modeling algorithm is *Latent Dirichlet Allocation* (LDA) [91], which models topics as a distribution of words, and represents documents as a mixture of topics. Given a collection of documents, LDA automatically discovers a pre-defined number of topics present in the data via statistical analysis. These topics can be used, for example, for developing and validating keyword features for classification [34], or for finding linguistic markers of schizophrenia [56], depression, and other mental health problems [32, 33, 35, 87, 92]. Although topic modeling is most often fully unsupervised, topic modeling algorithms may use domain knowledge to guide the discovered topics. For example, Yazdavar et al. [45] seed LDA with PHQ-9 categories to discover new terms relevant to each category.

Clustering is another method to find patterns or topics in text data. In clustering, text is compared and grouped ("clustered") by some measure of similarity. For example, word embeddings may be grouped based on their cosine distance to form clusters of related terms. As an example, Jackson et al. [13] created an ontology of terms related to mental illnesses by clustering word embeddings. Alternatively, text snippets may be clustered, as is the case with Althoff et al. [63], who used clustering to analyze counseling strategies in text message data.

For both topic modeling and clustering, the number of topics/clusters is a hyper-parameter that must be defined, and determining this number is more of an art than a science. Therefore, effective tuning of this hyper-parameter may require domain knowledge, rigorous methods for tuning, or both.

13.4 Applications of Natural Language Processing in Mental Health

In this section, we summarize the wide range of NLP applications within the mental health domain. These applications are summarized in Table 13.9 and discussed below.

13.4.1 Mental Illness Detection

The majority of applications of NLP for mental health has been for mental illness detection. Most work has focused on suicidality detection and depression detection. The goal of the application can broadly be divided into two task types. Yes/no type tasks seek to classify a post or user as either having the mental illness or not. Whereas scale type tasks seek to classify a post or user based on some scale of either being at risk for the mental illness, or the severity of the mental illness they are experiencing. The data sources vary as much as described in the Corpus Generation section, and the features used and analysis techniques vary as much as those described in the Data Processing section. Table 13.10 summarizes some of the work done using NLP for mental illness detection categorized by the mental illness they detect, data type and source, and type of the task. The "Note" column describes any unique characteristics of the referenced study.

Table 13.9 Application areas of NLP in mental health research and references for examples

Application		Example
Mental illness detection	Suicidality	[6, 8, 16, 32, 36–38, 43, 52, 53, 67, 93–98]
	Depression	[14, 41, 45–47, 51, 54, 99, 100]
	Post-traumatic stress disorder (PTSD)	[42, 43, 101, 102]
	Other	[21, 33, 34, 43, 55, 56, 64]
Symptom and severity extraction		[5, 10, 11, 21, 25–30, 103–105]
Lexicon and ontology construction		[10, 13, 34, 36, 44, 45, 50]
Knowledge discovery		[44, 63, 105–108]
Other applications		[7, 17, 58, 65, 66, 109–112]

Table 13.10 Overview of applications for mental illness detection

Reference	Mental Illness	Data Type	Data Source	Task Type	Note
[95]	Suicidality	Clinical	Psychiatry notes	Yes/no	
[8]	Suicidality	Clinical	EHR data	Yes/no	Focus on adults with autism spectrum disorder
[96]	Suicidality	Clinical	Emergency department and inpatient notes	Yes/no	Focus on adolescents
[67]	Suicidality	Combination	Clinical notes and Facebook posts	Scale	Focus on military personnel and veterans
[113]	Suicidality	Social media	Reddit	Scale	2019 CLPsych shared task
[37]	Suicidality	Social media	Reddit	Yes/no	Via answer generation on diagnostic questionnaires
[32]	Suicidality	Social media	Reddit	Yes/no	Transition from mental health discourse to suicidal ideation
[97]	Suicidality	Social media	Twitter	Other	Classified as 'suicidal ideation', 'reporting of a suicide', 'memorial', 'campaigning', and 'support'
[98]	Self-harm ideation	Social media	Online forum	Scale	
[14]	Depression	Clinical	EHR data	Yes/no	Found that models using NLP were superior to those relying on billing data alone
[99]	Depression	Clinical	Discharge summaries	Yes/no	
[45]	Depression	Social media	Twitter	Yes/no	Based on PHQ-9 symptoms persisting over time
[46]	Depression	Social media	Twitter	Yes/no	Included text and images
[41]	Depression	Social media	Twitter	Scale	
[100]	Depression	Social media	Twitter	Yes/no	Geographic, demographic, and seasonal patterns of depression reported by the Centers for Disease Control and Prevention (CDC)
[54]	Depression	Social media	Twitter	Yes/no	Post-partum depression, also predict the onset

Table 13.10 (continued)

Reference	Mental Illness	Data Type	Data Source	Task Type	Note
[47]	Depression	Social media	Facebook	Scale	Estimated based on the answers to a 100-item personality questionnaire
[101]	PTSD and depression	Social media	Twitter	Yes/no	2015 CLPsych shared task
[102]	PTSD and depression	Social media	Twitter	Yes/no	System description for 2015 CLPsych
[21]	Multiple	Clinical	Psychiatric notes	Yes/no	Novel use of the "History of mental illness" portion of psychiatric notes from CEGS N-GRID 2016 shared task data. Multi-label classification for 13 conditions: depression, bipolar disorder, anxiety spectrum disorders, obsessive compulsive disorders, obsessive compulsive spectrum disorder, attention deficit hyperactivity disorders, PTSD, eating disorders, dementia, complicated grief
[42]	Multiple	Social media	Twitter	Yes/no	PTSD, depression, bipolar disorder, and seasonal affective disorder
[43]	Multiple	Social media	Twitter	Yes/no	Suicide risk, anxiety, depression, eating disorder, panic attacks, schizophrenia, bipolar disorder, and PTSD
[33]	Multiple	Social media	Reddit	Yes/no	11 mental illness themes, including borderline personality disorder (BPD), bipolar disorder, schizophrenia, anxiety, depression, addiction, alcoholism, autism, opiates, self-harm and suicide watch
[34]	Multiple	Social media	Reddit	Yes/no	Classify posts into 20 DSM-5 categories

(continued)

Table 13.10 (continued)

Reference	Mental Illness	Data Type	Data Source	Task Type	Note
[55]	Multiple	Social media	Twitter	Yes/no	ADHD, generalized anxiety disorder, bipolar disorder, BPD, depression, eating disorders, obsessive compulsive disorder, PTSD, schizophrenia, and seasonal affective disorder
[56]	Schizophrenia	Social media	Twitter	Yes/no	
[64]	Autism Spectrum Disorder	Developmental evaluations	"The autism and developmental disabilities monitoring" network database	Yes/no	Novel data source which contains developmental evaluations from multiple health and educational sources

13.4.2 Symptom and Severity Extraction

Rather than detecting a mental illness outright, mental illness symptoms and their severity may be extracted from free-text and used to aid in diagnosis or to monitor patient progress. Track 2 of the 2016 the CEGS N-Grid shared tasks [5] focused on extraction of symptoms and their severity from neuropsychiatric clinical records, for which many novel solutions were developed [21, 25–30]. Outside of this shared task, Du et al. [103] investigated deep learning for recognizing suicide related psychiatric stressors from Twitter. They tackled this by identifying text spans referring to mentions of stressors. Leroy et al. [104] used a rule-based approach to extract 12 DSM criteria from EHRs based on descriptions of behaviors noted by the clinicians. Gorrell et al. [10] automatically extracted 11 negative schizophrenia symptoms (e.g., emotional withdrawal, poverty of speech, social withdrawal, etc.) from medical records. In a later study [105], they applied their approach to clinical notes of a large sample of patients with schizophrenia to build a system that assesses the relationship of negative symptoms with clinical outcomes. Jackson et al. [11] developed a system to extract symptoms of severe mental illness from clinical text, which cover 5 symptom domains, including: (1) positive symptoms, (2) negative symptoms, (3) disorganization symptoms, (4) manic symptoms, and (5) catatonic symptoms.

13.4.3 Lexicon and Ontology Construction

Lexicons and ontologies are discussed in greater detail in Chap. 7, but briefly, a lexicon is a set of terms and optionally their definitions. Whereas an ontology contains both a set of terms and the relations between them. Additionally, an ontology accounts for variation in term usage and often contains synonymous terms and abbreviations. Ontologies, such as the Unified Medical Language System (UMLS) [114] and its constituent ontologies such as ICD-9 and SNOMED CT often serve as keyword dictionaries for NLP tasks. They can be used to retrieve and filter relevant documents, identify relevant sections of a document, or select keywords as features for machine learning. However, since term usage evolves over time and can vary by institution, these resources tend to be incomplete. As a result, building new lexicons and ontologies, or augmenting existing ones is an important NLP task.

Figure 13.9 illustrates the lexicon and ontology construction process. Yazdavar et al. [45] divide lexicon and ontology usage into top down and bottom up approaches. Top down approaches are lexicon/ontology driven. Keywords are manually identified from lexicons or ontologies and combined with domain expertise to create a keyword dictionary derived solely from pre-existing resources. In contrast, bottom up approaches are data-driven, and lexicons/ontologies are developed from the data alone. These approaches use unsupervised learning methods, such as clustering or topic modeling to discover hidden groupings of terms as clusters or latent topics. Descriptive terms within these topics or clusters are selected and used to create a set of data-derived keywords. Hybrid approaches combine top down and bottom up approaches in a variety of ways. The simplest approach is to combine top down derived keywords with bottom up derived keywords into a single set of keywords. More sophisticated methods "seed" the

Fig. 13.9 Lexicon and ontology construction methods

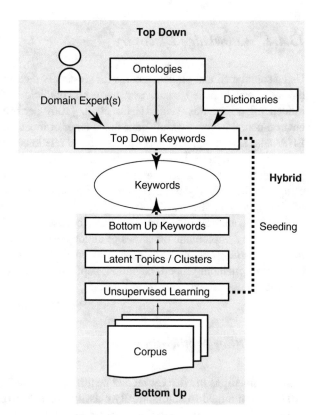

unsupervised learning method with ontology derived terms. The intuition is that these seeds give clusters or topics a starting point influenced by domain expertise from which to grow and find terms relevant to those starting seeds.

In their work, Yazdavar et al. develop a lexicon based on the PHQ-9 framework using a seed-based topic modeling method on Twitter data. Jackson et al. [13] find that SNOMED CT is not complete with respect to clinical symptoms, and semi-automatically augment it using terminology from clinical records. They apply clustering methods to classify new terms into one of nine symptom types: appearance/behavior, speech, affect/mood, thought, perception, cognition, insight, personality, and other. Gaur et al. [34] create a lexicon which is based on DSM-5 categories. They use several ontologies (ICD-10, SNOMED CT, DataMed [115, 116], and enriched Drug Abuse Ontology [117]) and combine them with social media derived keywords by finding n-grams and applying topic modeling to subreddits of interest. They later [36] develop a suicide risk severity lexicon using medical knowledge-bases and suicide ontologies combined with analysis of Reddit data. Saha et al. [44] semi-automatically create a drug list by manually listing drugs of interest, manually curating Wikipedia pages related to these drugs, and extracting brand names, generic names, and drug family information from the pages to create the final list. Gorrell et al. [10] manually create a keyword list of negative schizophrenia symptoms [118].

13.4.4 Knowledge Discovery

Using social media or clinical records for secondary data analysis can lead to the discovery of new knowledge such as patterns and predictors of mental health, or factors influencing it. In this vein, Heslin et al. [106] perform an analysis on socio-environmental factors that influence the number of inpatient days for psychosis using EHR data. Das et al. [107] perform a study on relations between cardiovascular disease and severe mental illness in ethnic minorities using EHR data. Deferio et al. [108] monitor and characterize off-label antidepressant use using EHR data. Patel et al. [105] identify negative symptoms leading to hospital admission and readmission of schizophrenia patients. Althoff et al. [63] discover the effectiveness of counseling strategies via analysis of text message based counseling conversations. Saha et al. [44] measure the symptomatic outcomes of antidepressant drug treatment by developing machine learning classifiers to detect psychopathological states associated with medicine intake, including mood, cognition, depression, anxiety, psychosis, and suicidal ideation in social media users over time.

13.4.5 Other Applications

Other applications in NLP for mental health include the 2016 CLPsych shared task [109], which aimed to automatically classify postings from a youth mental health forum into one of four severity labels: green, amber, red, or crisis. These labels indicate the risk of self-harm as indicated by the content of the posting. The goal was to support forum moderators by giving them a tool to prioritize their attention. Rumshisky et al. [7] built a predictive approach that infers psychiatric readmission based on the clinical content available in narrative discharge summaries. The goal was to facilitate the development of interventions that can reduce risks of early readmission. Klein et al. [58] developed a classification system for personal medication intake using Twitter data. Adekkanattu et al. [17] employed information extraction methods for extracting PHQ-9 scores from free text of EHRs. Kadra et al. [110] extracted details of antipsychotic prescriptions from structured fields and free-text narratives of EHRs. Sohn et al. [111] extracted adverse drug events from clinical narratives of psychiatry and psychology patients. Lyalina et al. [112] automatically identified phenotypic signatures of neuropsychiatric disorders from clinical narratives. They identified UMLS concepts in clinical narratives and searched for enriched codes and associations among codes that were representative of autism, bipolar disorder, and schizophrenia. Pestian, et al. [65] train a classifier to distinguish between authentic and fake suicide notes. Later [66], they held a shared task focused on automatic identification of positive and negative term sentiment in suicide notes, for which an annotated corpus was made publicly available.

13.5 NLP in Mental Health Practice

Within the clinical domain, NLP has been identified as an integral component in the Learning Healthcare System (LHS) [119] for both analytics, and real-time support [120]. Even though mental health is increasingly being recognized as a key to overall well-being [24], there are very few examples of NLP for improving mental health in practice. The majority of the work involves NLP for improved information retrieval [10, 12] (see Corpus Generation section). Integration of NLP into LHS for real-time clinical decision support or knowledge discovery has received limited development in the broader clinical domain [120], and nearly no development in the mental health domain. Kaggaal et al. [120] provide a description of how they incorporate NLP into an LHS, and describe potential applications and challenges they faced within the broader clinical domain. This can serve as a guide and inspiration for novel applications of NLP for mental health.

Outside of the clinical domain, there are also just a few examples of NLP for mental health practice. Applications have primarily focused on research and observational studies. This has produced considerable evidence that information derived from NLP in social media and other non-clinical sources can indicate the mental status at the message/post, personal, and population levels [2]. However, developing effective intervention strategies has proven challenging both methodologically and ethically. Barak and Grohl [121] provide an overview of intervention strategies up to the year 2011. These strategies include psycho-educational websites, conversational agents, online counseling, online support groups, blogs, SMS and text messaging therapies, and potential future directions such as virtual reality.

Psycho-educational interventions aim to provide patients with information about their illness, techniques to treat their illness, and the resources available to help them [121]. They have been shown to have positive therapeutic value [122] for disorders such as depression and anxiety [123, 124], eating disorders [125], smoking and alcohol consumption [126, 127]. Future directions of such strategies include using natural language generation (NLG) to personalize education. Personalization has been shown to increase effectiveness of educational intervention [121]. It has been widely adopted for marketing purposes, but remains to be applied for mental health related intervention strategies.

Psycho-educational interventions are an example of a one-way communication intervention strategy. A message is sent to a user, but the user cannot send a message back. Two-way communication intervention strategies have also been explored. These are more interactive and involve sending messages back and forth between patient and care provider. Examples include conversational agents [128], text messaging [129, 130], online counseling [131], and online support groups [132]. Most of these strategies don't involve NLP, and are therefore out of the scope of this chapter. They can, however be useful once an at risk patient or population is identified via social media or other means. For a review of text messaging as an intervention strategy, see Fjeldsoe et al. [130], and a review of the effectiveness of online support groups, see Griffiths et al. [132]. Methods that do use NLP tend to use NLG for personalizing automated communication. For example, Aguilera and Munoz [128] created an online virtual agent that incorporates NLG to help people recover from depression in their homes. Bauer et al. [129] use automated text message (SMS) conversations to support cognitive behavioral therapy.

13.6   Challenges, Limitations, and Ethical Considerations

13.6.1   Challenges

Although NLP in the mental health domain has shown great success and shows future promise, there are several challenges confronting its application. Selection bias is a particular concern when using social media data, since these data favor people who use social media [32, 45] and who publicly talk about their mental illness or medication intake [44]. This is particularly relevant for studies in depression, where social withdrawal may occur. In general, social media only captures what the patients choose to share; as a result, researchers may not see the whole picture of the patient [44] or of the population. How representative are samples drawn from social media [45]? This question also extends to biases related to demographics in social media. In many social media studies, age and gender statistics are not accounted for and may influence results [33]. Yazdavar et al. [46] indicate that demographic information is critical, specifically because "women are diagnosed with depression twice as often as men", but "suicide rates for men are three to five times higher than compared to women". Additionally, "signs and triggers of depression vary for different age groups", and therefore systems may be biased, and may not generalize well to different demographic groups.

In addition to the inherent bias in demographics represented in social media, selection bias may be introduced in other ways. For example, retrieving data using certain keywords can introduce a bias [11]. This potential bias may influence EHR data draws as well. In addition to data biases, Ernala et al. [133] identify methodological problems with mental health related social media research. They find that predictive models built on social media data may produce strong internal validity with respect to the samples drawn, but have frequently poor external validity with respect to the actual mental health of patients. They suggest that the models used may be invalid, and that the diagnostic signals are not measuring the actual mental health of the patients, but instead may be measuring other behaviors which may or may not be truly indicative of a particular diagnosis. Chancellor et al. [134] indicate a need for model interpretability.

13.6.2 Ethical Considerations

User agreements most often have few, if any restrictions on how data from social media is used, and since social media research is often considered observational, these studies often forego the requirement of ethics committees [134]. As such, ethical considerations for biases, data collection, and algorithm design are responsibilities of the researcher. Benton et al. [135] provide an overview of ethical research protocols for health related social media research, which covers a broad range of important topics relevant to this field. Chancellor et al. [134] present a more narrowly focused perspective, and focus solely on social media for mental health research. They create a taxonomy of ethical concerns, which include consent at scale, considerations for minority or vulnerable populations, discrimination, emotional vulnerability, maintaining online community integrity, a need for privacy, protection, and anonymization, questions of when and how to intervene, and the role of clinicians. Many of these concerns are echoed by other authors. Guntuku et al. [39] stress the need for privacy, stating that users may be surprised by how much mental health related information can be "gleaned from their digital traces". Due to the stigmas associated with mental health this information may engender discrimination. They suggest data protection and ownership frameworks are needed, and transparency about what health indicators are derived and why they are derived is critical. This potential for discrimination is elaborated by Saha et al. [44], who state that negative consequences of their work are possible, specifically discrimination by insurance companies or potential for misinterpretation of their study by users. Choudhury et al. [32] reiterate the importance of privacy, and in their study remove personally identifiable information by de-identifying and paraphrasing samples before reporting them in their paper. They [32] further suggest that intervention strategies require more research, stating that it could erode online community integrity and damage the perception of social media platforms as a "safe place for seeking support". Lastly, Guntuku et al. [39] describe the need for privacy and a need for "clear guidelines on mandated reporting" in their work concerning mental illness and depression detection.

13.7　Conclusions

This chapter provided an overview of NLP in mental health research and practice. We discussed corpus generation, data processing, and methods of text analysis, and provided example applications within the mental health domain. Typical sources of data include electronic health records and social media. These data sources provide different perspectives and complementary information. Text data is processed by first preprocessing to clean and normalize the data, followed by featurization, which extracts features used in its analysis. Analysis may be rule-based or machine learning based (supervised or unsupervised), and is dependent on the intended application. Applications can be grouped into four major categories: text classification, information extraction, lexicon and ontology construction, and knowledge discovery, each of which produce distinct results. No matter the application it is important to be aware of potential limitations and ethical considerations, in particular biases in the data, and to respect patients and their privacy. NLP plays an important role in mental health informatics, and provides the unique ability to extract information from and analyze unstructured text data. This information complements other disciplines to give a more complete view of the mental health of a patient or a population.

References

1. Abbe A, Grouin C, Zweigenbaum P, Falissard B. Text mining applications in psychiatry: a systematic literature review. Int J Methods Psychiatr Res. 2016;25(2):86–100.
2. Calvo RA, Milne DN, Hussain MS, Christensen H. Natural language processing in mental health applications using non-clinical texts. Nat Lang Eng. 2017;23(5):649–85.
3. Perera G, Broadbent M, Callard F, Chang CK, Downs J, Dutta R, et al. Cohort profile of the South London and Maudsley NHS Foundation Trust biomedical research Centre (SLaM BRC) case register: current status and recent enhancement of an electronic mental health record-derived data resource. BMJ Open. 2016;6(3):e008721.
4. Meystre SM, Savova GK, Kipper-Schuler KC, Hurdle JF. Extracting information from textual documents in the electronic health record: a review of recent research. Yearb Med Inform. 2008;17(01):128–44.
5. Filannino M, Stubbs A, Uzuner Ö. Symptom severity prediction from neuropsychiatric clinical records: overview of 2016 CEGS N-GRID shared tasks track 2. J Biomed Inform. 2017;75:S62–70.
6. Walsh CG, Ribeiro JD, Franklin JC. Predicting risk of suicide attempts over time through machine learning. Clin Psychol Sci. 2017;5(3):457–69.

7. Rumshisky A, Ghassemi M, Naumann T, Szolovits P, Castro V, McCoy T, et al. Predicting early psychiatric readmission with natural language processing of narrative discharge summaries. Transl Psychiatry. 2016;6(10):e921.
8. Downs J, Velupillai S, George G, Holden R, Kikoler M, Dean H, et al. Detection of suicidality in adolescents with autism spectrum disorders: developing a natural language processing approach for use in electronic health records. In: AMIA annual symposium proceedings. vol. 2017. American Medical Informatics Association, Bethesda; 2017. p. 641.
9. Anderson HD, Pace WD, Brandt E, Nielsen RD, Allen RR, Libby AM, et al. Monitoring suicidal patients in primary care using electronic health records. J Am Board Family Med. 2015;28(1):65–71.
10. Gorrell G, Roberts A, Jackson R, Stewart R. Finding negative symptoms of schizophrenia in patient records. In: Proceedings of the Workshop on NLP for medicine and biology associated with RANLP 2013, pp 9–17
11. Jackson RG, Patel R, Jayatilleke N, Kolliakou A, Ball M, Gorrell G, et al. Natural language processing to extract symptoms of severe mental illness from clinical text: the clinical record interactive search comprehensive data extraction (CRIS-CODE) project. BMJ Open. 2017;7(1):e012012.
12. Fernandes AC, Cloete D, Broadbent MT, Hayes RD, Chang CK, Jackson RG, et al. Development and evaluation of a de-identification procedure for a case register sourced from mental health electronic records. BMC Med Inform Decis Mak. 2013;13(1):71.
13. Jackson R, Patel R, Velupillai S, Gkotsis G, Hoyle D, Stewart R. Knowledge discovery for deep Phenotyping serious mental illness from electronic mental health record. F1000Research. 2018;7:210.
14. Perlis R, Iosifescu D, Castro V, Murphy S, Gainer V, Minnier J, et al. Using electronic medical records to enable large-scale studies in psychiatry: treatment resistant depression as a model. Psychol Med. 2012;42(1):41–50.
15. Murphy SN, Mendis M, Hackett K, Kuttan R, Pan W, Phillips LC, et al. Architecture of the open-source clinical research chart from informatics for integrating biology and the bedside. In: AMIA annual symposium proceedings. vol. 2007. American Medical Informatics Association, Bethesda; 2007. p. 548.
16. Barak-Corren Y, Castro VM, Javitt S, Hoffnagle AG, Dai Y, Perlis RH, et al. Predicting suicidal behavior from longitudinal electronic health records. Am J Psychiatr. 2016;174(2):154–62.
17. Adekkanattu P, Sholle ET, DeFerio J, Pathak J, Johnson SB, Campion Jr TR. Ascertaining depression severity by extracting patient health questionnaire-9 (PHQ-9) scores from clinical notes. In: AMIA annual symposium proceedings. vol. 2018. American Medical Informatics Association, Bethesda; 2018. p. 147.
18. U S Dept of Labor EBSA. The Health Insurance Portability and Accountability Act (HIPAA); 2004. http://purl.fdlp.gov/GPO/gpo10291.
19. Stubbs A, Uzuner Ö. Annotating longitudinal clinical narratives for de-identification: the 2014 i2b2/UTHealth corpus. J Biomed Inform. 2015;58:S20–9.
20. Stubbs A, Filannino M, Uzuner Ö. De-identification of psychiatric intake records: overview of 2016 CEGS N-GRID shared tasks track 1. J Biomed Inform. 2017;75:S4–S18.
21. Tran T, Kavuluru R. Predicting mental conditions based on "history of present illness" in psychiatric notes with deep neural networks. J Biomed Inform. 2017;75:S138–48.
22. Uzuner Ö. Recognizing obesity and comorbidities in sparse data. J Am Med Inform Assoc. 2009;16(4):561–70.
23. Uzuner Ö, Goldstein I, Luo Y, Kohane I. Identifying patient smoking status from medical discharge records. J Am Med Inform Assoc. 2008;15(1):14–24.
24. Uzuner Ö, Stubbs A, Filannino M. A natural language processing challenge for clinical records: research domains criteria (RDoC) for psychiatry. J Biomed Inform. 2017;75:S1–3.
25. Goodwin TR, Maldonado R, Harabagiu SM. Automatic recognition of symptom severity from psychiatric evaluation records. J Biomed Inform. 2017;75:S71–84.

26. Rios A, Kavuluru R. Ordinal convolutional neural networks for predicting RDoC positive valence psychiatric symptom severity scores. J Biomed Inform. 2017;75:S85–93.

27. Posada JD, Barda AJ, Shi L, Xue D, Ruiz V, Kuan PH, et al. Predictive modeling for classification of positive valence system symptom severity from initial psychiatric evaluation records. J Biomed Inform. 2017;75:S94–S104.

28. Liu Y, Gu Y, Nguyen JC, Li H, Zhang J, Gao Y, et al. Symptom severity classification with gradient tree boosting. J Biomed Inform. 2017;75:S105–11.

29. Scheurwegs E, Sushil M, Tulkens S, Daelemans W, Luyckx K. Counting trees in random forests: predicting symptom severity in psychiatric intake reports. J Biomed Inform. 2017;75:S112–9.

30. Clark C, Wellner B, Davis R, Aberdeen J, Hirschman L. Automatic classification of RDoC positive valence severity with a neural network. J Biomed Inform. 2017;75:S120–8.

31. Obar JA, Wildman SS. Social media definition and the governance challenge-an introduction to the special issue. Telecommun Policy. 2015;39(9):745–50.

32. De Choudhury M, Kiciman E, Dredze M, Coppersmith G, Kumar M. Discovering shifts to suicidal ideation from mental health content in social media. In: Proceedings of the 2016 CHI conference on human factors in computing systems. New York: ACM; 2016. p. 2098–110.

33. Gkotsis G, Oellrich A, Velupillai S, Liakata M, Hubbard TJ, Dobson RJ, et al. Characterisation of mental health conditions in social media using informed deep learning. Sci Rep. 2017;7:45141.

34. Gaur M, Kursuncu U, Alambo A, Sheth A, Daniulaityte R, Thirunarayan K, et al. Let me tell you about your mental health!: Contextualized classification of reddit posts to dsm-5 for web-based intervention. In: Proceedings of the 27th ACM international conference on information and knowledge management. New York: ACM; 2018. p. 753–62.

35. Shen JH, Rudzicz F. Detecting anxiety through reddit. In: Proceedings of the fourth workshop on computational linguistics and clinical psychology – from linguistic signal to clinical reality; 2017, pp 58–65

36. Gaur M, Alambo A, Sain JP, Kursuncu U, Thirunarayan K, Kavuluru R, et al. Knowledge-aware assessment of severity of suicide risk for early intervention. In: The world wide web conference. New York: ACM; 2019. p. 514–25.

37. Alambo A, Gaur M, Lokala U, Kursuncu U, Thirunarayan K, Gyrard A, et al. Question answering for suicide risk assessment using reddit. In: 2019 IEEE 13th International Conference on Semantic Computing (ICSC). Newport Beach, CA: IEEE; 2019. p. 468–73.

38. Kavuluru R, Ramos-Morales M, Holaday T, Williams AG, Haye L, Cerel J. Classification of helpful comments on online suicide watch forums. In: Proceedings of the 7th ACM international conference on bioinformatics, computational biology, and health informatics. New York: ACM; 2016. p. 32–40.

39. Guntuku SC, Yaden DB, Kern ML, Ungar LH, Eichstaedt JC. Detecting depression and mental illness on social media: an integrative review. Curr Opin Behav Sci. 2017;18:43–9.

40. Paul MJ, Dredze M. You are what you tweet: analyzing twitter for public health. In: Fifth international aaai conference on weblogs and social media; 2011

41. De Choudhury M, Gamon M, Counts S, Horvitz E. Predicting depression via social media. In: Seventh international AAAI conference on weblogs and social media; 2013

42. Coppersmith G, Dredze M, Harman C. Quantifying mental health signals in Twitter. In: Proceedings of the workshop on computational linguistics and clinical psychology: From linguistic signal to clinical reality; 2014, pp 51–60

43. Benton A, Mitchell M, Hovy D. Multi-task learning for mental health using social media text. arXiv preprint arXiv:171203538. 2017

44. Saha K, Sugar B, Torous J, Abrahao B, Kcman E, De Choudhury M. A social media study on the effects of psychiatric medication use. Proceedings of the International AAAI Conference on Web and Social Media. 2019;13:440–51.

45. Yazdavar AH, Al-Olimat HS, Ebrahimi M, Bajaj G, Banerjee T, Thirunarayan K, et al. Semi-supervised approach to monitoring clinical depressive symptoms in social media. In:

Proceedings of the 2017 IEEE/ACM international conference on advances in social networks analysis and mining 2017. New York: ACM; 2017. p. 1191–8.

46. Yazdavar AH, Mahdavinejad MS, Bajaj G, Romine W, Monadjemi A, Thirunarayan K, et al. Fusing visual, textual and connectivity clues for studying mental health. arXiv preprint arXiv:190206843. 2019

47. Schwartz HA, Eichstaedt J, Kern ML, Park G, Sap M, Stillwell D, et al. Towards assessing changes in degree of depression through facebook. In: Proceedings of the workshop on computational linguistics and clinical psychology: from linguistic signal to clinical reality; 2014, pp 118–125

48. Homan CM, Lu N, Tu X, Lytle MC, Silenzio V. Social structure and depression in TrevorSpace. In: Proceedings of the 17th ACM conference on Computer supported cooperative work & social computing. New York: ACM; 2014. p. 615–25.

49. Cavazos-Rehg PA, Krauss MJ, Sowles SJ, Connolly S, Rosas C, Bharadwaj M, et al. An analysis of depression, self-harm, and suicidal ideation content on Tumblr. Crisis. 2016

50. Strapparava C, Mihalcea R. Learning to identify emotions in text. In: Proceedings of the 2008 ACM symposium on Applied computing; 2008, pp 1556–1560

51. Nguyen T, Phung D, Dao B, Venkatesh S, Berk M. Affective and content analysis of online depression communities. IEEE Trans Affect Comput. 2014;5(3):217–26.

52. Li A, Huang X, Hao B, O'Dea B, Christensen H, Zhu T. Attitudes towards suicide attempts broadcast on social media: an exploratory study of Chinese microblogs. PeerJ. 2015;3:e1209.

53. Masuda N, Kurahashi I, Onari H. Suicide ideation of individuals in online social networks. PloS One. 2013;8(4):e62262.

54. De Choudhury M, Counts S, Horvitz EJ, Hoff A. Characterizing and predicting postpartum depression from shared facebook data. In: Proceedings of the 17th ACM conference on Computer supported cooperative work & social computing. New York: ACM; 2014. p. 626–38.

55. Coppersmith G, Dredze M, Harman C, Hollingshead K. From ADHD to SAD: Analyzing the language of mental health on Twitter through self-reported diagnoses. In: Proceedings of the 2nd workshop on computational linguistics and clinical psychology: from linguistic signal to clinical reality; 2015, pp 1–10

56. Mitchell M, Hollingshead K, Coppersmith G. Quantifying the language of schizophrenia in social media. In: Proceedings of the 2nd workshop on Computational linguistics and clinical psychology: from linguistic signal to clinical reality; 2015, pp 11–20.

57. MacAvaney S, Desmet B, Cohan A, Soldaini L, Yates A, Zirikly A, et al. RSDD-Time: Temporal annotation of self-reported mental health diagnoses. arXiv preprint arXiv:180607916. 2018

58. Klein A, Sarker A, Rouhizadeh M, O'Connor K, Gonzalez G. Detecting personal medication intake in Twitter: an annotated corpus and baseline classification system. BioNLP. 2017;2017:136–42.

59. Culotta A. Towards detecting influenza epidemics by analyzing twitter messages. In: Proceedings of the first workshop on social media analytics. New York: ACM; 2010. p. 115–22.

60. Paul MJ, Dredze M. A model for mining public health topics from twitter. Health. 2012;11(16–16):1.

61. Jamnik MR, Lane DJ. The use of Reddit as an inexpensive source for high-quality data. Pract Assess Res Eval. 2017;22:1–10.

62. De Choudhury M. Role of social media in tackling challenges in mental health. In: Proceedings of the 2nd international workshop on Socially-aware multimedia. ACM, New York; 2013. p. 49–52.

63. Althoff T, Clark K, Leskovec J. Large-scale analysis of counseling conversations: an application of natural language processing to mental health. Trans Assoc Comput Linguist. 2016;4:463–76.

64. Maenner MJ, Yeargin-Allsopp M, Braun KVN, Christensen DL, Schieve LA. Development of a machine learning algorithm for the surveillance of autism spectrum disorder. PLoS One. 2016;11(12):e0168224.

65. Pestian J, Nasrallah H, Matykiewicz P, Bennett A, Leenaars A. Suicide note classification using natural language processing: A content analysis. Biomed Infor Insights. 2010;3:BII–S4706.
66. Pestian JP, Matykiewicz P, Linn-Gust M, South B, Uzuner O, Wiebe J, et al. Sentiment analysis of suicide notes: a shared task. Biomed Infor Insights. 2012;5:BII–S9042.
67. Thompson P, Bryan C, Poulin C. Predicting military and veteran suicide risk: Cultural aspects. In: Proceedings of the workshop on computational linguistics and clinical psychology: from linguistic signal to clinical reality; 2014, pp 1–6
68. Ferrucci D, Lally A. UIMA: an architectural approach to unstructured information processing in the corporate research environment. Nat Lang Eng. 2004;10(3–4):327–48.
69. Divita G, Carter ME, Tran LT, Redd D, Zeng QT, Duvall S, et al. v3NLP Framework: tools to build applications for extracting concepts from clinical text. eGEMs. 2016;4(3):1228.
70. Manning C, Surdeanu M, Bauer J, Finkel J, Bethard S, McClosky D. The Stanford CoreNLP natural language processing toolkit. In: Proceedings of 52nd annual meeting of the association for computational linguistics: system demonstrations; 2014. pp 55–60
71. Toutanova K, Klein D, Manning CD, Singer Y. Feature-rich part-of-speech tagging with a cyclic dependency network. In: Proceedings of the 2003 Conference of the North American chapter of the association for computational linguistics on human language technology-volume 1. Association for computational Linguistics; 2003. pp 173–180.
72. Chen D, Manning C. A fast and accurate dependency parser using neural networks. In: Proceedings of the 2014 conference on empirical methods in natural language processing (EMNLP); 2014. pp 740–750
73. Chapman WW, Bridewell W, Hanbury P, Cooper GF, Buchanan BG. A simple algorithm for identifying negated findings and diseases in discharge summaries. J Biomed Inform. 2001;34(5):301–10.
74. Aronson AR, Lang FM. An overview of MetaMap: historical perspective and recent advances. J Am Med Inform Assoc. 2010;17(3):229–36.
75. Mikolov T, Sutskever I, Chen K, Corrado GS, Dean J. Distributed representations of words and phrases and their compositionality. In: Advances in neural information processing systems; 2013. pp 3111–3119
76. Pennington J, Socher R, Manning C. Glove: global vectors for word representation. In: Proceedings of the 2014 conference on empirical methods in natural language processing (EMNLP); 2014. pp 1532–1543
77. Pyysalo S, Filip G, Moen H, Salakoski T, Ananiadou S. Distributional semantics resources for biomedical text processing
78. Devlin J, Chang MW, Lee K, Toutanova K. Bert: Pre-training of deep bidirectional transformers for language understanding. arXiv preprint arXiv:181004805. 2018
79. Peters ME, Neumann M, Iyyer M, Gardner M, Clark C, Lee K, et al. Deep contextualized word representations. arXiv preprint arXiv:180205365. 2018
80. Rosenthal S, Nakov P, Kiritchenko S, Mohammad S, Ritter A, Stoyanov V. Semeval-2015 task 10: Sentiment analysis in twitter. In: Proceedings of the 9th international workshop on semantic evaluation (SemEval 2015); 2015, pp 451–463
81. Nakov P, Ritter A, Rosenthal S, Sebastiani F, Stoyanov V. SemEval-2016 task 4: Sentiment analysis in Twitter. In: Proceedings of the 10th international workshop on semantic evaluation (semeval-2016); 2016, pp 1–18
82. Rosenthal S, Farra N, Nakov P. SemEval-2017 task 4: Sentiment analysis in Twitter. In: Proceedings of the 11th international workshop on semantic evaluation (SemEval-2017); 2017. pp 502–518
83. Baccianella S, Esuli A, Sebastiani F. Sentiwordnet 3.0: an enhanced lexical resource for sentiment analysis and opinion mining. LREC. 2010;10:2200–4.
84. Nielsen FÅ. A new ANEW: Evaluation of a word list for sentiment analysis in microblogs. arXiv preprint arXiv:11032903. 2011
85. Tausczik YR, Pennebaker JW. The psychological meaning of words: LIWC and computerized text analysis methods. J Lang Soc Psychol. 2010;29(1):24–54.
86. Pennebaker JW, Boyd RL, Jordan K, Blackburn K. The development and psychometric properties of LIWC2015; 2015

87. Resnik P, Garron A, Resnik R. Using topic modeling to improve prediction of neuroticism and depression in college students. In: Proceedings of the 2013 conference on empirical methods in natural language processing; 2013, pp 1348–1353

88. Viani N, Yin L, Kam J, Alawi A, Bittar A, Dutta R, et al. Time expressions in mental health Records for Symptom Onset Extraction. In: Proceedings of the ninth international workshop on health text mining and information analysis; 2018, pp 183–192.

89. Kim Y Convolutional neural networks for sentence classification. arXiv preprint arXiv:14085882. 2014

90. Vaswani A, Shazeer N, Parmar N, Uszkoreit J, Jones L, Gomez AN, et al. Attention is all you need. In: Advances in neural information processing systems; 2017, pp 5998–6008

91. Blei DM, Ng AY, Jordan MI. Latent dirichlet allocation. J Mach Learn Res. 2003;3(Jan):993–1022.

92. Resnik P, Armstrong W, Claudino L, Nguyen T, Nguyen VA, Boyd-Graber J. Beyond LDA: exploring supervised topic modeling for depression-related language in Twitter. In: Proceedings of the 2nd workshop on computational linguistics and clinical psychology: from linguistic signal to clinical reality; 2015, pp 99–107.

93. Braithwaite SR, Giraud-Carrier C, West J, Barnes MD, Hanson CL. Validating machine learning algorithms for twitter data against established measures of suicidality. JMIR Mental Health 2016 May;3(2):e21. Available from: http://mental.jmir.org/2016/2/e21/.

94. Haerian K, Salmasian H, Friedman C. Methods for identifying suicide or suicidal ideation in EHRs. In: AMIA annual symposium proceedings, vol. 2012. Chicago: American Medical Informatics Association; 2012. p. 1244.

95. Fernandes AC, Dutta R, Velupillai S, Sanyal J, Stewart R, Chandran D. Identifying suicide ideation and suicidal attempts in a psychiatric clinical research database using natural language processing. Sci Rep. 2018;8(1):7426.

96. Bhat HS, Goldman-Mellor SJ. Predicting adolescent suicide attempts with neural networks. arXiv preprint arXiv:171110057. 2017;

97. Burnap P, Colombo W, Scourfield J. Machine classification and analysis of suicide-related communication on twitter. In: Proceedings of the 26th ACM conference on hypertext & social media. New York: ACM; 2015. p. 75–84.

98. Cohan A, Young S, Yates A, Goharian N. Triaging content severity in online mental health forums. J Assoc Inf Sci Technol. 2017;68(11):2675–89.

99. Zhou L, Baughman AW, Lei VJ, Lai KH, Navathe AS, Chang F, et al. Identifying patients with depression using free-text clinical documents. Stud Health Technol Inform. 2015;216:629–33.

100. De Choudhury M, Counts S, Horvitz E. Social media as a measurement tool of depression in populations. In: Proceedings of the 5th annual ACM web science conference. New York: ACM; 2013. p. 47–56.

101. Coppersmith G, Dredze M, Harman C, Hollingshead K, Mitchell M. CLPsych 2015 shared task: depression and PTSD on Twitter. In: Proceedings of the 2nd workshop on computational linguistics and clinical psychology: from linguistic signal to clinical reality; 2015, pp 31–39

102. Preotiuc-Pietro D, Sap M, Schwartz HA, Ungar L. Mental illness detection at the world well-being project for the CLPsych 2015 shared task. In: Proceedings of the 2nd workshop on computational linguistics and clinical psychology: from linguistic signal to clinical reality; 2015, pp 40–45

103. Du J, Zhang Y, Luo J, Jia Y, Wei Q, Tao C, et al. Extracting psychiatric stressors for suicide from social media using deep learning. BMC Med Inform Decis Mak. 2018;18(2):43.

104. Leroy G, Gu Y, Pettygrove S, Galindo MK, Arora A, Kurzius-Spencer M. Automated extraction of diagnostic criteria from electronic health records for autism spectrum disorders: development, evaluation, and application. J Med Internet Res. 2018;20(11):e10497.

105. Patel R, Jayatilleke N, Broadbent M, Chang CK, Foskett N, Gorrell G, et al. Negative symptoms in schizophrenia: a study in a large clinical sample of patients using a novel automated method. BMJ Open. 2015;5(9):e007619.

106. Heslin M, Khondoker M, Shetty H, Pritchard M, Jones PB, Osborn D, et al. Inpatient use and area-level socio-environmental factors in people with psychosis. Soc Psychiatry Psychiatr Epidemiol. 2018;53(10):1133–40.

107. Das-Munshi J, Ashworth M, Gaughran F, Hull S, Morgan C, Nazroo J, et al. Ethnicity and cardiovascular health inequalities in people with severe mental illnesses: protocol for the E-CHASM study. Soc Psychiatry Psychiatr Epidemiol. 2016;51(4):627–38.

108. Deferio JJ, Levin TT, Cukor J, Banerjee S, Abdulrahman R, Sheth A, et al. Using electronic health records to characterize prescription patterns: focus on antidepressants in nonpsychiatric outpatient settings. JAMIA Open. 2018;1(2):233–45.

109. Milne DN, Pink G, Hachey B, Calvo RA. Clpsych 2016 shared task: triaging content in online peer-support forums. In: Proceedings of the third workshop on computational linguistics and clinical psychology; 2016. p. 118–127.

110. Kadra G, Stewart R, Shetty H, Jackson RG, Greenwood MA, Roberts A, et al. Extracting antipsychotic polypharmacy data from electronic health records: developing and evaluating a novel process. BMC Psychiatry. 2015;15(1):166.

111. Sohn S, Kocher JPA, Chute CG, Savova GK. Drug side effect extraction from clinical narratives of psychiatry and psychology patients. J Am Med Inform Assoc. 2011;18(Supplement_1):i144–9.

112. Lyalina S, Percha B, LePendu P, Iyer SV, Altman RB, Shah NH. Identifying phenotypic signatures of neuropsychiatric disorders from electronic medical records. J Am Med Inform Assoc. 2013;20(e2):e297–305.

113. Zirikly A, Resnik P, Uzuner O, Hollingshead K. CLPsych 2019 shared task: predicting the degree of suicide risk in Reddit posts. In: Proceedings of the Sixth Workshop on Computational Linguistics and Clinical Psychology; 2019. p. 24–33.

114. Bodenreider O. The unified medical language system (UMLS): integrating biomedical terminology. Nucleic Acids Res. 2004;32(Suppl_1):D267–70.

115. Chen X, Gururaj AE, Ozyurt B, Liu R, Soysal E, Cohen T, et al. DataMed–an open source discovery index for finding biomedical datasets. J Am Med Inform Assoc. 2018;25(3):300–8.

116. Ohno-Machado L, Sansone SA, Alter G, Fore I, Grethe J, Xu H, et al. Finding useful data across multiple biomedical data repositories using DataMed. Nat Genet. 2017;49(6):816–9.

117. Cameron D, Smith GA, Daniulaityte R, Sheth AP, Dave D, Chen L, et al. PREDOSE: a semantic web platform for drug abuse epidemiology using social media. J Biomed Inform. 2013;46(6):985–97.

118. Liu Q, Woo M, Zou X, Champaneria A, Lau C, Mubbashar MI, et al. Symptom-based patient stratification in mental illness using clinical notes. J Biomed Inform. 2019;98:103274.

119. Friedman C, Rubin J, Brown J, Buntin M, Corn M, Etheredge L, et al. Toward a science of learning systems: a research agenda for the high-functioning learning health system. J Am Med Inform Assoc. 2015;22(1):43–50.

120. Kaggal VC, Elayavilli RK, Mehrabi S, Pankratz JJ, Sohn S, Wang Y, et al. Toward a learning health-care system–knowledge delivery at the point of care empowered by big data and NLP. Biomed Inform Insights. 2016;8:S37977–BII.

121. Barak A, Grohol JM. Current and future trends in internet-supported mental health interventions. J Technol Hum Serv. 2011;29(3):155–96.

122. Ritterband LM, Gonder-Frederick LA, Cox DJ, Clifton AD, West RW, Borowitz SM. Internet interventions: in review, in use, and into the future. Prof Psychol Res Pract. 2003;34(5):527.

123. Spek V, Cuijpers P, Nyklcek I, Riper H, Keyzer J, Pop V. Internet-based cognitive behaviour therapy for symptoms of depression and anxiety: a meta-analysis. Psychol Med. 2007;37(3):319–28.

124. Donker T, Griffiths KM, Cuijpers P, Christensen H. Psychoeducation for depression, anxiety and psychological distress: a meta-analysis. BMC Med. 2009;7(1):79.

125. Neve M, Morgan PJ, Jones P, Collins C. Effectiveness of web-based interventions in achieving weight loss and weight loss maintenance in overweight and obese adults: a systematic review with meta-analysis. Obes Rev. 2010;11(4):306–21.

126. Bewick BM, Trusler K, Barkham M, Hill AJ, Cahill J, Mulhern B. The effectiveness of web-based interventions designed to decrease alcohol consumption – a systematic review. Prev Med. 2008;47(1):17–26.

127. Myung SK, McDonnell DD, Kazinets G, Seo HG, Moskowitz JM. Effects of web-and computer-based smoking cessation programs: meta-analysis of randomized controlled trials. Arch Intern Med. 2009;169(10):929–37.
128. Aguilera A, Muñoz RF. Text messaging as an adjunct to CBT in low-income populations: a usability and feasibility pilot study. Prof Psychol Res Pract. 2011;42(6):472.
129. Bauer S, Percevic R, Okon E, Meermann R, Kordy H. Use of text messaging in the aftercare of patients with bulimia nervosa. Eur Eat Disord Rev: The Professional Journal of the Eating Disorders Association. 2003;11(3):279–90.
130. Fjeldsoe BS, Marshall AL, Miller YD. Behavior change interventions delivered by mobile telephone short-message service. Am J Prev Med. 2009;36(2):165–73.
131. Grohol JM. Online counseling: a historical perspective; 2004.
132. Griffiths KM, Calear AL, Banfield M. Systematic review on internet support groups (ISGs) and depression (1): do ISGs reduce depressive symptoms? J Med Internet Res. 2009;11(3):e40.
133. Ernala SK, Birnbaum ML, Candan KA, Rizvi AF, Sterling WA, Kane JM, et al. Methodological gaps in predicting mental health states from social media: Triangulating diagnostic signals. In: Proceedings of the 2019 CHI conference on human factors in computing systems, vol. 2019. New York: ACM. p. 134.
134. Chancellor S, Birnbaum ML, Caine ED, Silenzio V, De Choudhury M. A taxonomy of ethical tensions in inferring mental health states from social media. In: Proceedings of the conference on fairness, accountability, and transparency. New York: ACM; 2019. p. 79–88.
135. Benton A, Coppersmith G, Dredze M. Ethical research protocols for social media health research. In: Proceedings of the first ACL workshop on ethics in natural language processing; 2017. p. 94–102.

Chapter 14
Information Visualization in Mental Health Research and Practice

Harry Hochheiser and Anurag Verma

Abstract Understanding the complex relationships between a range of disparate types of data including (but not limited to) clinical signs and symptoms, socio-economic statuses, and environmental exposures is an ongoing struggle for researchers, administrators, clinicians, public health experts, and patients who struggle to use data to understand mental health. Information visualization techniques combining rich displays of data with highly responsive user interactions allow for dynamic exploration and interpretation of data to gain otherwise unavailable insights into these challenging datasets. To encourage broader adoption of visualization techniques in mental health, we draw upon research conducted over the past thirty years to introduce the reader to the field of interactive visualizations. We introduce theoretical models underlying information visualization and key considerations in the design of visualizations, including understanding user needs, managing data, effectively displaying information, and selecting appropriate approaches for interacting with the data. We introduce various types of mental health data, including survey data, administrative data, environmental data, and mobile health data, with a focus on focus on data integration and the use of predictive models. We introduce currently available open-source and commercial tools for visualization. Finally, we discuss two outstanding challenges in the field: uncertainty visualization and evaluation of visualization.

Keywords Information visualization · Visual analytics · Uncertainty · Evaluation User interaction · Design

H. Hochheiser (✉)
University of Pittsburgh, Pittsburgh, PA, USA
e-mail: harryh@pitt.edu

A. Verma
University of Pennsylvania, Philadelphia, PA, USA
e-mail: anuragv@upenn.edu

© Springer Nature Switzerland AG 2021
J. D. Tenenbaum, P. A. Ranallo (eds.), *Mental Health Informatics*, Health
Informatics, https://doi.org/10.1007/978-3-030-70558-9_14

14.1 Introduction

Even for relatively "simple" processes and diseases, our ability to make sense of large health related data sets has long been eclipsed by the complexity of those data. Most biological processes involve thousands of genes and proteins and tens of thousands of interactions in detailed pathways influenced by environmental factors, presenting challenges in our abilities to convert data into knowledge. Mental and behavioral processes are even more complex—involving a nearly infinite number of social, emotional, cognitive, and biological processes, all interacting in complex ways. From the earliest days of science, visualization has been a key strategy for managing this complexity. Although early anatomical sketches and hand-drawn phylogenetic trees may have given way to complex genome-scaled wall-sized displays [1], the underlying motivation hasn't changed: well-designed graphical representations allow us to use our powerful visual system to identify trends, make connections, see patterns, and move from data to understanding.

Visualization can be broadly defined as the use of graphical display techniques to aid understanding of data. Well-constructed visualizations often draw both on scientific understandings of the human visual system and ways to leverage artistic and design sensibilities to turn complex data into attractive displays that foster understanding and insight. Historically, the term "scientific visualization" has been used to refer to representations of physical data such as anatomic entities, geographic features, weather systems, while "information visualization" has been used to refer to representations of data lacking obvious interpretation. For example, a visualization of functional magnetic resonance imaging (fMRI) data indicating activation levels in different brain regions would most logically be a scientific visualization based on a 3D map of a human brain, while the graphical representation of a dataset linking genetic mutations and behavioral symptoms would be an example of information visualization.

Building on a long history of graphs, charts, and static graphical representations, information visualization emerged as a field in the early 1990s [2], as the increased availability of powerful and inexpensive graphical displays brought the possibility of rapid data interaction, or *interactive data visualization*, to commodity desktop computers. Advances in academic research and commercial product development have spurred the use of visualization in several domains, ranging from basic research to consumer applications. Visualization products are also being used across all phases of the data interpretation process—from initial cleansing and exploration of raw data to robust visualization of well-curated data.

Although the application of information visualization in mental health has been limited to date, success stories in other fields suggest substantial opportunities for use by researchers, clinicians, and patients challenged with the interpretation of diverse and complex datasets. Building on successful techniques used in cancer research, basic researchers might use displays linking genetic variations with neural pathway disruptions and mental or behavioral phenotypes to understand molecular

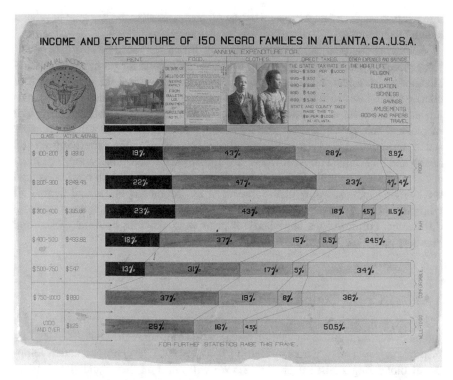

Fig. 14.1 W.E.B Dubois' depiction of income and expenses of 150 African American and negro families in Atlanta in 1900 [2] (Library of Congress)

mechanisms implicated in specific types of mental or behavioral dysfunction. Clinicians might use temporal views of patient data—depicting both individuals and cohorts—to understand the longitudinal trajectories of various mental health syndromes. Mobile apps and other consumer-facing tools might use visualization to help individuals understand their own mental health and how it is impacted by physical activity, diet, and environmental factors.

An early example of the use of visualization in mental health can be found in a graphical representation of what we now might call "social determinants of health", prepared by W.E.B. DuBois for the "Exhibition of American Negroes", held at the Exposition Universelle in Paris in 1900 (Fig. 14.1) [3]. Dubois' evocative use of stacked bar charts concisely illustrates the financial burden of rent, food, clothing, taxes, and other expenses (including education, art, amusements, and any health care), stratified across seven income brackets and augmented by details of tax rates and diet. Although DuBois did not tie this visualization directly to mental health, companion graphs detailing occupations, population distribution, migration, marriage rates, and other social factors paint a detailed picture of African American life at the turn of the twentieth century. Combining disparate datasets to provide insight into a broad range of factors related to mental health remains the key goal of mental health visualization.

Achieving this goal will require addressing difficulties faced by efforts in genetics, genomics, phenotyping, and other health domains with longer histories of visualization, with a few wrinkles thrown in for good measure. Like investigators of cancer and other medical conditions, mental health informaticians will be challenged by the need to integrate detailed molecular and cellular data not only with mental and behavioral data, but also with interpersonal, environmental, and broader social and cultural data. Our understanding of the phenomena underlying mental health and their interactions, however, are arguably less well-understood. The intricacies of the human brain, difficulties in diagnosis of mental health conditions, and the evolving understanding of the impact of environmental and social factors all complicate issues. As we will see, visualization can play a role in addressing these difficulties. Fortunately, a large body of prior work provides both theoretical and practical guidance.

14.2   A Crash Course in Information Visualization

Interactive information visualization research first took off in the 1990s [4], drawing inspiration from earlier works by Bertin [5], Tukey [6], Cleveland [7], and developers of pioneering statistical graphs [8]. We will build on this foundational work, using theoretical taxonomies to describe how users might think about data and visualizations through *cognitive models* [4, 6, 9, 10], the *tasks* [11, 12] that might be addressed through interactive visualization, and the *interaction techniques* [13, 14] used to browse, navigate, and otherwise control data displays. (These and related tools are defined in Table 14.1.) Together, these topics will provide an introductory roadmap for contextualizing existing tools, and identify new opportunities. Additional details expanding on this necessarily brief introduction can be found in excellent texts on information visualization, including (but not limited to) those by Ward et al. [15], Spence [16], and Ware [10].

Two caveats limit the scope of this discussion. First, much of the recent work in interactive data visualization has often been described under the rubric of "visual analytics", a term used to encompass the data preparation, analysis, and communication processes involved in the use of interactive tools to interpret complex data, often in coordination with machine learning techniques (described in Chapter 10) [17, 18]. For the purpose of this brief chapter, we will not dwell on the distinctions between visual analytics and information visualization. As with other prior work in information visualization, we limit our scope to abstract data types lacking in any known, physical realization, thus leaving visualization of anatomic data through imaging modalities to others.

Table 14.1 Glossary

Term	Definition/Example
Data visualization	The use of graphical techniques to encode attributes of data items and relationships between those items, as a means of facilitating the interpretation of those data.
Interaction techniques	The combination of user-controls for providing input to computer applications, and the semantics, or interpretation of those actions. Examples might include drawing a rectangular box around a map region to "zoom into" that area.
Interactive data visualization	Data visualizations combined with appropriate interaction techniques, as opposed to static views printed on paper or on non-editable displays.
Information visualization	Interactive data visualizations of abstract data sets, as opposed to scientific visualizations of entities with known spatial organizations, such as brain images.
Information visualization systems	Functional tools or products combining visualization designs, interaction techniques, and means of accessing data sets to use in those visualizations.
Visual analytics	The data preparation, analysis, and communication processes involved in the use of interactive tools to interpret complex data, often in coordination with machine learning techniques.
Cognitive models	Descriptions of the thought processes and representations involved in the use of an interactive tool. Often used to determine how to design visualization and related interactions to best meet user needs.
Tasks	The goals that a user hopes to accomplish when using a visualization. Tasks are often defined in terms of questions that might be asked about the data set as a whole or about specific items(s).
Machine learning	The use of computational and statistical techniques to develop models capable of classifying data items, identifying clusters, or otherwise enabling inferences about unseen data.
Dimensionality-reduction	Mathematical techniques for converting very high-dimensionality data to lower-dimensionality representations, usually for depiction in a two- or three-dimensional space for display on a screen or on a printed page.
Electronic health records (EHR)	A digital version of patient medical history, administrative clinical data stored by provider over time.
SNPs	Single nucleotide polymorphisms (SNPs) represent a difference in nucleotide at certain section of the DNA. They are commonly referred as SNPs (pronounces "snips")
GWAS	Genome-wide association study (GWAS) is a statistical approach to study association between common genetic variants (thousands to millions) across the genome and a phenotype of interest.
PheWAS	Phenome-wide association study (PheWAS) is a statistical approach to study association between a selected list of genetic variants and collection of phenotypes (hundreds to thousands).

14.2.1   Why Visualization?

Interactive visualizations are perhaps most powerful in the early stages of a research effort when researchers are struggling to make sense of complex, unruly datasets. Often considered a component of the broader process of exploratory data analysis [19, 20], visualization is useful for examining broad trends and relationships, assessing data quality, generating preliminary models of underlying phenomena, and (ideally) generating relevant hypotheses suitable for exploration in controlled experiments. Put more simply, visualization is useful when we do not know what questions to ask—a situation that is likely familiar to many working at the intersection of mental health and informatics.

Information visualization approaches use a combination of informative data displays and data manipulation techniques to support interactive data exploration. Data displays are generally selected to fit the data types—layouts that work for temporal data might not be so useful for tabular data. Interaction techniques generally combine direct manipulation approaches (i.e., clicking or dragging directly on elements of the display) with familiar graphical user interface (GUI) widgets or touch screen manipulations. Both aspects of visualization design are discussed in more detail below.

But first, a motivational example. An exploration of the potential use of mental illness terms extracted from clinical notes to stratify patients based on symptom similarity illustrates some of the issues associated with the application of visualization in mental health informatics. Noting the challenges associated with identifying patients with syndromic mental health diagnoses like schizophrenia, Liu et al. [21] attempted to use terms found in clinical notes to stratify patients. Specifically, they developed a list of symptoms associated with schizophrenia and extracted terms on the list from clinical notes describing patients diagnosed with schizophrenia. Based on these terms, they used mathematical approaches to model topics found in the notes [22] and to embed the resulting patient descriptions in a two-dimensional space [23]. The two-dimensional embedding enables visualization of the similarity between patients within each "topic" identified by the topic analysis, for different numbers of topics. These displays clearly show that relatively clear distinctions between patients described by a small number of topics become less clear as the number of topics increases (Fig. 14.2), perhaps suggesting that increased granularity of description might increase the difficulty of classifying patients.

These two-dimensional scatterplots can be very useful tools for understanding data distributions, but they suffer from the information loss associated with any *dimensionality-reduction* techniques. Overcoming these limitations is one of the goals of *information visualization systems*. (Definitions of these terms and others in Table 14.1.) Designers of these tools might attempt to design displays capable of showing relationships between multiple visualizations, perhaps through multiple views, each displaying relationships between multiple visual representations of the data. These views might be linked through interactive controls supporting manipulation and exploration of data, using computational power to increase the potential for data plots to go beyond showing static pictures to supporting active interrogation

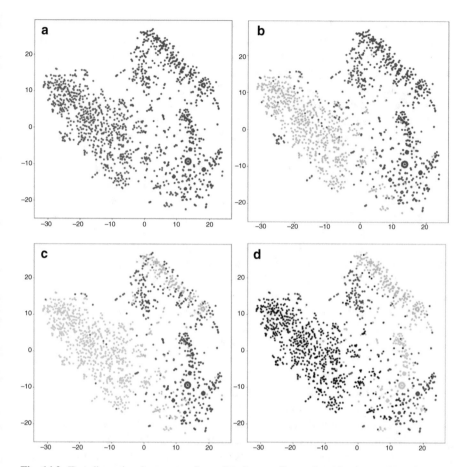

Fig. 14.2 Two-dimensional representations of patient profiles, colored by the number of topics. When two topics are used, the patients appear to separate into two well-defined groups (**a**). As the number of topics increases to three (**b**), four (**c**), and five (**d**), the cohorts become more intermingled, suggesting that additional detail in diagnoses might complicate distinguishing between patients. Figures courtesy of J. Tenenbaum, based on an analysis by Liu et al. [21]

of data. To see how this might be done, we must discuss both the *tasks* that might be supported by visualization tools and how designers might go about designing effective visualizations.

14.2.2   Visualization Tasks

Several theoretical models have been developed to describe the open-ended process of using visualization to understand new and unfamiliar sets of data. For example, the *Knowledge crystallization* model suggests that visualization might help in the identification of key attributes of a problem, the discovery of values for those attributes, and in the subsequent (and iterative) refining of relevant questions [4]—a process also known as *sensemaking* [9]. For example, a researcher exploring patterns associated with depression in a selected patient cohort might initially discover a few psychosocial indicators common to affected patients, and identify values for each of those indicators for each patient in the set. In subsequent exploration, this might in turn lead them to identify additional attributes of interest, perhaps including symptoms commonly associated with specific medical conditions, nutritional deficits, or relevant socio-economic indicators.

Task models provide insight into how visualization tools can best meet the goal of building an understanding of an unfamiliar data set. Perhaps most famously, Shneiderman's *Visual Information Seeking Mantra* suggests the importance of combining *overviews* for understanding data distribution with *features* for narrowing down to specific subsets and finally for an in-depth examination of data items—"Overview first, zoom and filter, then details-on-demand." [11] Anyone who's used an online map tool to go from a city-level view to find a specific type of restaurant, and then clicked on the provided link to see reviews can appreciate the utility of this approach.

Amar and Stasko took a different approach, focusing on a more specific set of 10 low-level tasks [24], and added tools for computing and re-arranging data for the three categories in the Visual Information Seeking Mantra. Although some mappings between the tasks are direct, others are more implicit. For example, even if not explicitly designed to do so, a visual overview might facilitate the identification of extreme values and determination of ranges (Table 14.2).

Although these models provide a preliminary framework for understanding visualization tasks, they only scratch the surface. Yi and colleagues proposed a different perspective, identifying seven types of interactions (Table 14.3) [13]. Related works have used the exploration of the user's perceptual processes to refine task descriptions [12, 26]; suggested additional tasks related to the process of collaborative data interpretation, including annotation, provenance tracking, and data sharing [27]; and linked low-level user interactions to higher-level goals [28]. Specialized task taxonomies have been developed for specific domains, including the evolution of networks [29]; both general [30] and temporal [31] graph visualization; multidimensional rankings [32]; and geovisualization [33], among others.

The embedding of patient profiles in a low-dimensional space (Fig. 14.2) provides an illustration of how some of these tasks might be supported by a visualization tool. Overviews are given by the scatterplots' depictions of the points in the 2-D space. Similarly, color codes support clustering, correlating, and finding anomalies. Other tasks such as filtering or retrieving details on demand might require interactive widgets. However, none of this task support comes "for free"—the scatterplot layouts, color codes for topic groups, and any controls that might be added to support interactive engagement with the data are all a result of careful visualization design.

Table 14.2 Comparison between the Visual Information Seeking Mantra and low-level tasks

Visual Information Seeking Mantra (Shneiderman, 1996) [11]	Low-level tasks (Amar and Stasko, 2005) [24]	Examples
Overview	Find extremum	Which patients are the most/least physically active?
	Determine range	What are the lowest and highest scores of these patients on the mini-mental state exam? [25]
	Characterize distribution?	What is the distribution of the expression levels of this protein in these samples
Zoom and filter	Filter	Which patients are over 70 years of age?
Details on demand	Retrieve value	What is the expression level of this gene in that sample?
	Compute derived value	What is the average number of daily interpersonal contacts for individuals in this cohort?
	Sort	Order patients by frequency of physical activity (# events/week)
	Find anomalies	Which participants had unexpected relationships between physical activity and self-reported Well-being?
	Cluster	Which participants are similar to this one?
	Correlate	What is the correlation between metabolites and protein expression for these patients?

Table 14.3 Categories of information visualization tasks, as defined by Yi and colleagues [13]

Task	
Select	Mark something as interesting
Explore	Show me something else
Reconfigure	Show me a different arrangement
Encode	Show me a different representation
Abstract/elaborate	Show me more or less detail
Filter	Show me something conditionally
Connect	Show me related items

14.2.3 Building Visualizations

Task frameworks suggest what researchers might hope to accomplish with visualizations, but they do not address *how* this might be done. Developing novel and increasingly powerful tools in support of these tasks is a goal of visualization research. Once again, experience from previous work can prove useful, in the form of models for the process of designing visualization tools [16, 34–36]. Although these models provide differing perspectives, several key steps are critical to the success of visualization efforts.

14.2.3.1 Understanding User Needs and Goals

Also referred to as "domain problem and data characterization" [35], the first step in building a visualization is often to build detailed models of the likely users of a system, the domains in which they work, and the goals that they would hope to accomplish with a visualization. Building on contextual interviewing [37] and related techniques developed in the human-computer interaction literature [19, 38], these user-centered activities use close observation and interaction with potential users to inform the design of tools that will ideally be well-suited to meet identified needs. Insights gained through such efforts might influence the terminology used in the visualization tools, the types of data items and relationships that are displayed, and the interactions that are supported. Thinking back to our 2-dimensional representation of schizophrenia patients (Fig. 14.2), a tool to be used by a researcher for identifying subpopulations in a larger sample might be designed to provide clinicians and researchers the ability to view cohorts of patients, to compare them against each other, and to visualize differential outcomes over time. A very different tool based on the same dataset might be used by patients to see how they and their family members resembled or differed from others with similar diagnoses. This patient-facing tool might provide a display that focused on reduced complexity, using lay (as opposed to scientific) descriptions of symptoms and diagnoses, and focusing on individual instances rather than overall patterns.

14.2.3.2 Preparing Data

As with many other data science efforts [39], visualization work involves a good amount of behind-the-scenes effort. Data cleansing, normalization of textual labels, converting continuous to discrete values (or vice-versa), and efforts familiar to data analysts might be accompanied by additional considerations specific to visualization design. Patient ages, for example, might be kept as continuous values if they are to be used as an axis in a 2D scatterplot, or discretized into 10-year ranges if colors are to be used to represent ages. Additional transformations might include converting data to formats most amenable to processing by visualization systems. This may entail data tables [4], graphs or trees [34], or some other representation of one of the data types to be discussed below. Some projects might require the imputation of missing values or dimensionality reduction through methods such as the 2D embedding used in the schizophrenia data example described above (Fig. 14.2). In the simplest case, the endpoint of this process is a collection of items, each with some number of attributes. More complex datasets may involve relationships between items of different types, with each relationship potentially being described by attributes of its own.

14.2.3.3 Displaying Data

Sometimes referred to as "visualization abstraction" [34] or "visual mapping" [4], the design of the displays at the heart of information visualizations involves deciding how data items and their attributes will be displayed. A simplified version of this design process breaks down into three design phases: the selection of a guiding visual metaphor, arranging items in space and using visual properties to encode attribute values.

Selection of a guiding visual metaphor is a fancy way of saying, "what sort of visualization are you going to use"? At its most basic, this question asks you to consider the types of data in your dataset, how they relate to each other, and how you might want to display those data visually to best support key questions. For analyses focused on near-continuous values, such as exploring the relationship between an individual's age and their average daily time spent on social media, you might use a traditional 2D scatterplot, with one primary value on each axis, perhaps coloring points by the individual's gender (Fig. 14.3a). This basic scatterplot might be enhanced by histograms displaying the distribution of values on each of three main dimensions (Fig. 14.3b). That same dataset might also be represented instead in terms of five-year age ranges, with values for each age range plotted in vertical lanes (Fig. 14.3c), or as the number of items gets larger, bar charts (Fig. 14.3d) or violin plots (Fig. 14.3e) or other displays capable of showing data distributions.

For hierarchical data, potentially including broad classes of mental health phenomena and their decomposition into progressively more specific phenomena, a tree diagram with general classes on the top or left progressing toward more specific options on the bottom or right (Fig. 14.4).

The use of space to encode information is key to many, but not all, visualizations. For bar charts and scatterplots, the location in the axes naturally convey values such as age, frequency of social media use, etc., with the lower-left corner often corresponding to the lowest value of attributes, which increase to the upper-right. In tree diagrams, the position might be used to depict the relationships between items, with more general items on the top/left vs. the bottom/right.

Other approaches might forego the use of location to encode data, opting instead for visual clarity. Network diagrams, including depictions of relationships between people, are often depicted as node-link diagrams rendered through so-called "force-directed" algorithms [40] that use simulated physical mechanisms based on the relative weights of connections between nodes to "push" or "pull" those nodes closer together or further apart, in the hopes of identifying a comprehensible layout (Fig. 14.5). Also referred to as graph diagrams, these network visualizations can be used to display almost any sort of relationships—including mechanistic views of relationships between genes, molecules, diseases, and symptoms; interpersonal networks identifying interactions between individuals in a community; bibliographic

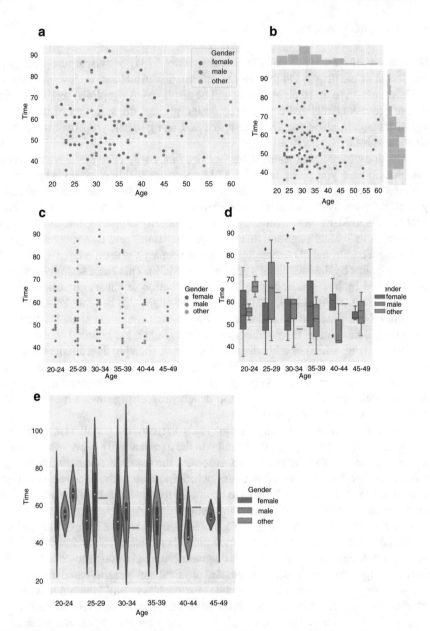

Fig. 14.3 Multiple displays of synthetic data relating social media use (in minutes/day) to the age of the user. (**a**) A basic scatterplot with age on the x-axis and minutes/day on the y-axis colored by gender. (**b**) an alternative scatterplot augmented with histograms showing the distribution of the age and minutes/day variables. (**c**) A view of individuals binned by age in 5-year ranges, with multiple columns dividing each bin by gender. In this view, each point is plotted explicitly. (**d**) A box and whisker plot, showing the median value (horizontal line), 1st and 3rd inter-quartile-range (bottom and top of boxes), extreme ranges (1.5 IQRs from the first and 3rd), and extreme points (beyond 1.5 IQRs). (**e**) A violin plot, showing the ranges given in the box plot, with the horizontal extent of each lane showing the distribution of values

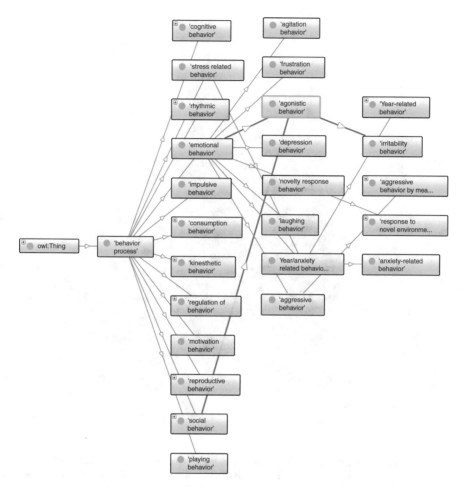

Fig. 14.4 A rendering of a subset of the human phenotype ontology [40], as displayed by the OntoGraf visualization in the Protégé [41] ontology development tool. Descendants of the top-level concept "behavior process" are shown in the third column with subclasses of "emotional behavior" and "agonistic behavior" shown in subsequent columns. Mousing over "agonistic behavior" causes incoming relationships to be highlighted in bold, emphasizing the dual inheritance nature of "agonistic behavior," which is both an "emotional behavior" and a "social behavior"

networks of literature co-citation and related topics, and countless others. Visual attributes can be used to encode additional detail—for example, by using the *size* of a node to indicate the importance of an entity, the *thickness* of edges (the lines between nodes) to indicate strength of associations, and *colors* of either nodes or edges to indicate categorical grouping. Despite their strengths, network diagrams can be hard to work with, as thousands of connections that might be possible even with a moderately-sized dataset of hundreds of items can lead to difficulties in interpreting very large graphs (colloquially known as "hairballs"). A large body of prior visualization work has resulted in many creative approaches to improving the comprehensibility of large network datasets [43, 44].

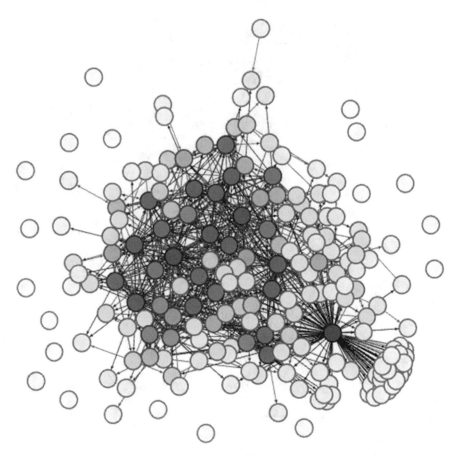

Fig. 14.5 An example of a force-directed network, involving 981 connections between 200 individuals who discussed mental disorders on a health-related social network. Measures of the connectivity properties of the nodes and online social activity were correlated with recovery [42]

Although these examples are exclusively focused on locating objects on a two-dimensional plane, visualizations in higher dimensions are certainly possible. One of the pioneering early papers in the field—"Information visualization using 3D interactive animation"—combined a variety of three-dimensional projected views with interactions designed to move data points in space to reveal those that would otherwise have been distorted [2]. So-called "zooming" visualizations combine an (x,y) placement for each item with a magnification factor, creating a "stack" of objects that can be displayed at different scales [45], just like an small overview of a large image or map file might be placed alongside a large view zoomed in to show detail. These higher-dimensionality displays should be used with care, as the additional value-added might be more than offset by increased difficulties in navigating these more complex spaces.

Encoding Attribute Values Having placed data items in space, the visualization designer will likely move next to the question of how each item—or each relationship—should be displayed. Almost any aspect of the rendering can be used to convey information about each item: color, shape, size, orientation, texture, and other so-called *retinal variables* can be used to encode dimensions of the data objects [5]. Some mappings, such as using the size of an object to represent a continuous attribute or a color to a nominal variable, may be relatively familiar. However, careful design is necessary, as inappropriate encodings can cause confusion.

Layouts and visual properties are often chosen to maximize the utilization of available space, the number of dimensions displayed, and the clarity of the resulting depiction. Careful choice of layouts and visual encodings can embed several dimensions in a single plot, with coordinated interactions between multiple representations of a single data set increasing the number of dimensions that can be included [46]. Similarly, work on graph drawing has explored layout algorithms designed to reduce clutter and increase the comprehensibility in complex graphs such as the example shown in Fig. 14.5 [47]. Although the number of different ways to combine colors, shapes, sizes, other properties to encode data in a 2-D space may seem daunting, a large body of prior experience provides guidance [10, 16, 48, 49].

Referring back to the patient profiles displayed in Fig. 14.2, we can see that each patient is represented by a dot, with two to five colors used to indicate the topic groupings in panels A-D, and the (x,y) position used to indicate the patient's location in the reduced-dimensionality 2-D space. Given additional details about each patient that might be extracted from the clinical records used to generate these embedding, we might ask how alternative views might encode additional information. For example, we might plot patient age on the x-axis and body-mass index on the y-axis, to explore relationships between topics and key demographic and health factors. This view might keep the color-coding of the two topics while using the size of each patient's dot to provide a measure of the frequency or severity of mental health issues. Although this new proposed view might be helpful for some goals, it might come at the cost of losing the clear separation between topics found in Fig. 14.2. This tradeoff exemplifies a tradeoff familiar to visualization developers: for many non-trivial datasets, we find that no single view can meet all, or even most, needs. Bridging this gap often requires a combination of multiple views of a dataset and interactive techniques for exploring and manipulating those views.

Creating effective and clear displays of scientific data requires a combination of careful consideration of the underlying data, clear scientific and statistical thinking, and an understanding of basic design principles. Done poorly, static graphs can lead to suboptimal or even potentially misleading data presentations [50, 51]. Problematic graph designs include bar graphs with non-zero baselines, which exaggerate small differences; scatter plots that use the radius (and not the area) of a point to indicate a magnitude, thus exaggerating differences (as the area grows with the square of the radius); bar charts providing relatively simple summaries of distributions, as opposed to richer displays of individual data points [52, 53]; odds-ratio displays that present zero-based (as opposed to one) values on a linear (as opposed to logarithmic scale), thus making an odds-ratio of 2 seem much larger than an odds-ratio of 0.5 [54]; and many others. Aspiring designers of information visualization displays will need to understand basic design principles: the books of Edward Tufte provide an excellent introduction [8, 55–57]. To avoid all-too-frequent difficulties with color selection, e.g. non-color-blind-friendly palettes, tools such as colorbrewer [58] (available at www.colorbrewer2.org) should be used to select color palettes whenever possible.

14.2.3.4 Interacting with Data

Appropriate data layouts are necessary, but not sufficient, for successful interactive visualization. Without techniques for interacting with the data, visualization is just a pretty picture on a screen. It is only when we begin to leverage the interaction capabilities associated with modern graphical user interfaces and touch screens that visualization tools become truly engaging and enabling. Appropriate interactions can transform a visualization into an engaging tool for exploring complex data, as users can explore different perspectives on data, use filters to restrict displays to data of interest, search and browse for answers, and potentially even turn data analysis into a social activity [59, 60].

Information visualization interaction techniques stem from the long history of the *direct manipulation* user interfaces familiar to any user of modern computing tools. Unlike the command-line based interfaces of the 1980s and earlier that required typed commands with complex syntax, direct manipulation interfaces rely on graphical displays, mouse-controlled pointers (and later touch-based input) for direct control of items on the screen, and a variety of graphical widgets, including buttons, scrollbars, and more complex tools for selecting items and values and for initiating or stopping tasks. These operations are "rapid, incremental, and reversible" [61], with minimal syntax and reduced need for error messages, as input values were tightly controlled by the graphical widgets.

These principles inform the design of interactions for information visualization tools. When using a scatterplot display containing many points (Fig. 14.2), one might click-draw a rectangle to select a subset of points of interest. Zoom and pan controls might similarly be used to navigate around the space, using interactions familiar to anyone who has used an online map. For a network display (Fig. 14.5), users might click on nodes to highlight connected nodes, or even drag nodes to new positions to reconfigure (Table 14.3). In any display, selecting a data point can lead to the display of all of the attributes of interest—"details on demand" [11].

In the spirit of direct manipulation, all of these approaches emphasize interacting with the display whenever possible. Direct interactions eliminate the division between input and output, allowing users to click or select directly on the table or graph displaying the data in question. Compared to earlier generations of textual interfaces based on complex commands, these interfaces reduce the effort required for manipulation of the data and freeing the user to focus on the key task of interest—learning from the data. When possible, operations for rescaling, resizing, zooming, or filtering, should be implemented as 'dynamic queries", providing rapid (<100 ms) updates on each interaction event, giving users the impression of interactive and animated data [62].

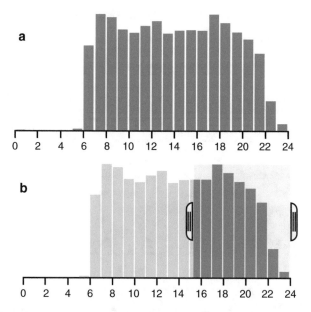

Fig. 14.6 An illustration of a double-thumb slider. (**a**) A histogram shows the frequency of flight departure times throughout the day. (**b**) To focus on late afternoon flights, the user has drawn a rectangular region starting from approximately 3 pm until midnight. This box acts as a graphical query: flights within this time interval remain selected, while others are filtered from the current result set. Handles on the vertical edges of the region act can be dragged to the left or the right to expand the region included in the result set. The entire box can be dragged to move the selected window over different time ranges (source: https://square.github.io/crossfilter/)

Interacting directly with the data might break down somewhat for high-dimensional datasets. As only a subset of possible dimensions might be visible at any given time, traditional (or slightly enhanced) widgets might be used to choose which dimensions are shown in a scatterplot or to filter displayed values to show only those items matching some range of values or categories in an unseen dimension. Another popular approach, first developed by Tweedie et al. in the Attribute Explorer [63], involves using multiple histograms, each capturing the frequency of values of an attribute. Each of these histograms can then be used as a selector, through a double-thumbed scrollbar (Fig. 14.6) used to limit values to a selected subset of ranges. As values are constrained based on a filter in one dimension, all histograms are dynamically revised to show the distribution of values across the selected subset. Concurrent filters on multiple attributes form a conjunctive query—a process known as *cross-filtering* (Fig. 14.7).

Cross-filters are a special case of a more generalized technique for using multiple perspectives on a dataset to overcome the limitations of any given display. *Coordinated views* combine multiple visualizations of a given dataset, generally showing different attributes, with linked interactions showing relationships between

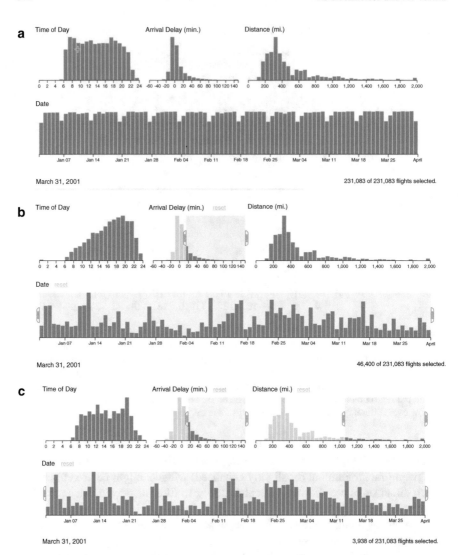

Fig. 14.7 An illustration of a cross-filtering interface. Histograms for each of four variables (time of day, arrival delay, distance, and date), also act as input filters. As a filter is adjusted to restrict the range of values included based on the current dimension, histograms for the other dimensions are dynamically adjusted with each mouse movement to display the distribution of the remaining items across the other dimensions. (**a**) The complete dataset, containing 231,083 flights. (**b**) A filtered dataset, with arrival delays restricted to those of 20 minutes or more. Note that flights with longer delays tend to happen more frequently later in the day. (**c**) Further restriction to flights of more than 1100 miles suggests longer flights with longer delays occur at similar frequencies throughout the day. (Source: https://square.github.io/crossfilter/)

the views. Thus, mousing over or clicking on an item in one view might cause that same item to be highlighted in all other available views, enabling visualization of that item in comparison to others, through multiple perspectives. Other possibilities include the mouse-over selection of several items, a technique known as *brushing*. Returning to the psychological case study previously described (Fig. 14.2), we might imagine coordinating the two-dimensional plot with views providing histograms of patients by age or by diagnosis count, or perhaps with a network view showing patients related by shared diagnostic codes or symptoms. For additional examples of coordinated views, see Figs. 14.8 and 14.16.

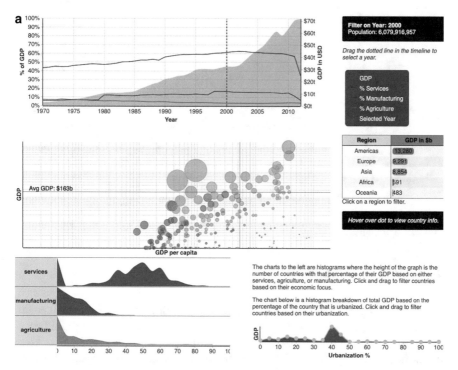

Fig. 14.8 Coordinated views of national economic data from the world bank. (**a**) An unfiltered view of economic data with graphs listing GDP by time (top), GDP vs. GDP per capita, and a histogram of the number of countries with different levels of services, manufacturing, and agriculture. (**b**) Filtering the view to the countries in the midrange of services shows a flatter and lower-level of overall GDP, while also removing some of the countries on the higher-end of both GDP and GDP per capita. (source: https://drarmstr.github.io/chartcollection/examples/worldbank_example.html)

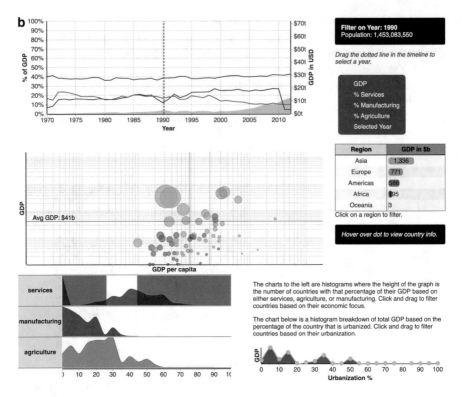

Fig. 14.8 (continued)

14.3 Mental Health Data

Visualization approaches might be applied to several data sources for mental health information (Fig. 14.9), including population and provider-based surveys for prevalence estimates and clinical databases containing patient-level data such as electronic health records (EHRs). Each of these data types brings opportunities for visualization.

14.3.1 Survey and Psychometric Instrument Data

In medicine, clinicians and researchers have access to a multitude of instruments and technologies for objectively measuring clinical phenomena. In mental health and the behavioral sciences, psychometric instruments are the primary method for obtaining objective, standard measures of mental and behavioral phenomena (see also Chap. 9). A psychometric instrument is a structured, pre-defined procedure for collecting standardized, quantifiable data about some mental or behavioral

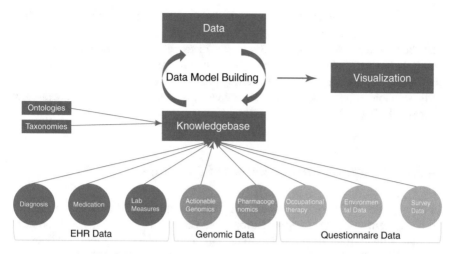

Fig. 14.9 Mental health data sources and workflow to build visual analytic models. This figure is adapted from Boyd et al.'s [65] proposed work on visual approaches for electronic health record data. The circles below represent different sources of data related to mental health. The integration of these data sources into a single knowledgebase is critical to deriving insights related to mental health using visual analytics. Further, data standardization and transformation using ontologies and taxonomies would help build a reproducible common data model. Lastly, data modeling approaches can refine the raw data to knowledge for visualization

phenomena, and is formally defined as "a set of stimuli administered to an individual or a group under standard conditions to obtain a sample of behavior for assessment" [66]. Psychometric instruments include structured interviews, inventories, rating scales, surveys, questionnaires, tasks, and checklists. These instruments are developed using formal statistical methods and are often used to obtain a standard measure of some latent, i.e., not directly observable, phenomenon.

Psychometric instruments are widely accepted tools in the field of mental health and the behavioral sciences. Stakeholders in diverse roles across the health enterprise routinely perform a variety of activities related to psychometric instruments to achieve a variety of goals. Researchers use psychometric instruments to acquire knowledge about the nature of mental and behavioral phenomena. It is used to obtain information about the nature and severity of symptoms, and about patient exposures, living environments, and to select appropriate treatments. They also use them to monitor patients' response to treatment, and to detect potential adverse reactions.

Federally funded survey programs collect several mental health data points related to the prevalence of disorders. Standardized mental health instruments used for data collection provides structured data, which can be modeled for visualization. For example, the National Health Interview Survey (NHIS) uses the K-6 instrument which collects the history of mental health care [67]. Similarly, the Behavioral Risk Factor Surveillance System (BRFSS) [68] and the National Health and Nutrition Examination Survey (NHANES) collected data using the patient health questionnaire (PHQ-9) [69] instrument, to diagnose several mental health disorders efficiently. These questionnaires collect not only the history of mental health but also the severity of the disorders. Bar charts, histograms, and trend graphs showing changes over time, often segmented by demographic groupings [70], are often used to visualize these data. As familiar starting points, these approaches can be particularly valuable when linked with alternative presentations in a coordinated-view framework (Figs. 14.6, 14.7 and 14.8).

14.3.2   Electronic Health Record (EHR) Data

In the past decade, EHRs have been implemented as integral components across all health centers in the USA and Europe (see Chapter 16) [71, 72]. EHRs contain a vast amount of data about both individual patients and local patient populations. Patient data typically include family history, social history, and medical history; presenting problems and signs and symptoms identified for each encounter, as well as results of laboratory tests, imaging, physical exams, and neuropsychological exams. EHRs contain mental health information in both structured (diagnosis codes, lab measures, medications, questionnaires) and unstructured (patient notes) data formats [73]. EHRs also provide data about providers and the care delivery practices of the organization maintaining the EHR. For example, EHRs contain information about the volume and types of conditions treated by a provider or the organization, as well documentation, prescribing, and ordering patterns. In larger health systems, EHRs may also contain data about the clinical decision support features built into the EHR for conditions for which a patient is being treated, as well as details related to physician "override" of decision support recommendations.

Approaches to visualizing EHR and administrative data often rely on the temporal nature of the data, using timelines to indicate key events and diagnoses [74]. Furthermore, sophisticated algorithms are developed to build data models from unstructured data (patient notes) [75–78], and to use temporal displays to visualize the resulting data [79, 80].

14.3.3   Genetic Data

Genetics plays an essential role in understanding the development of disease risk. Unlike certain diseases where risks can be identified by genetic variation in one or two genes such as cystic fibrosis, mental health disorders risks are much more complex [81, 82]. There are hundreds of genetic variations across the genome that are shown to be associated with mental health disorders. The application of visualization to genomics and genetics data has been the subject of substantial work over the past 20 years. Visualization efforts in this domain include gene expression *heatmaps*, networks of interacting proteins, annotated genetic sequences, and many others, as summarized in recent reviews [83, 84]. A common data visualization technique used to depict results in genome-wide association studies (GWAS) are *Manhattan plots*—scatterplots with location of genetic variations (commonly referred as single nucleotide polymorphisms or SNPs, pronounced "snips") on the chromosome are shown on x-axis and p-value on the y-axis (Fig. 14.10-I). These plots provide a way to detect SNPs significantly associated with a disease. To further understand the role of a specific SNP or genomic region requires an integration of additional information which can add complexity to visualization. LocusTrack, Haploview, and similar tools have focused on visualization of GWAS results (Fig. 14.10) [85], and provide support for multiple types of annotations. These tools have become standards in the GWAS analysis pipeline [87].

Similar approaches have been used to provide insight into pharmacogenomics data by comparing drugs and relevant variants [88]. Bihlmeyer et al. provide an example of the use of network visualizations to understand gene expression and genome-wide association data related to Alzheimer's disease, including network visualizations of genes in relevant pathways [89]. In the past decade, electronic health record (EHR) linked biobanks have enabled a powerful way of investigating genetic association of SNPs with hundreds of diseases in a study population, also known as *phenome-wide association study* (PheWAS). PheWAS-View,

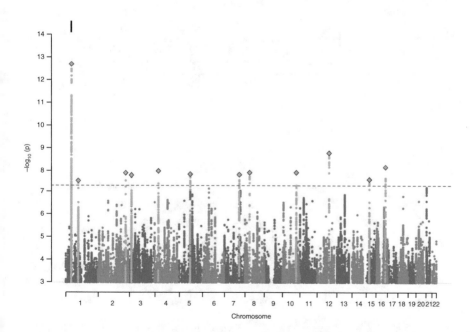

Fig. 14.10 (I) Common visual representation of GWAS results known as Manhattan plot. (II) GWAS result visualization from LocusTrack (**a**) publicly available GWAS schizophrenia results, (**b**) genes from the region of interest, and (**c**) genomic annotations [85]. (III) A network of diseases created from genetic association results from EHR-based PheWAS [86]

II

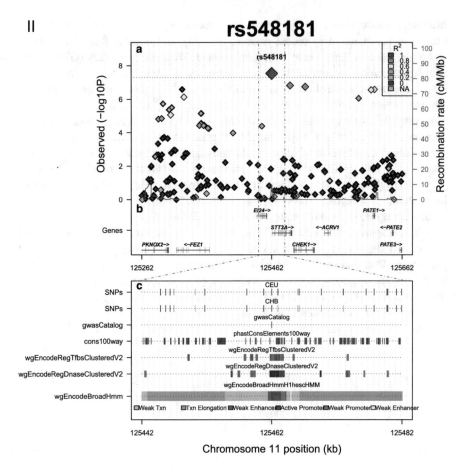

III

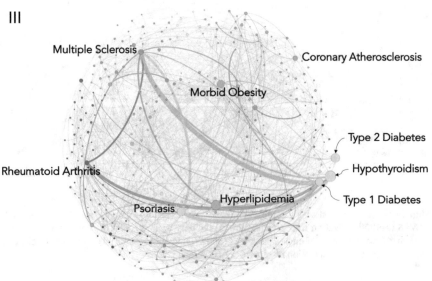

Fig. 14.10 (continued)

Synthesis-View, PheGWAS are some tools to create visual summaries from these complex data. Network based approaches (such as graph theory) have been implemented to create maps of diseases using findings from EHR-based genetic studies (Fig. 14.10-III).

14.3.4   Environmental Data

Although EHRs are an invaluable resource for mental health researchers with a longitudinal representation of an individual's health, EHRs typically contain limited data about important features of a person's physical, sociocultural, and interpersonal environments. Several studies demonstrate a link between features of physical environments and mental health, including green space, noise, air pollution, weather, and housing conditions [90]. These environmental conditions can be risk or resilience factors in the development of mental health conditions. Data on environmental variables are often collected by state and federal agencies and stored in a publicly accessible database. Geographical mapping of an individual's address to longitude and latitude is being used to integrate EHR data with environmental exposures [91]. Further, geospatial analysis of diseases, medication, and environmental exposure can determine the risk of different exposures on various mental health conditions. Applications of visualization to environmental data have included communication of risks of environmental exposures [92], the use of maps to visualize relationships between locations of liquor stores and socioeconomic factors on alcohol expenditures [93], and network visualizations describing relationships between environmental factors associated with schizophrenia [94].

14.3.5   Mobile Health Data

Over the past decade, mobile technologies have become an integral part of society, not only opening new possibilities for patients to track health, but also placing these technologies at their fingertips. The mobile app space is flooded with health-related apps capable of tracking mental health symptoms, providing self-help interventions, passively collecting data, and building relevant cognitive skills, [95, 96] Mobile apps can provide data in real-time, providing tremendous potential in developing preventive interventions related to mental health. Example applications include star plots for visualizing stress-related physiological signals collected by a mobile device (Fig. 14.11) [97], visualization of smart-watch data together with user interactions and text entries for tracking mental health status (Fig. 14.12) [98], and other patient-oriented mobile health applications designed to support mental health treatment (Fig. 14.13) [99].

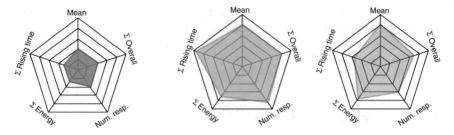

Fig. 14.11 Star plots indicating skin conductance measures during three phases of activity (relax, stress, and recovery) associated with mental stress. Each star plot shows 5 dimensions of skin conductance activity, through a point on each scale indicating the magnitude of the measurement. The resulting shape provides an overview of the various magnitudes, enabling easy comparison between the results at the different phases (figure from Holzinger, et al. Al. 2013 [97], © IFIP)

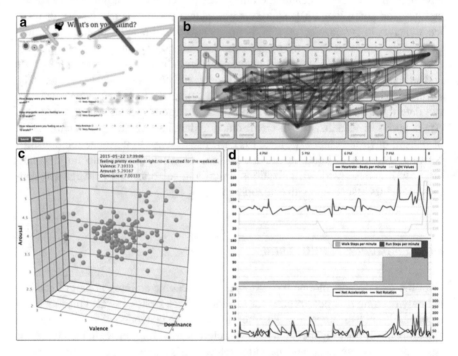

Fig. 14.12 A web application displaying interaction data with a web-based tool for mental health monitoring, combining (**a**) mouse-movement and (**b**) keyboard interaction traces for text entry of mood depictions with (**c**) a 3-D display of analyses of input texts and (**d**) scrollable timeline views of physiological measurements collected by a wearable device [98]

14.3.6   Using Data and Predictive Models in Mental Health Visualization

Understanding a patient's complete mental health status requires access to different data variables such as past medical history, prescriptions, laboratory test results, patient's access to healthcare, and socioeconomic status. Dashboards providing

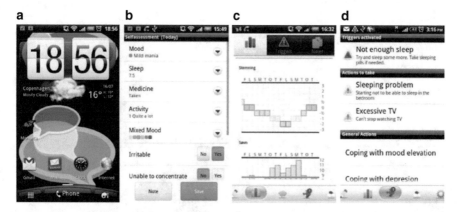

Fig. 14.13 Views of a mobile application for mental disorder treatment, including (**a**) a background illustrating patient-specific factors, (**b**) a form for self-reporting of patient status, (**c**) a visualization of historical data, and (**d**) patient feedback (figure used with permission) [99]

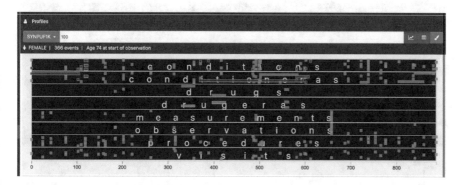

Fig. 14.14 Longitudinal EHR profile view in OHDSI ATLAS, including a stacked layout of observations recorded in different domains, placed on the x-axis based on the number of days from the first observation. Some rows (conditions, drugs, measurements, observations, procedures, and visits), use gray squares to represent individual events, while others (condition_eras and drug_eras) use rectangles extending in the horizontal direction to indicate states that persist over a specified time interval. The dashboard tool also has a feature to highlight events. For example, the events highlighted in red are observations of major depressive disorder (MDD) on different visits and prescribed medications for MDD are represented in orange

high-level overviews through multiple displays are proving to help navigate through complex information to extract trends and knowledge about the data.

The design and view of dashboards will vary based on the target audience and the most relevant metrics of the data. Some dashboards are designed for exploratory views of the data. The OHDSI (observational health data science and informatics) program [100] developed the ATLAS dashboard, which lets the user explore different views of the data. Users can interactively build a patient-specific dashboard to see longitudinal trends in data. For example, Fig. 14.14 shows a longitudinal view of patients' health history, with the highlight event option of the dashboard used to color code the event of interest— in this case, the diagnosis of major depressive disorder

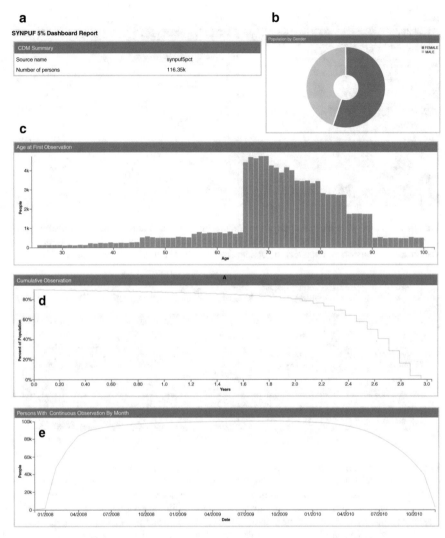

Fig. 14.15 Cohort view in OHDSI ATLAS. The dashboard showcases different views of data metrics for a defined cohort. (**a**) Textual summary of the sample size of the cohort. (**b**) Doughnut plot to view cohort by gender. (**c**) A histogram plot to display the distribution of cohort age at the first observation event. (**d**) A line graph represents the distribution of time observed in the cohort with the number of years on the x-axis and percent population on the y-axis. (**e**) Lastly, visual representation (line plot) of the number of people with an observation by month between 2008 and 2010

and prescription of related drugs. The other features of ATLAS include building cohorts on specific sets of questions and creating multiple alternative views of data.

Cohort views summarizing patterns and trends over populations can be useful for stratification and subpopulation identification. An ATLAS view of a cohort of patients with major depressive disorder (MDD) is given in Fig. 14.15. The default view of the dashboard shows general demographic information in different graphs

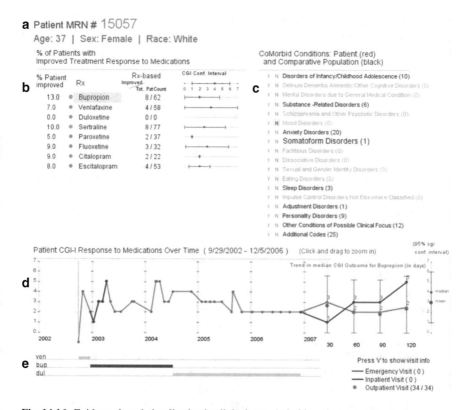

Fig. 14.16 Evidence-based visualization in clinical care. A dashboard prototype to display a comparative view of a patient's depression treatment and knowledge from patients with similar treatment. (**a**) Patient's demographics. (**b**) Displaying evidence of treatment response for different depression medications and improvements in patients on the clinical global impressions (CGI) scale for mental health status. (**c**) A view of the similarity between the patient's reported comorbidities in comparison to other patients on similar treatment. (**d**) A display of both the longitudinal view of the patient's treatment history and projected trends of the CGI metric if the patient were to be prescribed bupropion. Coordinated interactions link the various views [64]

such as population by gender (pie chart), age at first observation of MDD (bar chart), and the number of observations by month (line chart). There are several other predefined views available to drill down in the dataset and generate dashboard reports for visit occurrences, drug prescription, surgical procedures, lab measurements, and observational data, among others.

Using data streams from different domains has become imperative for decision making for clinical care. Although visualization can facilitate cross-sectional views of different data metrics in dashboards, displays of raw data might obscure patterns and trends of interest. Prediction machine-learning models can turn these raw data into knowledge for effective intervention and preventive care [101]. Mane et al. proposed VisualDecisionLinc (VDL), which demonstrates an effective way to visualize patients' treatment response to antidepressants [64] (Fig. 14.16). Particularly, displaying the metric of treatment response and comorbid conditions from other patients can help in identifying the best treatment regimen for the patient. Predictive modeling has several known applications in mental health, such as adverse drug reactions [102], prognostics [103], disease progression [104], and treatment efficacy [105], among others.

14.4   Current State and Outstanding Challenges

Advances in visualization research show multiple paths to greater use of visualization across multiple fields, with opportunities for application in mental health informatics. Stand-alone tools designed to meet specific needs can lower the cost of entry into the use of visualizations. For example, the Cytoscape network visualization tool has gained widespread adoption through its use of a plug-in architecture that has enabled numerous domain-specific customizations [106, 107].

Integration into common data analysis tools has also been proven to be a successful strategy, as in the UpSet set visualization tool [108], which was retooled as UpSetR [109], a package for the popular statistical analysis environment. Similarly, the vis-JS2jupyter tool [110] integrates network visualizations with widely-used Jupyter scientific notebooks. An alternative line of research has focused on the development of tools to ease the creation of interactive visualizations. The introduction of the D3 (data-driven-documents) [111] Javascript library in 2011 was a notable step forward in the expressivity of web-based tools for creating visualizations with Javascript, scalable vector graphics (SVG), and HTML. Subsequent efforts have extended this model to provide greater performance and functionality [112, 113].

These advances from the research world are complemented by commercial offerings providing cloud-based advanced visualization techniques. Specialized tools such as ESRI's ArcGIS geographic information systems (www.esri.com) and general-purpose tools such as SpotFire (www.tibco.com) and Tableau (www.tableau.com) offer powerful capabilities that might be particularly appealing to researchers and organizations who are not well-equipped to develop systems "from scratch", and have the funding to be able to purchase commercial software licenses.

As efforts described throughout this volume continue to increase the volume and the use of well-structured mental health data, the application of visualization to mental health problems will almost certainly become more commonplace. However, we can also expect to see that these efforts will struggle with two key challenges faced by previous efforts: handling of uncertainty, and rigorous evaluation of visualization systems.

14.4.1   Uncertainty

Uncertainties, especially in health care data, can create gaps in knowledge and hence, potential misinterpretation. In the mental health domain of health care, uncertainties have been found to arise in selecting the best course of action for a patient; determining whether a provider is appropriate for a given role; and in evaluating the impact of external, possibly unpredictable events [114]. Uncertainties can also arise from systematic, but poorly understood variations in care patterns. For example, Agniel et al. show biases of physician's practice are often overlooked when using EHR data for data modeling. They found that "hour of the day, the day of the week and the amount of time between consecutive tests is more predictive of three-year survival than the actual value of the test" [115]. Similar questions may arise when trying to infer the timing of events from the clinical text, with relative timing ("for the past several weeks", or "since the loss of their job") making histories of critical events difficult to reconstruct with any certainty.

Uncertainties in exactly what is being described provide further complications. Symptoms, diagnoses, environmental influences, and social factors are all relevant in describing a person's mental health. However, unlike medical conditions, such as infectious disease, neoplasm, or internal bleeding, that might be confirmed by laboratory tests, imaging studies, and direct measurement of well-quantified phenomena such as blood pressure, mental health conditions and symptoms are often less directly observable, requiring expert clinical interpretation. Consequently, symptom and diagnosis "data" in mental health is less likely to represent a pure signal, and typically includes noise (including error) introduced by both measurement technologies and clinical reasoning. Given the many sources of potential ambiguity, how can visualization systems best handle uncertainties of causative factors, symptoms, and diagnoses?

As these challenges are not unique to mental health, a number of efforts have attempted to systematize approaches for visualization in the face of uncertainty. Skeels, et al. defined a classification of three core levels of uncertainty, adapted in Table 14.4 below to apply to mental health informatics. It comprises measurement precision at the base, followed by completeness and finally inference, with each subsequent level building on those that came before. Credibility and disagreement were noted as additional factors that can occur at any of the three levels [116].

Despite these and other efforts into understanding uncertainty visualization, there is no single simple answer to the question of how uncertainty should be displayed. The specific needs of any given combination of data, users, and tasks will likely influence choices of which uncertainty should be displayed, and how. Identifying appropriate approaches will likely continue to be complicated by evaluation challenges, as discussed below.

Table 14.4 Skeel's Taxonomy of Uncertainty [116]

Dimension	Definition	Example
Measurement precision	Variations in measurements or assessments	Variability in patients' assessments of symptom severity
Completeness	Extent of the availability of data, relative to a complete data set	Omissions of data on specific clinical episodes, or from specific providers
Inference	Uncertainty regarding results of predictions, modeling, or other summative analyses	Differences in clinicians' expectations of impact for a given therapy for a specific patient

14.4.2 Evaluation

Evaluation is a long-standing challenge in visualization research. Ideally, evaluation studies would enable comparisons between tools or techniques to determine which work best, for which tasks, thus informing future designs. Traditional human-computer interaction research efforts might conduct empirical user studies to compare quantitative metrics such as task completion time or error rates observed with different designs [38]. Unfortunately, such measures often fail to capture the complexities of visualization tasks (Table 14.2)—when one is trying to correlate items, or find anomalies, what does it mean to be done? When the goal is to build understanding, is faster necessarily better?

These questions have led to an active body of an investigation into the development of rigorous methods for evaluating visualizations (Table 14.5). North and colleagues proposed the measurement of insights gained while using a tool, showing that insight measurements confirm the results of traditional task measurements while also adding a novel perspective [119, 120]. Other proposed approaches involve in-depth case studies [121]; expert reviews [122], possibly involving heuristic guidelines [123]; combined design and validation models that tie system validation to design goals [35, 36]; and development of quality metrics [117]. Although these approaches do not provide the quantitative comparisons associated with

Table 14.5 Selected approaches to evaluation in visualization

Dimension	Description
Measurement of insights gained	Quantification of factors or insights learned during use of a tool. Allows the possibility of quantitative comparison between tools or approaches, but clear definition of what constitutes an insight might be elusive.
In-depth case studies	Longitudinal observation and engagement with expert users as they use tools and interpret data. Provides deep insights into mental models, approaches for using and interpreting visualizations. Can inform redesign and enhancement. Valuable, but expensive.
Expert reviews	Knowledgeable experts, including those with visualization/interaction expertise and problem domain experts, provide detailed critiques of design elements and suitability to task, often with reference to published heuristic design goals.
Combined design and validation models	End-to-end approaches that combine multiple design processes at increasing levels of specificity (including domain/problem characterization; data/operation abstractions; interaction design; and algorithm design) with a series of evaluations aimed specifically at each aspect of the design process [35, 36].
Development of quality metrics	Quantifiable assessments of aspects of a system design with respect to specified combinations of datasets, users, and tasks. Examples might include clutter reduction or the identification of relations between dimensions [117].
Assessment of user engagement	Surveys to measure the extent to which users were interested in voluntarily using a tool, for an extended period of time, for a particular reason, and with a valued outcome [118].

comparative user studies, they do build on the substantial experience of other efforts in visualization evaluation. Other efforts have attempted to assess user engagement [118], although the nature of exactly what that means and how it is measured has been the subject of some debate [124]. Consistent with broader trends toward greater attention to rigor and reproducibility, investigators have also proposed approaches for the development of replication studies in visualization evaluation [125].

14.5 Conclusion

The translation of new ideas into practice is a challenge in many fields, including information visualization. Although interactive tools and ubiquitous infographics exploit principles developed in the more than 30-year history of the field, many interesting ideas from the early days of the field have not made the leap to common use. The current maturity of information visualization at the time of the emergence of mental health informatics suggests exciting opportunities for both fields.

Just as with earlier efforts, effective application of visualization to mental health data will require a combination of the problem- and user-centered perspectives. Challenges in harmonizing, managing, and interpreting data will likely continue to feed the development of ontologies, data models (Chap. 7), analytic approaches, and visualization tools. In all cases, careful attention to specific user tasks and goals, particularly through the frameworks discussed above, will be vital to the construction of successful systems. Consideration of the differing perspectives of clinicians, researchers, patients, caregivers, and other key constituencies will be critical to ensuring alignment between goals and designs. Exploration of the possibilities may lead to new insights informing research, patient self-management, and clinical care.

References

1. Ruddle RA, Fateen W, Treanor D, Sondergeld P, Ouirke P Leveraging wall-sized high-resolution displays for comparative genomics analyses of copy number variation. In 2013 IEEE Symposium on Biological Data Visualization (BioVis). 2013. p. 89–96. https://doi.org/10.1109/BioVis.2013.6664351.
2. Robertson GG, Card SK, Mackinlay JD. Information visualization using 3D interactive animation. Commun ACM. 1993;36:57–71.
3. Dubois WEB. [The Georgia Negro] Income and expenditure of 150 Negro families in Atlanta, Ga., USA.
4. Readings in information visualization: using vision to think. San Francisco: Morgan Kaufmann Publishers; 1999.
5. Bertin J. Semiology of graphics: diagrams, networks, maps. Madison: The University of Wisconsin Press; 1983.
6. Friedman JH, Stuetzle W, John W. Tukey's work on interactive graphics. Ann Stat. 2002;30:1629–39.

7. Cleveland WS. Elements of graphing data. Monterey, CA: Wadsworth Advanced Books and Software; 1985.
8. Tufte ER. The visual display of quantitative information. Cheshire: Graphics Press; 1986.
9. Russell DM, Stefik MJ, Pirolli P, Card SK. The cost structure of sensemaking. In: Proceedings of the INTERACT '93 and CHI '93 conference on human factors in computing systems. New York: ACM; 1993. p. 269–76. https://doi.org/10.1145/169059.169209.
10. Ware C. Information visualization: perception for design. Amsterdam: Elsevier; 2012.
11. Shneiderman B The eyes have it: a task by data type taxonomy for information visualizations. In Proceedings 1996 IEEE symposium on visual languages. 1996. p. 336–343. https://doi.org/10.1109/VL.1996.545307.
12. Amar R, Stasko J BEST paper: a knowledge task-based framework for design and evaluation of information visualizations. In IEEE symposium on information visualization. 2004. p. 143–150. https://doi.org/10.1109/INFVIS.2004.10.
13. Yi, J. S., Ah-Kang, Y. a & Stasko, J. Toward a deeper understanding of the role of interaction in information visualization. IEEE Trans Vis Comput Graph. 13, 1224–1231 (2007).
14. Tory M, Moller T. Human factors in visualization research. IEEE Trans Vis Comput Graph. 2004;10:72–84.
15. Ward MO, Grinstein G, Keim D, Grinstein G, Keim D. Interactive data visualization: foundations, techniques, and applications. 2nd ed. Boca Raton, FL: A K Peters/CRC Press; 2015. https://doi.org/10.1201/b18379.
16. Spence R. Information visualization: an introduction. Incorporated: Springer Publishing Company; 2014.
17. Thomas JJ, Cook KA. A visual analytics agenda. IEEE Comput Graph Appl. 2006;26:10–3.
18. Keim DA, et al. Visual analytics: definition, process, and challenges. In: Information visualization. Heidelberg: Springer; 2008. https://doi.org/10.1007/978-3-540-70956-5_7.
19. Tukey JW. Exploratory data analysis. Reading, MA: Addison-Wesley; 1977.
20. Du Toit S, Steyn G, Stumpf R. Graphical exploratory data analysis. Berlin: Springer-Verlag; 1986.
21. Liu Q, et al. Symptom-based patient stratification in mental illness using clinical notes. J Biomed Inform. 2019;98:103274.
22. Blei DM, Ng AY, Jordan MI. Latent Dirichlet allocation. J Mach Learn Res. 2003;3:993–1022.
23. van der Maaten L, Hinton G. Visualizing Data using t-SNE. J Mach Learn Res. 2008;9:2579–605.
24. Amar R, Eagan J, Stasko J. Low-level components of analytic activity in information visualization. In: Proceedings of the proceedings of the 2005 IEEE symposium on information visualization 15. Minneapolis, MN: IEEE Computer Society; 2005. https://doi.org/10.1109/INFOVIS.2005.24.
25. Pangman VC, Sloan J, Guse L. An examination of psychometric properties of the mini-mental state examination and the standardized mini-mental state examination: implications for clinical practice. Appl Nurs Res. 2000;13:209–13.
26. Amar RA, Stasko JT. Knowledge precepts for design and evaluation of information visualizations. IEEE Trans Vis Comput Graph. 2005;11:432–42.
27. Heer J, Shneiderman B. Interactive dynamics for visual analysis. Commun ACM. 2012;55:45–54.
28. Brehmer M, Munzner T. A multi-level typology of abstract visualization tasks. IEEE Trans Vis Comput Graph. 2013;19:2376–85.
29. Ahn J, Plaisant C, Shneiderman B. A task taxonomy for network evolution analysis. IEEE Trans Vis Comput Graph. 2014;20:365–76.
30. Lee B, Plaisant C, Parr CS, Fekete J-D, Henry N. Task taxonomy for graph visualization. In: Proceedings of the 2006 AVI workshop on BEyond time and errors: novel evaluation methods for information visualization 1–5. New York: ACM; 2006. https://doi.org/10.1145/1168149.1168168.
31. Kerracher N, Kennedy J, Chalmers K. A task taxonomy for temporal graph visualisation. IEEE Trans Vis Comput Graph. 2015;21:1160–72.

32. Gratzl S, Lex A, Gehlenborg N, Pfister H, Streit M. LineUp: visual analysis of multi-attribute rankings. IEEE Trans Vis Comput Graph. 2013;19:2277–86.
33. Roth RE. An empirically-derived taxonomy of interaction primitives for interactive cartography and Geovisualization. IEEE Trans Vis Comput Graph. 2013;19:2356–65.
34. Chi EH. A taxonomy of visualization techniques using the data state reference model. In IEEE symposium on information visualization 2000. INFOVIS 2000. PRO 69–75 (2000). https://doi.org/10.1109/INFVIS.2000.885092.
35. Munzner T. A nested model for visualization design and validation. IEEE Trans Vis Comput Graph. 2009;15:921–8.
36. Meyer M, Sedlmair M, Quinan PS, Munzner T. The nested blocks and guidelines model. Inf Vis. 2015;14:234–49.
37. Beyer H, Holtzblatt K. Contextual design: defining customer-centered systems. Cambridge, MA: Morgan Kaufmann; 1998.
38. Lazar J, Feng JH, Hochheiser H. Research methods in human-computer interaction. Cambridge, MA: Morgan Kaufmann; 2017.
39. ClowdFlower. Data science report. 2016. http://visit.crowdflower.com/rs/416-ZBE-142/images/CrowdFlower_DataScienceReport_2016.pdf.
40. Human Phenotype Ontology. Nucleic acids research. Oxford: Oxford Academic; 2017. https://academic-oup-com.pitt.idm.oclc.org/nar/article/45/D1/D865/2574174
41. Musen MA. The protégé project: a look back and a look forward. AI Matters. 2015;1:4–12.
42. Ma X, Sayama H. Mental disorder recovery correlated with centralities and interactions on an online social network. PeerJ. 2015;3
43. Beck F, Burch M, Diehl S, Weiskopf D. A taxonomy and survey of dynamic graph visualization. Comput. Graph. Forum. 2017;36:133–59.
44. Gibson H, Faith J, Vickers P. A survey of two-dimensional graph layout techniques for information visualisation. Inf Vis. 2013;12:324–57.
45. Bederson BB. The promise of zoomable user interfaces. Behav Inf Technol. 2011;30:853–66.
46. Weaver C. Cross-filtered views for multidimensional visual analysis. IEEE Trans Vis Comput Graph. 2010;16:192–204.
47. di Battista G, Eades P, Tamassia R, Tollis IG. Graph drawing: algorithms for the visualization of graphs. Upper Saddle River, NJ: Prentice Hall PTR; 1998.
48. Mackinlay J. Automating the Design of Graphical Presentations of relational information. ACM Trans Graph. 1986;5:110–41.
49. Cleveland WS, McGill R. Graphical perception and graphical methods for analyzing scientific data. Science. 1985;229:828–33.
50. Cooper RJ, Schriger DL, Close RJH. Graphical literacy: the quality of graphs in a large-circulation journal. Ann Emerg Med. 2002;40:317–22.
51. Pastore M, Lionetti F, Altoè G. When one shape does not fit all: a commentary essay on the use of graphs in psychological research. Front Psychol. 2017;8
52. Drummond GB, Vowler SL. Show the data, don't conceal them. J Physiol. 2011;589:1861–3.
53. Weissgerber TL, Milic NM, Winham SJ, Garovic VD. Beyond Bar and line graphs: time for a new data presentation paradigm. PLoS Biol. 2015;13:e1002128.
54. Hosseinpoor AR, AbouZahr C. Graphical presentation of relative measures of association. Lancet. 2010;375:1254.
55. Tufte ER. Visual explanations: images and quantities, evidence and narrative. Cheshire: Graphics Press; 1997.
56. Tufte ER. Envisioning information. Cheshire: Graphics Press; 1990.
57. Tufte ER. Beautiful evidence. Cheshire: Graphics Press; 2006.
58. Harrower M, Brewer CA. ColorBrewer.org: An online tool for selecting colour schemes for maps. Cartogr J. 2003;40(1):27–37.
59. Wattenberg M. Baby names, visualization, and social data analysis. In IEEE symposium on information visualization, INFOVIS 2005. 2005. p. 1–7. https://doi.org/10.1109/INFVIS.2005.1532122.

60. Wattenberg M, Kriss J. Designing for social data analysis. IEEE Trans Vis Comput Graph. 2006;12:549–57.
61. Shneiderman B. Direct manipulation: a step beyond programming languages. Computer. 1983;16:57–69.
62. Shneiderman B. Dynamic queries for visual information seeking. IEEE Softw. 1994;11:70–7.
63. Tweedie L, Spence B, Williams D, Bhogal R. The attribute explorer. In: Conference companion on human factors in computing systems. New York: ACM; 1994. p. 435–6. https://doi.org/10.1145/259963.260433.
64. Mane KK, et al. VisualDecisionLinc: a visual analytics approach for comparative effectiveness-based clinical decision support in psychiatry. J Biomed Inform. 2012;45:101–6.
65. Boyd AD, Young C, Matayakul M, Dieter MG, Pawola LM. Developing visual thinking in the electronic health record. Stud Health Technol Inform. 2017;245:308–12. https://doi.org/10.3233/978-1-61499-830-3-308.
66. Silverman W. Frequently performed psychological tests. In: Walker HK, Hall WD, Hurst JW, editors. Clinical methods: The history, physical, and laboratory examinations. 3rd ed. Boston: Butterworths; 1990. Chapter 208. PMID: 21250163.
67. Fowler FJ. The redesign of the National Health Interview Survey. Public Health Rep Wash DC. 1996;1974(111):508–11.
68. Nelson DE, Holtzman D, Bolen J, Stanwyck CA, Mack KA. Reliability and validity of measures from the behavioral risk factor surveillance system (BRFSS). Soz Praventivmed. 2001;46(Suppl 1):S3–42.
69. Centers for Disease Control and Prevention. General Information about the NHANES 2003–2004 laboratory methodology and public data files; 2006.
70. Tomitaka S, et al. Item response patterns on the patient health Questionnaire-8 in a nationally representative sample of US adults. Front Psych. 2017;8:251.
71. Boonstra A, Versluis A, Vos JFJ. Implementing electronic health records in hospitals: a systematic literature review. BMC Health Serv Res. 2014;14:370.
72. Evans RS. Electronic health records: then, now, and in the future. Yearb Med Inform. 2016;Suppl 1:S48–61.
73. Castillo EG, Olfson M, Pincus HA, Vawdrey D, Stroup TS. Electronic health Records in Mental Health Research: a framework for developing valid research methods. Psychiatr Serv. 2015;66:193–6.
74. Rind A, et al. Interactive information visualization to explore and query electronic health records. Found. Trends® Human–Computer Interact. 2013;5:207–98.
75. Kaur H, et al. Automated chart review utilizing natural language processing algorithm for asthma predictive index. BMC Pulm Med. 2018;18:34.
76. Assale M, Dui LG, Cina A, Seveso A, Cabitza F. The revival of the notes field: leveraging the unstructured content in electronic health records. Front Med. 2019;6:66.
77. Sheikhalishahi S, et al. Natural language processing of clinical notes on chronic diseases: systematic review. JMIR Med Inform. 2019;7:e12239.
78. Barrett N, Weber-Jahnke JH. Applying natural language processing toolkits to electronic health records – an experience report. Stud Health Technol Inform. 2009;143:441–6.
79. Yuan Z, Finan S, Warner J, Savova G, Hochheiser H. Interactive exploration of longitudinal cancer patient histories extracted from clinical text. JCO Clin. Cancer Inform. 2020;4:412–20. https://doi.org/10.1200/CCI.19.00115.
80. Hirsch JS, et al. HARVEST, a longitudinal patient record summarizer. J Am Med Inform Assoc. 2015;22:263–74.
81. Demkow U, Wolańczyk T. Genetic tests in major psychiatric disorders—integrating molecular medicine with clinical psychiatry—why is it so difficult? Transl Psychiatry. 2017;7:e1151.
82. Gandal MJ, et al. Shared molecular neuropathology across major psychiatric disorders parallels polygenic overlap. Science. 2018;359:693–7.
83. Nusrat S, Harbig T, Gehlenborg N. Tasks, techniques, and tools for genomic data visualization. Comput. Graph. Forum. 2019;38:781–805.

84. O'Donoghue SI, et al. Visualization of biomedical data. Annu Rev Biomed Data Sci. 2018;1:275–304.
85. Cuellar-Partida G, Renteria ME, MacGregor S. LocusTrack: integrated visualization of GWAS results and genomic annotation. Source Code Biol Med. 2015;10:1.
86. Verma A, et al. Human-disease phenotype map derived from PheWAS across 38,682 individuals. Am J Hum Genet. 2019;104:55–64.
87. George G, et al. PheGWAS: a new dimension to visualize GWAS across multiple phenotypes. bioRxiv. 2019; https://doi.org/10.1101/694794.
88. Dalabira E, et al. DruGeVar: an online resource triangulating drugs with genes and genomic biomarkers for clinical pharmacogenomics. Public Health Genomics. 2014;17:265–71.
89. Bihlmeyer NA, et al. Novel methods for integration and visualization of genomics and genetics data in Alzheimer's disease. Alzheimers Dement J Alzheimers Assoc. 2019;15:788–98.
90. Helbich M. Mental health and environmental exposures: an editorial. Int J Environ Res Public Health. 2018;15:2207.
91. Xie S, Greenblatt R, Levy MZ, Himes BE. Enhancing electronic health record data with geospatial information. AMIA Jt Summits Transl Sci Proc AMIA Jt Summits Transl Sci. 2017;2017:123–32.
92. Ramirez-Andreotta MD, et al. Improving environmental health literacy and justice through environmental exposure results communication. Int J Environ Res Public Health. 2016;13:690.
93. Andrew L, Jane L, Martin C, Scott L. Original quantitative research exploring and visualizing the small-area-level socioeconomic factors, alcohol availability and built environment influences of alcohol expenditure for the City of Toronto: a spatial analysis approach. Health Promot Chronic Dis Prev Can Res Policy Pract. 2019;39:15–24.
94. Isvoranu A-M, Borsboom D, van Os J, Guloksuz S. A network approach to environmental impact in psychotic disorder: brief theoretical framework. Schizophr Bull. 2016;42:870–3.
95. Sort A. The role of mHealth in mental health. mHealth. 2017;3:1–1.
96. Chandrashekar P. Do mental health mobile apps work: evidence and recommendations for designing high-efficacy mental health mobile apps. mHealth. 2018;4:6.
97. Holzinger A, Bruschi M, Eder W. On interactive data visualization of physiological low-cost-sensor data with focus on mental stress. In: Cuzzocrea A, Kittl C, Simos DE, Weippl E, Xu L, editors. Availability, reliability, and security in information systems and HCI. Berlin: Springer; 2013. p. 469–80. https://doi.org/10.1007/978-3-642-40511-2_34.
98. Kamdar MR, Wu MJ. Prism: a data-driven platform for monitoring mental health. In: Biocomputing 2016. Singapore: World Scientific; 2015. p. 333–44. https://doi.org/10.1142/9789814749411_0031.
99. Gravenhorst F, et al. Mobile phones as medical devices in mental disorder treatment: an overview. Pers Ubiquitous Comput. 2015;19:335–53.
100. Observational health data sciences and informatics. The book of OHDSI.
101. Becker D, et al. Predictive modeling in e-mental health: a common language framework. Internet Interv. 2018;12:57–67.
102. Zhao J, Henriksson A, Asker L, Boström H. Predictive modeling of structured electronic health records for adverse drug event detection. BMC Med Inform Decis Mak. 2015;15(Suppl 4):S1.
103. Webb CA, et al. Personalized prognostic prediction of treatment outcome for depressed patients in a naturalistic psychiatric hospital setting: a comparison of machine learning approaches. J Consult Clin Psychol. 2020;88:25–38.
104. Bhagwat N, Viviano JD, Voineskos AN, Chakravarty MM, Alzheimer's Disease Neuroimaging Initiative. Modeling and prediction of clinical symptom trajectories in Alzheimer's disease using longitudinal data. PLoS Comput Biol. 2018;14:e1006376.
105. Lee Y, et al. Applications of machine learning algorithms to predict therapeutic outcomes in depression: a meta-analysis and systematic review. J Affect Disord. 2018;241:519–32.
106. Shannon P, et al. Cytoscape: a software environment for integrated models of biomolecular interaction networks. Genome Res. 2003;13:2498–504.

107. Agg B, et al. The EntOptLayout Cytoscape plug-in for the efficient visualization of major protein complexes in protein-protein interaction and signalling networks. Bioinformatics. 2019;35(21):4490–2. https://doi.org/10.1093/bioinformatics/btz257.
108. Lex A, Gehlenborg N, Strobelt H, Vuillemot R, Pfister H. UpSet: visualization of intersecting sets. IEEE Trans Vis Comput Graph. 2014;20:1983–92.
109. Conway JR, Lex A, Gehlenborg N. UpSetR: an R package for the visualization of intersecting sets and their properties. Bioinforma Oxf Engl. 2017;33:2938–40.
110. Rosenthal SB, et al. Interactive network visualization in Jupyter notebooks: visJS2jupyter. Bioinforma Oxf Engl. 2018;34:126–8.
111. Bostock M, Ogievetsky V, Heer J. D^3 Data-Driven Documents. IEEE Trans Vis Comput Graph. 2011;17:2301–9.
112. Satyanarayan A, Moritz D, Wongsuphasawat K, Heer J. Vega-lite: a grammar of interactive graphics. IEEE Trans Vis Comput Graph. 2017;23:341–50.
113. Satyanarayan A, Russell R, Hoffswell J, Heer J. Reactive Vega: a streaming dataflow architecture for declarative interactive visualization. IEEE Trans Vis Comput Graph. 2016;22:659–68.
114. Pomare C, Ellis LA, Churruca K, Long JC, Braithwaite J. The reality of uncertainty in mental health care settings seeking professional integration: a mixed-methods approach. Int J Integr Care. 2018;18:13.
115. Agniel D, Kohane IS, Weber GM. Biases in electronic health record data due to processes within the healthcare system: retrospective observational study. BMJ. 2018;361:k1479. https://doi.org/10.1136/bmj.k1479.
116. Skeels M, Lee B, Smith G, Robertson GG. Revealing uncertainty for information visualization. Inf Vis. 2010;9:70–81.
117. Behrisch M, et al. Quality metrics for information visualization. Comput Graph Forum. 2018;37:625–62.
118. Hung Y-H, Parsons P. Assessing user engagement in information visualization. In: Proceedings of the 2017 CHI conference extended abstracts on human factors in computing systems. New York: ACM; 2017. p. 1708–17. https://doi.org/10.1145/3027063.3053113.
119. North C. Toward measuring visualization insight. IEEE Comput Graph Appl. 2006;26:6–9.
120. North C, Saraiya P, Duca K. A comparison of benchmark task and insight evaluation methods for information visualization. Inf Vis. 2011;10:162–81.
121. Shneiderman B, Plaisant C. Strategies for evaluating information visualization tools: multi-dimensional in-depth long-term case studies. In: Proceedings of the 2006 AVI workshop on beyond time and errors: novel evaluation methods for information visualization. New York: ACM; 2006. p. 1–7. https://doi.org/10.1145/1168149.1168158.
122. Tory M, Moller T. Evaluating visualizations: do expert reviews work? IEEE Comput Graph Appl. 2005;25:8–11.
123. Wall E, et al. A heuristic approach to value-driven evaluation of visualizations. IEEE Trans Vis Comput Graph. 2019;25:491–500.
124. Saket B, Endert A, Stasko J. Beyond usability and performance: a review of user experience-focused evaluations in visualization. In: Proceedings of the sixth workshop on beyond time and errors on novel evaluation methods for visualization. New York: ACM; 2016. p. 133–42. https://doi.org/10.1145/2993901.2993903.
125. Sukumar PT, Metoyer R Towards designing unbiased replication studies in information visualization. In 2018 IEEE evaluation and beyond – methodological approaches for visualization (BELIV) 93–101. 2018. https://doi.org/10.1109/BELIV.2018.8634261.

Chapter 15
Big Data: Knowledge Discovery and Data Repositories

Sumithra Velupillai, Katrina A. S. Davis, and Leon Rozenblit

Abstract "Big Data" is a concept that has been used in the last 10–15 years to describe the increasing complexity and amount of data available at scale in organizations and companies—data that often requires novel computational techniques and methods to generate knowledge. Compared to other health domains, mental health is influenced by a greater variety of factors, such as those related to mental, interpersonal, cultural, environmental, and biological phenomena. Thus, knowledge discovery in mental health research can involve a broad variety of data types and therefore data resources, including medical, behavioral, administrative, molecular, 'omics', environmental, financial, geographic, and social media repositories. Moreover, these varied phenomena interact in more complex ways in mental health and illness than in other domains of health so knowledge discovery must be open to this complexity. In this chapter, we outline the main underlying concepts of the "big data" paradigm and examine examples of different types of data repositories that could be used for mental health research. We also provide an example case study for developing a data repository, outlining the key considerations for designing, building, and using these types of resources.

Keywords Big data · Knowledge discovery · Data repositories · Mental health informatics · Knowledge bases

S. Velupillai (✉) · K. A. S. Davis
Department of Psychological Medicine, Institute of Psychiatry, Psychology & Neuroscience, King's College London, London, UK
e-mail: sumithra.velupillai@kcl.ac.uk; katrina.davis@kcl.ac.uk

L. Rozenblit
Prometheus Research, an IQVIA Business, New Haven, CT, USA
e-mail: leon.rozenblit@iqvia.com

© Springer Nature Switzerland AG 2021
J. D. Tenenbaum, P. A. Ranallo (eds.), *Mental Health Informatics*, Health Informatics, https://doi.org/10.1007/978-3-030-70558-9_15

15.1   What Is "Big Data": The Big Part, the Data Part?

"Big Data" is a term that has been used in the last 10–15 years to describe not only the increase in the volume and complexity of data available in organizations, but also the novel computational techniques and methods needed to derive knowledge from the data. One formal definition for "Big Data" was published by De Mauro, Greco and Grimaldi in 2016: "Big Data is the Information asset characterized by such a High Volume, Velocity and Variety to require specific Technology and Analytical Methods for its transformation into Value." [1] Big data is often described in terms of the 'Vs' that characterize it: *Volume, Velocity,* and *Variety. Volume* refers to the size of datasets [2]. *Velocity* refers to the dynamic nature of the data, meaning that it might be rapidly changing and may require frequent updates to retain value. *Variety* refers to data complexity. Data complexity can mean heterogeneity of data elements in a dataset (e.g., timestamps, codes, text, images, etc.), of types of data (e.g., genomic, clinical, behavioral, administrative), or of code systems (LOINC, ICD, SNOMED, RxNORM)—any of which can make the work of deriving meaning from the combined data more convoluted.

In healthcare, particularly for mental health, the 'Big Data' paradigm has been recognized to have great potential [2–5]. Scientific publications in this field have been increasing since 2003 (Figs. 15.1 and 15.2). It is expected that this paradigm and the concept of 'Big Data' will continue to evolve as will likely applications to mental health informatics research.

Compared to other health domains, mental health conditions are currently classified less by underlying mechanisms of pathology, and more by symptom patterns (see Chap. 5). While it is universally known that mental health and illness are influenced by complex relationships between mental, interpersonal, environmental, and biological factors [6] the nature of these relationships has been elusive. Knowledge discovery in mental health depends on greater insight into relationships between these disparate phenomena. This requires access to a range of data sources

Fig. 15.1 Search results from PubMed (as of 29 Sept 2019); keywords "big data" and 'big data" and "mental health"

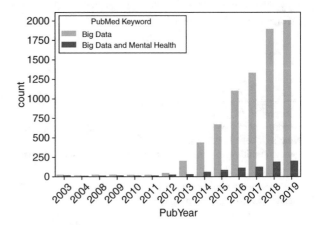

Fig. 15.2 PubMed search results on a logarithmic scale, including the search for 'informatics' for comparison

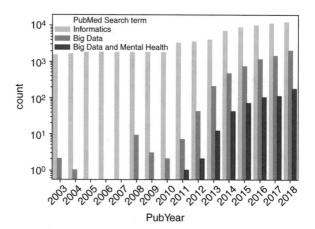

including medical, administrative, molecular, 'omics', environmental, socio-economic, geographic, and social media repositories [7–9].

How to decide what constitutes 'Big' (*Volume*), dynamic (*Velocity*) and varied (*Variety*) depends on, and is relative to, each clinical research question or problem, as well as to data availability. For instance, many relevant research problems in mental health research might relate to rare diseases (e.g. conversion disorder, certain types of psychosis) or rare outcomes (e.g. suicide, birth defects). In this this context "big data" can mean data that is very complex and difficult to work with, even if it is not necessarily large (Volume). It could be complex because data sources are scattered across healthcare institutions and need to be mapped and linked, and require complex analytical methods. The need for specialized infrastructures, computational tools and methods to analyze this type of data is perhaps the key component of the big data paradigm, and what makes it distinct from other approaches to research.

15.2 Methods and Paradigms

Compared to other research methodologies, the big data paradigm is often more exploratory, and data driven. Knowledge discovery typically means that one applies computational and statistical methods that are designed to identify previously unknown patterns in the data, thus leading to a hypothesis-*generating* approach. This contrasts with a hypothesis-*testing* approach, where theory and *a priori* knowledge drives the question framing, study design and research methodology choices (see Fig. 15.3). More recently, intermediate and mixed approaches have also emerged to synergistically combine the best of the two contrasting modes [10].

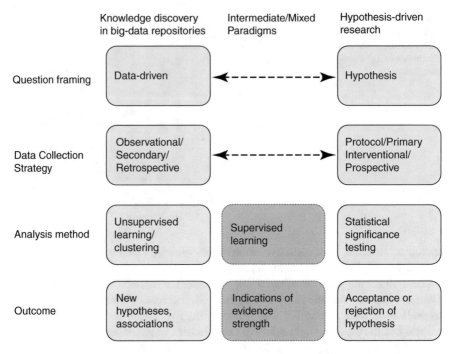

Fig. 15.3 The columns represent different research paradigms, and the rows different stages in the research process. The text in the boxes provides examples of activities and methods for each stage under the different paradigms. Note that a given dataset may fall at different points in the spectrum throughout its lifecycle- data collected through a hypothesis-driven protocol may later be used for knowledge discovery through secondary analysis, sometimes in combination with other datasets

Analytical and computational methods that are applied within the big data paradigm may range from simple statistical association to complex machine learning (ML) algorithms (see Chap. 10). Depending on the nature of the data in a data repository, several methods may need to be combined and applied to the data. For example, complex variables (e.g., images, natural language) often need to be converted to simpler structured variables that can then be used for further analysis. Machine learning algorithms that can natively deal with the complexity of the underlying data (e.g., multimodal learning algorithms) may also need to be applied. Machine learning and data mining algorithms (Chap. 10) are used to develop classification models and predictive models: they automatically identify patterns in the data by converting it so that the data can be modelled computationally. These algorithms are usually divided into two main groups: *supervised* and *unsupervised*. In supervised machine learning, the data has labels, e.g. diagnostic codes or assessment scores. The algorithm uses labeled training data to produce a model that can predict a label on new, unseen data. In unsupervised learning, the data has no labels, and the algorithm tries to identify inherent patterns in the data, e.g. clusters or other groupings.

15.2.1   Essential Elements for Big Data Repositories

Some key elements are essential to the utility of big data repositories: appropriate governance, technical infrastructure, and metadata.

15.2.1.1   Governance

The first aspect that needs to be in place in order for a big data repository to be of value is appropriate governance models. Governance models outline how the data in a repository can and should be used to comply with national and organizational regulations. This is particularly important in mental health research and other clinical research fields, where the data may contain sensitive, identifiable information. There are many different models for this, ranging from repositories that are completely open and where identifiable information has been removed, to repositories that are strongly guarded in secure environments and where access to the data is restricted to approved users. Data that poses any privacy risks is usually only made available under Data Use Agreements (DUAs) that specify how the data may be used and that require the user to take steps to ensure protection of participant or patient privacy.

In general, individuals providing data to a research repository give informed consent for the storage and use of that data, but rules and regulations are quite complex and vary from region to region. In many cases, data that have been stripped of all identifying information may be used for research without explicit consent. In some cases, Institutional Review Boards (IRBs), the entities responsible for reviewing research proposals within a given institution for ethical standards, may grant a "waiver of consent," allowing research to be performed without consent. In the context of retrospective data mining studies, these usually apply when there is minimal potential risk to the individual and when the research could not feasibly be carried out without such a waiver.

Technical Infrastructure

The core element of IT infrastructures for any data repository is handling data: data storage, management, and information models (the representation that specifies the types, relations and constraints of data) in databases. This can be designed and administered in different ways, with two emerging directions described as either "centralized" or "federated." *Centralized* systems are locally maintained and organized, sharing a central framework; they generally involve moving data to a common location (often at the level of physical storage on the same platform) and protecting the boundaries with common privacy and security processes and safeguards. In contrast, *federated* solutions leave the data in place stored in physically and logically separate individual systems; instead, integration is achieved by creating common query interfaces that serve as an abstraction layer to link the individual systems for different information needs. As an example of a centralized approach, some Nordic countries have longstanding population databases to which all hospitals are mandated to provide data, which can be linked to an individual with a unique personal identifier [11]. Federated models, on the other hand, can allow the data to stay owned by the healthcare management organizations, but leveraged together for secondary use, like the Mental Health Research Network [12] that brings together 13 centers and records from approximately 12.5 million people.

The process of accessing the data in a central system involves running a query against the common data store. In contrast, in federated systems, a query is typically passed to the common query layer, where it is broken up into pieces, with each piece sent to the appropriate source system. The results of the different query-pieces are then combined and returned to the user, as if coming from a single central system. Of course, the results will be limited by whatever constraints the common query interface imposes—for example, it's not uncommon for such systems to only return counts of cases, but not the detailed case attributes. In general, the federated approach can impose some additional technical complexity, but it can also solve a very important, and sometimes otherwise intractable problem in data governance: it allows different organizations to retain local control of their data while exposing the local data assets to limited forms of computation (e.g., counting cases) that are defined by the federated query interface.

A productive approach to increasing the utility of data in a federated model is to map the data to one of the established common data models (CDMs), which are standardized models for organizing and representing data across different repositories. For example, the Observational Medical Outcomes Partnership (OMOP) [13] is a CDM increasingly used for representing data from electronic health record (EHR) systems, transforming the content to a standardized format that can then be used for further analytics- see Fig. 15.4. Another example is the National Patient-Centered Clinical Research Network (PCORnet) [14] in which a CDM has been developed to enable further research capability of data repositories [15]. In clinical research, Clinical Data Interchange Standards Consortium (CDISC) has developed a set of common data models [16]. For instance, the Clinical Data Acquisition Standards Harmonization (CDASH) is a model for data collection, the Analysis Data Model (AdaM) for analysis, and the Operational Data Model (CDISC-ODM) for data exchange, that can help harmonize data collected by different clinical trials or investigator-initiated studies [17].

Other important aspects of technical infrastructure include ensuring appropriate compute capacity, software environments, backup procedures, firewalls, user access protocols, etc. There have been significant advances in the development of distributed, high-performance computing environments in recent years. Distributed environments allow for efficient processing of large datasets as well as deploying complex algorithms that a single computer or server would take much longer time to run. These enable more powerful processing for increasingly complex machine learning algorithms and may also support real-time processing. Hadoop [18], released by the Apache Software Foundation under an open source license, was one

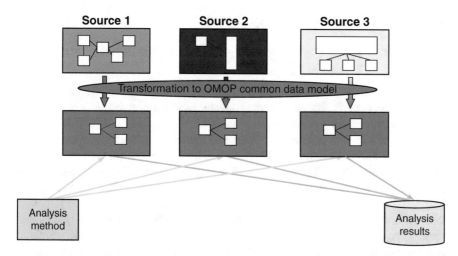

Fig. 15.4 Mapping disparate data sources to a Common Data Model such as OMOP enables federated analysis across data sources. (From https://www.ohdsi.org/data-standardization/the-common-data-model/)

of the earliest examples, and is still widely used. Other examples include Spark [19], Hive [20], Flink [21] and Kafka [22]—with each optimized for different properties, e.g., efficient in-memory processing, streaming data, etc. Novel developments also include technical solutions for virtual warehousing, where linkage of various data sources with different ownership and structure is enabled without moving the data to a central location (providing technical methods for the federated approach described above), as well as Platform-as-a-Service (PaaS) delivery models, which are complete virtual development and deployment environments, i.e. building and maintaining the infrastructure is done by the cloud environment provider, not the data repository owner.

Metadata

For data repositories to be useful and manageable, the raw data needs to also be organized and documented in a way that enables would-be users to understand the data—what it represents and how it was collected or created. Metadata, or data about the data, is essential to characterizing the content in a repository by adding a layer (or several layers) of information about the data itself. For instance, one layer of metadata in a data repository is structural, in that it defines the elements and their relations in the database itself, such as the tables and columns. Other metadata layers might represent descriptive information to enable searching and extracting information, e.g. disease area or protocol type in a research database. Metadata models are particularly important for mapping and linking different data repositories. To ensure the utility of any data repository, the data structure, contents, meaning, and provenance must be well documented and, as much as possible, follow appropriate standards.

15.3 Big Data and Data Repositories

15.3.1 The FAIR Guiding Principles

Since the late 2010s, there has been a movement towards "open science" that has grown into an expectation from funding agencies and major publishing outlets [23]. The intellectual starting point for this movement was the so-called "reproducibility crisis"—that is, the failure for published findings made by one group to be reproduced and published by another. There are numerous reasons for lack of reproducibility of research [24]. The "open science" paradigm addresses two of them, namely a lack of transparency in the methods and transparency of the data. One thing that individual researchers can do to make their own work "reproducible" is to ensure that methods and data are available alongside any results. However, publishing these in an *ad hoc* or non-curated manner may be insufficient for other people to make use of them. A group of stakeholders came together to formalize a set of guiding principles for researchers to enhance data sharing and reuse [25]. These guiding principles, published in 2016, were summed up by the acronym "FAIR"—Findable, Accessible, Interoperable and Reusable. *Findable* entails ensuring that data are assigned a globally unique and persistent identifier, described with rich metadata, and indexed in a searchable resource. *Accessible* involves using open, standardized protocols for data retrieval purposes, allowing for authorization when necessary, and metadata that persists even if the data are no longer available. *Interoperable* means that the repository should use a formal and standardized knowledge representation model, using standardized vocabularies that themselves follow FAIR principles. Ensuring that a repository is *reusable* means that it should be free from reuse restrictions, and released with clear usage licenses, with rich details around the content of the data in compliance with relevant community standards (see also Chap. 7).

Repositories are often created to store and allow recall of discrete sets of data for transparency and reproducibility. Curated repositories provide a way to satisfy these aims by following FAIR principles [26]. However, once a repository has been used for these purposes, it can have a secondary purpose: for further knowledge discovery using big data approaches [27].

15.4 Secondary Usage

The use of electronic health records as data repositories for research stands somewhat in contrast to the curated model for data repositories. "Learning Health Systems" (LHS), described in detail in Chap. 1, rely on data collected through clinical care to inform and enable research, which in turn informs practice. One key attribute of an LHS is that new data is captured as an integral by-product of the care experience [28]. In this paradigm, each patient encounter may be considered a data point from which to glean new knowledge. Modern EHR systems create opportunities for knowledge discovery using data collected as a by-product of clinical care, rather than as a research artifact.

This approach to knowledge discovery using EHR data is sometimes referred to as "secondary use" to distinguish it from the primary use of EHR data in support of care delivery, health system administration, and billing. Note, however, that EHR data alone are rarely sufficient as a data source to answer research questions about a specific disease or practice area. Understanding the difficulties with using EHR data for research directly help illuminate the benefits of more traditional data repositories. Unlike EHRs, data repositories do the hard work of organizing data for one or more research uses. When they are successful, they dramatically reduce the time necessary to "wrangle and clean" the data prior to using it to answer a research question. When they are exceptionally successful, they allow data to be used for many kinds of related research questions, many of which couldn't have been anticipated by the original designers of the data repository. Thus, data repositories are likely to remain in high demand even as our health systems move to further embrace EHRs and their secondary use in research.

15.4.1 Biobanks

Biobanks are large collections of biological and medical data, such as blood samples and blood pressure, on a group or groups of individuals that provide a platform for study of health science (see also Multi-Modal Data Repositories below). The UK Biobank for example, holds information and samples from 500,000 volunteers from England, Wales, and Scotland that are available to any researcher (for a small fee) to use for projects for the public good [29].

15.5 Categories of Data and Data Repositories

Data Repositories of big data come in many forms. Virtually any of the kinds of data that can be used to acquire biomedical or healthcare knowledge can be used in big data paradigms. However, unlike most other forms of research, the researcher working with repositories will usually have had very little input into the collection or organization of the data. Here we discuss the kinds of data that have been organized into repositories to which big-data methods have been applied. In the tables that follow in this chapter we have listed a variety of big data resources that have been, or could be, used to carry out knowledge discovery, categorized by the type of data and the resource type. In so doing, we have used an existing categorization of resources [30]. These categories are: (1) initiatives—activities or groups creating, collecting or cataloging data for research (I); (2) platforms—applications that enable a researcher to search for data sets (P); (3) datasets—specific data resulting from a study or created for a processing challenge (D); (4) studies—the processes that collect data from individuals or individual points to create the datasets (S).

Quite commonly, big data resources have characteristics of more than one type. For mental health, types of data repositories that have been developed and used include some that have been developed specifically for the study one particular disease, such as Genetic Links to Anxiety and Depression [31] or RADAR-MDD [32], both of which are primarily aimed at understanding recurrent depression in people living in the UK and Europe. Others are broader, and these tend to cover larger populations and data types, such as the Psychiatric Genomic Consortium [33] that has input from studies around the world and the AllofUs biobank that is collecting data to study all aspects of health and wellbeing [34]. Some repositories are easier to understand, because the data has been selected and organized, which we refer to as "curated", while some require expert knowledge or tools to search, but may be more convenient to store data as they have fewer rules. For example, a dictionary is highly curated, but the world-wide web is not. Big data repositories may comprise many different types of data—in some cases one at a time, and in others integrating many together.

15.5.1 Refined Scientific Knowledge: Publication Databases and Specialist Databases

Databases of refined scientific knowledge often have as their unit of reference the publications or records of scientific studies, which are curated with metadata to enable consistency and easy searching (see Table 15.1). Clinicians and researchers use these sorts of databases every day for both searching for specific studies and for carrying out systematic searches of a research topic. Publication databases are one type of refined scientific knowledge data repositories. There are several types of publication databases, each one covering some scope of medical knowledge from broad to specific. The best known of this is the Medline database, which evolved from the "Index Medicus", published by the US National Library of Medicine (NLM) since 1879 to index published literature of medical interest. Since 1997, Medline has been available to search online though the PubMed application. It currently has over 25 million citations indexed from 5200 journals, 85% of which have an abstract [47], and are also indexed by a bespoke hierarchical thesaurus known as Medical Subject Headings (MeSH) [48]. More specialist repositories, such as PsycINFO® [36] for behavioral and social science publications, will be highly tuned to the storage and recall of specific publications. Use of big data paradigms has enabled new uses of this data [49]. These have particular value in looking for potentially unanticipated patterns [50]. They have proved to be particularly useful in considering transdiagnostic patterns and comorbidity [51] by looking beyond the contents of publications to the patterns of the entire corpus, which often features publications in multiple disciplines and across multiple classes of disorders.

Table 15.1 Refined scientific knowledge repositories. As well as internal patterns, these databases are mined for information to analyze external datasets

Big data repository class	Type				Examples
	I	P	D	S	
Publication repositories			X		PubMed (accessing Medline) [35]
			X		PsycINFO [36]
Repositories for findings of OMICs studies (genomic, transcriptomic (RNA), epigenetic, proteomic and metabolomic)	X	X			Genomics: Online Mendelian inheritance of man (OMIM) [37]
	X				Web-based gene set analysis toolkit (WEBGestalt) combines many gene-based knowledge sources into a toolkit to extract value from genomics data [38]
Pharmacological and drug binding repositories	X	X			Medicines: DrugBank [39]
	X	X			Side effect resource (SIDER) [40] for medicines
	X				Neuroscience information framework [41] has an integrated search function across a range of different brain-related data sources
Research instruments—Psychometrics properties and in-vivo performance in various populations	X				ETS—Educational Testing Service's TestLink database [42]
	X				HaPI—Health and Psychosocial Instruments [43]
	X				MMY-TIP—mental measures yearbook with tests in print [44, 45]
	X	X			PsycTESTS® (American Psychological Association) [46]

More specialized repositories are tuned for storing and searching for specialized content. Types: Initiative (I), Platform (P), Dataset (D), Study (S)

Instead of, or as well as, publications, some findings will be recorded in other databases specialized to the study type. For example DrugBank is a database of drug binding data reported elsewhere [39] and PharmGKB is a curated database of pharmacogenetic interaction knowledge [52]. One study integrated a database on the molecular structure and interactions of medicines with one on side-effects to predict side-effects of psychiatric medication [53]. The same technique also has potential for drug repurposing and drug design [54].

15.5.2 Biological Data

Many big data repositories have been developed to store biological data either with or without other types of data (see Table 15.2). Databases of -omic data, where omics refers to a specific study in biology, as shown in Table 15.3 and described in more detail in Chapter 11. Imaging data, and data from wearable devices (see Chap. 17) without phenotypic data is of little use for knowledge discovery in mental health in itself. However, these data can be used for designing and training algorithms. The

Table 15.2 Biological data repositories

Big data repository class	Type				Name
	I	P	D	S	
Omics data (genomic, transcriptomic (RNA), epigenetic, proteomic and metabolomic)			X		South Asian Genomes and Exomes (SAGE)- a publicly available database of whole genome sequences from Asia [66]
	X		X		omicsDI [67] offers an integrated search across several more specific -omics repositories
Neuroimaging data (structural, functional and connectome)	X		X	X	Human Connectome Projects and the Connectome Coordination Facility [68]
		X	X		OpenNEURO for sharing MRI, MEG, EEG, iEEG and EcoG data [69]
			X	X	UK biobank imaging brain MRI data [70] and genetic data [71]

These repositories can be used to design and train algorithms to process future linked data. Data in such repositories can help with replication studies, as part of a strategy for delivering FAIR research, where the results are Findable, Accessible, Interoperable and Reusable. Types: Initiative (I), Platform (P), Dataset (D), Study (S)

Table 15.3 "Omics" are fields of study in biology

Scale	Name	Studies	Repository (example of)
Molecular	Genomics	DNA	Nucleic acid sequence
	Transcriptomics	RNA	Sequence read archive (SRA) [55] Gene activity/function: Gene expression omnibus (GEO) [56]
	Proteomics	Protein	Proteomics IDEntifications (PRIDE) Database [57] Proteome Xchange [58]
Processes	Metabolomics	Small-molecular signatures of reactions	Metabolomics workbench [59] MetaboLights [60]
Function	Pharmacogenomics	Drug action	Pharmacogene variation consortium (PharmVar) [61]
	Psychogenomics	Behavioral phenotypes mapped to genetic variations	National Institute for Mental Health (NIMH) Data Archive [62]

algorithms can then process and summarize results in a way that makes future biologic data from linked datasets, such as biobanks, more tractable. Examples can be seen in the use of the UK Biobank imaging and genetic data. Large numbers of brain MRI and genomes were made available as part of the UK Biobank process, resulting in a massive resource for which full processing would test the capacity of most research institutes. However, researchers have used this alongside machine learning to develop rules that allow, for example, the relative thickness of areas of the cortex to be accurately and automatically measured from brain MRI pictures

[63, 64] and copy-number variant sites in the genome to be identified [65]. These processes can then be used to probe the relationship between these features and disease using other clinical and research datasets.

Specialized tools such as WebGestalt [38] for genetic information and the Neuroscience Information Framework (NIF) [41] for brain-related information use specialized knowledge databases and biologic data repositories to add value to each resource. For instance, a team described performing a *reverse GWAS* for depression. A genome-wide association study (GWAS) usually starts from a trait or phenotype to find the genetic differences, but this team reversed the process and used WebGestalt to describe biologically significant subtypes of depression on the basis of the genetic differences seen between individuals [72].

15.5.3   *Behavioral Data*

Of particular interest for mental health and illness research are records of behavior, which may be derived from interactions with social media, computers, wearable devices, and mobile phones. Table 15.4 gives some examples of the types of data that have been used in research to date. Traditional research on behavior would use self-reported or informant-reported observations captured on questionnaires or observation schedules. In the digital era there is potential for passive data collection of physical activity (accelerometer in wearable device), location data (geolocation on phone), voice data (from phone conversations) and facial features (from video data). These Big Data streams bring many of the challenges from the 'Vs' (Volume, Velocity, Variety), and innovative processing methods are often used.

Table 15.4 Behavioral data repositories

Big data repository class	Type				Examples
	I	P	D	S	
Self-reports Informant observations	X				The Audio/Visual Emotion Challenge, e.g. AVEC 2018 [73]
Accelerometry and geolocation from phones and wearables	X			X	RADAR MDD: Using wearables to find a signature for depression relapse [32, 74]
Geolocation Voice data Video data Virtual data trails, such as social media interaction		X	X	X	Twitter: e.g. detecting stigma in social media posts [75] & looking at the US county-level geographical association of emotions in twitter posts and early mortality [76] Reddit: e.g. classifying mental health-related posts [77] & studying how the language of comments influences risk to suicidal ideation [78]

Such repositories have potential for continuous signal streams, needing high processing capabilities. Virtual data trails may include otherwise excluded populations (e.g. those not accessing care as they are well), but will be selective based on usage of platforms. Types: Initiative (I), Platform (P), Dataset (D), Study (S)

An example of a data processing opportunity came about through the accelerometer data from 100,000 participants in the UK Biobank cohort study. These wrist-worn sensors recorded motion in three dimensions 100 times a second (100 Hz) for seven days—over 60 million data-points for each person. The purpose of the motion capture was to assess activity and sleep in UK Biobank participants but processing such data on this scale had not been done before. Two techniques were developed. One team had video recording from a subset of those with accelerometers, which they manually coded, then processed using machine learning methods to pick out the accelerometer signature for activities of interest [79]. Another team summarized the data based on periodicity indicating circadian rhythms in the participants [80].

Elsewhere, the challenge of processing speech and video to detect emotion has been tackled in part with a set of research community challenges called the Audio/Visual Emotion Challenge (AVEC). AVEC brings together programmers from different fields into teams that are given a problem and a training set, and compete to develop the best prototype solutions over a limited time [81]. The scope of research may be expanded beyond just research volunteers into population-level mental health research through the use of virtual data trails. For instance, web searches related to suicide have been associated with trends in suicide over place and time [82], Twitter has been used to look at attitudes towards mental health [75] and Reddit used to look at associations between social support and mental health [78].

There are practical and ethical considerations around use of behavioral data, particularly for mental health research. Public consultations have shown people are wary about technology that tries to infer mental health states, such as speech processing, in a way that they are not about physical health [83]. What's more, use of data in the public domain may be legally acceptable, but social media users have expressed discomfort at their text being used for research [84]. A further limitation is culture-specificity of content. For example, one study in Chinese social media found risk factors for suicidal behavior not seen in English-language studies [85]. Studies may need to be repeated in cross-culturally representative databases before findings are generalized. For more on these topics, see Chaps. 13 and 18 on Natural Language Processing and Ethical, Legal and Social Issues, respectively.

15.5.4   Clinical Administrative Data Repositories

Clinical administrative databases come in two broad types, as shown in Table 15.5. The first, exemplified by the Nordic health registers, are collected for public health monitoring, have very wide coverage of the population (aiming to be universal), and some go back many decades. The second, collected primarily for billing and reimbursement, track healthcare usage more narrowly, and can be subject to bias from reimbursement policies [94]. These repositories have some distinctive characteristics. The scale of these databases has several advantages. They can include people who may not volunteer for research, detect rare outcomes, and have the statistical power to look at subgroups in the population. Use of this data can give answers to

Table 15.5 Clinical administrative data repositories

Big data repository class	Type				Examples
	I	P	D	S	
Health-care usage often linked to other administrative data			X		Nordic health registers from Denmark, Finland, Iceland, Norway, and Sweden [11]
			X		ICES database, Ontario, Canada [86]
			X		Western Australia administrative databases [87]
Medication adverse reaction databases	X	X	X		World Health Organization Programme for international drug monitoring: "VigiAccess" [88]
Reimbursement databases			X		Clalit Health Service, Israel [89] Longitudinal Health Insurance Database of Taiwan [90]
		X	X		Centers for Medicare & Medicaid Services Database [91]
		X	X		PharMetrics (owned by IMS health, now IQVIA) [92] Market Scan [93]

These repositories contain data on health-care usage and spontaneous reporting. Large numbers enable detection of rare events, effects of small size, and effects in specific subpopulations; biases can be introduced due to the population covered by databases (e.g., eligible for Medicaid vs privately insured) and reimbursement policies. Types: Initiative (I), Platform (P), Dataset (D), Study (S)

highly clinically relevant questions, for example, in clarifying who is at risk of antidepressant-related suicidal behavior and from which medications [95].

The distinctive characteristics also have some implications, particularly with respect to the quality of the data. It is important to remember that the data is entered for administrative or regulatory purposes, and subject to the fashions and influences of time and place. These may be particularly important for mental health in contrast with many physical disorders, where signs and symptoms are more clear-cut. For mental disorders, there are frequently barriers in seeking help, receiving a diagnosis, and getting treatment. And changes in these barriers may impact administrative-dependent statistics, which may look like changes in prevalence [96]. For instance UK statistics show that while the numbers of people with symptoms of depression has stayed more-or-less the same over time, the numbers with an administrative code of depression went down, and the numbers treated with an antidepressant went up [97, 98]. One can imagine a similar effect in the US based on changes in reimbursement for different diagnostic codes. Another consideration related to the characteristics of the data for efficient use of these databases is understanding that the coding systems that are used in the structured part of the clinical records are complex and are based on disease classifications (ontologies) that differ between settings and change over time. Figure 15.5 uses the example of what might be labelled as recurrent depression over time (from ICD-9 to ICD-10) and between settings (secondary care using ICD-10 and primary care using SNOMED-CT). The change in the WHO's International Classification of Disease (ICD) from ICD-9 to ICD-10

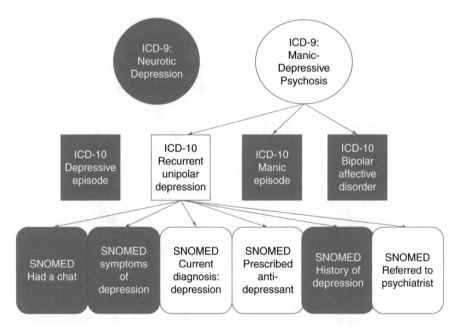

Fig. 15.5 Representing severe recurrent depression in the International Classification of Disease (ICD) versions 9 and 10, and Systematized Nomenclature of Medicine Clinical Terms (SNOMED-CT)

altered the way mood disorders are classified, due to ideological shifts in the classification of psychopathology. These changes mean that one-to-one mapping of concepts is not possible. To the coding of disease states using ICD-10, other coding languages add risk states, reasons for clinical encounter and management. The Systematized Nomenclature of Medicine Clinical Terms (SNOMED-CT) is a widely used, multilingual, computer processable ontology—but has a complex hierarchy structure, making the creation of a comprehensive list of codes to represent a disease in SNOMED a huge task. In Fig. 15.5, a clinician has noted the current depressive episode, prescription and referral for a patient, but a colleague might have instead coded the history of recurrent depression, or specific symptoms of depression. The choice of coded items is quite variable and non-specific codes (e.g. "Had a chat" SNOMED ID: 183093006) are very common. Researchers are encouraged to consult the clinicians and coders who use the language, as well as looking for established code lists.

Another clinical administrative database where the unit of analysis is not a patient but a medication is formed by spontaneous reporting of adverse events associated with medication, the largest of which is the World Health Organization Program for International Drug Monitoring central database, which gathers information from 123 countries, and has over 10 million reports [88, 99].

15.5.5 *Electronic Health Records*

Electronic health records (EHRs) contain the information entered by clinicians and administrators on a day-to-day basis in clinical care. Having evolved from systems of paper notes, they are meant to support clinical practice. EHR information can be structured, as in assessment forms, lab results, diagnostic or medication codes, as well as unstructured, as medical notes written in free text. They are not designed for research use, but can be used for research purposes with certain caveats in place [100] (see Table 15.6).

While administrative databases carry summary information about health episodes, as required by the entity housing the registry, EHRs go beyond this,

Table 15.6 Electronic Health Records (EHRs)

Big data repository class	Type				Examples
	I	P	D	S	
Electronic health records (structured info)			X		The Health Improvement Network (THIN), UK [116] Clinical Practice Research Database (CPRD), UK [117]
		X		X	Using data QUEST electronic data-sharing architecture [118], hosted by the University of Washington Institute of translational health sciences (ITHS), design a tool that looks for variations between providers based on coded encounters
		X			Canadian Primary Care Sentinel Surveillance Network [119]
Electronic health records (with natural language processing, NLP)	X	X			Virtual data warehouses with data from multiple HMOs such as the Mental Health Research Network, USA [12]
			X		Individual health maintenance organizations (HMOs) • Veterans Affairs [120] • Mayo Clinic [121], USA
			X		Individual hospitals with EHR
Linked EHR databases		X			Local and shared clinical repositories • Finding free-text psychosocial concepts in primary care data from a clinic in Ontario that predicted emergency room use [122] • Investigating the geographical variation in acute involuntary psychiatric admissions using local-level data in the Netherlands [123]
		X	X		UK data repositories • Clinical records interactive search (CRIS) [124] • Adolescent Data Platform [125] at Secure Anonymous Information Linkage, SAIL [126]
	X				• Mental Health Data Science Scotland [127], which hosts and Scottish Schools Health and Wellbeing Improvement Research Network (SHINE) [128]

These contain data collected during the course of healthcare. Frequently rich in potential but not easy to interpret. Coverage will be limited to those accessing care. Types: Initiative (I), Platform (P), Dataset (D), Study (S)

containing more contextual information about each healthcare encounter, even when limited to coded data. A study comparing the Clalit claims database in Israel to structured information from electronic health records from the same encounter show incremental gains from the extra information [101]. Such gains may come at the cost of extra practical difficulties and issues of confidentiality that arise from accessing individuals' notes, although there are a number of governance and regulation models that can facilitate access while maintaining high ethical standards (see Chap. 22). Going beyond codes by including the full text of electronic notes in the registry can vastly increase the ability for identifying aspects of phenotypes that are either not frequently coded [102, 103] or are not included in current ontologies [104]. It also offers some of the best opportunities for capturing personal life events, such as bereavement or domestic abuse, that are vital for research involving social determinants of health [105]. For example, knowledge discovery techniques have been used in full-text EHR notes especially to explore patterns of symptoms and diagnosis [106, 107], predict risk of disorder or adverse events [108, 109] and explore disease correlations [110].

As EHR systems have become more widely used in healthcare, the potentials for using these within big data paradigms have increased. Recently, initiatives for integrating and linking EHR repositories from different healthcare institutions have been developed, such as the Informatics for Integrating Biology & the Bedside (i2b2) consortium and the Shared Health Research Information Network (SHRINE) [111, 112], which enable more comprehensive use of diverse EHR data with both more individuals included and different disciplines represented. These initiatives use the federated model described above. Another example is PopMedNet [113], a platform with the aim to enable distributed health data networks. Furthermore, EHR systems allow for the opportunity to merge daily healthcare with data-driven research in (almost) real time, to accelerate learning health system frameworks [114, 115]. As described above and in Chap. 1, these frameworks have the goal of providing continuous improvements in healthcare delivery by using the information generated by clinical practice to improve the care delivered to patients.

15.5.6   Linked Multi-Modal Data Repositories: Multiple Data Sources

Linking databases with different types of data offers immense opportunities to researchers and clinicians using big-data paradigms to acquire actionable knowledge by maximizing the variety and volume of data available for generating hypotheses, as shown in Table 15.7. For example, a system that integrated notes from different specialties breaks down the traditional information silos that have built up first through paper, then through lack of interoperability, to increase the variety of the data [136]. It is worth noting that all the data for a multi-modal data repository

Table 15.7 Multi-modal data repositories

Big data repository class	Type				Examples
	I	P	D	S	
Biobanks		X			UK Biobank [29] Veterans Affairs Million Veterans Programme [129] NIH biobank AllofUs is currently recruiting 1 million US citizens, aiming to actively recruit diverse populations, including those that have been historically underrepresented in biomedical research [34]
	X	X			Electronic medical records and genomics network (eMERGE) [130]
	X	X			Informatics for integrating biology and the bedside (i2b2) [111]
	X	X	X		NHS Scotland SHARE uses blood samples left over after routine procedures linked to NHS records [131]
Linked multi-modal data and disease-specific collaborations Psychiatric biobanks and bioresources	X	X			European autism intervention (EU-AIMS) [132]
	X	X	X	X	Simons Foundation research autism initiative (SFARI) [133] The Simons simplex collection (SSC)
	X	X	X		Common Mind Consortium [134]
	X		X		Genetic Links to Anxiety and Depression (GLAD) Study [31]
		X	X		NIMH Repository and Genomics Resource [135]

These repositories bring together cohorts of participants, each of whom share biological data, healthcare use and other data, for example from surveys and behavioral monitoring. Depending on the original consent, it may be possible to go back either to the cohort or specific groups of participants for further questions. Types: Initiative (I), Platform (P), Dataset (D), Study (S)

could sit in one place, or could sit in separate repositories linked by a virtual framework that allows integrated searching [137], using the "federated query" model describe above.

The potential for knowledge discovery about mental disorders expands greatly when there is more variety in data types, for instance linking a participants' clinical information (such as presence of psychotic illness or not) and other types of data [138], including biological or behavioral data. Thus, genetic data linked to self-reported diagnoses can generate hypotheses about the heritability of mental disorders [139], and prescription data linked with diagnostic codes can look for patterns to generate hypotheses about of efficacy and adverse events [94, 140, 141]. Predictive models usually perform better when different types of data of more and different kinds are linked together. For instance algorithms predicting treatment response for people with depression have been shown to be more accurate when they take into account more types of data [142] and a study looking at predictors of suicide in US soldiers found important predictors such as service history and criminal record, in addition to standard clinical information [143]. Linkage of clinical data to external datasets can also be used to include aspects of functioning missing from clinical data of healthcare encounters, as in this study using disability claims

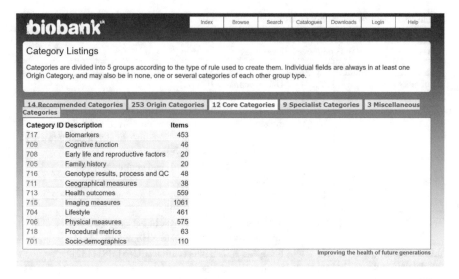

Fig. 15.6 Screenshot from the UK Biobank (Credit UK Biobank ©)

to explore absence from work [144] and in attempts to pool educational data about younger people, to look for early signs of mental disorder [145].

The linkage of detailed phenotypic data with -omics data, imaging data and detailed geographical data was formerly limited to small-scale cohort studies or surveys, which have led to the discovery of many features that confer risk of mental disorder, but each of small effect [146]. Very large samples are required to look at the interplay of these features. The UK Biobank for instance has enrolled 500,000 people who spent a half-day at an assessment center and gave blood for genomics, metabolomics and epigenetics; activity data and imaging data will be available on 100,000 each; a focused mental health questionnaire has been answered by 160,000. This information is linked to hospital registry data for all, and primary care data in a majority—and is searchable online (example in Fig. 15.6). Such data repositories are particularly useful for studies that look at associations between systems that are usually studied by different groups of researchers, such as metabolic phenotype with depression phenotype [147], and ripe for data mining for potential new bio-markers [148].

The field can benefit from participation in existing data repositories, but there are still limitations—and initiatives there to improve upon them. For example, UK Biobank has insufficient coverage of ethnic minorities to make any meaningful comparison between people of different backgrounds, or indeed to know whether findings even apply to individuals with ancestries other than the majority White European. The National Institute of Health in the USA has a bigger biobank called "AllOfUs" that has engaged minority communities to try to get coverage that will allow better studies of how ethnic background and associated factors affect mental health [149]. UK Biobank also has only a small share of questions on mental health and a restricted age range, but disease-specific biobanks such as the Genetic Links to Anxiety and Depression (GLAD) took advantage of a completely web-based platform to recruit people of all ages across the UK who had all experienced depression or an anxiety disorder. Finally, there are some studies that require an enormous number of observations to make discoveries, which has led to international collaborations to pool data like the Psychiatric Genomics Consortium [33].

Much of the work done on these linked databases is to try to generate hypotheses regarding potential etiology of mental disorders, and through this insight, to suggest potential treatment and prevention. For instance, considering comorbidities of mental disorders has suggested genes and proteins that may link them [110, 150] and the biologic basis of mental disorders is being investigated by the linking of genomic data to imaging data to mental and behavioral data [151]. Linking different kinds of psychosocial data can also help to understand health outcomes, such as linking personality traits to social behavior and self-harm [152] and to look at wider outcomes of mental disorder such as educational attainment [145] and occupation [153]. Conventional mental disorder diagnostic categories are usually used in knowledge discovery, but teams have also used data to suggest refinements to diagnostic categories—for instance the finding that immunology can be used to subtype Autism Spectrum Disorders—and these subtypes have an influence on clinical trajectory [154]. Others have gone beyond categories to look at transdiagnostic patterns and dimensional phenotypes [155]. This is greatly facilitated by extracting features from full text in electronic health records [103, 104].

15.5.7 Practical Challenges of Using Data Repositories for Mental Health Research

Different kinds of data collection methods may result in different biases. A distinction may be made between those research data sources where the participants are volunteers, and administrative data sources where data is used under provisions for the 'public good' in a massed and de-identified way. A volunteer cohort often has a selection bias towards the health-conscious and well-educated [156]. Administrative health data is commonly only routinely collected when the participant receives medical care—usually when they are unwell. This gives rise to an observation bias (attending medical care for one disorder makes documentation of another disorder more likely), which may need attention in analysis. A consideration of these and other source-specific biases is important in planning studies and interpreting results [157]. Two particularly pertinent considerations are *missingness* and *psychiatric diagnosis*.

Missingness Consider the situation where a researcher is interested in differences in psychiatric diagnosis in people from different racial groups. They may use an EHR repository and find a structured field for ethnicity, but they find that in over half of cases this is not completed. The researcher then discovers that someone has published a natural language processing application that extracts ethnicity information from free text, but it was developed on and designed for primary care notes rather than secondary care notes, so how the application will perform on this new data is unknown. There is the possibility to link the EHR to national census data (where regulations permit), but this only links in cases where the person has not relocated since the last census, and the census contains a different ethnicity classification than the EHR. The overall picture is not actually just missing data, but of multiple sub-optimal possibilities for ascertaining data, which the researcher has to navigate. While data missing at random is difficult enough, it is actually more likely that there will be different bias in the availability of each of these data types, which means that just using the cases with complete data is liable to reduce not only size, but representativeness of the whole. For example, the census data will be less likely to reflect students and people with insecure housing, who might make up important strata within the study.

Psychiatric Diagnosis There is a 'diagnosis' structured field in the EHR that is an ICD-10 code, but the researcher may find that since clinicians are obliged to complete this field as soon as they see someone in clinic, many cases are coded using "fudge codes" (such as F99—mental and behavioral disorder not otherwise specified). Using hospital discharge codes instead gives a more intelligible output, but restricting to people discharged from psychiatric hospitals will distort the sample to those who are most likely to be admitted—those who are perceived to be a risk to self or others. Ideally a researcher would like to know about the reliability of a discharge diagnosis through "validation studies", but as recent reviews testify [158, 159], the variability between sources of diagnosis, probably by hospital/clinician, and possibly by gender and ethnicity [160], mean that validation done in one cohort/database may not translate to another. There is also a documented phenomenon of a misclassification bias away from more stigmatizing diagnoses in administrative diagnoses [161]. Ultimately, databases may never be able to give that fully considered nuanced diagnostic formulation a clinical interview can give, and this can have consequences for research [162], so the researcher may have to embrace that uncertainty. The issue of diagnostic classification is particularly thorny when working across different cultures [163], so that extra considerations in research designs may be needed where this occurs [164].

15.6   Case Study: Developing a Big Data Registry/Repository

To understand the design constraints on research data repositories, it may be helpful to adopt the perspective of an entity (or entities) charged with developing and maintaining them. As an example, a task might be to develop a data repository of all data generated by research funded by the US National Institute of Mental Health, perhaps only on a single mental disorder, Autism Spectrum

Disorder (ASD). The only requirement is to store data about research participants or patients (not, for instance, data generated by wet-lab experiments on bacteria strains).

The first step is to conduct a **requirements analysis** to answer some basic questions to an adequate level of specificity. The goal of the analysis will be to develop a reasonably clear picture of the intended data uses, the expected data sources, and a vision for how to transform and store the data from the sources so that it supports the intended uses. This analysis should aim to answer (at least) the following questions:

- What are the intended data *uses*?
  - What kinds of research questions can the data answer?
  - Can prototypical analytics methods be articulated that are appropriate for the data?
  - Who are the expected users and what type of skills and knowledge relative to data use might they have?
  - Who are the important stakeholders in the data repository that may not be data users (e.g., the public, anyone providing funding, government oversight agencies, data sources, industry groups)? What does the repository need to show to keep these stakeholders informed and supportive?
  - Are there important privacy constraints on intended uses?
- What are the expected data *sources*?
  - What are the expected data types that will be supported? (E.g., limiting submissions to form-derived data, or more complex experimental results or raw sensor readings that may be submitted as large files).
  - What format are the sources most likely to provide the data in? How much variability is anticipated in data submission formats and content? How much uniformity can be enforced in data submission formats and content?
  - What data linking requirements (if any) are going to be enforced? Will research participants be linked across studies? How? Are there privacy constraints on linkage?
- What options are available for data transformation and storage that would support the intended uses?
  - What data models and architecture provide adequate representation for each intended data type (e.g. is a relational database sufficient? Can all data points and their relations be represented accurately)?
  - What mechanisms will be available to the data users to search and retrieve data of interest?

The requirements analysis should provide input into the next step: the design phase. One main area of tension in the design is likely to revolve around how strict vs. relaxed the data submission requirements might be, which is related to how highly "curated" the repository will become. Very relaxed requirements means anything goes in. It lowers the barrier to submission for data sources and reduces the cost of data validation for the repository. On the other hand, the result can be very difficult to use and may not support the intended data uses (such as one desideratum implied by our use case: aggregating analytic data sets across multiple studies).

Box 15.1 Constructing a Large Data Repository
What are the main design considerations?

- What are the data sources?
- What are the intended uses?
- Who are the intended users?
- How should the data be deposited and stored so that it supports the intended uses?

What are the main design dimensions?

- Data submission standards and quality requirements: Should they be easy or rigorous? Relaxed or tightly controlled?
- Data volume requirements: What are the characteristics of the data, and what implications do they have on requirements?
- Data governance: Under what conditions should/can data be made available? How many hoops does a potential data user have to jump through?

Box 15.2 Using a Large Data Repository
- Understand the data collection protocols
- Understand the large-scale data structure (the tables)
- Understand the fine-grained data structure (the columns, coding schemes)
- Learn to use cohort discovery tools, if available
- Identify a cohort of interest
- Apply for access
- Access a data set
- Run and review data quality reports and match against any data release notes
- Run exploratory analyses and verify that you understand each variable you plan to use
- Run actual analysis
- Contact original data acquisition team, if needed. Don't be shy.
- Publish and bask in glory
- Give credit

> **Box 15.3 Submitting Data to a Large Data Repository**
> - Understand the policies
> - Understand the data submission process
> - Complete forms (yes, many, many forms)
> - Generate the upload package
>   - Datasets
>   - Associated files
>   - Meta-data
> - Complete a test upload and review the validation error reports. Yes, many, many errors.
> - Fix data issues and resubmit. Rinse, repeat.
> - Bask in the warm glow of contributing to humanity's progress by expanding the shared pool of usable data

"Data Lakes" (defined as repositories capable of storing all of your structured and unstructured data without having to first impose any specific structure on that data) can easily become "Data Swamps" if care is not taken to curate what can flow in.

Unfortunately, the reversed approach, of a strictly curated registry with strict and extensive submission requirements, poses its own problems. It can create an insurmountable burden for data submission partners and can dramatically increase the cost of validation and meta-data management to make the data repository program financially unsustainable. To extend the earlier metaphor, if a "Data Lake" only admits the purest distilled water the result might be a mere trickle feeding a miniscule "Data Puddle." The wise designer must navigate this tension and the practical outcome is usually far from either extreme.

15.6.1 Who Develops Disease-Specific Data Repositories in Mental Health and Why?

There are several types of organizational entities that develop data repositories in mental health. Some of these are developed specifically for research purposes (e.g. a publication database), some are developed organically in an organization through daily practice or use (e.g. a reimbursement register), and some can be a combination of both (e.g. a linked EHR database). Government agencies, like the National Health Service (NHS) in the UK, or the National Institute of Mental Health (NIMH) in the US, produce, fund, or host data repositories of various types for research, policy information, and other purposes. Professional specialty societies such as the American Psychological Association (APA), or the American Academy of Neurology (AAN) also develop and host data repositories. Note that in the US professional specialty societies may have regulatory and financial incentives for developing data assets, e.g., to get society members reimbursement under the MIPS program. In other countries the incentives and players may be different.

Other examples include specific disease advocacy groups, such as the National Organization for Rare Disorders (NORD), the Anxiety and Depression Association of America (ADAA) [165], and the Simons Foundation Autism Research Initiative (SFARI). There are also academic research networks and research centers specifically focusing on certain diseases, such as the Autism Biomarker Consortium for Clinical Trials (ABC-CT).

More recently, online platforms of different types have also become important data repository sources for mental health. Some social media platforms have emerged focusing solely on mental health related topics where peer support is a main feature, e.g. platforms like PatientsLikeMe.com. Furthermore, online counseling services and internet-based cognitive behavioral therapy intrinsically generate data that could be used for knowledge discovery, though of course this approach calls for significant ethical and legal consideration.

For each of these types of repositories, it is important to consider who the stakeholders are, who might want the data and for what purpose, and understand the context in which it is developed. Moreover, depending on the context, it is also important to consider what the organizational or business models are underlying the repository and what the sustainability strategies are. Another contextual aspect that is important to consider with any data repository is the political context for the creation and maintenance of any resource, to understand strengths and limitations of the data.

15.7 Closing Thoughts: Opportunities and Challenges

We live in an era where the way mental health research is conducted can be transformed by novel combinations of technical infrastructure, data collection and availability, computational methods, and analytical approaches. Recent advances have opened unprecedented opportunities, but to truly reach a state of "reproducible" scientific practices and "open science" following the FAIR principles, certain aspects of knowledge discovery in these types of data repositories need special consideration.

Although most of the sources that are mentioned in this chapter are from developed countries, sufficient technology now exists in low and middle-income countries to collect data to enable them to benefit from data insights in order to create a learning health system. Data will come through conventional health information systems [166], community health workers [167] and demographic data through other agencies [168]. Infection and epidemics remain the most obvious aim of these systems, but developing countries also have a huge burden of non-communicable disease, including mental disorders, and use of data insights may decrease this burden and promote development [169, 170]. As mobile phones have become ubiquitous and technology an integral part of humanitarian response to disasters, data will become available on the most vulnerable populations on the globe who have been displaced through war and natural disaster, and could be used to help future responses.

Considerable challenges to using Big Data resources remain and must be tackled by both experienced and novice researchers working in the field. In fact, your work in this area will significantly impact how we take advantage of the opportunities and navigate the challenges. When working with data repositories and knowledge discovery methods, first consider the provenance of the data, which is often not collected with research in mind, or with a different type of research in mind. Second, consider that data collection, ingestion, and curation can inadvertently reduce to dichotomous outcomes what may be nuanced human traits or states. Then consider that linking between any two sources that were not initially designed to be linked is by no means simple or infallible.

The researcher who develops an approach to identify patterns in the data, or a predictive model based on retrospective data, often cannot interpret a finding unless they know where the data comes from, how it is collected, the limitations of repositories, and the underlying assumptions of the learning algorithms.

Despite the many remaining challenges, Big Data is growing in importance as an exceptionally exciting source of knowledge about mental health. We are confident that the growth will continue, and we hope yours will be among the many hands that will help overcome the challenges described above.

References

1. De Mauro A, Greco M, Grimaldi M. A formal definition of big data based on its essential features. Libr Rev. 2016;65:122–35.
2. Raghupathi W, Raghupathi V. Big data analytics in healthcare: promise and potential. Health Inf Sci Syst. 2014;2:3.
3. Gruebner O, Sykora M, Lowe SR, Shankardass K, Galea S, Subramanian SV. Big data opportunities for social behavioral and mental health research. Soc Sci Med. 2017;189:167–9.
4. McIntosh AM, Stewart R, John A, Smith DJ, Davis K, Sudlow C, et al. Data science for mental health: a UK perspective on a global challenge. Lancet Psychiatry. 2016;3:993–8.
5. Stewart R, Davis K. 'big data' in mental health research: current status and emerging possibilities. Soc Psychiatry Psychiatr Epidemiol. 2016;51:1055–72.
6. Russ TC, Woelbert E, Davis KAS, Hafferty JD, Ibrahim Z, Inkster B, et al. How data science can advance mental health research. Nat Hum Behav. 2019;3:24–32.
7. Khoury MJ, Ioannidis JPA. Big data meets public health. Science. 2014;346:1054–5.
8. Passos IC, Mwangi B, Kapczinski F. Big data analytics and machine learning: 2015 and beyond. Lancet Psychiatry. 2016;3:13–5.
9. Passos IC, Mwangi B, Kapczinski F, editors. Personalized psychiatry: big data analytics in mental health [Internet]. Springer International Publishing, Berlin; 2019 [cited 2019 Sep 24]. Available from: https://www.springer.com/gb/book/9783030035525
10. Hulsen T, Jamuar SS, Moody AR, Karnes JH, Varga O, Hedensted S, et al. From big data to precision medicine. Front Med (Lausanne). 2019;6:34.
11. Furu K, Wettermark B, Andersen M, Martikainen JE, Almarsdottir AB, Sørensen HT. The Nordic countries as a cohort for Pharmacoepidemiological research. Basic Clin Pharmacol Toxicol. 2010;106:86–94.
12. Mental Health Research Network [Internet]. [cited 2020 May 15]. Available from: http://hcsrn.org/mhrn/en/
13. OMOP common data model – OHDSI [Internet]. [cited 2020 Aug 12]. Available from: https://www.ohdsi.org/data-standardization/the-common-data-model/

14. PCORnet [Internet]. The national patient-centered clinical research network. [cited 2020 Aug 12]. Available from: https://pcornet.org/

15. PCORnet common data model forum [Internet]. GitHub. [cited 2020 Aug 12]. Available from: https://github.com/CDMFORUM

16. Standards | CDISC [Internet]. [cited 2020 Sep 11]. Available from: https://www.cdisc.org/standards

17. Hume S, Aerts J, Sarnikar S, Huser V. Current applications and future directions for the CDISC operational data model standard: a methodological review. J Biomed Inform. 2016;60:352–62.

18. Apache Hadoop [Internet]. [cited 2020 Aug 11]. Available from: https://hadoop.apache.org/

19. Apache Spark™ – Unified Analytics Engine for Big Data [Internet]. [cited 2020 Aug 11]. Available from: https://spark.apache.org/

20. Apache Hive TM [Internet]. [cited 2020 Aug 11]. Available from: https://hive.apache.org/

21. Apache Flink: Stateful Computations over Data Streams [Internet]. [cited 2020 Aug 11]. Available from: https://flink.apache.org/

22. Apache Kafka [Internet]. Apache Kafka. [cited 2020 Aug 11]. Available from: https://kafka.apache.org/

23. Martone ME, Garcia-Castro A, VandenBos GR. Data sharing in psychology. Am Psychol. 2018;73:111–25.

24. Baker M. 1,500 scientists lift the lid on reproducibility. Nature News. 2016;533:452.

25. Wilkinson MD, Dumontier M, IJJ A, Appleton G, Axton M, Baak A, et al. The FAIR Guiding Principles for scientific data management and stewardship. Scientific Data. 2016;3:160018.

26. Recommended Data Repositories | Scientific Data [Internet]. [cited 2020 May 15]. Available from: https://www.nature.com/sdata/policies/repositories

27. Hesse BW. Can psychology walk the walk of open science? Am Psychol. 2018;73:126–37.

28. Gremyr A, Malm U, Lundin L, Andersson A-C. A learning health system for people with severe mental illness: a promise for continuous learning, patient coproduction and more effective care. Digital Psychiatry Taylor & Francis. 2019;2:8–13.

29. UK Biobank [Internet]. [cited 2020 May 15]. Available from: https://www.ukbiobank.ac.uk/

30. Tenenbaum JD, Bhuvaneshwar K, Gagliardi JP, Fultz Hollis K, Jia P, Ma L, et al. Translational bioinformatics in mental health: open access data sources and computational biomarker discovery. Brief Bioinformatics. 2019;20:842–56.

31. Genetic links to anxiety and depression study – GLAD study [Internet]. [cited 2020 May 15]. Available from: https://gladstudy.org.uk/

32. Matcham F. Barattieri di san Pietro C, Bulgari V, de Girolamo G, Dobson R, Eriksson H, et al. remote assessment of disease and relapse in major depressive disorder (RADAR-MDD): a multi-Centre prospective cohort study protocol. BMC Psychiatry. 2019;19:72.

33. What is the PGC? [Internet]. Psychiatric Genomics Consortium. [cited 2020 May 15]. Available from: https://www.med.unc.edu/pgc/

34. The all of us research program investigators. The "All of Us" Research Program. N Engl J Med. 2019;381:668–76.

35. pubmeddev. Home – PubMed – NCBI [Internet]. [cited 2020 May 15]. Available from: https://www.ncbi.nlm.nih.gov/pubmed/

36. PsycInfo – APA Publishing | APA [Internet]. https://www.apa.org. [cited 2020 May 15]. Available from: https://www.apa.org/pubs/databases/psycinfo/index

37. OMIM – Online Mendelian Inheritance in Man [Internet]. [cited 2020 May 15]. Available from: https://omim.org/

38. Liao Y, Wang J, Jaehnig EJ, Shi Z, Zhang B. WebGestalt 2019: gene set analysis toolkit with revamped UIs and APIs. Nucleic Acids Res. 2019;47:W199–205.

39. Wishart DS, Feunang YD, Guo AC, Lo EJ, Marcu A, Grant JR, et al. DrugBank 5.0: a major update to the DrugBank database for 2018. Nucleic Acids Res. 2018;46:D1074–82.

40. SIDER side effect resource [Internet]. [cited 2020 May 15]. Available from: http://sideeffects.embl.de/

41. NIF | Welcome... [Internet]. [cited 2020 May 15]. Available from: https://neuinfo.org/
42. ETS Educational Testing Service's TestLink database [Internet]. [cited 2020 May 18]. Available from: https://www.ets.org/test_link/about/
43. HaPI Database [Internet]. Behavioral Measurement Database Services. [cited 2020 May 18]. Available from: https://www.bmdshapi.com/hapidatabase/
44. Mental Measurements Yearbook with Tests in Print [Internet]. [cited 2020 May 18]. Available from: https://www.ovid.com/product-details.10631.html
45. Mental Measurements Yearbook | Buros Center for Testing | Nebraska [Internet]. [cited 2020 May 18]. Available from: https://buros.org/mental-measurements-yearbook
46. PsycTESTS – APA Publishing [Internet]. https://www.apa.org. [cited 2020 May 18]. Available from: https://www.apa.org/pubs/databases/psyctests/index
47. MEDLINE®: Description of the Database [Internet]. [cited 2019 Oct 25]. Available from: https://www.nlm.nih.gov/bsd/medline.html
48. Medical Subject Headings – Home Page [Internet]. [cited 2019 Oct 25]. Available from: https://www.nlm.nih.gov/mesh/meshhome.html
49. Abbe A, Grouin C, Zweigenbaum P, Falissard B. Text mining applications in psychiatry: a systematic literature review. Int J Methods Psychiatr Res. 2016;25:86–100.
50. Smalheiser NR. Informatics and hypothesis-driven research. EMBO Rep. 2002;3:702.
51. Gonzalez-Mantilla AJ, Moreno-De-Luca A, Ledbetter DH, Martin CL. A cross-disorder method to identify novel candidate genes for developmental brain disorders. JAMA Psychiat. 2016;73:275–83.
52. PharmGKB [Internet]. PharmGKB. [cited 2020 May 15]. Available from: https://www.pharmgkb.org/
53. Bean DM, Wu H, Iqbal E, Dzahini O, Ibrahim ZM, Broadbent M, et al. Knowledge graph prediction of unknown adverse drug reactions and validation in electronic health records. Sci Rep [Internet]. 2017 [cited 2019 Oct 29];7. Available from: https://www.ncbi.nlm.nih.gov/pmc/articles/PMC5703951/
54. So H-C, Chau CK-L, Chiu W-T, Ho K-S, Lo C-P, Yim SH-Y, et al. Analysis of genome-wide association data highlights candidates for drug repositioning in psychiatry. Nat Neurosci. 2017;20:1342–9.
55. Home – SRA – NCBI [Internet]. [cited 2020 May 15]. Available from: https://www.ncbi.nlm.nih.gov/sra
56. Barrett T, Wilhite SE, Ledoux P, Evangelista C, Kim IF, Tomashevsky M, et al. NCBI GEO: archive for functional genomics data sets--update. Nucleic Acids Res. 2013;41:D991–5.
57. PRIDE – Proteomics Identification Database [Internet]. [cited 2020 May 15]. Available from: https://www.ebi.ac.uk/pride/archive/
58. Deutsch EW, Csordas A, Sun Z, Jarnuczak A, Perez-Riverol Y, Ternent T, et al. The ProteomeXchange consortium in 2017: supporting the cultural change in proteomics public data deposition. Nucleic Acids Res. 2017;45:D1100–6.
59. Metabolomics Workbench: Home [Internet]. [cited 2020 May 15]. Available from: https://www.metabolomicsworkbench.org/
60. MetaboLights – Metabolomics experiments and derived information [Internet]. [cited 2020 May 15]. Available from: https://www.ebi.ac.uk/metabolights/
61. PharmVar [Internet]. [cited 2020 May 15]. Available from: https://www.pharmvar.org/
62. NDA [Internet]. [cited 2020 May 15]. Available from: https://nda.nih.gov/
63. Alfaro-Almagro F, Jenkinson M, Bangerter NK, Andersson JLR, Griffanti L, Douaud G, et al. Image processing and quality control for the first 10,000 brain imaging datasets from UK biobank. NeuroImage. 2018;166:400–24.
64. Vidaurre D, Abeysuriya R, Becker R, Quinn AJ, Alfaro-Almagro F, Smith SM, et al. Discovering dynamic brain networks from big data in rest and task. NeuroImage. 2018;180:646–56.
65. Kirov G, Kendall K, Rees E, Escott-Price V, Hewitt J, Thomas R, et al. The Uk biobank: a resource for Cnv analysis. Eur Neuropsychopharmacol. 2017;27:S491.

66. Hariprakash JM, Vellarikkal SK, Verma A, Ranawat AS, Jayarajan R, Ravi R, et al. SAGE: a comprehensive resource of genetic variants integrating South Asian whole genomes and exomes. Database [Internet]. 2018 [cited 2020 May 15];2018. Available from: https://academic.oup.com/database/article/doi/10.1093/database/bay080/5067958

67. OmicsDI: Home [Internet]. [cited 2020 May 15]. Available from: https://www.omicsdi.org/database

68. Connectome – Homepage [Internet]. [cited 2020 May 15]. Available from: https://www.humanconnectome.org/

69. A free and open platform for sharing MRI, MEG, EEG, iEEG, and ECoG data – OpenNeuro [Internet]. [cited 2020 May 15]. Available from: https://openneuro.org/

70. Imaging data | UK Biobank [Internet]. [cited 2020 May 15]. Available from: https://www.ukbiobank.ac.uk/imaging-data/

71. Genetic data | UK Biobank [Internet]. [cited 2020 May 15]. Available from: https://www.ukbiobank.ac.uk/scientists-3/genetic-data/

72. Dahl A, Cai N, Ko A, Laakso M, Pajukanta P, Flint J, et al. Reverse GWAS: using genetics to identify and model phenotypic subtypes. PLoS Genet. 2019;15:e1008009.

73. Avec 2018 [Internet]. [cited 2020 May 15]. Available from: https://sites.google.com/view/avec2018

74. Major Depressive Disorder | RADAR-CNS [Internet]. [cited 2020 May 15]. Available from: https://www.radar-cns.org/about/conditions/major-depressive-disorder

75. Robinson P, Turk D, Jilka S, Cella M. Measuring attitudes towards mental health using social media: investigating stigma and trivialisation. Soc Psychiatry Psychiatr Epidemiol. 2019;54:51–8.

76. Eichstaedt JC, Schwartz HA, Kern ML, Park G, Labarthe DR, Merchant RM, et al. Psychological language on twitter Predicts County-level heart disease mortality. Psychol Sci. 2015;26:159–69.

77. Gkotsis G, Oellrich A, Velupillai S, Liakata M, Hubbard TJP, Dobson RJB, et al. Characterisation of mental health conditions in social media using informed deep learning. Sci Rep. 2017;7:45141.

78. Choudhury MD, Kiciman E. The language of social support in social media and its effect on suicidal ideation risk. Proceedings of the International Conference on Web and Social Media (ICWSM-17) [Internet]. AAAI; 2017. Available from: https://www.microsoft.com/en-us/research/publication/language-social-support-social-media-effect-suicidal-ideation-risk/

79. Willetts M, Hollowell S, Aslett L, Holmes C, Doherty A. Statistical machine learning of sleep and physical activity phenotypes from sensor data in 96,220 UK biobank participants. Sci Rep. 2018;8:1–10.

80. Lyall LM, Wyse CA, Graham N, Ferguson A, Lyall DM, Cullen B, et al. Association of disrupted circadian rhythmicity with mood disorders, subjective wellbeing, and cognitive function: a cross-sectional study of 91 105 participants from the UK biobank. Lancet Psychiatry. 2018;5:507–14.

81. Tasnim M, Stroulia E. Detecting depression from voice. In: Meurs M-J, Rudzicz F, editors. Advances in artificial intelligence. Springer International Publishing, Berlin; 2019. p. 472–478.

82. Gunn JF, Lester D. Using google searches on the internet to monitor suicidal behavior. J Affect Disord. 2013;148:411–2.

83. Royal S. Machine learning: what do the public think?; the Royal Society's public dialogue on machine learning. London, UK: Royal Society; 2017. p 92. Available from: https://royalsociety.org/~/media/policy/projects/machine-learning/publications/public-views-of-machine-learning-ipsos-mori.pdf

84. Conway M, O'Connor D. Social media, big data, and mental health: current advances and ethical implications. Curr Opin Psychol. 2016;9:77–82.

85. Cheng Q, Li TM, Kwok C-L, Zhu T, Yip PS. Assessing suicide risk and emotional distress in Chinese social media: a text mining and machine learning study. J Med Internet Res. 2017;19:e243.

86. ICES Data [Internet]. [cited 2020 May 15]. Available from: https://www.ices.on.ca/Data-and-Privacy/ICES-data
87. Data Linkage WA [Internet]. Data Linkage WA. [cited 2020 May 15]. Available from: https://www.datalinkage-wa.org.au/
88. VigiAccess [Internet]. [cited 2020 May 15]. Available from: http://www.vigiaccess.org/
89. Data – Clalit Research Institute [Internet]. [cited 2020 May 15]. Available from: http://clalitresearch.org/about-us/our-data/
90. Longitudinal Health Insurance Database of Taiwan [Internet]. [cited 2020 May 15]. Available from: https://nhird.nhri.org.tw/en/
91. Research, Statistics, Data & Systems | CMS [Internet]. [cited 2020 May 15]. Available from: https://www.cms.gov/Research-Statistics-Data-and-Systems/Research-Statistics-Data-and-Systems
92. Welcome to IQVIA – A New Path to Your Success Via Human Data Science [Internet]. [cited 2020 May 15]. Available from: https://www.iqvia.com/
93. IBM MarketScan Research Databases – Overview [Internet]. 2020 [cited 2020 May 15]. Available from: https://www.ibm.com/products/marketscan-research-databases
94. Thesmar D, Sraer D, Pinheiro L, Dadson N, Veliche R, Greenberg P. Combining the power of artificial intelligence with the richness of healthcare claims data: opportunities and challenges. PharmacoEconomics. 2019;37:745–52.
95. Miller M, Swanson SA, Azrael D, Pate V, Stürmer T. Antidepressant dose, age, and the risk of deliberate self-harm. JAMA Intern Med. 2014;174:899–909.
96. Goldberg PD, Goldberg D, Huxley DP, Huxley P. Mental illness in the community: the pathway to psychiatric care. London: Routledge; 1980.
97. John A, McGregor J, Fone D, Dunstan F, Cornish R, Lyons RA, et al. Case-finding for common mental disorders of anxiety and depression in primary care: an external validation of routinely collected data. BMC Med Inform Decis Mak. 2016;16:35.
98. Spiers N, Qassem T, Bebbington P, McManus S, King M, Jenkins R, et al. Prevalence and treatment of common mental disorders in the English national population, 1993–2007. Br J Psychiatry. 2016;209:150–6.
99. Bate A, Lindquist M, Edwards IR. The application of knowledge discovery in databases to post-marketing drug safety: example of the WHO database. Fundam Clin Pharmacol. 2008;22:127–40.
100. Hersh WR, Weiner MG, Embi PJ, Logan JR, Payne PRO, Bernstam EV, et al. Caveats for the use of operational electronic health record data in comparative effectiveness research. Med Care. 2013;51:S30–7.
101. Zeltzer D, Balicer RD, Shir T, Flaks-Manov N, Einav L, Shadmi E. Prediction accuracy with electronic medical records versus administrative claims. Med Care. 2019;57:551–9.
102. Richard M, Aimé X, Krebs M-O, Charlet J. Enrich classifications in psychiatry with textual data: an ontology for psychiatry including social concepts. Stud Health Technol Inform. 2015;210:221–3.
103. Velupillai S, Suominen H, Liakata M, Roberts A, Shah AD, Morley K, et al. Using clinical natural language processing for health outcomes research: overview and actionable suggestions for future advances. J Biomed Inform. 2018;88:11–9.
104. Jackson R, Patel R, Velupillai S, Gkotsis G, Hoyle D, Stewart R. Knowledge discovery for Deep Phenotyping serious mental illness from Electronic Mental Health records [version 2; referees: 2 approved with reservations]. F1000Research. 2018;7:210.
105. Weissman MM, Pathak J, Talati A. Personal life events-a promising dimension for psychiatry in electronic health records. JAMA Psychiatry. 2019;77(2):115–6.
106. Lyalina S, Percha B, LePendu P, Iyer SV, Altman RB, Shah NH. Identifying phenotypic signatures of neuropsychiatric disorders from electronic medical records. J Am Med Inform Assoc. 2013;20:e297–305.
107. Coleman KJ, Stewart C, Waitzfelder BE, Zeber JE, Morales LS, Ahmed AT, et al. Racial/ethnic differences in diagnoses and treatment of mental health conditions across healthcare systems participating in the mental Health Research network. Psychiatr Serv. 2016;67:749–57.

108. Huang SH, LePendu P, Iyer SV, Tai-Seale M, Carrell D, Shah NH. Toward personalizing treatment for depression: predicting diagnosis and severity. J Am Med Inform Assoc. 2014;21:1069–75.
109. Eriksson R, Werge T, Jensen LJ, Brunak S. Dose-specific adverse drug reaction identification in electronic patient records: temporal data mining in an inpatient psychiatric population. Drug Saf. 2014;37:237–47.
110. Roque FS, Jensen PB, Schmock H, Dalgaard M, Andreatta M, Hansen T, et al. Using electronic patient records to discover disease correlations and stratify patient cohorts. PLoS Comput Biol. 2011;7:e1002141.
111. i2b2: Informatics for integrating biology & the bedside [Internet]. [cited 2020 May 15]. Available from: https://www.i2b2.org/
112. SHRINE – Open. Catalyst [Internet]. [cited 2020 Aug 11]. Available from: https://open.catalyst.harvard.edu/products/shrine/
113. Brown J. Popmednet (Pmn) [Internet]. Zenodo; 2018 [cited 2020 Aug 11]. Available from: https://zenodo.org/record/1400722
114. Deans KJ, Sabihi S, Forrest CB. Learning health systems. Semin Pediatr Surg. 2018;27:375–8.
115. Horwitz LI, Kuznetsova M, Jones SA. Creating a learning health system through rapid-cycle, Randomized testing. N Engl J Med. 2019;381:1175–9.
116. Network THI. Home I THIN Data [Internet]. [cited 2020 May 15]. Available from: https://www.the-health-improvement-network.com
117. Clinical Practice Research Datalink I CPRD [Internet]. [cited 2020 May 15]. Available from: https://www.cprd.com/
118. Welcome to Data QUEST I dataquest.iths.org [Internet]. [cited 2020 May 15]. Available from: https://dataquest.iths.org/
119. Canadian Primary Care Sentinel Surveillance Network [Internet]. [cited 2020 May 15]. Available from: https://cpcssn.ca/
120. VA Informatics and Computing Infrastructure (VINCI) [Internet]. [cited 2020 May 15]. Available from: https://www.hsrd.research.va.gov/for_researchers/vinci/
121. Medical Informatics – Department of Health Sciences Research – Medical Informatics [Internet]. Mayo Clinic. [cited 2020 May 15]. Available from: https://www.mayo.edu/research/departments-divisions/department-health-sciences-research/medical-informatics
122. A proof of concept for assessing emergency room use with primary care data and natural language processing. Abstract – Europe PMC [Internet]. [cited 2020 May 15]. Available from: https://europepmc.org/article/med/23223678
123. Braam AW, van Ommeren OWHR, van Buuren ML, Laan W, Smeets HM, Engelhard IM. Local geographical distribution of acute involuntary psychiatric admissions in subdistricts in and around Utrecht, the Netherlands. J Emerg Med Elsevier. 2016;50:449–57.
124. Clinical Record Interactive Search (CRIS) [Internet]. [cited 2020 May 15]. Available from: https://www.maudsleybrc.nihr.ac.uk/facilities/clinical-record-interactive-search-cris/
125. Home – Adolescent Mental Health Data Platform [Internet]. [cited 2020 May 15]. Available from: https://www.adolescentmentalhealth.uk/
126. SAIL Databank – The Secure Anonymised Information Linkage Databank [Internet]. [cited 2020 May 15]. Available from: https://saildatabank.com/
127. Home I Mental Health Data Science Scotland [Internet]. [cited 2020 May 15]. Available from: https://mhdss.ac.uk/
128. SHINE – Schools Health and Wellbeing Improvement Research Network [Internet]. [cited 2020 May 15]. Available from: https://shine.sphsu.gla.ac.uk/
129. Million Veteran Program (MVP) [Internet]. [cited 2020 May 15]. Available from: https://www.research.va.gov/mvp/
130. Welcome to eMerge > Collaborate [Internet]. [cited 2020 May 15]. Available from: https://emerge-network.org/
131. Researchers I Register4Share [Internet]. [cited 2020 May 15]. Available from: http://www.registerforshare.org/researchers

132. EU-AIMS – European Autism Interventions – A Multicentre Study for Deve [Internet]. [cited 2020 May 15]. Available from: https://www.eu-aims.eu/
133. SFARI | Simons Foundation Autism Research Initiative [Internet]. SFARI. [cited 2020 May 15]. Available from: https://www.sfari.org/
134. CommonMind Consortium Knowledge Portal – syn2759792 [Internet]. [cited 2020 May 15]. Available from: https://www.synapse.org/#!Synapse:syn2759792/wiki/69613
135. Home | NRGR [Internet]. [cited 2020 May 15]. Available from: https://www.nimhgenetics.org/
136. Dentler K, ten Teije A, de Keizer N, Cornet R. Barriers to the reuse of routinely recorded clinical data: a field report. Stud Health Technol Inform. 2013;192:313–7.
137. Huser V, Cimino JJ. Desiderata for healthcare integrated data repositories based on architectural comparison of three public repositories. AMIA Annu Symp Proc. 2013;2013:648–56.
138. Weber GM, Mandl KD, Kohane IS. Finding the missing link for big biomedical data. JAMA. 2014;311:2479–80.
139. Tung JY, Do CB, Hinds DA, Kiefer AK, Macpherson JM, Chowdry AB, et al. Efficient replication of over 180 genetic associations with self-reported medical data. PLoS One. 2011;6:e23473.
140. Hayes JF, Marston L, Walters K, Geddes JR, King M, Osborn DPJ. Lithium vs. valproate vs. olanzapine vs. quetiapine as maintenance monotherapy for bipolar disorder: a population-based UK cohort study using electronic health records. World Psychiatry. 2016;15:53–8.
141. Ouchi K, Lindvall C, Chai PR, Boyer EW. Machine learning to predict, detect, and intervene older adults vulnerable for adverse drug events in the emergency department. J Med Toxicol. 2018;14:248–52.
142. Lee Y, Ragguett R-M, Mansur RB, Boutilier JJ, Rosenblat JD, Trevizol A, et al. Applications of machine learning algorithms to predict therapeutic outcomes in depression: a meta-analysis and systematic review. J Affect Disord. 2018;241:519–32.
143. Kessler RC, Warner CH, Ivany C, Petukhova MV, Rose S, Bromet EJ, et al. Predicting suicides after psychiatric hospitalization in US Army soldiers: the Army study to assess risk and resilience in Servicemembers (Army STARRS). JAMA Psychiat. 2015;72:49–57.
144. Gaspar HA, Baskin II, Marcou G, Horvath D, Varnek A. Stargate GTM: bridging descriptor and activity spaces. J Chem Inf Model. 2015;55:2403–10.
145. Downs JM, Ford T, Stewart R, Epstein S, Shetty H, Little R, et al. An approach to linking education, social care and electronic health records for children and young people in South London: a linkage study of child and adolescent mental health service data. BMJ Open [Internet]. 2019 [cited 2019 Oct 31];9:e024355. Available from: https://bmjopen.bmj.com/content/9/1/e024355
146. Iniesta R, Stahl D, McGuffin P. Machine learning, statistical learning and the future of biological research in psychiatry. Psychol Med. 2016;46:2455–65.
147. Brailean A, Curtis J, Davis K, Dregan A, Hotopf M. Characteristics, comorbidities, and correlates of atypical depression: evidence from the UK biobank mental health survey. Psychol Med. 2019:1–10.
148. Zhou Y, Zhao L, Zhou N, Zhao Y, Marino S, Wang T, et al. Predictive big data analytics using the UK biobank data. Sci Rep [Internet]. 2019 [cited 2019 Oct 21];9:6012. Available from: https://www.ncbi.nlm.nih.gov/pmc/articles/PMC6461626/
149. National Institutes of Health (NIH). All of us [Internet]. [cited 2020 May 15]. Available from: https://allofus.nih.gov/
150. Hofmann-Apitius M, Alarcón-Riquelme ME, Chamberlain C, McHale D. Towards the taxonomy of human disease. Nat Rev Drug Discov. 2015;14:75–6.
151. Thompson PM, Stein JL, Medland SE, Hibar DP, Vasquez AA, Renteria ME, et al. The ENIGMA consortium: large-scale collaborative analyses of neuroimaging and genetic data. Brain Imaging Behav. 2014;8:153–82.
152. Shaw RJ, Cullen B, Graham N, Lyall DM, Mackay D, Okolie C, et al. Living alone, loneliness and lack of emotional support as predictors of suicide and self-harm: seven-year follow up of the UK Biobank cohort. medRxiv. 2019;19008458.

153. Kyaga S, Landén M, Boman M, Hultman CM, Långström N, Lichtenstein P. Mental illness, suicide and creativity: 40-year prospective total population study. J Psychiatr Res. 2013;47:83–90.

154. Kohane IS. An autism case history to review the systematic analysis of large-scale data to refine the diagnosis and treatment of neuropsychiatric disorders. Biol Psychiatry. 2015;77:59–65.

155. McCoy TH, Castro VM, Hart KL, Pellegrini AM, Yu S, Cai T, et al. Genome-wide association study of dimensional psychopathology using electronic health records. Biol Psychiatry. 2018;83:1005–11.

156. Fry A, Littlejohns TJ, Sudlow C, Doherty N, Adamska L, Sprosen T, et al. Comparison of sociodemographic and health-related characteristics of UK biobank participants with those of the general population. Am J Epidemiol. 2017;186:1026–34.

157. Davis KAS, Cullen B, Adams M, Brailean A, Breen G, Coleman JRI, et al. Indicators of mental disorders in UK biobank—a comparison of approaches. Int J Methods Psychiatr Res. 2019;28:e1796.

158. Larvin H, Peckham E, Prady SL. Case-finding for common mental disorders in primary care using routinely collected data: a systematic review. Soc Psychiatry Psychiatr Epidemiol. 2019;54:1161–75.

159. Davis KAS, Sudlow CLM, Hotopf M. Can mental health diagnoses in administrative data be used for research? A systematic review of the accuracy of routinely collected diagnoses. BMC Psychiatry. 2016;16:263.

160. Davis K, Bashford O, Jewell A, Shetty H, Stewart R, Sudlow C, et al. The validity of selected mental health diagnoses in English hospital episode statistics using data linkage to clinical records interactive search at South London and Maudsley. 2019.

161. Davis KAS, Bashford O, Jewell A, Shetty H, Stewart RJ, Sudlow CLM, et al. Using data linkage to electronic patient records to assess the validity of selected mental health diagnoses in English hospital episode statistics (HES). PLoS One. 2018;13:e0195002.

162. Cai N, Revez JA, Adams MJ, Andlauer TFM, Breen G, Byrne EM, et al. Minimal phenotyping yields genome-wide association signals of low specificity for major depression. Nat Genet Nature Publishing Group. 2020;52:437–47.

163. Summerfield D. How scientifically valid is the knowledge base of global mental health? BMJ. 2008;336:992–4.

164. Kohrt BA, Rasmussen A, Kaiser BN, Haroz EE, Maharjan SM, Mutamba BB, et al. Cultural concepts of distress and psychiatric disorders: literature review and research recommendations for global mental health epidemiology. Int J Epidemiol. 2014;43:365–406.

165. Sign Up to Help: Patient Registries | Anxiety and Depression Association of America, ADAA [Internet]. [cited 2020 May 15]. Available from: https://adaa.org/sign-help-patient-registries

166. Ahuja S, Mirzoev T, Lund C, Ofori-Atta A, Skeen S, Kufuor A. Key influences in the design and implementation of mental health information systems in Ghana and South Africa. Global Mental Health [Internet]. 2016 [cited 2019 Oct 31];3:e11. Available from: https://www.cambridge.org/core/journals/global-mental-health/article/key-influences-in-the-design-and-implementation-of-mental-health-information-systems-in-ghana-and-south-africa/DD11E388FB2FFE1E2E7C9D9DF2885E99

167. Buehler B, Ruggiero R, Mehta K. Empowering community health workers with technology solutions. IEEE Technol Soc Mag. 2013;32:44–52.

168. McIntyre D, Muirhead D, Gilson L. Geographic patterns of deprivation in South Africa: informing health equity analyses and public resource allocation strategies. Health Policy Plan. 2002;17:30–9.

169. Nugent R, Bertram MY, Jan S, Niessen LW, Sassi F, Jamison DT, et al. Investing in non-communicable disease prevention and management to advance the sustainable development goals. Lancet. 2018;391:2029–35.

170. Semrau M, Evans-Lacko S, Alem A, Ayuso-Mateos JL, Chisholm D, Gureje O, et al. Strengthening mental health systems in low- and middle-income countries: the emerald programme. BMC Med. 2015;13:79.

Chapter 16
Electronic Health Records (EHRS) and Other Clinical Information Systems in Mental Health

Tyler Anne Hassenfeldt and Ross D. Martin

Abstract Adoption of cutting-edge information technology (IT) practices has lagged behind in healthcare as compared to other industries, negatively impacting patient safety and provider efficiency. While federal legislation has helped push through broader use of electronic health records (EHRs) in medical settings, the same incentives have not yet been provided within mental health care. We summarize pertinent legislation and the resulting funding initiatives and changes to healthcare delivery (e.g., accountable care organizations [ACOs], the patient-centered medical home [PCMH]). Although there are many safety and quality benefits to EHRs, drawbacks remain, particularly related to concerns about privacy of patient data. Additionally, providers cite burnout and cost as reasons for their reluctance to adopt EHRs in their practice. Finally, we discuss the market share for EHR vendors in medical and mental health settings and additional uses for EHRS outside of clinical care.

Keywords Electronic health records (EHRs) · Health information exchange (HIE) Personal health records (PHRs) · Mental health · Patient safety

T. A. Hassenfeldt (✉)
Department of Psychiatry and Behavioral Sciences, Duke University School of Medicine, Durham, NC, USA

Duke Center for Autism and Brain Development, Durham, NC, USA
e-mail: tyler.hassenfeldt@duke.edu

R. D. Martin
360 Degree Insights, LLC, Clarksville, MD, USA
e-mail: ross@360degreeinsights.com

© Springer Nature Switzerland AG 2021
J. D. Tenenbaum, P. A. Ranallo (eds.), *Mental Health Informatics*, Health Informatics, https://doi.org/10.1007/978-3-030-70558-9_16

16.1   Introduction

Health information technology (Health IT)—particularly electronic health records (EHRs) and health information exchange (HIE; Table 16.1)—are transforming how healthcare providers, patients, and payers create, store, access, and exchange clinical information. Especially in the last 10 years, EHR adoption has become significantly more widespread in the United States. However, the transition from paper records to electronic ones has not been without its challenges. Traditional methods for managing care delivery—including in the mental health field—do not yet fully leverage the promise of information on demand. Additionally, the sharing of information across silos remains a challenge for regulatory, privacy, business, financial, and inertial reasons. In this chapter, we explore the evolution of EHRs, health information exchange, personal health records (PHRs), and other clinical information systems and how these systems have changed the way mental health care services are delivered in the United States, including their transformational effects and the challenges that remain.

Anyone who has spent time talking with providers and patients about health system reform and information technology will inevitably hear someone ask the question, "Why is it that, for the last 40 years, I've been able to go to an ATM anywhere in the world and get money out of my local bank account but I still can't get my medical records to show up in the hospital across the street?" In a 2009 speech, President Obama quoted Newt Gingrich as saying, "we do a better job tracking a FedEx package in this country than we do tracking patients' health records." [2]

It does seem that healthcare, when compared with any other industry in the US, is desperately behind the information technology adoption curve. Even as the adoption of EHRs has grown dramatically in the last 20 years, there are still many processes that rely on paper, fax, and phone when all other aspects of human interactions have been augmented with electronic data flow. One can examine the drivers of IT adoption in other industries and compare them with those in healthcare to better understand why significant inefficiencies in information flow persist in healthcare.

The traditional fee-for-service (FFS) payment model, as an example, is a primary inhibitor for clinical data flow. As we discuss below, individual providers and healthcare systems have a disincentive to share information when FFS dominates.

Table 16.1 Network definitions from NAHIT [1]

Term	NAHIT definition
Health information exchange (HIE)	The electronic movement of health-related information among organizations according to nationally recognized standards
Health information organization (HIO)	An organization that oversees and governs the exchange of health-related information among organizations according to nationally-recognized standards
Regional health information organization (RHIO)	A health information organization that brings together health care stakeholders within a defined geographic area and governs health information exchange among them for the purpose of improving health and care in that community

Chart review or analysis of results ordered by another provider would likely not be reimbursable, even if additional testing were unnecessary and could be burdensome to the patient. When there is no reimbursement for delivering imaging or laboratory data to another provider or for receiving the data, there is instead a financial incentive to simply repeat a test. Providers also cite privacy and information security concerns as reasons to limit sharing data (see "EHR Disadvantages" section below).

16.1.1 Historical Perspective

The 2000s were a turning point in propelling the Health IT field forward in the US (see Fig. 16.1 for timeline of important dates). Beginning in 2004, national attention became increasingly focused on the safety and quality improvements that could be realized through EHRs and health information exchange, building the foundation for the dramatic Health IT investments that were to come.

In April 2004, given increasing healthcare costs and their impact on medical systems and the nation as a whole, President George W. Bush signed Executive Order 13335, which challenged the healthcare system to design and implement EHRs for all Americans by 2014. This order also formed the United States Department of Health & Human Services (DHHS) Office of the National Coordinator for Health Information Technology (ONC). From 2005 to 2010, the American National Standards Institute (ANSI) managed the Healthcare Information Technology Standards Panel (HITSP) with funding from the ONC to promote healthcare interoperability by harmonizing Health IT standards, particularly leveraging the standards from HL7, the National Council for Prescription Drug Programs (NCPDP), ANSI, and X12 among others. These Interoperability Specifications covered many domains such as laboratory results reporting, biosurveillance, consumer access to medical records, emergency response, and quality reporting [3]. These interoperability specifications led the way to certification programs for EHRs.

The National Alliance for Health Information Technology (NAHIT) operated from 2002 to 2009 with the purpose of creating best practices and a more standardized Health IT industry [4]. NAHIT defined three primary benefits to HIE systems: (1) care coordination at the provider and system levels, (2) increased understanding and autonomy for consumers related to their own health information, and (3) improved public health initiatives due to high quality aggregate data [1].

16.1.2 Federal Initiatives Related to Health IT

In 2009, as the world experienced the most significant economic recession since the Great Depression, the US Congress passed into law the Health Information Technology for Economic and Clinical Health (HITECH) Act as part of the

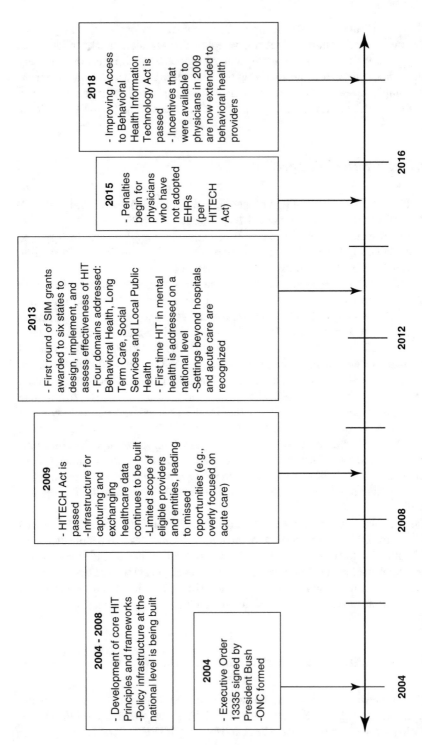

Fig. 16.1 Timeline of important dates in Health IT

American Recovery & Reinvestment Act of 2009 [5]. HITECH provided incentives for the "meaningful use" of EHRs among hospitals and physicians as well as penalties for not adopting EHRs beginning in 2015. The HITECH incentive program, however, excluded certain mental health care professionals (particularly non-physician advanced practice providers [APPs]). This focus primarily on physicians and acute care hospitals led to a missed opportunity to provide the same Health IT infrastructure for behavioral health providers. The resulting lag in the adoption of EHRs in mental health care prevented behavioral healthcare consumers from receiving the same safety and quality benefits afforded those accessing care in an EHR-supported medical setting.

The HITECH Act also included a positive change to the Health Insurance Portability and Accountability Act (HIPAA). Specifically, this provision allowed consumers to request a copy of their electronic health information, including having this data sent to the consumer's preferred repository, such as a PHR. The HITECH Act included $564 million in grant funding for statewide health information exchange (HIE) with a minimum of $800,000 for every state and territory in the US. While some HITECH-funded programs were able to accelerate HIE through these grants, many failed to deliver substantive change during the course of the grant program as EHR adoption was still low and the traditional funding of healthcare largely created disincentives for sharing data [6]. A national study of data from 2008 to 2014 indicated that 75% of hospitals in the United States had adopted at least a simple EHR, but that smaller and more rural hospitals lagged behind [7]. More recent data from 2019 suggests that up to 96% of acute-care hospitals in the US now use EHRs [8].

The introduction of the Affordable Healthcare Act (ACA) in 2012 was a landmark change to the delivery of healthcare services. Several new models for behavioral healthcare delivery were ushered in with ACA, including the introduction of accountable care organizations (ACOs) and the patient-centered medical home (PCMH) [9].

16.1.3   ACOs and PCMHs

ACOs are tasked with providing care for a specific set of consumers (e.g., everyone living in a specific region; see Fig. 16.2 for a sample ACO structure). ACOs bring together a player and a group of providers (usually including at least one hospital and primary and specialty care providers) to serve this population of consumers [9]. While there are critics of the ACO model, proponents suggest that this model could introduce more standardized models of care, improve HIE interoperability, and cut costs for both payers and providers [9] by better aligning the incentives that promote better quality care and care coordination. Where the fee for service model disincentivizes data sharing, ACO and PCMH models rely on complete, accurate, and timely exchange of clinical data between providers. Their adoption can therefore catalyze improvements to Health IT and HIE.

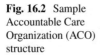

Fig. 16.2 Sample
Accountable Care
Organization (ACO)
structure

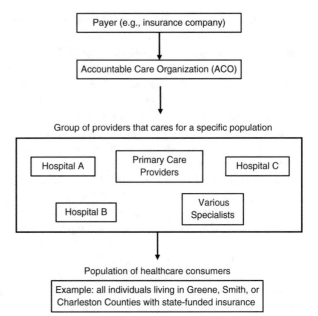

PCMHs tend to operate on a smaller scale than ACOs, but with a similar goal of caring for consumers with acute and chronic medical and psychological illnesses. PCMHs specifically integrate medical and behavioral healthcare in the same setting, with a strong emphasis on building up the consumer's relationship with their primary care provider. Interdisciplinary teamwork and strong care coordination are also integral pieces of the PCMH. Initially, consumers who were receiving mental health care perceived their mental health provider as their primary healthcare provider. The PCMH model evolved out of this concept by bringing routine preventative care and care for comorbid medical conditions into the established mental health care relationships. This model is intended to improve patient care and bring cost savings, but remains an emerging model with more investigation needed to determine which populations would most benefit from this delivery system [9]. Specific integration of behavioral healthcare (including mental health, substance use, and stressful life events) is crucial in order to optimize the quality of care, the patient experience, and financial feasibility for healthcare institutions [10].

Early research suggests that the PCMH system is a promising model, but there are challenges to implementation. A national study from 2006 to 2008 of 36 independent physical practices transitioning to the PCMH model found the time to implementation to be much lengthier than expected, with challenges including provider reluctance to adapt to new roles and poor HIE interoperability [11]. As for ACOs, HIE systems between medical and behavioral healthcare providers will be critical to improve communication across disciplines in care teams.

16.1.3.1   The State Innovation Models (SIM) Initiative

In 2013, CMS created State Innovation Models (SIM) grants, representing a new era at the intersection of Health IT and behavioral healthcare. Whereas the HITECH Act initially left behavioral healthcare providers out of the incentives for HIE system adoption, the SIM grants included behavioral health as one of their key focuses. In the first round of grants in 2013, CMS awarded $33 to $45 million to each of six states: Arkansas, Maine, Massachusetts, Minnesota, Oregon, and Vermont [12]. The main goal of these grants was implementation of value-based care and improved HIE systems. Many of the states implemented ACOs, PCMH models, or both. These grants were an initial step towards broadening Health IT beyond hospitals and medical professionals. In addition to behavioral health, the other domains that these grants focused on included long-term care, social services, and local public healthcare.

While several states found improvements in healthcare utilization, cost savings, and quality of care, other states did not change or worsened in these metrics [12]. Among many possible causes for these differences includes the highly different healthcare landscapes between these states prior to receiving the SIM grants. These grants were implemented over a period of 3.5–5 years. A summary of findings in 2018 indicated both improvements to the Health IT landscape during this time as well as several remaining challenges. Specifically, healthcare providers reported "use of, and perceived value from, admission, discharge, and transfer notifications" and consumers indicated that their providers followed up with them more post-hospitalization. In contrast, providers stated their concerns related to costs and poor interoperability for different types of healthcare providers and health-related data [9].

It was clear to legislators that additional laws and regulations were needed to advance healthcare interoperability. In December 2016, President Barack Obama signed the twenty-first Century Cures Act (Cures Act) into law [13]. This sweeping legislation included requirements for the Centers for Medicare and Medicaid Services (CMS) to create new rules for interoperability and patient access—especially targeting industry practices that were considered to be "information blocking," which impede the appropriate flow of healthcare data to patients and their providers. Final changes to the act (CMS Interoperability and Patient Access Act final rule [CMS-9115-F] [14]) were completed on March 6, 2020 and focused on improving interoperability as well as consumers' ability to access and control their own health information. These rules are intended to support semantic interoperability—that is, the content retains its original meaning when moving from one domain to another—a goal that remains challenging as terminologies continue to evolve rapidly. This rule also focused on promoting the use of application programming interfaces (APIs) that can make it easier for developers to more rapidly make connections between systems by using protocols published by the EHR vendors and provider organizations.

The final rule included several important regulations related to CMS-regulated payers and their use of APIs [13, 15]. Consumers must have electronic access to their encounter and claims information, including cost (e.g., through an EHR portal or pushed to a PHR). Subsets of clinical data must be exchanged, at the consumer's request, so that they are able to bring their data with them if they change payers. To support a more seamless exchange of electronic health information, the final rule largely restricted information blocking, or practices that interfere with the exchange of consumer health data (with several exceptions) [16]. In an effort to improve care coordination and promote HIE, providers will be required to send notifications of a patient's hospital admission, discharge, or transfer to other providers involved in the patient's care.

The frequency at which payers exchange information about consumers who are eligible for both Medicaid and Medicare ("dually eligible") was increased from monthly to daily in order to improve quality of care and accurate billing. Provider information must be made publicly available through an API in order to help consumers find providers to meet their needs. A list of providers and healthcare institutions that do not attest to certain interoperability requirements and who do not provide their digital contact information in a national database will be publicly available for consumers to review and make decisions related to their choice of provider. Initially, health institutions were given 6 months to come into compliance with these new regulations; however, the COVID-19 public health emergency led to an extension being granted for an additional 6 months to come into compliance.

Although behavioral health information technology did not receive the same level of support as was provided to acute care through the HITECH Act incentives, in October 2018, the Substance Use–Disorder Prevention that Promotes Opioid Recovery and Treatment (SUPPORT) for Patients and Communities Act [17] was signed into law. This law is focused on increasing access to substance use disorder treatment and prevention services. Section 6001 includes a provision that authorizes the Center for Medicare and Medicaid Innovation to test models to provide incentive payments to behavioral health providers for adopting electronic health records technology and for using that technology to improve the quality and coordination of care. As of this writing, no announcement about these test incentive programs has been forthcoming from CMS.

16.1.4   Overview of EHRs

NAHIT defined an EHR as "an electronic record of health-related information on an individual that conforms to nationally recognized interoperability standards and that can be created, managed, and consulted by authorized clinicians and staff across more than one healthcare organization" [1]. Distinguishing features of an EHR are its *interoperability* (e.g., ability to interact with other EHRs) and its standardization. It is important to note that the health information in the record itself is a separate concept from the health record *system*, which "supplies and performs the functions enabling information in the record to be used for various purposes" [1]. EHRs are organized and maintained by health care professionals. Some EHRs provide portals where consumers can access their personal data which has been collected by a provider or payer in the EHR. However, it is important to note that this is a consumer-accessible portion of the EHR, and *not* truly a PHR [1].

EHRs can be based on a local server, cloud-based, or managed as a hybrid of locally maintained and cloud-based repositories and services. Local server-based EHRs may be more easily adopted by larger health organizations which have more expansive IT resources and personnel, whereas cloud-based options are especially appealing to smaller organizations, including private practices [18]. Additionally, EHR vendors are increasingly tailoring their offerings to niche services and providers can choose to invest in EHRs of varying complexities—from basic functions to those with more complex "add-on" features [18].

EHRs can serve several purposes, including compliance, billing, and clinical functions. It is important to note that these functions may be at odds with each other and do not guarantee the best medical care for a patient. The Center for Information Technology Leadership (CITL) has long researched and analyzed the costs and benefits of healthcare informatics frameworks [19]. Thoughtful design of EHRs could have a valuable impact on their usability and increased efficiency. The user interface must be easy to navigate and visually appealing enough to be useful to the provider and/or consumer. Visualization, the visual presentation of the underlying data, is an important aspect of HIE design. Data visualization can also be thought of as the iterative process of knowledge being transformed from the underlying content into the user interface (see Chap. 14) [20].

Medical data is arguably unique from other datasets and therefore requires specific functions in its software and in its data visualization; EHRs must have multi-operator functionality with increasing awareness of consumer visualization and efficiency needs [20]. Kopanitsa and colleagues suggest that rather than user interfaces being directly modeled after healthcare providers' previous hard copy records, they need to be updated using modern design techniques and more intuitive, workflow-friendly graphical user interfaces (GUIs) [20]. For example, a recent study of providers at University of California, San Francisco (USCF) Health found that combining internal and external clinical data in the same tab of an EHR, rather than requiring providers to search out external information in another tab, increased provider use of the EHR [21].

16.1.4.1   Landscape of EHRs Across Medical and Mental Health Care

According to Health IT market research company KLAS, as we enter the 2020s, most large (>500 bed) healthcare organizations in the United States have chosen an EHR for their entire healthcare system that they intend to continue with moving forward [22]. Epic systems corporation (Epic) and Cerner corporation (Cerner) have an 85% combined share of the EHR market in these large hospitals, as well as a 54% share of smaller acute care hospitals (<100 beds; see Table 16.2) [22]. Epic is considered the market leader with 58% of the large hospitals (27% for Cerner), with a much narrower margin for acute care hospitals (28% Epic, 26% Cerner) [22].

Table 16.2 Current market share of EHRs in United States Hospitals, 2018 [22]

	Large hospitals (>500 beds, n = not reported)	Acute Care Hospitals (<100 beds, n = 5447)
Epic	58%	28%
Cerner	27%	26%
Allscripts	6%	6%
MEDITECH	4%	16%
CPSI	0%	9%
MEDHOST	0%	4%
Athenahealth	0%	2%

Other systems have lost market share in recent years, with hospitals that switch away from Cerner or Allscripts often looking to Epic [22]. Healthcare systems tend to gravitate towards the system used by other systems who are geographically close to them for better data sharing among regional systems [23]. This trend points out how far we have yet to go to achieve true vendor-agnostic interoperability. Regional dominance of a single system can have some disadvantages, however; providers and institutions should be able to have autonomy in their choice of an EHR vendor in order to avoid selecting an EHR that represents the lowest common denominator for the region rather than the best alignment with the institution's needs. Additionally, EHR customers should be able to change vendors at will and relatively easily, in order to ensure that their needs are being met even as they change. Vendor lock-in can make switching EHR vendors a prohibitively expensive proposition.

The EHR market for office-based practices is significantly more diverse. As of 6/25/2020, 636 unique EHR products have been certified to at least one certification criteria for the 2015 Edition of the ONC's EHR functional requirements [24]. This number has dropped significantly from the 1380 products certified to at least one certification criteria under the 2014 Edition. Unsurprisingly, the EHR market has experienced significant consolidation as the meaningful use incentive program has concluded.

16.1.4.2 Common EHR Vendors in the Mental Health Field

In 2018, KLAS reported on usage and product quality of behavioral health EHRs, including products related to mental healthcare, intellectual and developmental disabilities (IDDs), and substance use. Behavioral health EHRs were used primarily in outpatient settings or private practice (78% of those surveyed) or intensive outpatient/residential day programs (62%). Other settings that used these EHR systems included inpatient residential treatment centers (42%) and acute psychiatric settings (22%; see Fig. 16.3) [28, 60]. According to KLAS, customers were generally unsatisfied with vendor offerings for behavioral health-specific EHRs.

A 2020 version of this report found continued widespread disappointment by providers and healthcare administrators, often due to software difficulties, slow

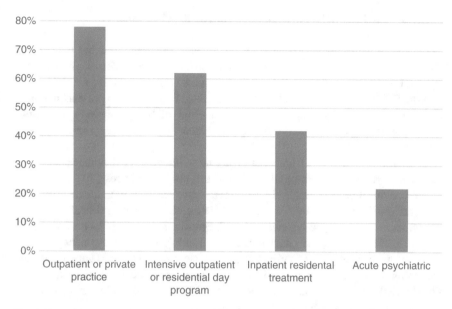

Fig. 16.3 Settings using behavioral health-specific EHRs [25, 26]

customer service response times, and under-delivery on proposed developments [27]. Some improvements had been made by specific vendors, such as faster response time to customer service difficulties and improved training on how to use the EHR. Most EHR users indicated they did not have plans to change EHRs, due to the limited market of viable and affordable alternatives. The most highly rated behavioral health EHRs included Credible (Behavioral Health Enterprise Software), Qualifacts (CareLogic EHR), and Cerner (Millenium Behavioral Health). One behavioral health-specific EHR, Valant, only operates in outpatient settings and has become popular with private practice behavioral healthcare providers [27]. Valant was designed by a psychiatrist and is praised for being user-friendly and for the high-quality training provided for professionals.

Epic's behavioral health components were newly released as of 2018 and limited customer satisfaction data was available; early reactions from customers indicated that additional licensing costs to add-on this behavioral health component to Epic's medical EHRs was a barrier to adoption [28]. Although Epic is identified as a market leader for its medical EHR, KLAS states in its 2020 report that "While both Epic and MEDITECH offer behavioral health-specific modules, most Epic and MEDITECH EMR [electronic medical record] customers meet their behavioral health needs by using a third-party system or customizing the standard EMR." [27] As mental-health specific EHRs become increasingly popular, vendors have created divergent information models that lack standardization [29]. Additionally, peer-reviewed literature on mental health-specific EHRs remains limited.

16.1.4.3 Medical EHRs with Behavioral Health Components

Many EHRs were created specifically for medical providers, making their use in mental health care settings difficult. Mental health care providers seek to fix this problem in multiple ways, such as by using a medical EHR next to a mental health-specific EHR or building mental health-specialized features into a pre-existing medical EHR. Providers are working towards unified EHRs, particularly in settings where mental health care services are embedded in medical (e.g., primary care) settings.

A qualitative study of 11 practices engaging in integrated behavioral health care indicated three main areas of need for these types of practices [30]. Behavioral health providers who were hired into primary care settings often created data that were not easily captured by the existing EHR, such as behavioral health notes or results from standardized behavioral health questionnaires. This lack of standardization made extracting the data for analysis and quality improvement purposes difficult. Additionally, fully unified templates were not available, which impeded the teams' ability to complete tasks together (e.g., shared care plans, joint notes). Finally, EHRs were not compatible with other EHRs or with tablets that were used to complete patient screenings or questionnaires.

Given these restrictions, clinicians in integrated teams often were forced to create workarounds, which were still rather clunky. Efficiency was decreased by many of these workarounds, including duplicate data entry (double documentation), free-standing manual data entry systems, scanning data into the EHR manually (which could not then be further analyzed or manipulated), or relying on patient or provider recall when access to records was unavailable [30].

After 2–3 years of experimentation, these practices (which had each been given $150,000 total over 3 years) yielded three main solutions. Practices either upgraded their EHRs, customized their EHR templates, or moved to a unified EHR. Customized EHR templates were time-consuming and could be expensive and required collaboration between HIT and behavioral health care professionals. Five of the 11 practices upgraded their EHRs, but these upgrades were costly and not covered by their study funding. Four of these practices were in the process of exploring or transitioning to a unified EHR. The unified EHR allows behavioral health templates to be built and embedded within the medical EHR, allowing behavioral health-specific data points that can be extracted and combined with medical and administrative data for analysis. These results suggest that the ideal unified EHR would be built with input from medical and behavioral health care professionals to support communication, care coordination, and other joint tasks of the integrated team [30]. The lack of true EHR interoperability, however, continues to exacerbate the challenge of creating seamless workflow among providers on disparate systems.

16.1.5   The Proposed Value of EHRs

A primary benefit of EHRs for mental health is the potential to enhance clinical care and care coordination both between providers within the same institution and among providers from separate healthcare institutions, all of which can lead to improvements in patient safety and the quality of care provided.

Mental health professionals, especially those in private practice who are responsible for making EHR selection decisions, cite a variety of benefits to switching from paper records to EHRs. Specifically, some of these benefits include care coordination between various types of healthcare providers, EHRs taking up less physical space in an office than file cabinets of paper records, ease of sharing records with approved parties, time savings through template-based documentation, and time saving from reducing 'phone tag' with patients and their providers. A unique aspect of EHR security cited was the ability to track who has accessed records and when [31, 32]. Other providers cited as benefits of the EHR in mental health practices the ability to receive fast updates for a patient returning to care after time away, the convenience of being able to access the EHR from home or while traveling, fewer lost paper records, and the ability of other providers on the same team to provide care in case the treating provider is unavailable [33].

16.1.5.1   Patient Safety and Quality of Care

A variety of valuable features that increase patient safety and the quality of care can be built into an EHR, including clinical decision support (CDS) systems. Algorithms alert providers prior to clinical decision-making to ensure that criteria for ordering a medication or procedure have been met fully and appropriately. Despite its potential, research on the benefits of CDS systems has produced variable results [34], suggesting that more research about the benefits of CDS systems is needed.

A number of barriers remain to useful, efficient, and accurate CDS use. An expert panel [35] identified a number of unintended drawbacks to CDS systems, including problems with both content and presentation. Related to content problems, CDS systems often replace human labor; however, panelists reported discovering that the importance of verification by a staff member had been undervalued and was not easily replaced by the CDS system. Additionally, alerts that are irrelevant to that situation at hand, redundant or repetitive, distracting, or stemming from poorly designed algorithms (or poor quality data) are barriers to good decision-making [34, 35]. Overall, increased CDS automation can create the threat of users becoming overly dependent on CDS systems. CDS systems cannot account for what they do not know and should be used in a consultative fashion rather than as a replacement for clinical decision making.

Other challenges exist related to CDS system presentation, including forced binary decision-making that does not account for 'gray areas,' fields that are populated automatically (but erroneously), and typographical errors [35]. Additionally, users may suffer from "alert fatigue," the phenomenon of being inundated with alerts that eventually leads to ignoring them altogether [35]. Positively, use of another safety feature, computerized physician order entry (CPOE), was a leading contributor to reduced length of stay and mortality at the hospital level, although differences were found by unit and room [25].

Despite the challenges discussed above, CDS systems can be implemented successfully. Other examples of CDSs include drug interaction and dosing alerts, alerts of suitability for specific patients (due to pregnancy, allergies, pre-existing conditions, etc.), reminders for patient follow up, and warnings for data submission deadlines [36]. The volume of patient data that is captured by EHRs can also be transformed into improved CDS algorithms, as described in Chap. 1.

An important challenge for the future development of CDS will be finding ways to facilitate routine or required care by decreasing the number of barriers or 'clicks' that stand in the way (Fig. 16.4). Fewer clicks reinforce behaviors; healthcare administrators can pre-determine the specific provider behaviors they wish to encourage and work with EHR and third-party app designers to make the system as supportive as possible to these projects.

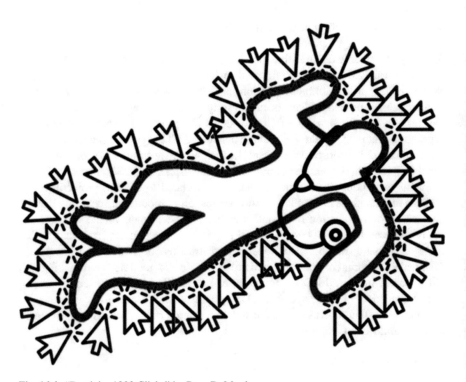

Fig. 16.4 "Death by 1000 Clicks" by Ross D. Martin

16.1.5.2 Improved Efficiency

Inefficient usage of medical services comprises a large percentage of healthcare costs in the United States, numbering into the hundreds of billions of dollars per year [26]. These inefficiencies include unnecessary imaging and procedures, hospital admissions, and surgeries. Incentivized by the HITECH Act, healthcare institutions have increasingly attempted to implement HIE systems as a direct solution to combat unneeded procedures and rising healthcare costs through care coordination and information sharing [26]. If the required information is easily accessible by the healthcare provider at the point of care, unnecessary tests and procedures can be avoided, along with any associated risks or side-effects of those procedures.

The sharing of relevant health information among providers through HIE systems has been found to reduce costs in both emergency department (ED) and outpatient settings. In the ED, HIE system use has been associated with a reduced number of laboratory tests and imaging, including ultrasounds, chest x-rays, and computed tomography (CT) scans [37, 38]. In the outpatient setting, HIE use was associated with reduced repetition of therapeutic medical procedures, but not diagnostic procedures [26].

HIEs and CDS systems improve efficiency by reducing administrative costs and reducing healthcare utilization costs. For example, finding a datum is faster and easier through use of a search function in an EHR than searching paper files by hand. Clerical staff time can be better utilized if healthcare providers enter data into the EHR accurately, enabling helpful searches. Messaging tools allow a freer flow of information between provider and patient and among providers.

Online scheduling, appointment reminders, and virtual check-in processes are simple tools that can improve a consumer's likelihood of keeping an appointment (or reducing their no-show rate). Virtual scheduling and check-in capabilities can also serve to minimize contact between patients and staff during the COVID-19 pandemic and at other times when infection control is particularly important, such as when a patient is immunocompromised. Clinical activities that require frequent patient interactions also benefit from the use of EHRs. Rather than having a patient come into the healthcare office daily or weekly for maintenance checks, providers can use the EHR to complete routine check-ins with the patient (e.g., smoking cessation, monitoring of medical devices), thereby saving significant time and finances on the part of both the provider and patient and decreased long-term healthcare costs through prevention [19].

Application functions are "functions that allow patients to manage their own health and participate in two-way data exchanges (transactions) with health entities" [19] and are a critical aspect of EHRs. Examples of application functions include scheduling appointments, requesting prescription renewals, completing questionnaires prior to an appointment, or even completing live telehealth appointments.

In the mid-2010s, two important Health IT initiatives emerged. Fast Healthcare Interoperability Resources (FHIR)® (pronounced "fire") [39], first proposed in 2011, was developed by a group of volunteers led by Grahame Grieve at the standards organization Health Level Seven International (HL7)® [40] as a means for EHRs to communicate with third-party apps. FHIR provides a mechanism for software developers to create tools that are able to 'speak' to EHRs more easily and for the transmission of data from one EHR to another. Its core advantage compared with prior interoperability efforts is that it uses protocols (such as HTTP or hypertext transfer protocol) familiar to millions of web application developers instead of proprietary or healthcare-specific coding methods. In contrast to prior standardization efforts, HL7 FHIR has enjoyed relatively rapid adoption by the Health IT developer community. A primary strength is that no complicated infrastructure is required to send or receive messages, as it is built on basic web technologies. It does not "solve" interoperability, but it has led to a proliferation of solutions built on HL7 FHIR protocols.

The CDS Hooks specification [41] is an emerging approach to dynamically embedding clinical decision support rules within a clinician's workflow (see Fig. 16.5). CDS Hooks APIs support the synchronous, workflow-triggered CDS calls that leverages HL7 FHIR [41]. On triggering an API, several different CDS responses (called "CDS cards") are returned, including simple text ("information card"), a suggested action ("suggestion card"), or a link to an application ("app link card"). CDS Hooks enable an EHR user to leverage the knowledge of the system to improve patient care with context-relevant tools such as presenting medication history or reviewing potential drug-drug interactions while lowering the cost of implementation by creating standardized data connectors (or hooks) that enable the independent development of CDS capabilities.

Used with permission of Professor Kenneth D. Mandl, Director, Computational Health Informatics Program, Boston Children's Hospital, Boston, MA.

Another initiative that has accelerated innovation in Health IT is the Substitutable Medical Apps, Reusable Technologies (SMART) initiative [42]. In 2009, Mandl

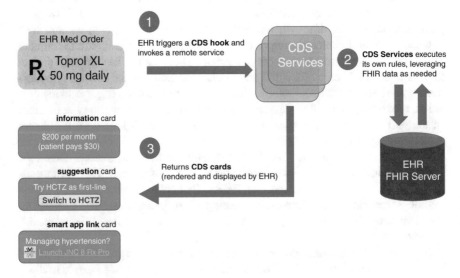

Fig. 16.5 CDS Hooks [41]

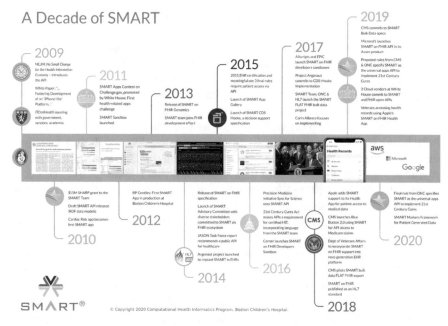

Fig. 16.6 A Decade of SMART [42]

and Kohane proposed the creation of a platform for the sharing of data-driven clinical applications—an "app store" for healthcare [43]. After an initial $15M grant from the ONC, the first draft SMART API was published.

Given the strong alignment between the SMART and FHIR initiatives, the project teams began collaborating in earnest in 2013 and released the first "SMART on FHIR" specification in 2014 (Fig. 16.6) [42]. SMART on FHIR enables providers and even consumers to determine which apps they would like to use on top of their existing EHR. Joshua Mandel, project lead, describes the technologies' complementary functions as this: "FHIR provides a standard set of data models or resource definitions to say, 'Here is how we can represent a medication or a problem or an allergy.' And SMART builds on that to say, 'Here's how we can plug an app into the EHR that uses those standard types of data.'" [44].

Used with permission of Professor Kenneth D. Mandl, Director, Computational Health Informatics Program, Boston Children's Hospital, Boston, MA.

16.1.5.3 EHR Disadvantages

Drawbacks still remain to the EHR, particularly in health care professionals' perception of their utility. In interviews with community behavioral health providers, when asked about barriers to efficient implementation of EHRs, 100% of providers mentioned privacy/security of patient data, 75% stated staff reluctance, and 59% reported quality of care as components of the system that would suffer [45]. Others report costs (both up-front and recurring) and physician reluctance as additional barriers [7].

Provider burnout has also been studied as related to the burden of learning and using an EHR. An article by Fortune magazine and Kaiser Health News [8] entitled "Death by 1,000 Clicks" critiqued many drawbacks related to EHRs and their creation and dispersion, including medical errors leading to patient harm, insurance fraud, user burnout, and cover-ups of safety and quality issues. While the exact nature of the relationship between EHR use and burnout is still being investigated, Schulte and Fry point to several EHR difficulties for providers, including the cognitive switch between speaking with a patient while entering data into a computer, the significant amounts time on a shift (and after hours) that is taken up by EHR documentation, difficulty making EHR improvements due to provider differences in how they practice, and the sheer number of clicks and lengths of notes within the EHR.

In a study of 87 primary care providers, self-reported non-proficiency with an academic health system's EHR was correlated with more time spent using the EHR outside of regular clinic hours [46]. As suspected, providers who spent more time in the EHR after hours also had higher self-reported emotional exhaustion scores on a standardized inventory. However, there was no relationship with EHR use or the number of messages received in the EHR and self-reported clinician cynicism. Given that exhaustion and cynicism are both considered factors in the concept of burnout, study authors summarized that clinicians were "overwhelmed by volume but still engaged in their work." This is an important area for additional future research related to possible differences between provider perception of workload and its relationship to 1) more objective measures of workload from EHR productivity data and 2) clinician wellbeing.

16.1.5.4 Secondary Uses for EHRs

Research Uses

A mutually beneficial relationship exists between clinical and research data, which work together to improve patient care and boost scientific discovery (see Chap. 1). HIE systems have provided enormous amounts of patient data which can be used to create "big data" research studies which can refine clinical practice (see Chap. 15). Big datasets are vast datasets which are produced at increasing speeds and manipulated in increasingly creative ways (coined in the 1990s by IT consulting company Gartner based on "data volume, velocity, and variety" as defining properties) [47]. Big data can also refer to unique methodologies used to organize and analyze these data [48].

Massive data sets can be overwhelming to analyze, and several improvements are needed as healthcare data scientists move forward. Both mathematical and statistical methods must be harnessed, data and data exploration tools should be shared more freely amongst researchers, and greater acceptance of novel data uses must occur [49]. Increased financial investment would also be necessary to build operationality for this type of data-sharing [49]. As a step in this direction, national funding sources are increasingly requiring healthcare institutions to commit to provide open access to their de-identified patient data [49]. Additionally, 90% of the United States' EHR vendors (as well as the top five largest healthcare systems) have signed the ONC interoperability pledge, which commits institutions and vendors to higher standards of care and increased transparency and consumer access [50].

It is also imperative that researchers increase the integration of complex patients into studies and that data science skills are provided to healthcare trainees during their medical education [48]. Moving forward, the hope is to leverage big data (which can be collected through HIE) to create advances in 'precision medicine' as described in Chap. 1. This would introduce more predictability in patient outcomes based on their past medical history and allow diagnostic panels and treatments to be more highly tailored to each patient [48].

Learning Health Systems (LHS) and Quality Improvement (QI)

The clinical data captured in EHRs is essential to enabling learning health systems (LHS, see also Chap. 1). As IT has rapidly changed other aspects of life, its integration with healthcare has led to the creation of LHSs to improve patient care. The National Academy of Medicine (formerly the Institute of Medicine) defines LHS as when "science, informatics, incentives, and culture are aligned for continuous improvement and innovation, with best practices seamlessly embedded in the delivery process and new knowledge captured as an integral by-product of the delivery experience." [51]

LHSs are being used to automate previously used quality improvement (QI) systems and also open up the possibility of novel QI systems [52]. A deductive thematic analysis in the United Kingdom indicated six main types of methods for enabling an LHS, including intelligent automation, clinical decision support, predictive models, positive deviance, surveillance, and comparative effectiveness research [52]. Having de-identified patient data stored electronically opens up opportunities to ask QI questions that would otherwise be too time-intensive and costly to ask. In contrast, using reports pulled from the EHR can provide vital information to describe the current state of healthcare (e.g., how providers' time is spent, how many interactions a patient has with a provider, length of time spent with a patient) and can thereby fuel QI improvements. Without the EHR, and without having comparable EHR data available from peer institutions, these questions would be difficult to answer.

16.1.6 Personal Health Records (PHRs)

Similar to EHRs, PHRs also provide a place for health information to be stored and exchanged. However, rather than being prioritized for health care providers, PHRs are created for consumers. Information is contributed to a PHR from an EHR,

Fig. 16.7 EHR/PHR/
Other data source
connectivity

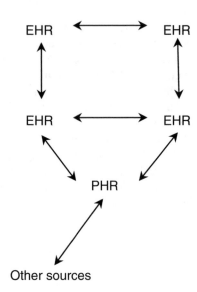

laboratory, connected medical devices, through manual entry, or from other sources. The distinguishing feature of PHRs is that the individual or their guardian or caregiver controls the data contained in the PHR and where it is directed [1] (see Fig. 16.7). Specifically, a PHR is defined as "an electronic record of health-related information on an individual that conforms to nationally recognized interoperability standards and that can be drawn from multiple sources while being managed, shared, and controlled by the individual." [1]

Consumers are able to access their health information and distribute this information to whomever they like. In contrast to EHRs, consumers are not required to maintain PHRs. PHRs can interface with EHRs from a health system, which can push EHR data to an individual's PHR. From there, the patient has the control and choice as to where the data goes. The relationship can be bidirectional as well, with consumers able to message providers or send various types of data through the PHR.

16.1.6.1 Types of PHRs

PHRs can be broken down further into categories, including provider-tethered, payer-tethered, and third-party PHRs [19], though this taxonomy may not be fully reflective of the current market. Provider-tethered PHRs are related to a specific healthcare organization or system and provide patient information that only stems from that specific institution, though they may also include data from other providers as records are shared. Payer-tethered PHRs may include a broader range of information, such as all healthcare visits completed by a consumer that were paid for by a specific insurance company, so they are not restricted to information from an individual provider organization.

Provider-tethered PHRs would not include information from outside that specific system, and payer-tethered PHR would not include health visits that were not paid for by that payer (e.g., out of pocket, paid for by another source, etc.) [19]. More recent advances in this field include interoperable PHRs and third-party PHRs. Interoperable PHRs involve the interaction and cooperation of multiple systems working together, while third-party PHRs are held by neither a specific healthcare system nor a payer. These third-party PHRs are, by necessity, reliant on the ability to extract patient data from EHRs via APIs or other integrations.

In the mid- to late-2000s, the concept of the PHR drew much interest, with both small and large tech companies trying their hand at creating an individually controlled and portable health record. Technology giants such as Apple, Google, and Microsoft have, at times, offered cloud-based PHRs, albeit with mixed success. Both Google Health (2008–2011) and Microsoft HealthVault (2007–2019) were eventually abandoned by their creators due to "low user adoption." [53] However, cloud-based PHRs (which can be accessed on any internet-connected device) remain appealing to consumers due to their low cost, ease of access, and scalability [54].

In contrast to the relatively low adoption of PHRs to date, the use of patient portals connected to a provider's EHR have become a common element of the Health IT landscape—largely due to the requirements for patient access to their records established under the HITECH Act's meaningful use incentive program. These portals have served a portion of the need that PHRs were intended to fill, but they are not PHRs as they are not under the patient's control and they provide access to the information in just one provider's EHR. This approach can perhaps work for people who spend their entire lives receiving health care services from a single health system, but with the US's mobile population and complex approach to healthcare financing and delivery, this scenario is rare at best. Patients with chronic and complex conditions report having as many as 20 or 30 separate logins to access the records offered by their many providers. A June 2020 blogpost by "ePatient Dave" deBronkart, a cancer survivor and Health IT expert, shows a video from a young patient advocate who is urging the Health IT to solve this problem now [55].

The ability to access a PHR on a computer, tablet, or smartphone, either through a Web browser or through a software application ("app"), is increasingly important to consumers in our highly interconnected world. Smartphones have been increasingly utilized for a variety of mental health-related causes, including tracking mood, sleep, and medication use, psychoeducation, biofeedback, virtual coaching, and social support—all the way up to full treatment sessions with a provider (see Chap. 17) [56]. With the rise of telemental health services, particularly in the context of the COVID-19 pandemic, one would expect to see even greater interest in PHR and patient data access technologies. PHRs can provide important support to these telehealth offerings, given that electronic health data can be shared with providers who are not in the same physical space as the consumer.

16.1.6.2 Drawbacks of PHRs

PHR utilization has not become as widespread as initially anticipated. Although many EHRs have portals where consumers can access their information, this tends to be a one-way process of data *access* rather than *exchange*. These portals are unlikely to be interoperable with other EHR portals; they are unable to be edited or commented upon by the consumer, and are not able to be easily collected and stored together in one place (such as for consumers seen at multiple healthcare institutions).

Concerns for PHRs include security of patient data, legal rights to access patient data, and equitable access to PHRs. Given the sensitive nature of topics discussed by mental health professionals and their patients (e.g., mental health diagnoses, psychosocial/family stressors, substance abuse, suicidality, legal issues), privacy and confidentiality are even more intensely important. For example, HIPAA has specific provisions related to mental health and substance use disclosures. While some provider documentation notes are able to be viewed by consumers in the PHR, some EHRs prevent mental health documentation from being shared with the patient due to their sensitive nature.

Conversations about informed consent between providers and consumers are integral to the success of health information exchange. Consumers have a right to know how their data is stored, protected, and shared. Additionally, if there is clinical or other data that the consumer is not privy to, this fact must be shared with them up front. The "Open Notes" movement is advocating for more transparency in notes, including sharing all medical notes with consumers and even asking consumers to collaborate on notes with their providers pre- and post-appointment [57].

An additional level of consideration must be used when working with pediatric populations, including consideration of at what age a child can take control of their own PHR and whether parents can continue to access to an adolescent's EHR (which could include sensitive information related to sexual activity, substance use, etc.) [58]. Finally, legal issues exist around HIE systems, related to meeting an organization's business needs (i.e., billing, insurance reimbursement), meeting legal requirements set by the government or accrediting bodies, and following other requirements set by a provider's employing institution.

In addition to the concerns described above, PHRs are not equally accessible to all consumers. A study of more than 3 million adults who received care from Kaiser Permanente (KP), the largest not-for-profit healthcare institution in the United States [59], indicated that 56% were registered to use the PHR (My Health Manager) which was integrated with the EHR (KP Health Connect). Consumers who identified as 'non-Hispanic white' were more likely to be registered than any other race/ethnicity, whereas those who identified their preferred written language as a language other than English were less likely to be registered. Other groups who were more likely to be registered included women, consumers aged 30 years or older, and those with more annual office visits. However, positively, health benefits accrued equally across race/ethnicity amongst registered consumers as compared to non-registered consumers.

16.1.7 Future Directions

Health IT and HIE technologies are both the enablers and the obstacles to realizing the vision of improved health and healthcare through a Learning Health System. Researchers and care provider entities must improve their collaborations in order to advance toward this goal. By working together, redundant studies could be eliminated, and the expertise of both groups leveraged. Not only should working groups include stakeholders from both clinical and research work, but data must be shared more freely between teams and across institutions, linking bench and clinical sciences and decreasing data silos while supporting appropriate role-based access [36]. To improve these collaborations, all clinical and research data creators and managers will need to more consistently use standardized clinical terminologies [36]— such as the International Classification of Disease (ICD), the International Health Terminology Standards Development Organization (SNOMED), and RxNorm—as well as messaging standards from organizations such as HL7, X12, and the National Council for Prescription Drug Monitoring Programs (NCPDP). The COVID-19 pandemic sharply increased the healthcare community's need for efficiency in collaboration and illustrates the importance of interoperability, particularly during a public health crisis.

16.1.8 Conclusion

Tremendous progress has been achieved in the Health IT industry in the past 20 years, including the introduction of EHRs and PHRs, the development of EHRs into broader interoperable networks (e.g., HIEs), and significant innovation in EHR content and user interfaces. Critical US legislation incentivized the widespread use of EHRs. Introduction of the ACA led to new delivery models within behavioral healthcare such as ACOs and PCMHs. EHRs have been leveraged for both clinical and research uses, and future advancement will necessitate increased collaboration between clinicians and scientists. It will be important to harness big data and novel statistical techniques to improve both basic science and clinical care. Challenges remain in the Health IT field related to the careful balancing of data sharing, data standardization, innovation, privacy, data security, and cost controls as we seek to advance clinical care, outcomes, and quality in healthcare.

References

1. The National Alliance for Health Information Technology. Report to the office of the national coordinator for health information technology on defining key health information technology terms. April 28, 2008.
2. Obama B. Address on health care reform to the American medical association. June 15, 2009.

3. American National Standards Institute. HITSP: Enabling healthcare operability. http://hitsp. org/default.aspx. Published 2020. Accessed 10 July 2020.
4. Monegain B. NAHIT is no more. Healthcare IT News. https://www.healthcareitnews.com/ news/nahit-no-more. Published August 18, 2009. Accessed 11 May 2020.
5. American Recovery and Reinvestment Act of 2009, Pub. L. No. 111–5. Sec. 2, Title XIII, Health Information Technology.
6. The Office of the National Coordinator for Health Information Technology. Health IT dashboard: ONC health information technology for economic and clinical health act grantee list. https://dashboard.healthit.gov/datadashboard/hitech-grantee-list.php Accessed 10 July 2020.
7. Adler-Milstein J, DesRoches CM, Kralovec P, et al. Electronic health record adoption in US hospitals: progress continues, but challenges persist. Health Aff. 2015;34(12):2174–80. https:// doi.org/10.1377/hlthaff.2015.0992.
8. Schulte F, Fry E. Death by 1,000 clicks: Where electronic health records went wrong. Kaiser health news and fortune magazine. https://khn.org/news/death-by-a-thousand-clicks/. Published March 28, 2019. Accessed 1 July 2020.
9. Nordal KC. Healthcare reform: implications for independent practice. Prof Psychol Res Pr. 2012;43(6):535–44. https://doi.org/10.1037/a0029603.
10. Miller BF, Ross KM, Davis MM, Melke SP, Kathol R, Gordon P. Payment reform in the patient-centered medical home: enabling and sustaining integrated behavioral health care. Am Psychol. 2017;72(1):55–68. https://doi.org/10.1037/a0040448.
11. Nutting PA, Crabtree BF, Miller WL, Stange KC, Stewart E, Jaen C. Transforming physician practices to patient-centered medical homes: Lessons from the national demonstration project. Health Aff. 2011;30(3):439–45. https://doi.org/10.1377/hlthaff.2010.0159.
12. RTI International for Centers for Medicare & Medicaid Services, Center for Medicare and Medicaid Innovation. State Innovation Models (SIM) Initiative Evaluation. December 2018.
13. The Office of the National Coordinator for Health Information Technology. ONC's cures act final rule. https://www.healthit.gov/curesrule/. Accessed 11 May 2020.
14. Centers for Medicare & Medicaid Services. CMS interoperability and patient access final rule. https://www.cms.gov/Regulations-and-Guidance/Guidance/Interoperability/index. Updated July 17, 2020. Accessed 20 July 2020.
15. Centers for Medicare & Medicaid Services Newsroom. Interoperability and patient access fact sheet. https://www.cms.gov/newsroom/fact-sheets/interoperability-and-patient-access-fact--sheet. Published March 9, 2020. Accessed 11 May 2020.
16. HealthIT.gov. Information blocking. https://www.healthit.gov/topic/information-blocking. Updated May 22, 2020. Accessed 13 June 2020.
17. Substance Use-Disorder Prevention that Promotes Opioid Recovery and Treatment for Patients and Communities Act. Public Law 115–271. October 24, 2018.
18. American Psychiatric Association. EHR: frequently asked questions. https://www.psychiatry.org/psychiatrists/practice/practice-management/health-information-technology/ehr-faq. Published 2020. Accessed 4 April 2020.
19. Kaelber D, Pan EC. The value of personal health record (PHR) systems. AMIA 2008 Symposium Proc. 2008:343–7.
20. Kopanitsa G, Hildebrand C, Stausberg J, Englmeier KH. Visualization of medical data based on EHR standards. Methods Inf Med. 2013;52:43–50. https://doi.org/10.3414/ME12-01-0016.
21. Adler-Milsten J, Wang D. The impact of transitioning from availability of outside records within electronic health records to integration of local and outside records within electronic health records. J Am Med Inform Assoc. 2020;27(4):606–12. https://doi.org/10.1093/jamia/ocaa006.
22. Tate C, Warburton P. US hospital EMR market share 2019: significant movement in every market sector. KLAS Research. https://klasresearch.com/report/us-hospital-emr-market-share-2019/1454. Published April 30, 2019. Accessed 27 May 2020.
23. Bryant M. Epic, cerner control 85% of large hospital EHR spaces, KLAS reports. Healthcare dive. https://www.healthcaredive.com/news/epic-cerner-control-85-of-large-hospital-ehr-space-klas-reports/553906/. Published May 2, 2019. Accessed 27 May 2020.

24. Certified Health IT Product List. Charts. https://chpl.healthit.gov/#/charts. Accessed 18 July 2020.
25. Lyons AM, Sward KA, Deshmukh VG, Pett MA, Donaldson GW, Turnbull J. Impact of computerize provider order entry (CPOE) on length of stay and mortality. J Am Med Inform Assoc. 2016;24(2):303–9. https://doi.org/10.1093/jamia/ocw091.
26. Eftekhari S, Yaraghi N, Singh R, Gopal RD, Ramesh R. Do health information exchanges deter repetition of medical services? ACM Trans Mange Inf Sys. 2017 Apr;8(1):8. https://doi.org/10.1145/3057272.
27. Blauer T, Despain J. Behavioral health EMR 2020: struggling market sees some changes in satisfaction. KLAS Research. https://klasresearch.com/report/behavioral-health-emr-2020/1676 Published March 2020. Accessed 27 May 2020.
28. Landi H. KLAS report: Behavioral health EHR vendors demonstrate poor performance. Healthcare Innovation Group – Clinical IT. https://www.hcinnovationgroup.com/clinical-it/news/13030788/klas-report-behavioral-health-ehr-vendors-demonstrate-poor-performance. Published October 16, 2018. Accessed 27 May 2020.
29. Ranallo PA, Kilbourne AM, Whatley AS, Pincus HA. Behavioral health information technology: from chaos to clarity. Health Aff. 2016;35(6):1106–13. https://doi.org/10.1377/hlthaff.2016.0013.
30. Cifuentes M, Davis M, Fernald D, Gunn R, Dickinson P, Cohen DJ. Electronic health record challenges, workarounds, and solutions observed in practices integrating behavioral health and primary care. J Am Board Fam Med. 2015 Sept–Oct;28(Suppl):S63–72. https://doi.org/10.3122/jabfm.2015.S1.150133.
31. Clay RA. What are the keys to a good electronic records system? Monitor Psychol. 2017 Jan; 48(1): 52. https://www.apa.org/monitor/2017/01/electronic-records
32. American Psychological Association. Electronic health record (EHR) choices: How early career psychologists can streamline their practice with electronic health records. https://www.apaservices.org/practice/update/2017/09-21/electronic-health-record. Published September 21, 2017. Accessed 4 April 2020.
33. Clay RA. The advantages of electronic health records. Monitor Psychol. 2012 May;43(5):72.
34. Miller A, Moon B, Anders S, Walden R, Brown S, Montella D. Integrating computerized clinical decision support systems into clinical work: A meta-synthesis of qualitative research. Int J Med Inform. 2015;84:1009–18. https://doi.org/10.1016/j.ijmedinf.2015.09.005.
35. Ash JS, Sittig DF, Campbell EM, Guappone KP, Dykstra RH. Some unintended consequences of clinical decision support systems. AMIA 2007 Symposium Proc. 2007;y7:26–30.
36. Castaneda C, Nalley K, Mannion C, et al. Clinical decision support systems for improving diagnostic accuracy and achieving precision medicine. J Clin Bioinforma. 2015;5(4) https://doi.org/10.1186/s13336-015-0019-3.
37. Yaraghi N. An empirical analysis of the financial benefits of health information exchange in emergency departments. J Am Med Inform Assoc. 2015;22:1169–72. https://doi.org/10.1093/jamia/ocv068.
38. Lammers EJ, Adler-Milstein J, Kocher KE. Does health information exchange reduce redundant imaging? Evidence from emergency departments. Med Care. 2014;52:227–34.
39. HL7 International. FHIR overview. https://www.hl7.org/fhir/overview.html. Published November 1, 2019. Accessed 15 June 2020.
40. HL7 International. http://www.hl7.org/. Accessed 20 June 2020.
41. HL7 & Boston Children's Hospital. CDS hooks. https://cds-hooks.org/. 2018. Accessed 20 June 2020.
42. Computational Health Informatics Program at Boston Children's Hospital. SMART Health IT. https://smarthealthit.org/. 2019. Accessed 20 June 2020.
43. Mandl KD, Kohane IS. No small change for the health information economy. N Engl J Med. 2009;360:1278–81. https://doi.org/10.1056/NEJMp0900411.
44. Hayhurst C. Everything you need to know about SMART on FHIR. Health tech insider. https://healthtechmagazine.net/article/2018/10/everything-you-need-know-about-smart-fhir-perfcon. Published October 30, 2018. Accessed 25 June 2020.

45. Shank N, Willborn E, PytlikZillig L, Noel H. Electronic health records: eliciting behavioral health providers' beliefs. Community Ment Health J. 2012;48:249–54. https://doi.org/10.1007/s10597-011-9409-6.
46. Adler-Milstein J, Zhao W, Willard-Grace R, Knox M, Grumbach K. Electronic health records and burnout: time spent on the electronic health record after hours and message volume associated with exhaustion but not with cynicism among primary care clinicians. J Am Med Inform Assoc. 2020;27(4):531–8. https://doi.org/10.1093/jamia/ocz220.
47. Laney D. Deja VVVu: Others claiming Gartner's construct for big data [blog post]. Gartner Blog Network [blog]. https://blogs.gartner.com/doug-laney/deja-vvvue-others-claiming-gartners-volume-velocity-variety-construct-for-big-data/ Published January 14, 2012. Accessed 26 April 2020.
48. Krumholz HM. Big data and new knowledge in medicine: The thinking, training, and tools needed for a learning health system. Health Aff. 2014;33(7):1163–70. https://doi.org/10.1377/hlthaff.2014.0053.
49. Krumholz HM, Terry SF, Waldstreicher J. Vital directions from the national academy of medicine: data acquisition, curation, and use for a continuously learning health system. J Am Med Assoc. 2016 Oct 25;316(6):1669–70.
50. HealthIT.gov. Interoperability pledge. https://www.healthit.gov/commitment. Accessed 26 April 26 2020.
51. National Academy of Medicine. The learning health system series. https://nam.edu/programs/value-science-driven-health-care/learning-health-system-series/. Published 2015. Accessed 26 April 2020.
52. Foley TJ, Vale L. What role for learning health systems in quality improvement within healthcare providers? Learn Health Syst. 2017;1:e10025. https://doi.org/10.1002/lrh2.10025.
53. Truong K. Microsoft HealthVault is officially shutting down in November. MedCityNews. https://medcitynews.com/2019/04/microsoft-healthvault-is-officially-shutting-down-in-november/. Published April 8, 2019. Accessed 20 May 2020.
54. Liu X, Liu Q, Peng T, Wu J. Dynamic access policy in cloud-based personal health record (PHR) systems. Inf Sci. 2017 Feb 10;379:62–81. https://doi.org/10.1016/j.ins.2016.06.035.
55. deBronkart D. ePatient-Dave: Democratizing healthcare. Morgan Gleason, 21, wins the second FHIR DevDays Patient Track. https://www.epatientdave.com/2020/06/24/morgan-gleason-21-wins-the-second-fhir-devdays-patient-track/. Published June 24, 2020. Accessed 1 July 2020.
56. Luxton DD, McCann RA, Bush NE, Mishkind MC, Reger GM. mHealth for mental health: integrating smartphone technology in behavioral healthcare. Prof Psychol Res Pr. 2011;42(6):505–12. https://doi.org/10.1037/a0024485.
57. Open Notes. https://www.opennotes.org/. Accessed 1 July 2020.
58. Nielsen BA. Confidentiality and electronic health records: keeping up with advances in technology and expectations for access. Clin Pract in Pediatr Psychol. 2015;3(2):175–8. https://doi.org/10.1037/cpp0000096.
59. Garrido T, Kanter M, Meng D, Turley M, Wang J, Sue V, Scott L. Race/ethnicity, personal health record access, and quality of care. Am J Manag Care. 2015;21(2):e103–13.
60. Blauer T, Christensen J. Behavioral health 2018: a first look at behavioral health EHR performance. KLAS Research. https://klasresearch.com/report/behavioral-health-2018/1264 Published September 2018. Accessed 27 May 2020.

Chapter 17
Informatics Technologies in the Diagnosis and Treatment of Mental Health Conditions

Wendy Marie Ingram, Rahul Khanna, and Cody Weston

Abstract Mental health conditions, unlike most other illnesses and disorders today, remain bereft of objective and conclusive physiological diagnostic tests. Classically, mental disorders are diagnosed, and treatment plans determined, based on extended interviews to collect patient reported symptoms and histories, careful evaluation by well-trained clinicians, and an often Odyssean journey to reach a satisfactory treatment plan. Mental health informatics technologies may change that. Both consumer and clinician facing technologies hold promise to revolutionize the detection and diagnosis, the prevention and treatment, and the coordination and continuity of care for those with mental health conditions. In this chapter we introduce and discuss the current state of informatics technologies as it relates to the diagnosis and treatment of mental health conditions. We also highlight outstanding issues and challenges.

Keywords Telehealth · Wearables · Smartphone based assessment · mHealth Mobile applications · Computerized psychometric assessment

W. M. Ingram (✉)
CEO, Dragonfly Mental Health, Research Scientist, Anesthesiology Department, Geisinger Health, Oakland, California, USA

R. Khanna
Consultant Psychiatrist & Honorary Fellow, Division of Mental Health, Austin Health, Department of Psychiatry, The University of Melbourne, Melbourne, Victoria, Australia
e-mail: Rahul.khanna@unimelb.edu.au

C. Weston
Psychiatry Department, Johns Hopkins School of Medicine, Baltimore, MD, USA
e-mail: Cweston5@jh.edu

© Springer Nature Switzerland AG 2021
J. D. Tenenbaum, P. A. Ranallo (eds.), *Mental Health Informatics*, Health Informatics, https://doi.org/10.1007/978-3-030-70558-9_17

17.1   Introduction

Mental disorders are typically diagnosed by first ruling out physical causes of symptoms through physical exams and laboratory testing, then performing in-depth psychological examination. The Diagnostic and Statistical Manual of Mental Disorders – 5 (DSM-5) is the most recent revision of the most widely accepted diagnostic criteria for psychological examination of mental illnesses [1]. It is used as part of a case formulation assessment that leads to a fully informed treatment plan for each patient. The DSM-5 is made up of three sections: I. Basics, II. Diagnostic Criteria and Codes, and III. Emerging Measures and Models. Within the second section lies the core of contemporarily defined and accepted mental disorders parsed into 22 different categories including Neurodevelopmental Disorders, Depressive Disorders, Feeding and Eating Disorders, and Personality Disorders, just to name a few. Trained mental health professionals such as social workers, psychologists, and psychiatrists can employ the Structured Clinical Interview for DSM-5 (SCID-5) in order to make systematic diagnoses for both clinical and research purposes [2, 3]. These semi-structured diagnostic interviews are available in a number of versions differing in detail and design, tailored for specific uses including clinical trials or research. SCID-5 interviews are thorough and typically take 30 to 90 minutes to complete, depending on the diagnosis being tested and the complexity of the patient's case. It is of note, however, that SCID-5 interviews are rarely used in non-research-related clinical practice [4, 5].

Despite the utilization of the methodical SCID-5 framework, there are many reasons that lead to inadequate care for patients with mental health conditions. Patients will often wait years after the onset of symptoms to seek treatment due in part to social stigma, restricted access to behavioral health specialists, and the complex nature of mental illnesses themselves [6]. Once a patient is seen, it is quite common for mental health clinicians to require multiple visits with a patient before determining a primary diagnosis and an appropriate treatment plan. The majority of symptoms of a mental health condition occur outside of office visits and may be masked within the clinical environment, intentionally or otherwise. In addition, epidemiological research has revealed that many "discrete" DSM-5 diagnoses co-occur in the same person (e.g. depression and anxiety, or attention deficit hyperactivity disorder and conduct disorder [7]). The complexity of mental health conditions, the diversity of presentation, and the severe shortage of mental health providers all contribute to many patients receiving shifting primary diagnoses over time as they interact with the health care system and are seen by increasingly specialized practitioners and/or as their condition worsens. For example, a diagnosis of bipolar disorder (BD), a serious mental illness, is often preceded by a diagnosis of depression, with a mean delay of 8.7 years [8–11]. Additionally, many mental health conditions are chronic and/or episodic in nature. Once a correct diagnosis is reached and an adequate treatment plan determined, many patients with mental illnesses will experience periods of remission where regular clinical observation is not required. During these times, continuity of care may lapse and it falls on the patient and their

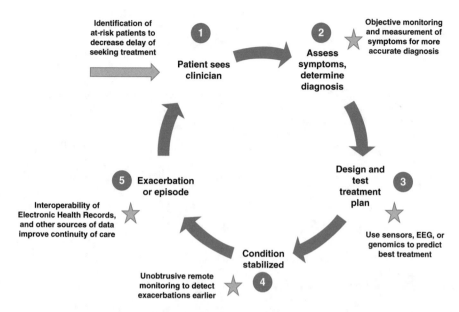

Fig. 17.1 Classical mental health treatment cycle and informatics technologies improvements. The classical mental health treatment cycle may be improved or augmented in many ways by informatics technologies. The blue arrows indicated the classical treatment cycle beginning with 1. Patient sees clinician and cycling through steps 2 through 5. Exacerbation or episode. The green arrow and stars indicate a selection of informatics technologies that could improve these steps in the process

personal support system to detect an exacerbation and reinitiate care [12]. When considered together, the above-mentioned issues lead to major challenges in detecting, diagnosing, preventing, treating, and coordinating continuity of care of mental health conditions. Fortunately, as depicted in Fig. 17.1 and described below, advances in mental health informatics may help address many of these issues through new research and application of informatics technologies [13].

17.2   Detection and Diagnosis

Arguably the largest problem in mental health is the delay of detection and accurate diagnosis of mental illness. In 2004, it was estimated that 80% of people with a lifetime DSM disorder had over a decade of delay between the onset of symptoms and initial contact with a mental health professional [14]. There now exist a multitude of both consumer and provider facing technologies that are helping to close that gap (Fig. 17.1, step 1). Consumers have direct access to several platforms and technologies that produce extensive amounts of data which can be leveraged using informatics methodologies to assist in early detection and more accurate diagnosis of mental health conditions (Fig. 17.2).

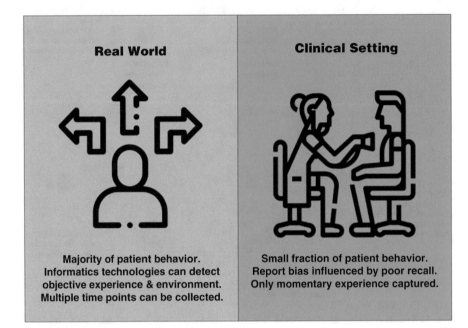

Fig. 17.2 Clinical Setting versus Real World. The clinical setting is limited by how much information can be gathered and how reliable that data is. Only a small fraction of patient behavior and experience can be assessed during clinical visit and is often influenced by problems with patient recall, especially when their mental health condition affects their cognitive ability or memory. The majority of patient experience occurs as the patient moves through the real world where informatics technologies such as wearables and smartphone applications can collect and synthesize objective behavioral and environmental information longitudinally

17.2.1 Consumer Facing Technologies

17.2.1.1 Wearable Devices

The most evident method of capturing behavioral data on free-moving, natural acting individuals involves wearable fitness trackers which contain accelerometers, global positioning system (GPS), and other types of data gathering equipment. These collect actigraphy data (or level of activity, including sleep patterns), location data and more. Direct to consumer and research grade actigraphy devices, most typically worn on the wrist, have been used to study sleep, activity, and movement disorders in ever more impressive detail [15–23]. Less well known are other wireless and wearable devices such as patches and clothing that allow for measurement and electronic transmittal of a variety of biometrics ranging from heartrate to interstitial fluid molecule monitoring [24–28]. Using wearable technology allows real-time objective assessment of patient behavior including sleep quality, eating and drinking behaviors, activity levels and psychomotor activity which can enhance and refine the detection and diagnosis of mental illnesses, likely a significant improvement over current methods involving predominantly patient reported experiences [29–31].

17.2.1.2   Smartphone Based Assessment

In addition to wearable technology, mobile phones allow for unprecedented measurement and analysis of activity, environment, mood state, and behavior at the
individual level. These advancements offer enormous potential for better characterizing symptoms and mechanisms of psychiatric disorders, as well as predicting
clinical severity and treatment response [30]. Presently it is estimated that 65% of
US adults have a smartphone allowing for the development and deployment of
applications capable of targeted or longitudinal psychiatric data collection. Global
activity can be tracked with GPS transmitters which have already been used to study
social behavior [32, 33] and food seeking [34, 35].

There are now over 10,000 smartphone-based applications providing various
mental health services with growing acceptability [36–40]. Many include validated
instruments for screening and symptom tracking, including the depression screener
Patient Health Questionnaire (PHQ-9) or the Generalized Anxiety Disorder 7-item
scale (GAD-7), while other mobile applications present screeners and resources for
self-evaluation and personal tracking such as the Center for Epidemiologic Studies
Depression Scale Revised (CESD-R) and Mood 24/7. In addition to measured or
reported information about individuals collected by smartphones, digital environmental sensors are also on the rise and allow the collection of data on noise, chemi-
cals, light, and weather-related environmental exposures [41–44]. The combination
of momentary or periodic assessments with passively collected smartphone-based
data holds even more promise to assist in detecting and monitoring psychiatric
symptomology. In the case of schizophrenia spectrum disorder, the metrics of distance traveled, time spent alone and time sitting still all were associated with
increased persecutory ideation (the delusion that includes the belief that they are
being or will be intentionally harmed) [45].

17.2.1.3   Social Media

One of the most data-rich sources for detecting mental health concerns is also one of
the most challenging: social media. For social, technical and ethical reasons, social
media data such as that derived from platforms like Twitter, Facebook, Reddit, Weibo
and Instagram have been found to be both promising and difficult to harness [46, 47]
(and see Chap. 13). Depression and suicidality have been preferentially studied leading to insights into sentiment, circadian signals, and pronoun usage being linked to
experience of mood disorder disturbance [48–59]. However studies of other disorders
such as autism, substance use disorder and eating disorders have demonstrated correlations with detectable signal in certain platforms and features in their data [60–63].

Utilization of social media text mining has also been employed to survey populations for concerning mental health deterioration following disasters [64]. There are
significant differences in social media usage between patients based on the severity
of their mental illness, however, which may affect studies employing this data to
detect and diagnose individuals [54]. Despite the promise of leveraging social media

data to detect and diagnose mental illnesses, it should also be noted that the use of these platforms may be contributing to mental distress or disorders themselves [65–69].

17.2.1.4 Implications for Mental Health Conditions

Thus far, individual-level moment-by-moment mood monitoring data has advanced our understanding of the temporal associations of different symptoms within mental disorders such as bipolar disorder, post-traumatic stress disorder, and anxiety disorders [70]. For example, a mood monitoring study of individuals with bipolar disorder found that chronic mood instability was more common than the diagnostic criteria of discrete episodes of mood variation [71]. Passive data from mobile phones can also increase our understanding of psychiatric disorders. Number and length of outgoing phone calls and text messages have been shown to be correlated with manic symptoms among individuals with bipolar disorder [72].

Complimentary studies using wearables in addition to self-reported mood data have elucidated potential underlying mechanisms of psychiatric disorders (Fig. 17.1, step 2). Individuals with borderline personality disorder demonstrated significant changes in diurnal physiology (i.e. sleep, activity and heart rate), which may exacerbate symptomatology and could prove to be useful targets for intervention [73]. Emotional processing has been shown to mediate the effects of antidepressants on mood, and early decrease in negative affective bias is considered an early marker of antidepressant efficacy [74]. In addition to the great wealth in knowledge generation about the diseases themselves through research, a crucial application of these consumer facing technologies is to improve detection and accurate diagnosis of disease (Fig. 17.3).

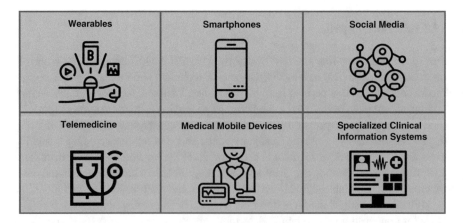

Fig. 17.3 Detection and diagnosis with informatics technologies. Wearables, smart phones, social media, telemedicine, medical mobile devices, specialized clinical information systems

17.2.2 Provider Facing Technologies

17.2.2.1 Computerized Psychometric Assessment

Recently, extensive research has been devoted to determining validity and reliability of web- and application-based psychometric assessments comparing against existing paper and in-person administered scales. Computerized psychometric assessments have generally been found equivalent to currently used methodologies, ranging from adolescent to geriatric populations [75–77]. These include psychometric assessments for mental illnesses and associated features such as anxiety, depression, schizophrenia, OCD, suicidal ideation, post-traumatic stress disorder, emotional disorders, cognitive disorders, and more [76, 78–88]. The benefits of utilizing validated computerized psychometric assessment are multifold. They save time for both clinicians and patients by being completed in a variety of settings, including by the patient in the comfort of their own home, before even scheduling an appointment. They can improve access to care for patients in settings that have behavioral health clinician shortages by effectively triaging patients, prioritizing patients with more severe or emergent conditions. In addition, it has been found that computerized adaptive testing, where each item is dynamically selected from a pool of items until a pre-specified measurement precision is reached, can actually improve the efficiency of testing while not losing reliability or validity [89–91].

17.2.2.2 Telemedicine

Access to specialized mental health clinicians that can reliably diagnose and treat mental health conditions is limited by both time and location. Telemedicine, the remote access to clinicians through digital technology, is particularly well suited to improve this aspect of the mental health field. Second only to radiologists, psychiatrists in 2019 were the most likely specialty to employ telemedicine to provide care to their patients (27.8%) [92]. Because psychiatrists rarely need to conduct physical exams of their patients in an outpatient setting, two-way video telemedicine allows for increased access to care that may not otherwise be possible, especially for populations in rural, underserved, and developing nations' communities [93–103]. Establishing a telemedicine practice, however, is not trivial and includes legal, technological, regulatory and billing issues that vary from state to state in the United States and from country to country worldwide [104, 105]. One of the barriers to the adoption of telemedicine is the resistance of clinicians themselves due to concern over developing trust and rapport with their patients as well as concerns over safety, security, and legal issues [105].

The 2019 novel coronavirus (COVID-19) global pandemic has played a transformative role in accelerating necessary rapid adoption of telepsychiatry resulting in both positive and negative consequences [106–115]. The pandemic itself has seriously and negatively impacted a large proportion of individuals' mental health [111,

116, 117]. Those with pre-existing mental health conditions were potentially impacted by not being able to be seen in person in order to refill prescriptions or address exacerbations in a timely manner, especially at the outset of the pandemic. The expansion of telepsychiatry was not instantaneous. It took a bit of time for rules to be suspended, allowing practitioners licensed in other states to provide services in areas that were in desperate need, and for practitioners and clinical systems to set up and adjust to the necessary infrastructure. However, following the growing pains of this sudden transition, clinicians that were previously reticent are now realizing unexpected benefits of telepsychiatry [118]. For example, outpatient psychiatry services at Johns Hopkins School of Medicine have reported that their no-show rates have dropped precipitously, and more patients can be seen each day per physician. Other psychiatric service lines, however, continue to be negatively impacted by the pandemic. Some inpatient units now require each patient to have their own room, essentially halving the number of beds available. Brain stimulation services including electroconvulsive therapy (ECT) and transcranial magnetic stimulation (TMS), are being delayed or rescheduled due to fear of contracting COVID-19. Altogether, it seems that the pandemic has one bright side in that the widespread adoption of telepsychiatry and reduced problematic regulation between states in the US may be here to stay, resulting in much needed improvements in access to care and reduced burden due to other disparities.

17.2.2.3 Mobile Medical Devices

Technological advances have led to the possibility of gathering even more sophisticated types of data that are relevant to mental health [119]. While not used in conventional diagnostic work ups of most mental disorders, research has demonstrated that many conditions are accompanied by clinically meaningful differences in brain structure and activity. Portable brain mapping is migrating from dedicated imaging facilities to the bedside and now into the community with mobile point-of-care MRI head and neck scanners, now FDA approved (example: hyperfine.io) [120]. Functional near infrared spectroscopy [121–124], portable EEG and telemetry applications [125–134], ultrasound imaging [135–137], and optical tomography [138–141] have all seen vast improvements in cost, portability, and accuracy. With increased portability and affordability, mobile medical devices will likely usher in a new era in biometric-based detection, diagnostics, and personalized care for mental health conditions (Fig. 17.1, step 3).

17.2.2.4 Specialized Clinical Information Systems

At the core of mental health informatics is the recognized value in collecting, storing, analyzing, and using specialized information. The collection of this information and its processing leads to improved understanding of community needs, prevalence, treatment response, and other beneficial insights valuable for planning and efficient detection. In 2005 the World Health Organization published a Mental Health Policy and Service Guidance Package specifically covering Mental Health Information Systems [142]. In this report, the authors conclude that general health information systems often fail to capture the data necessary for mental health purposes due to lack of adequate understanding of this branch of medicine. It was perhaps too early at that point, but a major missing piece in their report is the inclusion of mobile applications as a means of providing this specialized information systems for mental health [143]. Connecting primary and secondary care for mental health conditions, knowing when and where to refer patients, and efficiently diagnosing disorders may be fundamentally enhanced by informatics technology driven by mobile applications.

While still challenging, it is now easier than ever to securely connect smartphone based informatics systems to traditional electronic health records allowing for improved monitoring, management, and diagnosis of mental disorders [144–147]. Both electronic health records and smartphone-based applications are not without their challenges and concerns, however. Although there are thousands of mental health applications currently available, almost none provide scientific evidence that their systems properly diagnosis or improve outcomes among users [148–151], and there is evidence that consumers will largely not continue to use the apps when not enrolled in a clinical trial [152, 153]. Furthermore, patient perspectives on the privacy of their mental health information are complex and dynamic, requiring ardent patient engagement in the further development of mental health information systems and how they are used [154].

17.3　Prevention and Treatment

Informatics technology has applicability in prevention, treatment development, and therapeutic response prediction [70]. Individual-level digital monitoring, mental health information systems, and blending of these data are critically useful for the development of predictive algorithms that will allow for better prevention and treatment of mental health conditions, with increasing sensitivity to personalized medicine approaches (Fig. 17.4).

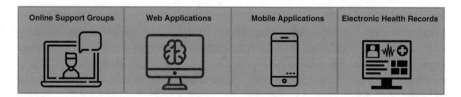

Fig. 17.4 Prevention and treatment. Online Support Groups, Web Apps, Mobile Apps, Electronic Health Records

17.3.1 Consumer and Provider Facing Technologies

17.3.1.1 Online Support Groups

As epidemiological studies reveal an increase in mental health conditions worldwide [155], the shortage of specialized clinicians and limited access to behavioral health care is driving many people to seek support online through disorder specific support groups [156]. International surveys have repeatedly demonstrated that an increasing number of people are seeking help through online support groups [157–161]. Interviews and content analysis reveal that people predominantly seek online support to avoid stigma and to gain immediate, compassionate emotional support, especially when in-person care is unavailable or inconvenient [162–171]. These groups have been used effectively by patients with many disorders, including postpartum depression, schizophrenia, eating disorders, and OCD. Many online support programs and groups are not designed, directed, or evaluated by clinical experts and thus may vary tremendously in their efficacy and safety for those using this modality in exclusion of professional psychiatric and/or psychological support. However, there are examples of clinically designed and distributed online support systems such as the recent Australian site "Moderated online social therapy for youth mental health." [172]

17.3.1.2 Web Based and Mobile Applications

The advent of smartphones and the near ubiquitous availability of internet access in modern times have allowed people unprecedented access to means of daily mental health monitoring and convenient access to resources and remote care. The ability to self-monitor and have applications alert health care providers allows for earlier detection of exacerbations, episodes, or deterioration in individuals which in turn allows for earlier and more effective intervention. Both consumer and provider facing web-based and mobile applications are already available and have been shown to be effective for conditions such as OCD [173, 174] and predicting antidepressant response [175]. A number of web-based and mobile application mental healthcare programs have emerged to meet the need for prevention, early detection, remote therapy, and medication management as well [39, 40, 176–180]. These hold promise for extending the reach of scarce providers into underserved areas and for reaching patients who are reluctant or unable to reach providers in traditional settings. In addition to stand-alone mobile treatment, smartphone based cognitive behavioral therapy (CBT) may also accelerate or support pharmacotherapy for illnesses like depression [181]. Given the time-intensive nature of traditional in-person CBT, this could greatly extend the reach of this intervention in areas with a limited supply of psychotherapists (Fig. 17.1, step 4).

Mobile app-based programs are increasingly available as force-multipliers for teaching wellness skills such as mindfulness and self-compassion and were effective at reducing psychological distress and improving mental well-being among various populations worldwide [182–184]. In addition to the use of self-report measures, smartphone-based applications have the advantage of collecting other forms of data (keystroke rate, activity data, vocal patterns) that can be used to better understand a person's day-to-day mental status. This can be especially useful in tracking symptoms in affective disorders, particularly bipolar disorder [39]. Prediction of future psychiatric manifestations is challenging with current tools, and accurate assessment could prevent significant harm in the form of risk-taking and suicidal behaviors if interventions were offered early. Despite the potential cost- and time-savings associated with adoption of mobile health technologies, psychiatric and psychological practices remain reluctant to adopt them due to lack of specific interest, challenges learning and deploying the technologies, and patient-reported difficulties using the tools [185]. Because mobile mental health applications are still relatively young as a field, there is limited regulatory oversight to differentiate safe and evidence-based interventions from others. This presents a significant barrier to adoption, as clear guidelines could confer legitimacy to rigorously developed applications and increase provider confidence [186] and clearly identify applications and programs that do not have an evidence base [187, 188]. While some efforts are being made to evaluate apps [189], there remains a need for more rigorous and widely accepted oversight and validation.

17.3.1.3   Coordination and Continuity of Care

Mental healthcare suffers from a severe lack of coordinated continuity of care [190–193]. Many studies suggest that patient outcomes would improve dramatically if coordination and continuity of care were enhanced [190–193]. Informatics technology could be the driving force behind such improvements [194] and yet continue to prove difficult to implement and bring to scale [195, 196]. Electronic health records (EHRs), sensors, digital technology and applications on wearable devices or smartphones have been tested in a variety of mental health conditions and shown promising results. However, interoperability issues and high initiation costs of these informatics technologies slow their adoption and deployment. An increase in implementation research may be useful in driving this domain forward (Fig. 17.1, step 5).

17.4   Ongoing Issues and Challenges

As is the case with any rapidly developing field, informatics technologies in the diagnosis and treatment of mental health conditions face several ongoing challenges. Some of these are conceptual and others practical. The conceptual issues relate to the nature and limits of psychiatric diagnoses themselves. Further, practical issues relate to clinician and patient acceptance, the latter of which raises equity and access challenges.

17.4.1 Contemporary Psychiatric Diagnostics

To understand the challenges and opportunities of informatics in mental health diagnostics and treatment, we must understand the status quo and its limits. Although structured and validated interviews and rating scales are common in research settings, contemporary clinicians primarily diagnose mental illnesses through information gained through patient self-report and observations made during the clinical interview [197]. This information is then considered in light of the operationalized diagnostic criteria as outlined in the Diagnostics and Statistical Manual (DSM, currently version 5) published by the American Psychiatric Association (APA) or from the International Classification of Diseases (ICD, current version 11, though the US still largely uses ICD-10) published by the World Health Organization. The two documents, both consensus-based, share substantial overlap in their approach to categorizing psychiatric illnesses based on observable symptom clusters. They have been purposefully agnostic regarding etiology since DSM-III (1980) and primarily aimed to increase inter-clinician diagnostic reliability. The DSM-5 'recognize[s] that the current diagnostic criteria for any single disorder will not necessarily identify a homogeneous group…available evidence shows that… validators [e.g. biomarkers] cross existing diagnostic boundaries but tend to congregate more frequently within and across adjacent DSM-5 chapter groups.' [198] As such, practical questions of utility remain the explicit primary aim of these documents [199]. Despite this limited aim, lacking a clear alternative, these manuals have come to be the basis of everything from treatment research to compensation and remuneration schemes. The disorder categories they describe have therefore becoming rarified in a way not originally intended.

The implications of this background for the application of informatics solutions for diagnosis and treatment are manifold. Firstly, machine learning techniques common for analyzing the dense data provided by novel tools expect a valid 'ground truth' to train on. If that ground truth is flawed, our conclusions risk being even more flawed. So just collecting more accurate, refined data using more sophisticated tools within the same paradigm risks making the current approach more entrenched, adding to the mass of signs and symptoms that can be sliced and diced into more diagnostic categories. It may provide more phenotypes, but we will not have any more insight into which phenotypes represent a clinically meaningful class of disorders (i.e., disorders with common etiologies that can be precisely targeted).

Further, although the informatics techniques described above may give a more accurate window into an illness state than retrospective self-report to a clinician, the latter is what most of the extant evidence base stands on. In fact, there is evidence that patients' everyday experience or physiological state and retrospective evaluation of mental states are distinct [200]. We therefore risk conflating distinct (if overlapping) illness states, adding to confusion and possibly hindering rather than helping to accurately and efficiently diagnose patients. To present an example, studies have correlated actigraphy profiles with a depressive episode [33]. Although exciting, it would not be correct to say that a person diagnosed in this way will have an identical clinical trajectory or treatment response to one diagnosed on classic self-report. The question of what the clinician should then do to intervene with such a patient remains open. The issue is akin to the proverbial 'incidentaloma' in physical medicine, where a lesion is detected incidentally on a scan, but the patient is otherwise asymptomatic. The classic case is that of the pituitary incidentaloma, where pituitary masses are being detected in large quantities in patients having a brain scan for other reasons. The extant literature may for example suggest that 80% of said lesions are fatal without treatment, however this is based on symptomatic patients. Several years, surgeries and active surveillance later, doctors now know most of these lesions follow a benign course and intervention was unnecessary or worse, detrimental [201].

We present these caveats not to discourage further advancement in this field but to prompt informed clinicians and informaticians to fully appreciate both the risks and potentials for emerging tools and analytic approaches. Rather than aiming to diagnose within existing paradigms, we must remember that diagnoses are not aims in themselves but are ultimately the means to making predictions about outcomes, specifically treatment outcomes. This broader aim does not necessarily need to travel the circuitous path of a DSM-5 diagnosis. Rather, purely objective data-driven analytics can be embedded within clinical trials alongside classic diagnostic and treatment approaches and aim to predict the ultimate outcomes directly. Doing so will not only help validate emerging technologies but also enhance clinician acceptance.

17.4.2 Clinician Acceptance

The issue of clinician acceptance is a challenge not restricted to informatics. Medicine is a conservative industry with good reason. The infamous startup mantra of 'move fast and break things' is ill-suited to high risk organizations, where 'first, do no harm' has held sway (in theory if not always in practice) for millennia. This conservatism however can sometimes have deadly consequences and several studies suggest the gap between research and widespread implementation in healthcare is seventeen years [202]. Demographic shifts alone, however, make the status quo untenable. By 2030, there is expected to be a worldwide shortage of 15 million health workers [203]. It is therefore crucial that informaticians and clinicians partner effectively to implement practical models of care.

Contemporary EHRs have been described by clinicians as an intruder between patient and clinician which slow workflows [204] and compromise rapport [205]. Clinicians who are involved in the development and customizing of the software are however more likely to be satisfied users [206]. Intuitive and customized interfaces are necessary yet insufficient. The technologies we describe in this chapter depend on large volume and high-quality data, yet data quality can only improve if informaticians can show value to the clinicians and patients entering the data. So although informatics has great potential for improved business intelligence [207] and resultant improvements in efficiency, revenue and reporting, such potential can only be realized by simultaneously bringing clinical value and cultivating stakeholder buy in.

Another barrier to clinician acceptance is a lack of training and remuneration [208, 209]. The ability to utilize consumer-grade technologies for diagnosis are a double-edged sword. On the one hand, this greatly expands the scale of diagnosis and intervention. On the other hand, it leaves clinical uses dependent on the whims of commercial actors which have a different set of priorities and regulation. Externalities like the Cambridge Analytica scandal of 2018 or the 2019 USA trade ban with Huawei, then the second largest smartphone manufacturer globally, are but two recent examples of events that can cause shifts in data availability for health analytics. Such events affect platform owners' policies around access, individual willingness to share their data and regulations that cover data and technology transfer [210]. Meanwhile, commercial incentives discourage open reporting of consumer device accuracy, making external validation crucial. A recent comparison of a range of consumer wearables with sleep diaries and research grade equipment showed both the steady improvements in accuracy but also wide divergence between devices [211]. For example, when examining their ability to distinguish lying in bed awake from sleep, mean percent error ranged from 11.6% to 31.6%. Further, proprietary software often does not allow extraction of raw data and manufacturers are not obligated to share any data pre-processing changes that may occur even between different firmware versions of the same device. Furthermore, at the clinician level, there also exists a lag in the appropriate remuneration for the use of emerging technologies in mental healthcare. To facilitate clinician adoption of new informatics technologies, training and education are required and cost precious time and money, often out of limited continuing education funds. Companies developing these technologies often target administrators within health care systems to purchase their products or license their software. Without proper training and onboarding of healthcare workers themselves [212], with appropriate compensation for their time, implementation and adoption are going to be impeded. In contrast to companies, researchers producing cutting edge developments in informatics technology generally lack the funding or infrastructure to translate scientific and algorithmic innovation to user-ready applications. Clinicians cannot be expected to invest their own time into incorporating informatics research innovations into their practice without extensive support. Additional focus on and funding for translation of informatics research to the clinical setting is required for these breakthroughs to reach patients and clinicians and realize their promised benefits [213].

17.4.3   Patient Acceptance, Access and Equity

Superficially, the popularity and volume of web-based treatments described above implies a high level of acceptance in the population. However, once the high global prevalence of mental illness is accounted for, these numbers still represent a small segment of those in need. Further, up to 94% of those downloading popular mental health apps stop using them within two weeks [153]. This suggests work is needed to provide value and enhance engagement. Co-development and living laboratory approaches, where multiple stakeholders including patients, clinicians, funders and developers work together, are one potential path forward [214].

Bringing informatics technologies for diagnosis and treatment to individuals with mental health conditions also raises several specific access challenges. There is a bidirectional relationship between poverty and mental illness [215], so patient-access to devices and the internet may be limited. In Australia, despite having the 10th highest average wage in the world, a study of schizophrenia sufferers published in 2020 showed that only 58% owned a smartphone and 30% had never accessed the internet from any device [216]. Both clinician- and patient-facing limits to access require resolution and often lie outside the boundaries of health departments or organizations. Further, specific symptoms like paranoid delusions may also impact patients' willingness to use informatics tools for diagnosis or treatment.

17.5 Summary and Conclusion

As we can see, informatics technologies have made great strides in bringing innovative approaches to mental health diagnoses and treatment. Some, like telemedicine and computerized psychometric testing, digitize existing validated approaches. Others, such as wearables and mobile medical devices, can provide insights hitherto impossible. These may allow us eventually to entirely leapfrog the extant diagnostic paradigms and help predict treatment outcomes and prognoses directly.

Though not insurmountable, several challenges remain before promising research outcomes can be translated to everyday care. One impediment is the uncertain validity of the current diagnoses as described in the DSM and ICD, an understanding of which is crucial for deriving useful insights from these novel tools. Beyond this, several clinician and patient-side factors must be addressed. On the clinician side, enhanced training, remuneration and transparency from technology vendors could enhance acceptance. Some of these may require regulatory changes to overcome proprietary concerns and encourage validation studies. For patients, more needs to be done to address limited engagement and the ethical and practical access and equity issues. A focus on co-development and re-thinking funding approaches may be helpful. Properly managed, the future for such technologies for diagnosis and treatment remains bright.

References

1. American Psychiatric Association. Diagnostic and statistical manual of mental disorders. 2013.
2. First, M., Williams, J., Karg, R. & Spitzer, R. L. Structured clinical interview for DSM-5 - research version. (2015).

3. First M, Williams J, Karg R, Spitzer RL. Structured clinical interview for dsm-5 disorders, clinician version. Washington, DC: American Psychiatric Association; 2016.
4. Osório FL, et al. Clinical validity and intrarater and test-retest reliability of the structured clinical interview for DSM-5 - clinician version (SCID-5-CV). Psychiatry Clin Neurosci. 2019;73:754–60.
5. Aboraya A. Do psychiatrists use structured interviews in real clinical settings? Psychiatry (Edgmont). 2008;5:26–7.
6. Wang PS, et al. Failure and delay in initial treatment contact after first onset of mental disorders in the National Comorbidity Survey Replication. Arch Gen Psychiatry. 2005;62:603–13.
7. Kessler RC, Chiu WT, Demler O, Walters EE. Prevalence, severity, and comorbidity of 12-month DSM-IV disorders in the National Comorbidity Survey Replication. Arch Gen Psychiatry. 2005;62:617.
8. Fritz K, et al. Is a delay in the diagnosis of bipolar disorder inevitable? Bipolar Disord. 2017;19:396–400.
9. Morselli PL, Elgie R, GAMIAN-Europe. GAMIAN-Europe/BEAM survey I--global analysis of a patient questionnaire circulated to 3450 members of 12 European advocacy groups operating in the field of mood disorders. Bipolar Disord. 2003;5:265–78.
10. Lish JD, Dime-Meenan S, Whybrow PC, Price RA, Hirschfeld RM. The National Depressive and manic-depressive association (DMDA) survey of bipolar members. J Affect Disord. 1994;31:281–94.
11. Hirschfeld RMA, Lewis L, Vornik LA. Perceptions and impact of bipolar disorder: how far have we really come? Results of the national depressive and manic-depressive association 2000 survey of individuals with bipolar disorder. J Clin Psychiatry. 2003;64:161–74.
12. Sahoo MK, Chakrabarti S, Kulhara P. Detection of prodromal symptoms of relapse in mania and unipolar depression by relatives and patients. Indian J Med Res. 2012;135:177–83.
13. Bader CS, Skurla M, Vahia IV. Technology in the assessment, treatment, and management of depression. Harv Rev Psychiatry. 2020;28:60–6.
14. Wang PS, Berglund PA, Olfson M, Kessler RC. Delays in initial treatment contact after first onset of a mental disorder. Health Serv Res. 2004;39:393–415.
15. Winnebeck EC, Fischer D, Leise T, Roenneberg T. Dynamics and ultradian structure of human sleep in real life. Curr Biol. 2018;28:49–59.e5.
16. Dy ME, et al. Defining hand stereotypies in Rett syndrome: a movement disorders perspective. Pediatr Neurol. 2017;75:91–5.
17. de Zambotti M, Baker FC, Colrain IM. Validation of sleep-tracking technology compared with Polysomnography in adolescents. Sleep. 2015;38:1461–8.
18. Lee I-M, et al. Accelerometer-measured physical activity and sedentary behavior in relation to all-cause mortality: the Women's health study. Circulation. 2018;137:203–5.
19. Areàn PA, Hoa Ly K, Andersson G. Mobile technology for mental health assessment. Dialogues Clin Neurosci. 2016;18:163–9.
20. Tedesco S, Barton J, O'Flynn B. A review of activity trackers for senior citizens: research perspectives, commercial landscape and the role of the insurance industry. Sensors (Basel). 2017;17:1277.
21. Espay AJ, et al. Technology in Parkinson's disease: challenges and opportunities. Mov Disord. 2016;31:1272–82.
22. Haubenberger D, et al. Transducer-based evaluation of tremor. Mov Disord. 2016;31:1327–36.
23. Ben-Zeev D, Scherer EA, Wang R, Xie H, Campbell AT. Next-generation psychiatric assessment: using smartphone sensors to monitor behavior and mental health. Psychiatr Rehabil J. 2015;38:218–26.
24. Heikenfeld J, et al. Accessing analytes in biofluids for peripheral biochemical monitoring. Nat Biotechnol. 2019;37:407–19.
25. Cui Y. Wireless biological electronic sensors. Sensors (Basel). 2017;17:2289.
26. Rahman, M. et al. Are we there yet? Feasibility of continuous stress assessment via wireless physiological sensors. ACM-BCB ... ... ACM Conference on Bioinformatics, Computational Biology and Biomedical, Washington, DC. 2014, pp 479–488.

27. Bruen D, Delaney C, Florea L, Diamond D. Glucose sensing for diabetes monitoring: recent developments. Sensors (Basel). 2017;17:1866.
28. Solovei D, Žák J, Majzlíková P, Sedláček J, Hubálek J. Chemical sensor platform for non-invasive monitoring of activity and dehydration. Sensors (Basel). 2015;15:1479–95.
29. Patel S, Saunders KE. Apps and wearables in the monitoring of mental health disorders. Br J Hosp Med (Lond). 2018;79(672–675)
30. Knight A, Bidargaddi N. Commonly available activity tracker apps and wearables as a mental health outcome indicator: a prospective observational cohort study among young adults with psychological distress. J Affect Disord. 2018;236:31–6.
31. Sandstrom GM, Lathia N, Mascolo C, Rentfrow PJ. Opportunities for smartphones in clinical care: the future of mobile mood monitoring. J Clin Psychiatry. 2016;77:e135–7.
32. Wahle F, Kowatsch T, Fleisch E, Rufer M, Weidt S. Mobile sensing and support for people with depression: a pilot trial in the wild. JMIR Mhealth Uhealth. 2016;4:e111.
33. Masud MT, et al. Unobtrusive monitoring of behavior and movement patterns to detect clinical depression severity level via smartphone. J Biomed Inform. 2020;103:103371.
34. Widener MJ, et al. Activity space-based measures of the food environment and their relationships to food purchasing behaviours for young urban adults in Canada. Public Health Nutr. 2018;21:2103–16.
35. Seto E, et al. Models of individual dietary behavior based on smartphone data: the influence of routine, physical activity, emotion, and food environment. PLoS One. 2016;11:e0153085.
36. BinDhim NF, et al. Depression screening via a smartphone app: cross-country user characteristics and feasibility. J Am Med Inform Assoc. 2015;22:29–34.
37. Bakker D, Kazantzis N, Rickwood D, Rickard N. Mental health smartphone apps: review and evidence-based recommendations for future developments. JMIR Ment. Heal. 2016;3:e7.
38. Murnane EL et al. Mobile manifestations of alertness: connecting biological rhythms with patterns of smartphone app use. MobileHCI Proc. … international Conference on Human-Computer Interaction with Mobile Devices and Services. Devices Serv. MobileHCI 2016. 2016 pp 465–477.
39. Matthews M, et al. Development and evaluation of a smartphone-based measure of social rhythms for bipolar disorder. Assessment. 2016;23:472–83.
40. Bauer AM, et al. Acceptability of mHealth augmentation of collaborative care: a mixed methods pilot study. Gen Hosp Psychiatry. 2018;51:22–9.
41. Reis S, et al. Integrating modelling and smart sensors for environmental and human health. Environ Model Softw with Environ data news. 2015;74:238–46.
42. Nicolini C, et al. Prototypes of newly conceived inorganic and biological sensors for health and environmental applications. Sensors (Basel). 2012;12:17112–27.
43. Donker T, et al. Smartphones for smarter delivery of mental health programs: a systematic review. J Med Internet Res. 2013;15:e247.
44. Marcano Belisario JS, et al. Comparison of self-administered survey questionnaire responses collected using mobile apps versus other methods. Cochrane Database Syst Rev. 2015;7:MR000042. https://doi.org/10.1002/14651858.MR000042.pub2.
45. Buck B, et al. Capturing behavioral indicators of persecutory ideation using mobile technology. J Psychiatr Res. 2019;116:112–7.
46. Wongkoblap A, Vadillo MA, Curcin V. Researching mental health disorders in the era of social media: systematic review. J Med Internet Res. 2017;19:e228.
47. Golder S, Ahmed S, Norman G, Booth A. Attitudes toward the ethics of research using social media: a systematic review. J Med Internet Res. 2017;19:e195.
48. Wongkoblap A, Vadillo MA, Curcin V. Modeling depression symptoms from social network data through multiple instance learning. AMIA Jt Summits Transl Sci proceedings AMIA Jt Summits Transl Sci. 2019;2019:44–53.
49. Ford E, Curlewis K, Wongkoblap A, Curcin V. Public opinions on using social media content to identify users with depression and target mental health care advertising: mixed methods survey. JMIR Ment. Heal. 2019;6:e12942.
50. Coppersmith G, Leary R, Crutchley P, Fine A. Natural language processing of social media as screening for suicide risk. Biomed Inform Insights. 2018;10:1178222618792860.

51. Du J, et al. Extracting psychiatric stressors for suicide from social media using deep learning. BMC Med Inform Decis Mak. 2018;18:43.
52. Eichstaedt JC, et al. Facebook language predicts depression in medical records. Proc Natl Acad Sci U S A. 2018;115:11203–8.
53. Merchant RM, et al. Evaluating the predictability of medical conditions from social media posts. PLoS One. 2019;14:e0215476.
54. Abu Rahal Z, Vadas L, Manor I, Bloch B, Avital A. Use of information and communication technologies among individuals with and without serious mental illness. Psychiatry Res. 2018;266:160–7.
55. Seabrook EM, Kern ML, Fulcher BD, Rickard NS. Predicting depression from language-based emotion dynamics: longitudinal analysis of Facebook and twitter status updates. J Med Internet Res. 2018;20:e168.
56. Mowery D, et al. Understanding depressive symptoms and psychosocial stressors on twitter: a corpus-based study. J Med Internet Res. 2017;19:e48.
57. Muzaffar N, et al. The Association of Adolescent Facebook Behaviours with symptoms of social anxiety, generalized anxiety, and depression. J Can Acad Child Adolesc Psychiatry. 2018;27:252–60.
58. Seabrook EM, Kern ML, Rickard NS. Social networking sites, depression, and anxiety: a systematic review. JMIR Ment. Heal. 2016;3:e50.
59. Won H-H, et al. Predicting national suicide numbers with social media data. PLoS One. 2013;8:e61809.
60. Hswen Y, Gopaluni A, Brownstein JS, Hawkins JB. Using twitter to detect psychological characteristics of self-identified persons with autism Spectrum disorder: a feasibility study. JMIR Mhealth Uhealth. 2019;7:e12264.
61. Kim SJ, Marsch LA, Hancock JT, Das AK. Scaling up research on drug abuse and addiction through social media big data. J Med Internet Res. 2017;19:e353.
62. Moessner M, Feldhege J, Wolf M, Bauer S. Analyzing big data in social media: text and network analyses of an eating disorder forum. Int J Eat Disord. 2018;51:656–67.
63. McCaig D, Bhatia S, Elliott MT, Walasek L, Meyer C. Text-mining as a methodology to assess eating disorder-relevant factors: comparing mentions of fitness tracking technology across online communities. Int J Eat Disord. 2018;51:647–55.
64. Gruebner O, et al. A novel surveillance approach for disaster mental health. PLoS One. 2017;12:e0181233.
65. Marino C, Gini G, Vieno A, Spada MM. The associations between problematic Facebook use, psychological distress and Well-being among adolescents and young adults: a systematic review and meta-analysis. J Affect Disord. 2018;226:274–81.
66. Turner PG, Lefevre CE. Instagram use is linked to increased symptoms of orthorexia nervosa. Eat Weight Disord. 2017;22:277–84.
67. Brailovskaia J, Margraf J, Köllner V. Addicted to Facebook? Relationship between Facebook addiction disorder, duration of Facebook use and narcissism in an inpatient sample. Psychiatry Res. 2019;273:52–7.
68. Saunders JF, Eaton AA. Snaps, Selfies, and shares: how three popular social media platforms contribute to the sociocultural model of disordered eating among young women. Cyberpsychol Behav Soc Netw. 2018;21:343–54.
69. Escobar-Viera CG, et al. For better or for worse? A systematic review of the evidence on social media use and depression among lesbian, gay, and bisexual minorities. JMIR Ment Heal. 2018;5:e10496.
70. Gillett G, Saunders KEA. Remote monitoring for understanding mechanisms and prediction in psychiatry. Curr Behav Neurosci Reports. 2019;6:51–6.
71. Simon J, Budge K, Price J, Goodwin GM, Geddes JR. Remote mood monitoring for adults with bipolar disorder: an explorative study of compliance and impact on mental health service use and costs. Eur Psychiatry. 2017;45:14–9.
72. Faurholt-Jepsen M, et al. Smartphone data as objective measures of bipolar disorder symptoms. Psychiatry Res. 2014;217:124–7.

73. Carr O, et al. Variability in phase and amplitude of diurnal rhythms is related to variation of mood in bipolar and borderline personality disorder. Sci Rep. 2018;8:1649.
74. Harmer CJ, Goodwin GM, Cowen PJ. Why do antidepressants take so long to work? A cognitive neuropsychological model of antidepressant drug action Br J Psychiatry. 2009;195:102–8.
75. Townsend L, et al. Development of three web-based computerized versions of the kiddie schedule for affective disorders and schizophrenia child psychiatric diagnostic interview: preliminary validity data. J Am Acad Child Adolesc Psychiatry. 2020;59:309–25.
76. Sharp C, et al. The incremental validity of borderline personality disorder relative to major depressive disorder for suicidal ideation and deliberate self-harm in adolescents. J Personal Disord. 2012;26:927–38.
77. Head J, et al. Use of self-administered instruments to assess psychiatric disorders in older people: validity of the general health questionnaire, the Center for Epidemiologic Studies Depression Scale and the self-completion version of the revised clinical interview Sch. Psychol Med. 2013;43:2649–56.
78. Gelenberg AJ. Using assessment tools to screen for, diagnose, and treat major depressive disorder in clinical practice. J Clin Psychiatry. 2010;71(Suppl E):e01.
79. Kim K, et al. Development of a computer-based behavioral assessment of checking behavior in obsessive-compulsive disorder. Compr Psychiatry. 2010;51:86–93.
80. Ventura J, Cienfuegos A, Boxer O, Bilder R. Clinical global impression of cognition in schizophrenia (CGI-CogS): reliability and validity of a co-primary measure of cognition. Schizophr Res. 2008;106:59–69.
81. Cahn-Hidalgo D, Estes PW, Benabou R. Validity, reliability, and psychometric properties of a computerized, cognitive assessment test (Cognivue®). World J. psychiatry. 2020;10:1–11.
82. Vincent, A. S., Fuenzalida, E., Beneda-Bender, M., Bryant, D. J. & Peters, E. Neurocognitive assessment on a tablet device: Test-retest reliability and practice effects of ANAM Mobile. Appl Neuropsychol Adult. 2019, pp 1–9. https://doi.org/10.1080/23279095.2019.1640698
83. Ivins BJ, Arrieux JP, Schwab KA, Haran FJ, Cole WR. Using rates of low scores to assess agreement between brief computerized neuropsychological assessment batteries: a clinically-based approach for psychometric comparisons. Arch Clin Neuropsychol. 2019;34:1392–408.
84. Bifulco A, et al. Web-based measure of life events using computerized life events and assessment record (CLEAR): preliminary cross-sectional study of reliability, validity, and association with depression. JMIR Ment. Heal. 2019;6:e10675.
85. Cano-Vindel A, et al. A computerized version of the patient health Questionnaire-4 as an ultra-brief screening tool to detect emotional disorders in primary care. J Affect Disord. 2018;234:247–55.
86. Eisen SV, et al. Development and validation of a computerized-adaptive test for PTSD (P-CAT). Psychiatr Serv. 2016;67:1116–23.
87. Loe BS, Stillwell D, Gibbons C. Computerized adaptive testing provides reliable and efficient depression measurement using the CES-D scale. J Med Internet Res. 2017;19:e302.
88. Erbe D, Eichert H-C, Rietz C, Ebert D. Interformat reliability of the patient health questionnaire: validation of the computerized version of the PHQ-9. Internet Interv. 2016;5:1–4.
89. Smits N, Cuijpers P, van Straten A. Applying computerized adaptive testing to the CES-D scale: a simulation study. Psychiatry Res. 2011;188:147–55.
90. Fliege H, et al. Evaluation of a computer-adaptive test for the assessment of depression (D-CAT) in clinical application. Int J Methods Psychiatr Res. 2009;18:23–36.
91. Becker J, et al. Functioning and validity of a computerized adaptive test to measure anxiety (A-CAT). Depress Anxiety. 2008;25:E182–94.
92. Robeznieks A. Which medical specialties use telemedicine the most? 2019. Available at: https://www.ama-assn.org/practice-management/digital/which-medical-specialties-use-telemedicine-most. Accessed 30 August 2020.
93. Fairchild RM, Ferng-Kuo S-F, Rahmouni H, Hardesty D. Telehealth increases access to Care for Children Dealing with Suicidality, depression, and anxiety in rural emergency departments. Telemed J E Health. 2020;26(11):1353–62. https://doi.org/10.1089/tmj.2019.0253.

94. Mehrotra A, et al. Rapid growth in mental health telemedicine use among rural Medicare beneficiaries. Wide Variation Across States Health Aff (Millwood). 2017;36:909–17.
95. Chakrabarti S. Usefulness of telepsychiatry: a critical evaluation of videoconferencing-based approaches. World J. psychiatry. 2015;5:286–304.
96. Gibson KL, et al. Conversations on telemental health: listening to remote and rural First nations communities. Rural Remote Health. 2011;11:1656.
97. Pignatiello A, et al. Child and youth telepsychiatry in rural and remote primary care. Child Adolesc Psychiatr Clin N Am. 2011;20:13–28.
98. Spaulding R, Cain S, Sonnenschein K. Urban telepsychiatry: uncommon service for a common need. Child Adolesc Psychiatr Clin N Am. 2011;20:29–39.
99. Hubley S, Lynch SB, Schneck C, Thomas M, Shore J. Review of key telepsychiatry outcomes. World J psychiatry. 2016;6:269–82.
100. Gardner JS, Plaven BE, Yellowlees P, Shore JH. Remote Telepsychiatry workforce: a solution to Psychiatry's workforce issues. Curr Psychiatry Rep. 2020;22:8.
101. Chipps J, Ramlall S, Mars M. A telepsychiatry model to support psychiatric outreach in the public sector in South Africa. Afr J Psychiatry. 2012;15:264–70.
102. Naskar S, Victor R, Das H, Nath K. Telepsychiatry in India – Where do we stand? A comparative review between global and indian telepsychiatry programs. Indian J Psychol Med. 2017;39:223–42.
103. Malhotra S, Chakrabarti S, Shah R. Telepsychiatry: promise, potential, and challenges. Indian J Psychiatry. 2013;55:3–11.
104. Abrams J, et al. Practical issues in delivery of clinician-to-patient telemental health in an academic medical center. Harv Rev Psychiatry. 2017;25:135–45.
105. Cowan KE, McKean AJ, Gentry MT, Hilty DM. Barriers to use of Telepsychiatry: clinicians as gatekeepers. Mayo Clin Proc. 2019;94:2510–23.
106. O'Brien M, McNicholas F. The use of telepsychiatry during COVID-19 and beyond. Ir J Psychol Med. 2020. pp 1–6. https://doi.org/10.1017/ipm.2020.54
107. Smith K, Ostinelli E, Macdonald O, Cipriani A. COVID-19 and Telepsychiatry: development of evidence-based guidance for clinicians. JMIR Ment. Heal. 2020;7:e21108.
108. Chen JA, et al. COVID-19 and telepsychiatry: early outpatient experiences and implications for the future. Gen Hosp Psychiatry. 2020;66:89–95.
109. Gautam M, Thakrar A, Akinyemi E, Mahr G. Current and future challenges in the delivery of mental healthcare during COVID-19. SN Compr Clin Med. 2020. pp 1–6. https://doi.org/10.1007/s42399-020-00348-3
110. Sheridan Rains L, et al. Early impacts of the COVID-19 pandemic on mental health care and on people with mental health conditions: framework synthesis of international experiences and responses. Soc Psychiatry Psychiatr Epidemiol. 2020; https://doi.org/10.1007/s00127-020-01924-7.
111. Talevi D, et al. Mental health outcomes of the CoViD-19 pandemic. Riv Psichiatr. 2020;55:137–44.
112. Liu S, et al. Online mental health services in China during the COVID-19 outbreak. Lancet Psychiatry. 2020;7:e17–8.
113. Ćosić K, Popović S, Šarlija M, Kesedžić I. Impact of human disasters and COVID-19 pandemic on mental health: potential of digital psychiatry. Psychiatr Danub. 2020;32:25–31.
114. Zhou X, et al. The role of Telehealth in reducing the mental health burden from COVID-19. Telemed J E Health. 2020;26:377–9.
115. Zhou J, Liu L, Xue P, Yang X, Tang X. Mental health response to the COVID-19 outbreak in China. Am J Psychiatry. 2020;177:574–5.
116. Hagerty SL, Williams LM. The impact of COVID-19 on mental health: the interactive roles of brain biotypes and human connection. Brain Behav Immun Heal. 2020;5:100078.
117. Vindegaard N, Benros ME. COVID-19 pandemic and mental health consequences: systematic review of the current evidence. Brain Behav Immun. 2020; https://doi.org/10.1016/j.bbi.2020.05.048.

118. Torous J, Jän Myrick K, Rauseo-Ricupero N, Firth J. Digital mental health and COVID-19: using technology today to accelerate the curve on access and quality tomorrow. JMIR Ment. Heal. 2020;7:e18848.

119. Byrom B, McCarthy M, Schueler P, Muehlhausen W. Brain monitoring devices in neuroscience clinical research: the potential of remote monitoring using sensors, Wearables, and Mobile devices. Clin Pharmacol Ther. 2018;104:59–71.

120. Nakamoto R, et al. Comparison of PET/CT with sequential PET/MRI using an MR-compatible Mobile PET system. J Nucl Med. 2018;59:846–51.

121. Peters J, Van Wageningen B, Hoogerwerf N, Tan E. Near-infrared spectroscopy: a promising Prehospital tool for Management of Traumatic Brain Injury. Prehosp Disaster Med. 2017;32:414–8.

122. Sakudo A. Near-infrared spectroscopy for medical applications: current status and future perspectives. Clin Chim Acta. 2016;455:181–8.

123. Kim HY, Seo K, Jeon HJ, Lee U, Lee H. Application of functional near-infrared spectroscopy to the study of brain function in humans and animal models. Mol Cells. 2017;40:523–32.

124. Fukuda K, Sato D. Cancellation method of signal fluctuations in brain function measurements using near-infrared spectroscopy. Conference proceedings: annual international conference of the IEEE engineering in medicine and biology society, 2018. pp 3302–3305.

125. Krigolson OE, Williams CC, Norton A, Hassall CD, Colino FL. Choosing MUSE: validation of a low-cost, portable EEG system for ERP research. Front Neurosci. 2017;11:109.

126. Neumann T, et al. Assessment of the technical usability and efficacy of a new portable dry-electrode EEG recorder: First results of the HOMEONE study. Clin Neurophysiol. 2019;130:2076–87.

127. Shou, G., Mosconi, M. W., Ethridge, L. E., Sweeney, J. A. & Ding, L. Resting-state Gamma-band EEG abnormalities in Autism. Conference proceedings: ... annual international conference of the IEEE engineering in medicine and biology society 2018. pp 1915–1918.

128. Hashemi A, et al. Characterizing population EEG dynamics throughout adulthood. eNeuro. 2016;3(6):ENEURO.0275-16.2016.

129. Ogino M, Mitsukura Y. Portable drowsiness detection through use of a prefrontal Single-Channel electroencephalogram. Sensors (Basel). 2018;18:4477.

130. Stopczynski A, Stahlhut C, Larsen JE, Petersen MK, Hansen LK. The smartphone brain scanner: a portable real-time neuroimaging system. PLoS One. 2014;9:e86733.

131. Sterr A, et al. Sleep EEG derived from behind-the-ear electrodes (cEEGrid) compared to standard Polysomnography: a proof of concept study. Front Hum Neurosci. 2018;12:452.

132. Sintotskiy G, Hinrichs H. In-ear-EEG - a portable platform for home monitoring. J Med Eng Technol. 2020;44:26–37.

133. Baker JT, Germine LT, Ressler KJ, Rauch SL, Carlezon WA. Digital devices and continuous telemetry: opportunities for aligning psychiatry and neuroscience. Neuropsychopharmacology. 2018;43:2499–503.

134. Radüntz T, Meffert B. User experience of 7 Mobile electroencephalography devices: comparative study. JMIR Mhealth Uhealth. 2019;7:e14474.

135. Desmidt T, et al. Ultrasound measures of brain Pulsatility correlate with subcortical brain volumes in healthy young adults. Ultrasound Med Biol. 2018;44:2307–13.

136. Imbault M, Chauvet D, Gennisson J-L, Capelle L, Tanter M. Intraoperative functional ultrasound imaging of human brain activity. Sci Rep. 2017;7:7304.

137. Provost J, et al. 3D ultrafast ultrasound imaging in vivo. Phys Med Biol. 2014;59:L1–L13.

138. Wheelock MD, Culver JP, Eggebrecht AT. High-density diffuse optical tomography for imaging human brain function. Rev Sci Instrum. 2019;90:051101.

139. Ferradal SL, et al. Functional imaging of the developing brain at the bedside using diffuse optical tomography. Cereb Cortex. 2016;26:1558–68.

140. Eggebrecht AT, et al. Mapping distributed brain function and networks with diffuse optical tomography. Nat Photonics. 2014;8:448–54.

141. Khan AF, Zhang F, Yuan H, Ding L. Dynamic activation patterns of the motor brain revealed by diffuse optical tomography. Conference proceedings: ... annual international conference of the IEEE engineering in medicine and biology society, 2019, pp 6028–6031.
142. The World Health Organization. The WHO mental health policy and service guidance package. 2005. Available at: https://www.who.int/mental_health/policy/essentialpackage1/en/. Accessed 30 August 2020.
143. de Silva PN. Use of appropriate technology to improve mental health service delivery. Br J Hosp Med (Lond). 2018;79:682–5.
144. Wang K, Varma DS, Prosperi M. A systematic review of the effectiveness of mobile apps for monitoring and management of mental health symptoms or disorders. J Psychiatr Res. 2018;107:73–8.
145. Ranallo PA, Kilbourne AM, Whatley AS, Pincus HA. Behavioral health information technology: from Chaos to clarity. Health Aff (Millwood). 2016;35:1106–13.
146. Bowens FM, Frye PA, Jones WA. Health information technology: integration of clinical workflow into meaningful use of electronic health records. Perspect Heal Inf Manag. 2010;7:1d.
147. Graber ML, Byrne C, Johnston D. The impact of electronic health records on diagnosis. Diagnosis (Berlin, Germany). 2017;4:211–23.
148. Larsen ME, et al. Using science to sell apps: evaluation of mental health app store quality claims. NPJ Digit Med. 2019;2:18.
149. Marshall JM, Dunstan DA, Bartik W. The digital psychiatrist: in search of evidence-based apps for anxiety and depression. Front Psych. 2019;10:831.
150. Grist R, Porter J, Stallard P. Mental health Mobile apps for preadolescents and adolescents: a systematic review. J Med Internet Res. 2017;19:e176.
151. Rathbone AL, Prescott J. The use of Mobile apps and SMS messaging as physical and mental health interventions: systematic review. J Med Internet Res. 2017;19:e295.
152. Fleming T, et al. Beyond the trial: systematic review of real-world uptake and engagement with digital self-help interventions for depression, low mood, or anxiety. J Med Internet Res. 2018;20:e199.
153. Baumel A, Muench F, Edan S, Kane JM. Objective user engagement with mental health apps: systematic search and panel-based usage analysis. J Med Internet Res. 2019;21:e14567.
154. Shen N, et al. Understanding the patient privacy perspective on health information exchange: a systematic review. Int J Med Inform. 2019;125:1–12.
155. Steel Z, et al. The global prevalence of common mental disorders: a systematic review and meta-analysis 1980–2013. Int J Epidemiol. 2014;43:476–93.
156. DeAndrea DC. Testing the proclaimed affordances of online support groups in a nationally representative sample of adults seeking mental health assistance. J Health Commun. 2015;20:147–56.
157. Bauer R, et al. International multi-site survey on the use of online support groups in bipolar disorder. Nord J Psychiatry. 2017;71:473–6.
158. Ali K, Farrer L, Gulliver A, Griffiths KM. Online peer-to-peer support for young people with mental health problems: a systematic review. JMIR Ment Heal. 2015;2:e19.
159. Townsend L, Gearing RE, Polyanskaya O. Influence of health beliefs and stigma on choosing internet support groups over formal mental health services. Psychiatr Serv. 2012;63:370–6.
160. Smith-Merry J, et al. Social connection and online engagement: insights from interviews with users of a mental health online forum. JMIR Ment Heal. 2019;6:e11084.
161. Williams A, Fossey E, Farhall J, Foley F, Thomas N. Going online together: the potential for mental health workers to integrate recovery oriented E-mental health resources into their practice. Psychiatry. 2018;81:116–29.
162. Beck SJ, Paskewitz EA, Anderson WA, Bourdeaux R, Currie-Mueller J. The task and relational dimensions of online social support. Health Commun. 2017;32:347–55.

163. Evans M, Donelle L, Hume-Loveland L. Social support and online postpartum depression discussion groups: a content analysis. Patient Educ Couns. 2012;87:405–10.
164. Välimäki M, Athanasopoulou C, Lahti M, Adams CE. Effectiveness of social media interventions for people with schizophrenia: a systematic review and meta-analysis. J Med Internet Res. 2016;18:e92.
165. Yip JWC. Evaluating the communication of online social support: a mixed-methods analysis of structure and content. Health Commun. 2020;35:1210–8.
166. Greiner C, Chatton A, Khazaal Y. Online self-help forums on cannabis: a content assessment. Patient Educ Couns. 2017;100:1943–50.
167. Mullen G, Dowling C, O'Reilly G. Internet use among young people with and without mental health difficulties. Ir J Psychol Med. 2018;35:11–21.
168. Finfgeld DL. Therapeutic groups online: the good, the bad, and the unknown. Issues Ment Health Nurs. 2000;21:241–55.
169. Stefanopoulou E, Lewis D, Taylor M, Broscombe J, Larkin J. Digitally delivered psychological interventions for anxiety disorders: a comprehensive review. Psychiatry Q. 2019;90:197–215.
170. Kendal S, Kirk S, Elvey R, Catchpole R, Pryjmachuk S. How a moderated online discussion forum facilitates support for young people with eating disorders. Health Expect. 2017;20:98–111.
171. McCormack A. Individuals with eating disorders and the use of online support groups as a form of social support. Comput Inform Nurs. 2010;28:12–9.
172. Andrews D, Foley M. Moderated online social therapy for youth mental health. (2020). Available at: http://most.org.au/.
173. Herbst N, et al. The potential of telemental health applications for obsessive-compulsive disorder. Clin Psychol Rev. 2012;32:454–66.
174. Andersson E, et al. Internet-based cognitive behaviour therapy for obsessive-compulsive disorder: a randomized controlled trial. Psychol Med. 2012;42:2193–203.
175. Jaworska N, de la Salle S, Ibrahim M-H, Blier P, Knott V. Leveraging machine learning approaches for predicting antidepressant treatment response using electroencephalography (EEG) and clinical data. Front Psych. 2018;9:768.
176. Economides M, et al. Long-term outcomes of a therapist-supported, smartphone-based intervention for elevated symptoms of depression and anxiety: Quasiexperimental, pre-Postintervention study. JMIR Mhealth Uhealth. 2019;7:e14284.
177. Wright JH, et al. Computer-assisted cognitive-behavior therapy for depression: a systematic review and meta-analysis. J Clin Psychiatry. 2019;80:18r12188.
178. Marcelle ET, Nolting L, Hinshaw SP, Aguilera A. Effectiveness of a multimodal digital psychotherapy platform for adult depression: a naturalistic feasibility study. JMIR Mhealth Uhealth. 2019;7:e10948.
179. Hull TD, Mahan K. A study of asynchronous Mobile-enabled SMS text psychotherapy. Telemed J E Health. 2017;23:240–7.
180. Mohr DC, et al. IntelliCare: an eclectic, skills-based app suite for the treatment of depression and anxiety. J Med Internet Res. 2017;19:e10.
181. Mantani A, et al. Smartphone cognitive behavioral therapy as an adjunct to pharmacotherapy for refractory depression: randomized controlled trial. J Med Internet Res. 2017;19:e373.
182. Mak WW, et al. Efficacy and moderation of Mobile app-based programs for mindfulness-based training, self-compassion training, and cognitive behavioral Psychoeducation on mental health: randomized controlled noninferiority trial. JMIR Ment. Heal. 2018;5:e60.
183. Renfrew ME, et al. A web- and Mobile app-based mental health promotion intervention comparing email, short message service, and videoconferencing support for a healthy cohort: randomized comparative study. J Med Internet Res. 2020;22:e15592.
184. Hafeman DM, et al. Assessment of a person-level risk calculator to predict new-onset bipolar Spectrum disorder in youth at familial risk. JAMA Psychiat. 2017;74:841–7.
185. Anastasiadou D, Folkvord F, Serrano-Troncoso E, Lupiañez-Villanueva F. Mobile health adoption in mental health: user experience of a Mobile health app for patients with an eating disorder. JMIR Mhealth Uhealth. 2019;7:e12920.

186. Terry NP, Gunter TD. Regulating mobile mental health apps. Behav Sci Law. 2018;36:136–44.
187. Stratton E, et al. Effectiveness of eHealth interventions for reducing mental health conditions in employees: a systematic review and meta-analysis. PLoS One. 2017;12:e0189904.
188. Ashford MT, Olander EK, Rowe H, Fisher JR, Ayers S. Feasibility and acceptability of a web-based treatment with telephone support for postpartum women with anxiety: randomized controlled trial. JMIR Ment. Heal. 2018;5:e19.
189. One mind psyber guide. Available at: https://onemindpsyberguide.org/about-psyberguide/. Accessed 31 August 2020.
190. Woodson TT, et al. Designing health information technology tools for behavioral health clinicians integrated within a primary care team. J Innov Heal informatics. 2018;25:158–68.
191. Gentles SJ, Lokker C, McKibbon KA. Health information technology to facilitate communication involving health care providers, caregivers, and pediatric patients: a scoping review. J Med Internet Res. 2010;12:e22.
192. Rantz M, et al. Enhanced registered nurse care coordination with sensor technology: Impact on length of stay and cost in aging in place housing. Nurs Outlook. 2015;63:650–5.
193. Roos E, Bjerkeset O, Steinsbekk A. Health care utilization and cost after discharge from a mental health hospital; an RCT comparing community residential aftercare and treatment as usual. BMC Psychiatry. 2018;18:363.
194. Baumel A, et al. Health technology intervention after hospitalization for schizophrenia: service utilization and user satisfaction. Psychiatr Serv. 2016;67:1035–8.
195. Arrieta MI, Foreman RD, Crook ED, Icenogle ML. Providing continuity of care for chronic diseases in the aftermath of Katrina: from field experience to policy recommendations. Disaster Med Public Health Prep. 2009;3:174–82.
196. Belling R, et al. Achieving continuity of care: facilitators and barriers in community mental health teams. Implement Sci. 2011;6:23.
197. Sadock, B., Sadock, V. & Ruiz, P. Chapter 2: Psychiatric interview, history, and mental status examination. in Kaplan & Sadock's concise textbook of clinical psychiatry, 4th ed. 2017.
198. American psychiatric association. Use of the manual. In Diagnostic and statistical manual of mental disorders. 2013.
199. Jablensky A. Psychiatric classifications: validity and utility. World Psychiatry. 2016;15:26–31.
200. Kahneman D, Riis J. Living, and thinking about it: two perspectives on life. In: Huppert F, Baylis N, Keverne B, editors. The science of well-being. Oxford: Oxford University Press; 2005. p. 285–304.
201. Boguszewski CL, de Castro Musolino NR, Kasuki L. Management of pituitary incidentaloma. Best Pract Res Clin Endocrinol Metab. 2019;33:101268.
202. Morris ZS, Wooding S, Grant J. The answer is 17 years, what is the question: understanding time lags in translational research. J R Soc Med. 2011;104:510–20.
203. Liu JX, Goryakin Y, Maeda A, Bruckner T, Scheffler R. Global Health workforce labor market projections for 2030. Hum Resour Health. 2017;15:11.
204. Pearce C, Trumble S, Arnold M, Dwan K, Phillips C. Computers in the new consultation: within the first minute. Fam Pract. 2008;25:202–8.
205. Kazmi Z. Effects of exam room EHR use on doctor-patient communication: a systematic literature review. Inform Prim Care. 2013;21:30–9.
206. Redd TK, et al. Variability in electronic health record usage and perceptions among specialty vs. primary care physicians. AMIA Annu Symp Proc. 2015;2015:2053–62.
207. Zheeng G, Zhang C, Li L. Bringing business intelligence to healthcare informatics curriculum. In: Proceedings of the 45th ACM technical symposium on Computer science education - SIGCSE '14. New York: ACM Press; 2014. p. 205–10. https://doi.org/10.1145/2538862.2538935.
208. Hilty DM, Chan S, Torous J, Luo J, Boland RJ. Mobile health, smartphone/device, and apps for psychiatry and medicine: competencies, training, and faculty development issues. Psychiatr Clin North Am. 2019;42:513–34.

209. Torous J, Chan S, Luo J, Boland R, Hilty D. Clinical informatics in psychiatric training: preparing Today's trainees for the already present future. Acad Psychiatry. 2018;42:694–7.
210. Gostin LO, Halabi SF, Wilson K. Health data and privacy in the digital era. JAMA. 2018;320:233–4.
211. Lee J-M, Byun W, Keill A, Dinkel D, Seo Y. Comparison of wearable trackers' ability to estimate sleep. Int J Environ Res Public Health. 2018;15:1265.
212. Thimbleby H Cybersecurity problems in a typical hospital (and probably all of them). Developing Safe Systems, Proceedings of the 25th Safety-Critical Systems Symposium, pp 415–439
213. Calvo RA, Dinakar K, Picard R, Christensen H, Torous J. Toward impactful collaborations on computing and mental health. J Med Internet Res. 2018;20:e49.
214. Schuurman D, Marez L. Living labs: a structured approach for implementing open and user innovation. 2015.
215. Rao G, Ridley M, Schilbach F, Patel V. Poverty and mental illness: Causal evidence. 2019.
216. Wong KTG, Liu D, Balzan R, King D, Galletly C. Smartphone and internet access and utilization by people with schizophrenia in South Australia: quantitative survey study. JMIR Ment. Heal. 2020;7:e11551.

Chapter 18
Ethical, Legal, and Social Issues (ELSI) in Mental Health Informatics

Vignesh Subbian, Hannah K. Galvin, Carolyn Petersen, and Anthony Solomonides

Abstract This chapter explores a wide range of ethical, legal, and social issues in mental health informatics. The topics covered are broadly categorized into four groups: (1) ethical issues related to artificial intelligence in mental healthcare, (2) issues related to mobile health and eHealth applications, (3) sociotechnical issues related to data sharing, advocacy, and genomics in mental health informatics, and (4) relevant laws and regulations including Health Insurance Portability and Accountability Act of 1996 (HIPAA), HIPAA Privacy Rule, HIPAA Security Rule, Confidentiality of Substance Use Disorder Patient Records, 21st Century Cures Act, General Data Protection Regulation, and California Consumer Privacy Act.

Keywords Biomedical ethics · Data sharing · Machine intelligence · Mental health · Privacy

V. Subbian (✉)
Department of Biomedical Engineering and Department of Systems and Industrial Engineering, The University of Arizona, Tucson, AZ, USA
e-mail: vsubbian@arizona.edu

H. K. Galvin
Cambridge Health Alliance, Cambridge, MA, USA
e-mail: hagalvin@challiance.org

C. Petersen
Division of Biomedical Statistics and Informatics, Mayo Clinic, Rochester, MN, USA
e-mail: Petersen.Carolyn@mayo.edu

A. Solomonides
Outcomes Research Network, Research Institute, NorthShore University HealthSystem, Evanston, IL, USA

© Springer Nature Switzerland AG 2021
J. D. Tenenbaum, P. A. Ranallo (eds.), *Mental Health Informatics*, Health Informatics, https://doi.org/10.1007/978-3-030-70558-9_18

18.1 Introduction

Ethical, Legal, and Social Issues (ELSI) of informatics in mental health differ from those in other clinical conditions in terms of stigma, trust, and agency in mental healthcare and research. In this chapter, we describe a range of issues in mental health informatics. The chapter begins with the role of stigma in sharing personal and health data with mental health practitioners and researchers. Subsequent sections present ethical issues related to digital health technologies including artificial intelligence (AI) based systems, mobile health (mHealth), social media, telepsychiatry, and other eHealth tools. Topics in these sections are presented using a micro-meso-macro analysis framework, where micro-level implications deal with individuals (e.g., patients, mental health care providers), meso-level implications primarily relate to organizations or systems (e.g., healthcare systems), and macro-level implications deal with society and populations at-large (e.g., mental health advocacy, which is also detailed in a section on its own). In addition to the micro-meso-macro framework, we draw upon traditional paradigms that rely on delineation between clinical research and practice, as well as more contemporary paradigms that foster integration of research and practice [1]. The chapter also addresses ELSI related to genomics and mental health informatics with a focus on better characterization of mental health disorders. Finally, the chapter ends with an overview of laws, regulations, and legal issues pertaining to the field (Table 18.1). Table 18.1 provides an overview of the chapter.

Table 18.1 Overview of ELSI topics in this Chapter

AI in Mental Health	Ethical issues at data-level
	Ethical issues in designing AI-based systems
	Ethical issues in deploying AI-based systems in practice
mHealth & eHealth applications for mental health	Passive data collection
	Telepsychiatry and Telemental health
	Virtual helpers and providers
Other key sociotechnical issues	Stigma and data sharing
	Mental health advocacy
	Genomics and mental health informatics
Law & Regulations	Health insurance portability and accountability act of 1996 (HIPAA)
	HIPAA privacy rule
	HIPAA security rule
	Confidentiality of substance use disorder patient records
	21st century cures act
	General data protection regulation (GDPR)
	California consumer privacy act (CCPA)

18.2   Stigma and Data Sharing

Being diagnosed with a mental health condition can be a very distressing experience for many people. The stigma attached to mental health-related diagnoses may emerge from the general population (public stigma), from institutions and their policies that limit opportunities of those with mental illness (structural), or internally from the patient themselves (self-stigma) [2]. Mental health stigma can reduce the likelihood that a person will seek care [3, 4]. If a person does seek care, interactions with health care professionals that reflect and/or imply stigma associated with mental illness also occur [5, 6], leading to further barriers to progress in therapy and healing. The isolation that people who have been diagnosed with a mental illness experience as a result of stigma does not necessarily go away with treatment; engagement between mental health professionals and people who have mental illness does not reduce stigma to the degree that social engagement with family and friends does [7].

Given the negative effects of stigma, one might expect people who have been diagnosed with mental health conditions to be reluctant to share their personal data. *After all,* one may be led to ask, *what benefit could there be in acknowledging the existence of a mental health condition, if it encourages contempt in others?* However, people diagnosed with a mental health condition have expressed a range of views about sharing personal information related to their diagnoses depending on the overall purpose, who collects the data, and what precautions are in place to ensure confidentiality.

When it comes to research, people are most comfortable sharing personal and health data with researchers who seek to improve the quality of care. In a questionnaire probing views about health information sensitivity and privacy, 82.5% of people seeking mental health services regarded mental health information as sensitive [8]. Almost as many (77.8%) reported a willingness to share mental health information with some or all clinicians, primarily because they believe it will improve their care, and nearly all were willing to share their information for research. In some cases, the capacity to consent to data sharing may be compromised at various points over the course of the mental health condition, a circumstance that adds a layer of complexity and perhaps uncertainty to interactions between researchers and potential participants. In a focus group setting, people using mental health services reported being willing to share health and socioeconomic data for research undertaken to improve treatment and health policy if investigators were transparent about how data would be used [9]. However, data sharing practices mattered to these focus group participants, who were less comfortable sharing data through digital applications than through paper records or other means. In a semi-structured interview setting, people with mental health conditions were generally supportive of health information exchange, but their extent of trust in sharing personal health information was dependent on their past care experiences with providers [10].

In addition, people using mental health services report positive views of data sharing through open data efforts such as OurDataHelps.org, an initiative launched to build suicide prevention tools [11]. Participants in semi-structured interviews reported altruism, and personal experience with mental health, suicide, and loss, as motivations to share personal data despite concerns about privacy and surveillance. Among family members of people who had committed suicide, data sharing was described as a way to make sense of a suicide and to take purposeful action in the aftermath of suicide. It is important to note that the risks associated with loss of privacy are different for family members than for people using mental health services themselves.

18.3   Ethical AI in Mental Healthcare

In this section, we outline ethical and social issues related to artificial intelligence (AI) technologies, including machine learning (ML) based tools, for mental health care in the following order: [1] ethical issues at the data-level, [2] ethical issues in designing AI-based systems, and [3] ethical issues in deploying and using AI-based systems in practice.

18.3.1   Ethical Issues at Data-Level

The classical framework of bias in computer systems [12] classifies biases and other issues as pre-existing (i.e., issues that pre-date the actual creation of the system), technical (i.e., issues that arise during design and development of AI-based systems), and emergent (i.e., issues that arise after the creation of the system). Pre-existing biases may originate from individuals or social institutions and enter a computer or AI-based system through explicit or implicit means, despite well-intentioned efforts. Such biases emerge particularly from historical data used to train AI-based systems, which are rarely independent of the social contexts. Rather, data related to previous events are embedded in sociotechnical contexts and represent the attitudes and practices of the society at-large from which the data are derived [13]. For example, if providers have historically prescribed higher doses of psychotropic medications for a certain group, then an AI-based system trained using such data is likely to recommend a similar high dosage for an individual from that group. Given that mental health disparities such as biased prescription and referral patterns are highly prevalent [14], it is important to identify the sources of biases and compensate for known biases during algorithm design and development [15]. Otherwise, pre-existing biases will propagate further and emerge in decisions and recommendations from AI-based systems. This raises macro-level questions: *What steps can data scientists and developers take to identify biases and to improve bias management practices? What steps can health systems take to select algorithms that mitigate biases and promote equitable care for all?*

18.3.2 Ethical Issues in Designing AI-Based Systems

While designing AI-based systems, it is important to avoid technical biases that might rise from misjudgments during model specification and evaluation. The conventional taxonomic way of categorizing mental disorders may not accurately represent the underlying disturbances [16], posing an important opportunity to specify and evaluate models in a responsible and rigorous manner. More specifically, the same biological disturbance may result in different psychological issues, while on the other hand, two different biological disturbances may result in similar psychological issues [17]. This complexity of mental health conditions calls for caution and more human involvement in the overall feature engineering process, including working closely with clinical domain experts, selecting appropriate target variables, and defining and labeling outcomes. Even though much of the feature engineering process (see Chap. 10) can be automated, it is an iterative, domain-specific, and creative process that is prone to technical biases. This raises meso-level questions: *Who should be involved in the feature engineering process and in what ways? What technical biases might arise from the process?* Additionally, it is important to ask similar questions during model evaluation because the performance (e.g., model error rates) may vary between patient groups [18].

18.3.3 Ethical Issues in Deploying AI-Based Systems in Practice

The fiduciary relationship between a person seeking healthcare services and a clinician is central to the practice of medicine, and even more critical in mental healthcare because of the sensitive nature of such conditions. This relationship is challenged when AI-based systems are deployed in clinical practice by the larger health system administration, even if care decisions are still made by individual mental health providers [19]. Furthermore, patients are rarely aware of the source of the clinician's judgement when AI-based tools are being used, for example, to assess risk of mental illness or make treatment decisions [20]. This raises the micro-level question: *How should a recommendation or prognosis from an AI-based system be shared with a person seeking help for a mental health condition?* We argue that it is important to convey the underlying source of care recommendations to patients, similar to how clinicians would justify and explain the need for a physical exam or an established questionnaire-based screening such as the Patient Health Questionnaire [21] for depression screening. This may be more challenging in mental healthcare than in general healthcare not only because of the belief that people with mental health conditions may not have the capacity to evaluate treatment options and make informed choices but also because explanations about recommendations from the AI-based system may further aggravate the clinical condition and lead to distress in some patients.

18.4 Mobile Health and eHealth Applications
for Mental Health

Mobile health (mHealth) apps targeted at mental health conditions (see Chap. 17 for more details) may focus on one or a number of areas: medication adherence; aggregation of self-reported or passively-collected data; medical reference for providers and/or patients; app-guided relaxation, stress management, hypnosis, meditation, or journaling; and provision of behavioral telehealth treatment either in real time or asynchronously, either with a live person, social media group or utilizing automated systems [22, 23].

For those apps that render clinical reminders or automated guidance, potential ethical and legal pitfalls arise if the app provides flawed output because of a technical issue or limitations in the software logic [22]. Similar risks exist for apps that aggregate data that are self-reported (e.g., data collected through a symptom tracker) or passively collected (e.g., data collected utilizing wearable devices for sleep disturbances). Additionally, these apps pose concerns related to the storage and transmission of such data, as well as the clinical responsibility for receiving it. While users may enter personal information into apps assuming the data are confidential, the Health Insurance Portability and Accountability Act of 1996 (HIPAA) protections often do not apply to health data shared with apps; patients should be made aware that data will likely be covered under HIPAA only after they are transmitted to a clinician (and even then, only those data that are under the clinician's control would likely be subject). Additionally, the Food and Drug Administration (FDA) exercises regulatory discretion over health-related apps considered to "promote a healthy lifestyle," such that little supervision is required for these types of apps [22]. As such, data may be vulnerable when it is stored on a third-party server, written to system logs in an insecure manner, or transferred via the Internet without appropriate protocols [24]. In a 2015 study of 79 mobile health apps certified by the United Kingdom National Health Service as being clinically safe and trustworthy, 89% transferred information online, 66% of which was not encrypted (none of the apps encrypted the data stored on the device). A significant number of these apps (20%) did not have a privacy policy to inform users about how and when their personal information would be collected, retained, or shared [25].

A key micro-level question confronting users of mental health services and tools is, *Can I trust mobile health apps and related tools to protect information about me?* Mental health apps that are developed and operated by commercial entities operate in a somewhat different environment than healthcare providers seeking the sharing of data for research. Among mental health apps, a dearth of privacy policies or "Terms and Conditions" agreements to provide transparency into data sharing practices is common. A market survey of mental health apps available in 2018 found 56, many of which requested permission to access device features, shared health information with an online community, or lacked a privacy policy describing how data would be collected and used [26]. A 2019 study analyzing data sharing and privacy policies of apps for mental health condition management and behavior change (e.g., smoking cessation) found that 69% had a privacy policy, and of these, 88% reported primary uses of data but only 64% reported secondary uses [27]. Data transmission to third parties was rampant, with 23 of the 25 apps that had a privacy policy doing so and 33 of all 36 apps sharing information with third parties. Eighty-one percent of apps transmitted data to Google and/or Facebook, but only 43% reported sharing data with Google and 50% reported sharing information with Facebook. In general, privacy policies failed to offer users an informed choice about whether to share mental health information. Another 2019 study evaluated the first 100 mental health apps from popular app stores and found that fewer than 20% of both iOS and Android apps had a privacy policy and no more than 15% had a Terms of Service agreement, despite the fact that app stores required apps to include both documents [28]. Among apps that did have such policies and/or terms, a majority of them were written at a post-secondary reading level, rendering them unclear to many potential users.

18.4.1 Passive Data Collection

Apps that passively collect data must balance the clinical utility with the concern for surveillance of the user and potentially anyone with whom the user comes in contact. Mental health apps have been found to frequently request permissions to access elements of a user's mobile device, including those considered to be "dangerous permissions," or areas that involve the user's private information or stored data [26]. Informed consent and appropriate access controls are essential [29], as certain types of data can be particularly sensitive. In a survey of 825 German citizens regarding their attitudes toward depression self-management apps, participants were particularly concerned about tracking of location via GPS and social interaction or communication [30]. However, even fully informing users and providing access controls may not be fully sufficient, as once a device has been converted into a sensor (for instance, by accessing the smartphone's microphone to record sound), bystanders may also be surveilled without their (or the user's) intent or knowledge [31–33].

If data are transmitted to a clinician, questions arise as to who is responsible for that information and follow-up. Many electronic health record (EHR) system workflows involve data transmission to office staff or work queues that may be unattended for hours. Should a patient complete a questionnaire or transmit passively collected data that indicates a need for urgent follow-up, health care organizations need guidance on how best to detect and manage such cases amongst the influx of data.

18.4.2 Telepsychiatry and Telemental Health

For those apps that connect users to live providers, such caregivers and vendors are subject to the same regulatory and cross-state licensure issues as traditional telemental health providers [34]. Patients should be made aware that some services may utilize "coaches" or other unlicensed providers, and should be cautioned to read the

Terms of Service (assuming they exist) carefully for such distinctions [22]. Improving education around caregiver qualifications as well as digital health literacy regarding how data can be collected and shared are both key for consumers to be protected in the health care ecosystem of the 21st century [35].

For providers, emergency management of patients who may live across the country or across the globe is also an important consideration, and it is essential to have procedures in place in anticipation of such events [34]. The complexity of these types of risk management strategies deepen with apps that utilize artificial intelligence in the form of a "virtual therapist." Although these types of chatbots may facilitate disclosure by patients who find their non-judgmental nature less threatening than communicating with a live person, they follow a pre-defined script and may not be able to understand a user's intent or respond to potentially acute or life-threatening symptoms [36].

18.4.3 Virtual Helpers and Providers

The pressure on healthcare providers to see a greater number of patients has resulted in the proliferation of "physician extenders"—nurse practitioners, physician's assistants, medical navigators, and others—so it is not difficult to imagine a future in which a virtual extender, i.e., an AI system, perhaps with a human-in-the-loop, is deployed as a line of first call for less risky mental health issues. Consequently, it is also possible to imagine the situation evolving into one in which the patient fails to distinguish between the virtual provider and a human provider. An early experiment along the lines of the Turing test was conducted by Weizenbaum with his program ELIZA (capitalization in the original). The program was designed to emulate a Rogerian therapist, whose essential technique is to mirror back to the patient, suitably transformed for grammar, any assertion or question by the patient:

> **Conversation between ELIZA program and patient**
> *Patient: I am not feeling so well today.*
> *ELIZA: So, you are not feeling so well today. Tell me more.*
> *Patient: ... ...*

When Weizenbaum's personal assistant (a human subject) was invited to try out the program, she entered into the spirit of the exercise but soon asked him to leave the room because she was revealing personal information she did not want to share with him [37]. In other words, ELIZA appeared to elicit a similar reaction a human therapist might expect from a patient.

There are various possible manifestations of AI in healthcare to be discussed. We shall classify them into minders, prostheses, caregivers, providers, and personhood, although these more or less informal categories are neither exhaustive nor mutually exclusive.

18.4.3.1 Minders

Minders are devices and "apps" that monitor and support an individual in some particular goal, such as to lose or maintain weight, resist an addictive behavior, live tolerably with a mood disorder or a chronic condition (e.g., diabetes, which may affect the state of mind), or adhere to medications. This raises a micro-level question: *How far is it acceptable for such a device or application to go in its allegedly benign effort to support the individual?* For instance, are intelligent bathroom scales allowed to "help" a person who is trying to lose weight with nudges, in the form of "little white lies" that encourage the dieter with good news or exaggerate the weight gain when they lose control—assuming that the network of devices and apps that include the scales can access sufficient intelligence to do this reliably?

18.4.3.2 Prostheses

Prostheses and implants present a more complex conundrum, especially those external appendages that are controlled directly by brain activity, but from our point of view, the case of artificial organs may be of greater interest. An artificial pancreas of sorts is already available [38]. What if an intelligent and interactive implant could release medication to control a bipolar disorder, taking into account not only the biochemistry of the individual, but also their interactions with the environment and physical manifestations of mood such as agitation, or exuberance, or depression? *Is it ethical to allow this artificial gland to dispense medication and modify dosage based on its own learning?* We must also consider whether it is ethical to create policies that prevent the use of such prostheses in individuals who can safely use them for other purposes such as management of blood glucose levels in diabetes.

18.4.3.3 Caregivers

A skilled nursing facility can be a challenging, and, for some, not a very rewarding place to work. The hours are long, the patients are often both incapacitated and depressed or angry at their condition, and sometimes they are uncooperative. Some of the care that needs to be provided is mundane and yet calls for patience. *Could it be that robotic assistants can do some of this work—without tiring or losing focus?* As the science progresses and designs improve, would they be able to assume more and more duties, ultimately undertaking duties normally reserved only for nursing staff? In the inexorable progression suggested by the foregoing, *how long before intellectually challenging roles, such as those of nurse practitioners and physician's assistants, may be at first shared and then undertaken by such robotic intelligences?* We suggest that the answers to these questions may be benign or troublesome, depending on the place and role of humans in such society.

18.4.3.4   Providers

From a clinical point of view, a provider supported by an AI system should be no more worrying than if the support is provided by an image processing service that annotates images for the pathologist's review: it is a technological enhancement of a¹ human faculty. An AI-based system, for example, may be able to generate a more complete and more robustly ranked and justified differential diagnosis than a provider working on their own. In the mental healthcare space between software and human, knowledge is acquired through communicative interactions such that a more accurate diagnosis is likely to be achieved. On the other hand, such human-in-the-loop configuration has a poor reputation because it can result in what has been pejoratively dubbed "fauxtomation", apparent automation of a task that in fact cannot be completed without human intervention.

18.4.3.5   Personhood and AI

From the earliest research in AI as a technology, an inherent goal has been the search *for synthetic intelligence* [39]. The broader philosophical implications of this phenomenon need not be considered at length here, but certain trends in the design of AI systems owe their momentum to the aspiration for a synthetic intelligence that may pass for human. Two such trends seem particularly pertinent in the case of mental health: one is the anthropomorphism (i.e., attribution of human characteristics into non-human entities) built into certain applications, and the second is the legal debate concerning the attribution of personhood to an AI system.

- *Anthropomorphism:* A designer or developer need not believe in a synthetic intelligence to adopt anthropomorphic avatars or personae as convenient human-machine interaction practice. On one hand, the suggestibility of humans has been repeatedly demonstrated in psychological experiments and is particularly potent in interaction with conversational agents such as ELIZA. On the other hand, the potential for a learning algorithm to be derailed in interaction and say, become abusive, was amply demonstrated by the Microsoft experiment with the chatbot Tay [40], which began issuing racist and misogynistic responses within 24 hours of being launched on Twitter. It can be argued that in at least certain mental health circumstances in which the patient is not well grounded in reality or may have suffered in an abusive environment, there is potential for the conversation to take an unexpected and counter-therapeutic turn.
- *Personhood:* Legal experts are already discussing parallels between AI and corporations for the attribution of personhood [41]. Given the rapid adoption of remote monitoring and motivational apps, depending on the ultimate resolution of the personhood debate, an imaginable future step in the mental health space may be an AI-based "guardian" for an ambulatory patient who does not have decisional capacity.

18.5   Mental Health Advocacy

Patient advocacy involves action by the people using healthcare services, their families, and others to ensure that the health care system is aware of the healthcare consumer's needs. It may involve activity related to treatment or research [42], and may be episodic or ongoing, depending upon the needs and goals of both the people using healthcare and the health care organizations themselves. During recent decades, increased openness to treating patients as partners has featured in mental healthcare, as in other areas of healthcare [43]. Sadly, some mental healthcare providers may wonder: *What can a person with a mental health condition bring to the healing process?* Similarly, some users of mental health services may ask: *How can I obtain value from treatment if clinicians do not work with me in a meaningful way?* Epistemic injustice, a social phenomenon that prevents a people from effectively arguing against inaccurate understandings of their lived experience, has proven to be a particular challenge for people diagnosed with a mental health condition [44]. For instance, people who have been diagnosed with mental illness may be perceived as unable to function without ongoing support or as lacking the capacity to make rational decisions. Such perceptions may make it difficult for them to be taken seriously as self-advocates. Despite historical concerns about people's ability to perceive their own psychological health realistically, participate meaningfully in care planning, and maintain progress made during treatment over years, individuals receiving mental health services have actively participated in patient engagement programs. For people with mental health conditions to effectively advocate for their treatment-related needs, this involvement requires digital health systems and tools tailored to individual needs that go beyond the patient portals and applications required by law, such as patient data access provisions in the 21st Century Cures Act: Interoperability, Information Blocking, and the ONC for Health IT Certification Program [45].

18.5.1   What Role Does Patient Advocacy Play in General?

Patient advocacy brings to the table the worldview of individuals as they perceive it, using their language and context [46]. Healthcare organizations seeking leadership or advocacy work by service users may directly solicit feedback (e.g., via electronic surveys), involve patients in design of treatment or other aspects of patient experience, seek patient perspective in hiring decisions, and include service users on staff or decision-making groups (e.g., advisory boards) [47, 48]. Within the research realm, funding agencies may involve patients in developing research programs and evaluating research proposals. Investigators may include patients and/or patient advocates in various ways (e.g., in study design and/or implementation, participant recruitment) to gain a broader view of proposed work, to increase the likelihood that individuals will agree to participate, or because research funders require direct patient involvement [49].

18.5.2   What Motivates Self-Advocacy in Mental Health?

People living with mental health conditions develop their own models to describe their situation and their own ways of managing their condition. People with mental health conditions who actively advocate for greater patient involvement in the healthcare system call themselves advocates, service users, survivors, and other roles. A primary goal of the service user/survivor movement is creating a new approach to research and treatment that acknowledge the importance of individuals' lived experience and takes into account such experience in setting target health outcomes and designing treatment [50].

18.5.3   How Do Mental Health Service Users and Advocates Bring Lived Experience to Mental Health Treatment?

Survivor research in mental health (also known as Mad Studies), a body of work describing mental health from the perspective of those who have been treated for mental illness, extends the foundation on which the current theory of mental illness diagnosis and treatment are based. Such studies rely upon qualitative methods, research partnerships between mental health service users, survivors and researchers, and allow for greater research control by service users than is the norm in most mental health research [51]. Survivor activism, in more moderate forms, has been recognized as user involvement or patient engagement [52].

Through the Icarus Project, for example, people living with mental health conditions, such as bipolar disorder, practice a broad range of wellness activities, alternative therapies, and creative arts with or without conventional psychiatric treatment to build their own model of care [53]. This approach is based on the idea that one's lived experience informs treatment and that valuing this lived experience can reduce the likelihood of psychiatric episodes, the need for rehospitalization, and alienation from society. Similarly, the Hearing Voices Movement has evolved as a way of valuing the experience of individuals who hear or previously heard voices (auditory verbal hallucinations) and facilitating interactions between mental health service users, survivors, and researchers [54]. By acknowledging hearing voices as a dimension of human experience, stigma is reduced, and individuals become empowered in their treatment.

Despite advocates' efforts to bring organized, scientific approaches to program development and implementation within the broader healthcare community, the credibility of advocacy work remains a question [52]. A number of systemic barriers to the meaningful inclusion of mental health service users in treatment planning and management have been identified, including lack of awareness of the value of including service users, slow progress for change, inadequate opportunities for participation, mental health stigma, and policy issues [55]. There is a need for guidelines that emphasize the importance of the patient's story as lived by the patient and support the clear elicitation of the patient's story as they assume greater responsibility for their treatment and progress [56]. There is also a need to recognize that there is no single "story" describing the experience of all patients, and that within treatment and/or research administration one patient cannot speak for an entire patient population [57]. These needs, coupled with privacy concerns, are an opportunity to develop and implement informatics solutions that will not only enable patient engagement and appropriate collection and use of their lived experiences, but also promote the care coordination across various providers, including mental health, primary care, and emergency care providers. This requires responsible sharing of highly sensitive, yet relevant information such as medical and mental health history and social determinants of health.

18.6 Genomics and Mental Health Informatics

According to the 2018 Report of the National Advisory Mental Health Council (NAMHC) Workgroup on Genomics [58], challenges presented to mental health disciplines include:

- To advance genetic investigations of paradigmatic disorders (schizophrenia, bipolar disorder, autism spectrum disorder) to understand their biology and genotype-phenotype relationships, and to advance the study of other apparently less heritable disorders; to study the genetic underpinnings of psychiatric conditions, to shed light on the biological significance of shared and unshared genetic risk;
- To broaden the human genomes under study to include those of multiple global populations;
- To gain deeper understanding of how the non-coding genome contributes to disease risk, and of how somatic mosaicism in the brain might influence psychiatric and neurodevelopmental disorders;
- To engage with other disciplines (neurobiology, psychology, and clinical disciplines) to ensure that genetic information is shared in forms that are useful and readily interpretable, and to ensure that genetic information that is applied to biological and phenotypic follow-up studies is derived from rigorous, well-powered studies that have been interpreted appropriately;
- To work with the biology community to develop and improve experimental systems, design principles, and computational tools for the conduct of meaningful and insightful follow-up studies of the highly polygenic risk factors that underlie common psychiatric disorders [58].

Genetic essentialism (the notion that the perceived genetic make-up determines an individual's identity and characteristics) and prognostic pessimism are crucial ethical issues that tend to shift attention from inequitable socio-economic, political, and cultural structures that influence mental health outcomes [59, 60]. There is real danger that a mental health diagnosis in an EHR becomes a persistent label and good reason to seek solutions to control when, where, by whom, and how that diagnosis may be viewed. The possibility that such a diagnosis may then be linked to a set of genomic findings multiplies the danger that the person may be seen by others as one whose future is already mapped out.

Prognostic pessimism, however, is a problem for the person with the condition even more than for the care provider or scientist. There is a narrow view of genomic testing that frames the individual as rational consumer, ready to be tested and "to prevent the onset of illness through proactive pharmacological treatments, preemptive interventions, and lifestyle changes, as well as [subject to] an obligation to act in relation to one's family and future, especially since genetics stresses heritability of disease from one generation to the next" [59]. From an informatics standpoint, it is the tools of shared decision-making and the shared health record that may support co-creation of the patient's history and offer the hope of a creative therapeutic alliance, in addition to advocacy and self-advocacy [43]. There are grounds to hope that carefully designed informatics tools, including those developed by patients [61], have the potential to support the therapeutic alliance.

A significant scientific goal for genomics in mental health is better characterization of psychiatric conditions. Phenotype-genotype associations have been successful in other areas of medicine, but the evidence in mental health is at best weak. Among plausible challenges for informatics encompassing genomics would be risk prediction for asymptomatic individuals, taking account of family history where possible, alongside the patient's circumstances and genome. However, the Genetic Information Nondiscrimination Act of 2008 (GINA) provides protection only in the domains of employment and health insurance coverage, but not disability or life insurance, or in mortgage and student loan eligibility [60], so that risk prediction could prove a double edged weapon for some, as well as for their close relatives. Nonetheless, population-level findings may be useful for planning in public health. All of this depends on adequate characterization of at least certain major disorders, such as autism, schizophrenia, bipolar disorder, and major depression, with confirmatory testing in the case of symptomatic patients to refine the characterization. To this end, the Research Domain Criteria (RDoC) framework provides a multidimensional framework for characterizing and studying mental disorders in the research context [62] (see Chap. 12). A similar approach is needed in clinical practice, along with sophisticated informatics tools, to better characterize individuals with mental health disorders.

18.7 Laws and Regulations

This section delineates regulations, ethical codes, and principles that are particularly pertinent to the field of mental health informatics and health information technology (HIT).

18.7.1 Health Insurance Portability and Accountability Act of 1996 (HIPAA)

In the United States, HIPAA was originally intended to improve health insurance coverage for employees between jobs as well as to combat waste, fraud, and abuse in health insurance and health care delivery. The original legislation includes "Administrative Simplification" provisions which require the Secretary of the Department of Health and Human Services to advance standards for the electronic exchange, privacy, and security of health information. These rules apply to "Covered Entities" (CE), which include health plans, health care clearinghouses, and any health provider who transmits health information in electronic form. They were later extended to "business associates", meaning any person or entity that performs certain functions or activities on behalf of, or provide services to, a CE for which the use or disclosure of Protected Health Information (PHI) [63] is required. Under HIPAA, healthcare organizations are free to share sensitive health information about individuals, including information about mental health conditions, with business associates for development of AI algorithms and technologies without the consent of individuals whose data are shared [64].

18.7.2 HIPAA Privacy Rule

The US Department of Health and Human Services (HHS) published the HIPAA Privacy Rule (December 2000, modified in August 2002) and Security Rule (February 2003), both of which were heavily informed by an interim report from the Institute of Medicine/National Academy of Sciences [65]. This 1997 report asserted that the benefits of electronic health information were being compromised by inadequate data protection. Of note, the Committee on Maintaining Privacy and Security in Health Care Applications of the National Information Infrastructure which authored the report emphasized the vulnerability of this patient information both within organizations and throughout the health care industry, as well as the role of patient concerns and expectations in addressing privacy and security issues. It recommended specific technical and organizational policies, practices and procedures – a framework which was eventually adopted into the HIPAA Security Rule of 2003 [65].

The HIPAA Privacy Rule defines "Protected Health Information" (PHI) as all "individually identifiable health information" held or transmitted by a covered entity (CE) in any form or media (electronic, paper, or oral). "Individually identifiable health information" is any information, including demographic data that relates to the individual's physical or mental health or condition (past, present, or future), the provision of health care to the individual, or the payment thereof (past, present or future).

The HIPAA Privacy Rule restricts use or disclosure of such information without the written authorization of the individual (or the individual's personal representative) except for the CE's own treatment, payment, and health care operations (TPO) activities and to another CE which has a relationship with the individual and where the PHI pertains to such activities regarding the individual. Additionally, disclosure is permitted to HHS when it is undertaking a compliance investigation, review, or enforcement action.

The HIPAA Privacy Rule includes a "Right of Access" provision, whereby individuals are granted access to their own PHI, with the following exceptions: psychotherapy notes, information compiled for legal proceedings, laboratory results to which the Clinical Laboratory Improvement Act prohibits access, or data held by specific research laboratories. CEs may deny access in situations in which a health care professional believes such access could harm the individual or another; in such cases, the individual has the right to have such denials reviewed for a second opinion by a licensed health care professional. Under HIPAA, individuals have the right to request that CEs amend their PHI when the information is inaccurate or incomplete. If the request is denied, CEs must provide a written denial and allow the individual to submit a statement of disagreement to be included in the medical record.

It is important to understand that under HIPAA, "psychotherapy notes" are defined as "notes recorded (in any medium) by a health care provider who is a mental health professional documenting or analyzing the contents of conversation during a private counseling session or a group, joint, or family counseling session and that are separated from the rest of the individual's medical record." HIPAA specifically excludes the following from this definition: "medication prescription and monitoring, counseling session start and stop times, the modalities and frequencies of treatment furnished, results of clinical tests, and any summary of the following items: Diagnosis, functional status, treatment plan, symptoms, prognosis, and progress to date" [66]. These elements may be part of a typical psychiatry or psychopharmacology note, and are not considered parts of a "psychotherapy note," which is subject to a strict definition under HIPAA, as above. The Privacy Rule does segment out true psychotherapy notes from TPO activities, requiring CEs to obtain an individual's authorization to use or disclose psychotherapy notes except for purposes of treatment within the CE who originated the note or for legal/compliance purposes [63].

18.7.3   HIPAA Security Rule

The HIPAA Security Rule was published several years after the enactment of HIPAA as a means to establish protection standards for a subset of PHI defined by the Privacy Rule; specifically, any *electronic* PHI (e-PHI) that is created, received, used, or maintained by a CE. Unlike the Privacy Rule, the Security Rule does not apply to PHI transmitted by other modalities like orally or in writing. The Security

Rule requires that CEs do all of the following through the implementation of appropriate administrative, technical, and physical safeguards [63]:

- Ensure the confidentiality, integrity, and availability of all e-PHI they create, receive, maintain, or transmit. "Confidentiality" means that e-PHI is not available or disclosed to unauthorized persons. "Integrity" denotes that e-PHI is not altered or destroyed in an unauthorized manner. "Availability" means that the e-PHI is accessible and usable on demand by an authorized person.
- Identify and protect against reasonably anticipated threats to the security or integrity of the information.
- Protect against reasonably anticipated, impermissible uses or disclosures.
- Ensure compliance by their workforce.

18.7.4 Confidentiality of Substance Use Disorder Records

HIPAA specifically protects psychotherapy notes, given the sensitivity of material that may be disclosed within the confines of the therapeutic relationship. Additionally, US regulations recognize substance use disorder (SUD) as worthy of further protections given the potential for the use of such information in administrative or criminal hearings. Therefore, in 1975, Title 42 of the Code of Federal Regulations Part 2: Confidentiality of Substance Use Disorder Patient Records (commonly referred to as "42 CFR Part 2") was first enacted to address concerns about the privacy of people with SUD. The law covers federally assisted Part 2 treatment programs, prohibiting them from disclosing information that would indicate an individual has or had a SUD without the person's written consent. It additionally specifies a set of requirements for such consent forms and that each disclosure must be accompanied by a notice prohibiting redisclosure without additional written consent as specified by the regulation [67].

As of the date of this publication, the U.S. Department of Health and Human Services Substance Abuse and Mental Health Services Administration (SAMHSA) is proposing to revise the legislation to enhance care for opioid use disorders (OUD) in response to the opioid epidemic and to facilitate better care coordination of all SUDs while maintaining confidentiality protections. Proposed changes include allowing people to consent to disclosure of treatment records to an entity rather than an individual recipient and the ability for opioid treatment programs to disclose data to a central registry as well as state prescription drug monitoring programs [68].

While HIPAA and 42 CFR Part 2 apply to all 50 states, when state-specific regulations provide for a stronger standard of authorization for disclosure of data, such regulations are not pre-empted by federal law. As of 2016, 14 states and the District of Columbia had requirements that applied to the records of people receiving mental health treatment from any provider in the state, and 23 additional states had requirements applying to records of people receiving mental health treatment through a state program [69, 70]. Many states additionally have specific laws authorizing minors to consent to mental health services and/or drug and alcohol counseling and medical care [71]. From an HIT perspective, these statutes are challenging to harmonize, as they vary widely in both requirements and definition of "mental health information".

18.7.5   21st Century Cures Act

Signed into law in December 2016, the 21st Century Cures Act addresses a wide range of issues affecting provision of mental health care as well as the use of informatics to do so, including:

- A charge to HHS to develop conditions of certification prohibiting health IT developers from "information blocking", a mandate for the National Coordinator of Health Information Technology (ONC) to convene stakeholders to develop a Trusted Exchange Framework and Common Agreement to support data exchange. However, the final rule published in 2020 allows for several exceptions from the information blocking provision and will likely need to be clarified by case law.
- Amendments to the Health Information Technology for Economic and Clinical Health (HITECH) Act intended to reduce regulatory or administrative burdens related to the use of EHR technology
- A charge for the HHS Office of Civil Rights to clarify HIPAA as it relates to supported decision making for mental health and substance abuse and to ensure that patients, caregivers, and providers have "adequate, accessible, and easily comprehensible resources regarding use and disclosure of protected health information" [72].

The law also included a number of provisions, not specifically related to informatics, to bolster the funding and treatment of mental health conditions and to combat the opioid epidemic.

18.7.6   Research Regulations

In regard to mental health and psychotropic drug research, US regulations have derived from *The Belmont Report*, published in 1979 by the National Commission for the Protection of Human Subjects of Biomedical and Behavioral Research. This Commission was charged by the U.S. National Research Act of 1974 with identifying the basic ethical principles underlying such research and developing guidelines to support compliance with these principles. This report emphasizes the ethical principles respect for persons (autonomy), beneficence, and justice [73], and served as the basis for the Federal Policy for Protection of Human Subjects, known as "the Common Rule," signed into law by HHS and 14 other Federal departments and agencies in 1991. The Common Rule outlines the basic provisions for Institutional Review Boards and the informed consent of research subjects; while the FDA is not included under the Common Rule, it is required to harmonize with it wherever permitted by law pertaining to its regulation of the clinical investigation of drugs, biologicals, and medical devices. The Rule has been revised several times, most recently in 2018, at which time the types of research that qualified for exemption were broadened, the structure and content of informed consent documents was changed, and changes to the IRB process for certain multi-center studies were put in place [74]. The boundaries of the Common Rule were tested by a Minnesota case in which a psychiatric inpatient was given the choice between involuntary commitment and enrollment in a clinical trial for FDA-approved drugs as part of his treatment plan. His 2004 suicide resulted in a state law prohibiting patients under emergency psychiatric hold or state commitment from participating in psychopharmacologic trials in order to protect against coercion [75].

It should be noted that current US federal law does not specifically provide for a *right* of privacy per se (other than the 4th Amendment right to be free from unreasonable searches and seizures); instead, HIPAA and subsequent legislation at the *macro* level created the *meso*-level infrastructure necessary to support secure transfer of data and afford patients the right to access and amend their records (at the *micro* level), except in instances where this may lead to harm of self or others. Given the nature of symptoms experienced by some people with mental health conditions, balancing the right to access one's own data under HIPAA with protection from harm may be a very delicate and nuanced balance indeed.

18.7.7   General Data Protection Regulation (GDPR)

In contrast, the European Union (EU) GDPR does provide EU citizens with such privacy rights. This law, which evolved from the existing set of European data protection rules set forth in the 1995 Data Protection Directive with the intention to address the challenges of data protection in this age of rapid technological development and globalization, came into effect on May 24, 2016. It gave companies a two-year transition period through May 2018 to bring their practices in line with the new rules [76]. The GDPR was founded on the principles that that protection of people in relation to the processing of personal data is a fundamental right, but not an *absolute* right, in that it must be balanced against other fundamental rights.

The GDPR concerns data that could be used to identify an individual. For such data, consent of the individual to whom the data pertains is required. This is defined as "a clear affirmative act [that is, a positive opt-in] establishing a freely given, specific, informed and unambiguous indication of the data subject's agreement to the processing of personal data relating to him or her." The regulation requires organizations to name any third parties who will rely on the consent, keep evidence of the consent, and allow for data subjects to easily withdraw their consent; it additionally prohibits making consent to processing data a precondition of service if doing so is not dependent for the performance of that service. The GDPR provides people a number of rights including the so-called "right to erasure" or "right to be forgotten", which allows individuals to request to have all of their personal information erased by the controller of such data. Finally, the GDPR acknowledges that children merit specific protection with regard to their personal data, such that consent for data processing must be granted by a parent or guardian for a child under age 16 years (13 years in some member states) and companies working with children are required to have systems in place to reasonably verify the age of individuals and obtain appropriate consent. Notably, however, the GDPR recognizes the need for minors to access confidential care, stating, "the consent of the holder of parental responsibility should not be necessary in the context of preventive or counselling services offered directly to a child."

18.7.8   California Consumer Privacy Act (CCPA)

In June 2018, the State of California enacted CCPA, which was heavily influenced by the GDPR. This law is the first U.S. attempt at a comprehensive data protection law and went into effect in 2020. It applies to for-profit entities that that do business within the state and which collect personal information about people in California. The regulation gives consumers the right to have access to the personal information collected about them, transparency into the sources from which the information is collected and the third parties with whom it is shared, the ability to opt out and to request that a business delete any personal information that has been collected [77].

While the CCPA specifically excludes protected health information (PHI) as defined by HIPAA, non-protected health information such as that in an individual's employment record from a short-term disability claim, de-identified PHI that can now be linked back to an individual, inferences that may have been drawn from PHI to create a new data set for marketing, or non-medical demographic data collected by a health IT vendor are covered. As such, this legislation extends protections to areas not previously covered by HIPAA and sets the stage for changes to be undertaken by companies with a California footprint that could affect wider practices nationwide.

18.8   Concluding Remarks

Ethical issues at the intersection of informatics and mental health are relatively more profound than other clinical domains. Modern digital health technologies including AI-based applications and the ubiquitous collection of a variety of data from individuals will continue to raise new ethical and legal challenges, particularly in the areas of privacy and individual rights [78]. The use of such technologies in mental healthcare need continuous assessment and governance to mitigate biases at all levels and ensure patient safety and well-being. Broad stakeholder involvement including individuals with lived experiences, technology developers and providers, clinicians, and policymakers is necessary for developing governance structures for ethical use of data and technology in mental healthcare.

18.9 Discussion Questions for Reader Consideration

- What steps can data scientists and developers take to identify biases in clinical and behavioral health data and improve bias management practices?
- What steps can health systems take to select algorithms that mitigate biases and promote equitable care for all?
- In what ways can mobile health technology benefit patients with behavioral health conditions to improve quality of care, clinical outcomes, and to decrease costs?
- What are some of the major ethical and legal concerns around the use of mobile health technology in behavioral health care?
- How can these concerns be addressed through legislation and further technological developments?
- In what ways does US HIPAA legislation serve to facilitate the care of patients with behavioral health conditions? In what ways may it pose concerns for these patients? For treating providers?
- In what ways could implementing health information technology to support HIPAA legislation contribute to disparities affecting patients with behavioral health conditions?
- What challenges do developers of health information technology face given the lack of harmonization in US state privacy laws?
- In what ways could the privacy rights afforded by the GDPR help to address any of the issues you identified in the three questions above? Where do gaps still exist both in patient care and in guiding technology development?

References

1. Faden RR, Kass NE, Goodman SN, Pronovost P, Tunis S, Beauchamp TL. An ethics framework for a learning health care system: a departure from traditional research ethics and clinical ethics. Hastings Cent Rep. 2013; https://doi.org/10.1002/hast.134.
2. Corrigan PW, Bink AB. The stigma of mental illness. In: Encyclopedia of mental health: second edition. Amsterdam: Elsevier; 2015. p. 230–4. https://doi.org/10.1016/B978-0-12-397045-9.00170-1.
3. Clement S, Schauman O, Graham T, et al. What is the impact of mental health-related stigma on help-seeking? A systematic review of quantitative and qualitative studies. Psychol Med. 2015;45(1):11–27. https://doi.org/10.1017/S0033291714000129.
4. Berry K, Sheardown J, Pabbineedi U, Haddock G, Cross C, Brown LJE. Barriers and facilitators to accessing psychological therapies for severe mental health difficulties in later life. Behav Cogn Psychother. 2019; https://doi.org/10.1017/S1352465819000596.

5. Ring D, Lawn S. Stigma perpetuation at the interface of mental health care: a review to compare patient and clinician perspectives of stigma and borderline personality disorder. J Ment Heal. 2019, March:1–21. https://doi.org/10.1080/09638237.2019.1581337.

6. Sukhera J, Chahine S. Reducing mental illness stigma through unconscious bias-informed education. MedEdPublish. 2016;5(2) https://doi.org/10.15694/mep.2016.000044.

7. Henderson C, Noblett J, Parke H, et al. Mental health-related stigma in health care and mental health-care settings. The Lancet Psychiatry. 2014;1(6):467–82. https://doi.org/10.1016/S2215-0366(14)00023-6.

8. Soni H, Grando A, Aliste MP, et al. Perceptions and preferences about granular data sharing and privacy of behavioral health patients. Stud Health Technol Inform. 2019;264:1361–5. https://doi.org/10.3233/SHTI190449.

9. Satinsky E, Driessens C, Crepaz-Keay D, Kousoulis AA. Mental health service users' perceptions of data sharing and data protection: A short qualitative report. J Innov Heal Informatics. 2018;25(4):239–42. https://doi.org/10.14236/jhi.v25i4.1033.

10. Shen N, Sequeira L, Silver MP, Carter-Langford A, Strauss J, Wiljer D. Patient privacy perspectives on health information exchange in a mental health context: qualitative study. JMIR Ment Heal. 2019;6(11):e13306. https://doi.org/10.2196/13306.

11. Sleigh J. Experiences of donating personal data to mental health research: an explorative anthropological study. Biomed Inform Insights. 2018;10:117822261878513. https://doi.org/10.1177/1178222618785131.

12. Friedman B, Nissenbaum H. Bias in computer systems. ACM Trans Inf Syst. 1996;14(3):330–47. https://doi.org/10.1145/230538.230561.

13. McCarthy MT. The big data divide and its consequences. Sociol Compass. 2016;10(12):1131–40. https://doi.org/10.1111/soc4.12436.

14. Snowden LR. Bias in mental health assessment and intervention: theory and evidence. Am J Public Health. 2003;93(2):239–43. https://doi.org/10.2105/AJPH.93.2.239.

15. Walsh CG, Chaudhry B, Dua P, et al. Stigma, biomarkers, and algorithmic bias: recommendations for precision behavioral health with artificial intelligence. JAMIA Open. 2020;3(1):9–15. https://doi.org/10.1093/jamiaopen/ooz054.

16. Bzdok D, Meyer-Lindenberg A. Machine learning for precision psychiatry: opportunities and challenges. Biol Psychiatry Cogn Neurosci Neuroimaging. 2018;3(3):223–30. https://doi.org/10.1016/j.bpsc.2017.11.007.

17. Huys QJM, Maia TV, Frank MJ. Computational psychiatry as a bridge from neuroscience to clinical applications. Nat Neurosci. 2016;19(3):404–13. https://doi.org/10.1038/nn.4238.

18. Chen IY, Szolovits P, Ghassemi M. Can AI help reduce disparities in general medical and mental health care? AMA J Ethics. 2019;21(2):E167–79. https://doi.org/10.1001/amajethics.2019.167.

19. Char DS, Shah NH, Magnus D. Implementing machine learning in health care – addressing ethical challenges. N Engl J Med. 2018; https://doi.org/10.1056/NEJMp1714229.

20. Martinez-Martin N, Dunn LB, Roberts LWI. It ethical to use prognostic estimates from machine learning to treat psychosis? AMA J Ethics. 2018;20(9):E804–11. https://doi.org/10.1001/amajethics.2018.804.

21. Martin A, Rief W, Klaiberg A, Braehler E. Validity of the brief patient health questionnaire mood scale (PHQ-9) in the general population. Gen Hosp Psychiatry. 2006;28(1):71–7. https://doi.org/10.1016/J.GENHOSPPSYCH.2005.07.003.

22. Armontrout J, Torous J, Fisher M, Drogin E, Gutheil T. Mobile mental health: navigating new rules and regulations for digital tools. Curr Psychiatry Rep. 2016; https://doi.org/10.1007/s11920-016-0726-x.

23. Radovic A, Vona PL, Santostefano AM, Ciaravino S, Miller E, Stein BD. Smartphone applications for mental health. Cyberpsychology, Behav Soc Netw. 2016; https://doi.org/10.1089/cyber.2015.0619.

24. S. Bhuyan S, Kim H, Isehunwa OO, et al. Privacy and security issues in mobile health: current research and future directions. Heal Policy Technol. 2017. https://doi.org/10.1016/j.hlpt.2017.01.004.

25. Huckvale K, Prieto JT, Tilney M, Benghozi PJ, Car J. Unaddressed privacy risks in accredited health and wellness apps: A cross-sectional systematic assessment. BMC Med. 2015; https://doi.org/10.1186/s12916-015-0444-y.

26. Parker L, Halter V, Karliychuk T, Grundy Q. How private is your mental health app data? An empirical study of mental health app privacy policies and practices. Int J Law Psychiatry. 2019;64:198–204. https://doi.org/10.1016/j.ijlp.2019.04.002.

27. Huckvale K, Torous J, Larsen ME. Assessment of the data sharing and privacy practices of smartphone apps for depression and smoking cessation. JAMA Netw open. 2019;2(4):e192542. https://doi.org/10.1001/jamanetworkopen.2019.2542.

28. Robillard JM, Feng TL, Sporn AB, et al. Availability, readability, and content of privacy policies and terms of agreements of mental health apps. Internet Interv. 2019;17 https://doi.org/10.1016/j.invent.2019.100243.

29. Mohr DC, Zhang M, Schueller SM. Personal sensing: understanding mental health using ubiquitous sensors and machine learning. Annu Rev Clin Psychol. 2017; https://doi.org/10.1146/annurev-clinpsy-032816-044949.

30. Hartmann R, Sander C, Lorenz N, Böttger D, Hegerl U. Utilization of patient-generated data collected through mobile devices: insights from a survey on attitudes toward mobile self-monitoring and self-management apps for depression. J Med Internet Res. 2019; https://doi.org/10.2196/11671.

31. Liddle J, Burdon M, Ireland D, et al. Balancing self-tracking and surveillance: legal, ethical and technological issues in using smartphones to monitor communication in people with health conditions. J Law Med. 2016.

32. Perez AJ, Zeadally S. Privacy issues and solutions for consumer wearables. IT Prof. 2018; https://doi.org/10.1109/MITP.2017.265105905.

33. Subbian V, Solomonides A, Clarkson M, et al. Ethics and informatics in the age of COVID-19: challenges and recommendations for public health organization and public policy. J Am Med Inform Assoc. July 2020. https://doi.org/10.1093/jamia/ocaa188.

34. Kramer GM, Luxton DD. Telemental health for children and adolescents: an overview of legal, regulatory, and risk management issues. J Child Adolesc Psychopharmacol. 2016; https://doi.org/10.1089/cap.2015.0018.

35. Segura Anaya LH, Alsadoon A, Costadopoulos N, Prasad PWC. Ethical implications of user perceptions of wearable devices. Sci Eng Ethics. 2018; https://doi.org/10.1007/s11948-017-9872-8.

36. Rucker M. Using AI for mental health effectively. https://www.verywellmind.com/using-artificial-intelligence-for-mental-health-4144239. Accessed November 23, 2019.

37. Weizenbaum J. ELIZA-A computer program for the study of natural language communication between man and machine. Commun ACM. 1966;9(1):36–45. https://doi.org/10.1145/365153.365168.

38. Cobelli C, Renard E, Kovatchev B. Artificial pancreas: past, present, future. Diabetes. 2011;60(11):2672–82. https://doi.org/10.2337/db11-0654.

39. Anderson J, Rainie L. Artificial intelligence and the future of humans. https://www.pewresearch.org/internet/2018/12/10/artificial-intelligence-and-the-future-of-humans/. Accessed September 6, 2020.

40. Schwartz O. In 2016, microsoft's racist chatbot revealed the dangers of online conversation – IEEE Spectrum. IEEE Spectrum. https://spectrum.ieee.org/tech-talk/artificial-intelligence/machine-learning/in-2016-microsofts-racist-chatbot-revealed-the-dangers-of-online-conversation. Published November 25, 2019. Accessed September 6, 2020.

41. Banteka N. Artificially Intelligent Persons. Houst Law Rev. 2020;58 https://doi.org/10.2139/ssrn.3552269.

42. NIMH. Alliance for research progress. https://www.nimh.nih.gov/outreach/alliance/index.shtml. Accessed May 30, 2020.

43. Galvin HK, Petersen C, Subbian V, Solomonides A. Patients as agents in behavioral health research and service provision: recommendations to support the learning health system. Appl Clin Inf. 2019;10(05):841–8. https://doi.org/10.1055/s-0039-1700536.

44. Fricker M. Powerlessness and social interpretation. Episteme. 2006;3:96–108. https://doi.org/10.3366/epi.2006.3.1-2.96.
45. 85 FR 25642 – 21st Century Cures Act: Interoperability, Information Blocking, and the ONC Health IT Certification Program; 2020:25642–25961.
46. Ciccarella A, Staley AC, Franco AT. Transforming research: engaging patient advocates at all stages of cancer research. Ann Transl Med. 2018;6(9):167. https://doi.org/10.21037/atm.2018.04.46.
47. Scholz B, Bocking J, Happell B. How do consumer leaders co-create value in mental health organisations? Aust Heal Rev. 2017;41(5):505–10. https://doi.org/10.1071/AH16105.
48. van de Bovenkamp HM, Zuiderent-Jerak T. An empirical study of patient participation in guideline development: exploring the potential for articulating patient knowledge in evidence-based epistemic settings. Heal Expect. 2015;18(5):942–55. https://doi.org/10.1111/hex.12067.
49. Newhouse R, Barksdale DJ, Miller JA. The patient-centered outcomes research institute: research done differently. Nurs Res. 2015;64(1):72–7. https://doi.org/10.1097/NNR.0000000000000070.
50. Newbigging K, Ridley J. Epistemic struggles: the role of advocacy in promoting epistemic justice and rights in mental health. Soc Sci Med. 2018; https://doi.org/10.1016/j.socscimed.2018.10.003.
51. Faulkner A. Survivor research and Mad Studies: the role and value of experiential knowledge in mental health research. Disabil Soc. 2017; https://doi.org/10.1080/09687599.2017.1302320.
52. Borsay A. Beyond the water towers: the unfinished revolution in mental health services 1985–2005. Br J Learn Disabil. 2006;34(3):193–4. https://doi.org/10.1111/j.1468-3156.2006.00409.x.
53. DuBrul SA. The icarus project: a counter narrative for psychic diversity. J Med Humanit. 2014;35:257–71. https://doi.org/10.1007/s10912-014-9293-5.
54. Corstens D, Longden E, McCarthy-Jones S, Waddingham R, Thomas N. Emerging perspectives from the hearing voices movement: implications for research and practice. Schizophr Bull. 2014;40(4):S285–94. https://doi.org/10.1093/schbul/sbu007.
55. Gee A, McGarty C, Banfield M. Barriers to genuine consumer and carer participation from the perspectives of Australian systemic mental health advocates. J Ment Heal. 2016;25(3):231–7. https://doi.org/10.3109/09638237.2015.1124383.
56. Morse AR, Forbes O, Jones BA, Gulliver A, Banfield M. Whose story is it? Mental health consumer and carer views on carer participation in research. Heal Expect. August 2019. https://doi.org/10.1111/hex.12954.
57. Daya I, Hamilton B, Roper C. Authentic engagement: a conceptual model for welcoming diverse and challenging consumer and survivor views in mental health research, policy, and practice. Int J Ment Health Nurs. 2019; https://doi.org/10.1111/inm.12653.
58. Report of the National Advisory Mental Health Council Workgroup on Genomics. https://www.nimh.nih.gov/about/advisory-boards-and-groups/namhc/reports/report-of-the-national-advisory-mental-health-council-workgroup-on-genomics.shtml#recommendations. Accessed December 8, 2019.
59. Kong C, Dunn M, Parker M. Psychiatric genomics and mental health treatment: setting the ethical agenda. Am J Bioeth. 2017;17(4):3–12. https://doi.org/10.1080/15265161.2017.1284915.
60. Ward ET, Kostick KM, Lázaro-Muñoz G. Integrating genomics into psychiatric practice. Harv Rev Psychiatry. 2019;27(1):53–64. https://doi.org/10.1097/HRP.0000000000000203.
61. Petersen C. Patient informaticians: turning patient voice into patient action. JAMIA Open. 2018;1(2):130–5. https://doi.org/10.1093/jamiaopen/ooy014.
62. Cuthbert BN, Insel TR. Toward the future of psychiatric diagnosis: the seven pillars of RDoC. BMC Med. 2013;11(1):126. https://doi.org/10.1186/1741-7015-11-126.
63. HIPAA for Professionals | HHS.gov. https://www.hhs.gov/hipaa/for-professionals/index.html. Accessed November 23, 2019.
64. Newman N. The costs of lost privacy: consumer harm and rising economic inequality in the age of Google. William Mitchell Law Rev. 2013;40:849–1611.

65. Committee on Maintaining Privacy and Security in Healthcare Applications of the National Information Infrastructure. For the record: institute of medicine report. Washington, DC: National Academies Press; 1997. https://doi.org/10.17226/5595.
66. Office of Civil Rights H. HIPAA Administrative Simplification Regulation Text; 2013.
67. 42 CFR 2 – Confidentiality of alcohol and drug abuse patient records; 1987.
68. HHS 42 CFR part 2 proposed rule fact sheet | HHS.gov. https://www.hhs.gov/about/news/2019/08/22/hhs-42-cfr-part-2-proposed-rule-fact-sheet.html. Accessed November 23, 2019.
69. State Health IT Privacy and Consent Laws and Policies. | HealthIT.gov. https://www.healthit.gov/topic/state-health-it-privacy-and-consent-laws-and-policies. Accessed November 23, 2019.
70. Office of the National Coordinator of Health Information Technology. State laws requiring authorization to disclose mental health information for treatment, payment, or healthcare operations. https://www.healthit.gov/sites/default/files/State Mental Health Laws Map 2 Authorization Required 9-30-16_Final.pdf. Accessed May 31, 2020.
71. Boonstra HD, Nash E. Minors and the right to consent to health care. Guttmacher Policy Rev. 2000;3(4).
72. 21st Century Cures Act: Interoperability, Information Blocking, and the ONC Health IT Certification Program, 85 FR 25642, https://www.federalregister.gov/documents/2020/05/01/2020-07419/21st-century-cures-act-interoperability-information-blocking-and-the-onc-health-it-certification. Published 2020. Accessed March 17, 2021.
73. The National Commission for the Protection of Human Subjects of, Biomedical and Behavioral Research. The belmont report; 1979.
74. U.S. Department of Health and Human Services. Revised common rule. https://www.hhs.gov/ohrp/regulations-and-policy/regulations/finalized-revisions-common-rule/index.html. Accessed May 31, 2020.
75. Lewellen N. Dan's [F]law: statutory failure to enforce ethical behavior in clinical drug trials. Minn Law Rev. 2016;99.
76. The European Parliament and the Council of the European Union. Regulation (EU) 2016/679 of the european parliament and of the council of 27 April 2016 on the protection of natural persons with regard to the processing of personal data and on the free movement of such data, and repealing Directive 95/46/EC (General Data Protection Regulation) (Text with EEA relevance). 2016.
77. Bill Text – AB-375 Privacy: personal information: businesses. https://leginfo.legislature.ca.gov/faces/billTextClient.xhtml?bill_id=201720180AB375. Accessed November 23, 2019.
78. Doraiswamy PM, London E, Varnum P, et al. Empowering 8 billion minds: enabling better mental health for all via the ethical adoption of technologies. NAM perspect. October 2019. https://doi.org/10.31478/201910b.

Chapter 19
The Future of Mental Health Informatics

Gregory K. Farber, Joshua A. Gordon, and Robert K. Heinssen

Abstract The current state of mental health informatics has been covered in the earlier chapters in this book. The focus of this chapter is on the future of this emerging field. First, a vision for that future is enumerated, imagining what an integrated approach to mental health informatics would be able to accomplish. Second, the harmonization of data across diverse mental health-relevant datasets is discussed. This is a significant obstacle to aggregating data from multiple laboratories that must be overcome. The need for training the informatics-savvy mental health research and healthcare workforce that will be required to achieve that vision is explored. Finally, a case study is presented showing what can be done using existing infrastructure and suggesting how a learning health care system can be built on top of that infrastructure.

Keywords Training · Learning health care system · Data archives · Data harmonization · Data analysis workflows

19.1 Envisioning an Ambitious Future

The brain is arguably the most important and complicated organ in the human body. Our understanding of the details by which the brain performs functions such as storing and recalling memories, enabling us to experience pleasure or misery, or acquiring knowledge and understanding are very rudimentary. A much more detailed understanding of the brain and the way the brain develops and changes in response

G. K. Farber (✉) · J. A. Gordon · R. K. Heinssen
National Institute of Mental Health, Rockville, MD, USA
e-mail: farberg@mail.nih.gov; joshua.gordon@nih.gov; rheinsse@mail.nih.gov

© Springer Nature Switzerland AG 2021   505
J. D. Tenenbaum, P. A. Ranallo (eds.), *Mental Health Informatics*, Health
Informatics, https://doi.org/10.1007/978-3-030-70558-9_19

to external stimuli is essential if we want to understand any of the illnesses that arise in the brain.

Our current understanding of the brain focuses on understanding the makeup of circuits of neurons or brain regions that act to perform certain functions (see [1–3] for some examples). The definition of the components of a circuit often depends on the experiments that are being done. Magnetic resonance imaging, for example, defines circuits at a scale that likely involves millions of neurons. Other experiments aim for much more detailed understanding of small numbers of neurons and other cells in the brain. Since there are more than 80 billion neurons in the human brain, each making connections to thousands of other cells in the brain, the reasons for our rudimentary understanding of the brain are obvious. This lack of understanding is the root cause behind the investment of the National Institute of Mental Health, many of our sister NIH Institutes, and many other funders, in basic neuroscience. Understanding the differences at the circuit level that result in mental illness is our current best hope to discover new treatments and improve existing treatments. The scale of circuits that are relevant to mental illness and the timescale for which we need to collect data from those circuits still is not clear. There is hope that circuits that involve very large numbers of cells might provide biomarkers and/or ways to monitor the results from different treatments. Such macro-circuits can be probed using techniques such as magnetic resonance imaging or electroencephalography and using clinical/phenotypic measures. However, understanding circuits at the micro-circuit or molecular level using tools from genomics, molecular biology, optics, and cellular electrophysiology is also needed, as described in Chaps. 8 and 11.

Mental illnesses, like many physical illnesses, are complex conditions, in which people with similar symptoms likely have different underlying biological causes of those symptoms. A good example of such a complex condition is diabetes. The biological causes of type 1 diabetes are quite different from those of type 2 diabetes. In that example, testing for the presence of the C-peptide of insulin provides a useful biomarker to distinguish the two subgroups [4]. Such complex diagnostic groups stand in stark contrast to relatively simple illnesses such as most viral or bacterial infection or deeply penetrant genetic diseases. For simple illnesses, the course of the disease is often similar in almost all individuals. As a result, treatments can be developed in a straightforward fashion once the underlying biology is understood (see Box 19.1). (SARS-CoV-2, the virus that causes COVID-19, is a notable exception— straightforward to diagnose, but remarkably heterogeneous in its course.)

Until recently, the Diagnostic and Statistical Manual of Mental Disorders (DSM) was the basis for assigning a patient to a diagnostic group in research studies and clinical trials. Recognizing that most DSM diagnostic categories represent a heterogeneous group of patients, NIMH believed this approach was constraining research, and introduced the Research Domain Criteria (RDoc) to support classifying mental disorders based on more refined dimensions of observable behavior and neurobiological measures at either the micro or macro circuit level [5]. This framework in combination with the new focus on mechanistic targets for pharmaceutical, device, and psychosocial treatment development [6] provides a way to help dissect complex conditions into more homogeneous groups, thereby isolating symptoms and mechanisms targeted by a specific treatment. It is the NIH's hope that when we have detailed molecular understanding of the causes of mental illness, this bottom up approach of starting with basic neuroscience and moving toward treatment will be used by all. However, until we have a more detailed understanding, we are left with the need to divide those with mental illness into groups using existing observations. RDoC seems to have allowed the research community to formulate experiments in ways that would not have been easy to do using the DSM. We hope it will continue to evolve into a framework that will be useful to the research community—especially those who are trying to think about new ways to find more homogeneous subpopulations that respond to a particular treatment.

Box 19.1 Simple Versus Complex Disorders
Examples of simple disorders in the brain include: Angelman's syndrome, Rett syndrome, and Williams syndrome.
Examples of complex disorders include: schizophrenia, depression, autism, and obsessive compulsive disorder.

Complex disorders pose challenges for scientists trying to understand or treat them. As suggested by the diabetes example, the first order of business is to figure out how many subgroups there really are. The situation is illustrated in Fig. 19.1. A drug or psychosocial intervention that is applied to a heterogeneous group may work on a cluster of patients but may fail for the majority in the diagnostic group. What options exist to figure out how many clusters there are?

One obvious approach to understanding complex diseases of the brain involves a bottom up approach. Diseases in this context might refer to the way the brain functions at birth or it could refer to the way that the brain changes as a result of environmental stimuli. Understanding how biology maps on to signs and symptoms of mental illnesses could provide a pathway towards refining diagnostic groups into clusters. Biological information of relevance could include information about how brain circuits in an individual are different from those who do not suffer from a mental illness or it might include information about how brain circuits have changed due to environmental risk factors. A level closer to the symptomatology may be measures of brain circuit function; circuits are thought to be the basic units in which the neural processing that guides behavior occurs. The scientific community has made a great deal of progress in understanding brain circuits in a number of model organisms (see [7] for an example in the visual system circuits), but the translation of that understanding to humans has proven difficult [8]. Recent efforts supported by programs like the U.S. National Institutes of Health BRAIN Initiative to develop new tools to probe circuits in both model organisms and in humans have accelerated our understanding [9], but there is still a great deal of work to be done before this bottom up approach to tackle mental illness can be used to understand and treat humans.

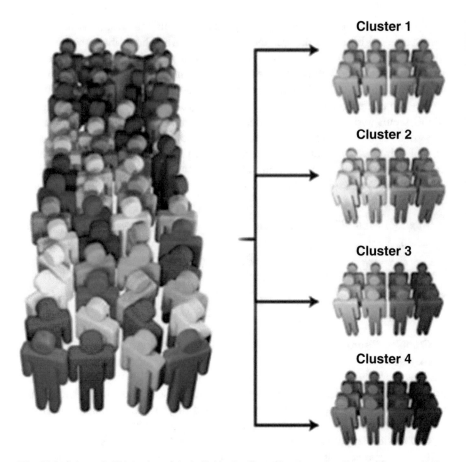

Fig. 19.1 Schematic Illustration of the individuals affected by a complex disease. Everyone in the initial population shares a common symptom. The clusters on the right are meant to suggest that there are four subpopulations, each with their own biological cause of this symptom. The sharing of colors in each cluster indicate that there is still heterogeneity even in a cluster

An alternative, top-down approach to clustering may prove to be clinically useful more rapidly. Using an approach that is agnostic to causes or neurobiology, researchers have been accumulating moderate sized datasets that include multimodal data, likely some combination of imaging, phenotypic and genomic data, from individuals with groups of mental illnesses. One consortium, the Bipolar-Schizophrenia Network on Intermediate Phenotypes (B-SNIP), pooled roughly one thousand people with psychosis, combining neurophysiological, cognitive, and symptom-based measurements. Clustering algorithms suggested that this group could be divided into three different biotypes [10]. Interestingly, these biotypes did not correspond to specific diagnoses; a replication study is currently underway. Another study used functional magnetic resonance imaging data from about 1000 individuals with depression [11]. Clustering based on resting state functional connectivity maps suggested four different types of brain maps in this sample; the different map types had different clinical characteristics. These early results suggest that even with current technologies, circuit-based measures hold the promise of being able to define clinically relevant subtypes of mental illnesses.

The NIMH vision for the future, however, goes beyond these early efforts. We can envision combining sophisticated bottom-up understanding of the biology of mental illnesses—encompassing genetic and environmental risk factors, and a deep circuit-based understanding of the mechanisms of behavior—with deep multimodal top-down phenotyping—including clinical, physiological, and anatomical measurements—to reveal the underlying structure of mental illness while simultaneously elucidating its mechanisms in sufficient detail to design personalized brain-based therapies. This might occur when informatics researchers suggest unexpected groupings of research participants. It is easy to imagine that the analysis of large data sets with harmonized data elements might uncover commonalities far outside of traditional diagnostic groups. The data harmonization should make the data amenable to artificial intelligence approaches. Data from mobile devices or other devices that allow wide ranging, inexpensive data collection may turn out to be essential for such computational experiments. Following the discovery of a group, detailed exploration using a bottom up approach may reveal common brain circuits that are altered. In short, we can envision mental health informatics truly transforming mental healthcare.

19.1.1 Essential Component 1: Datasets, Data Storage, and Workflows

What is needed for these informatics approaches to yield definitive solutions to the "clustering problem"? First and foremost, data are needed from a large number of human subjects. "Large" is meant to be vague. There is not enough information yet to estimate the size of the populations that will be needed, but the results from genomics studies in the brain suggest that data may be needed from tens of thousands of people [12]. If that really is true, it suggests that there may be a need to prioritize collecting data inexpensively using personal tracking devices and related data collection techniques. The Learning Health System (LHS), which leverages data collected in the course of clinical care, could play an important role in fulfilling this need (see Chap. 1). It is important to note that the data collected may not at first glance have any direct relevance to how the brain functions. Useful biomarkers just need to show a reliable correlation that allows assignment of research participants or patients to a cluster.

The data need to be well structured and ideally should be widely accessible. The actual data that might be useful for clustering is not at all clear. It seems likely that clinical assessments, self-report assessments, data from mobile technologies, genomics data, and data from various imaging technologies (EEG, MRI, eye tracking, PET) may all be useful. Hopefully, data that are inexpensive to collect will turn out to be useful. There are now many examples where citizen scientists and those who either have an illness or have family members with an illness have made important contributions to data analysis [13]. This suggests that restricting the availability of data just to researchers at academic institutions is not the most efficient pathway to solving the subgroup problem. Of course, making the data too widely available can raise important ethical issues [14] (see Chap. 18).

Wilkinson et al. [15] have described a set of guiding principles to make data Findable, Accessible, Interoperable, and Reusable (FAIR, Box 19.2 and Chap. 15). Making it possible for investigators to find data related to mental illness is not completely solved, but there has been some progress. One good starting point to find human subjects data related to mental health is the NIMH Data Archive (www.nda. nih.gov, NDA). That archive makes data available from more than 500,000 research subjects. dbGaP and associated NCBI archives provide a similar framework for storing genomics data as the BRAIN Initiative data archives do [16]. In addition to this small list, there are many other data archives that contain data useful for those trying to do research on mental illness [17]. Unfortunately, the infrastructure to easily locate all of the archives does not exist yet.

Box 19.2 Fair Principles

To be **findable**, data should have a persistent identifier(s), have rich metadata (data describing the data), and be registered or indexed in searchable resources. Finding the data is the first step in using it, and findability should be possible for both humans and computers.

Once a user finds data, they need to be **accessible**. This may include special authorization and authentication protocols for sensitive data. The metadata should be widely accessible even if the underlying sensitive data is restricted.

Interoperability refers to the ability to link data coming from multiple sources and to use standard workflows or analysis pipelines to analyze the data. The use of standard data collection methods by a research community can be a great aid in creating interoperable data sets.

Reusability really refers to the ability of someone who was not involved in the initial measurement of the data to use that data. The real test of reusability is for the secondary user to understand how the initial data were measured using information in the metadata and then reuse the data in a new way without having to consult with those who measured the data initially.

A second requirement to solve the clustering problem is data analysis workflows to effectively and appropriately analyze the data. Given the complexity of the data and of the brain, the need for a cadre of software developers and informaticians to collaborate with the mental health community (both researchers and citizen scientists) to deal with the data cannot be understated. There can be significant barriers to the two groups working together. Facilitating interdisciplinary research is not straightforward [18], but if there are sufficient incentives and a thoughtful framework those problems can be overcome.

The availability of cloud data storage and the ability to compute in the cloud on identical data using different data analysis workflows have started to make a significant difference in our understanding of the strengths and weaknesses of particular workflows [19]. Understanding the strengths and weaknesses of particular data analysis workflows is currently difficult since what appear to be subtle differences in starting parameters or even the sort of computational hardware that is used can make head to head comparisons difficult or impossible. Those problems can be solved by making standardized data sets available, allowing groups to instantiate their workflows on the same computational platform, and thereby create a platform to understand the strengths and weaknesses of different data analysis workflows. The combination of such an infrastructure along with the realization that data sets are too large to download will likely result in data sets being maintained in one location for the research community to analyze. We are not there yet, but such a world will protect against misuse of data much better than the current situation where the same data set is stored in dozens or hundreds of locations. That change cannot happen too quickly.

19.1.2   Essential Component 2: Harmonizing and Integrating across Datasets

For mental health informatics to achieve its potential will require large datasets encompassing a variety of data types. Already, data archives store prodigious amounts of data. One significant issue that needs to be overcome is the challenge of using data from different datasets.

One example of a sizeable data archive facing these challenges is the NIMH Data Archive, which has been accepting data for just over a decade [20]. Data from more than 1000 grant awards, and 200 publications, have been deposited. When data are deposited, the data are stored in a specific "data structure" defined by someone in the research community. For clinical or phenotypic data, such a data structure is usually a list of multiple questions. Each question has a set of allowable answers. Data structures can be described by data dictionaries, with the individual questions referred to in this context as data elements. Note that, as discussed in Chap. 7, many different terms are used in different informatics communities to describe what NIMH calls a data structure. These terms include "common data element (CDE)", "information model (IM)", "clinical element model (CEM)", etc.

It is truly shocking how many different clinical data collection instruments are in use in the mental health community. NDA currently has more than 2800 data structures which contain more than 260,000 individual questions. More data structures are defined every week. Clearly the number of different data structures measuring similar concepts is a major barrier to solving the cluster problem described above. When the data from one laboratory can't be easily linked to similar data from a different laboratory many researchers will give up any attempt at secondary data analysis rather than working through the tedious data wrangling that would be required to use the data. In FAIR terminology, data in mental health are not very interoperable (Fig. 19.2).

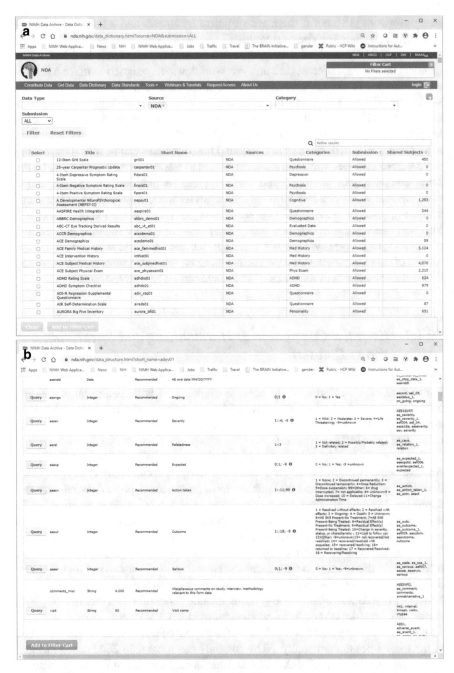

Fig. 19.2 Examples of "data structures" in the NIMH Data Archive. (**a**) shows the start of the alphabetical list of data structures/data dictionaries. (**b**) shows the Adverse Events data structure with some of the individual questions and the allowable range of values for those individual questions/data elements. A common data element would be a data structure that is widely used in a research community

How can this problem be solved? Defining a set of data structures that are meant to be used by all mental health researchers to collect basic data is one obvious solution [21], but it can be difficult to convince the research community to adopt those data structures without strong requirements from the funding agencies and/or the journals. The benefits of creating a basic set of data structures that would facilitate linking data sets from different laboratories probably outweighs the reluctance among the research community to adopt such measures, but an approach using carrots rather than sticks would be preferable. Developing a common information model [22] may also be possible but could be labor intensive. An additional benefit of having data structures that are widely used is that there would be a good pathway to improve those data structures as they were used by many laboratories in many different conditions. Currently, most mental health data structures are not widely enough used to get better over time.

The Human Connectome Program [23–26] provides an example of an approach that encourages harmonization using carrots rather than sticks. That project developed an MRI data collection protocol [27, 28] that had significant advantages in terms of signal to noise and time needed to collect data. The resulting dataset also had the advantage of being large. Without NIH requiring the use of that data collection protocol, many researchers and other large data collection efforts began to use it [29]. That experience suggests that when either a clear improvement in data collection technology or a large data set becomes available, researchers may modify their data collection plans to harmonize their study with existing data sets. In the Human Connectome case, it is not clear how much of this data harmonization was due to technology development versus the ability to use a large amount of new data, but discussions with researchers suggest both were factors. That experience suggests that NIMH and other funders could consider funding large uniform data collection efforts as a way to persuade the research community to adopt common data structures rather than require the use of certain data structures as a term of receiving grant funding.

One very important benefit to reusing data structures is that existing validation tools can then be used to improve the rigor and reproducibility of data collection. At the NDA, researchers are required to deposit data every 6 months. Those data are shared with the research community only at the end of a grant award or when a publication related to the data occurs. This six-month data deposition schedule helps researchers discover cases where the data they have collected is not consistent with the data structure that they themselves defined. It is rare when a research laboratory submits data for the first time and does not discover some unexpected issues. Correcting those issues close in time to when the data were collected improves the rigor and reproducibility of the science. The NDA validation tool [20] can be used separately from data deposition. In an ideal world, research labs would use the validation tool daily or weekly to catch and correct any issues, for example outliers or invalid values.

How should data harmonization be accomplished for data that have already been collected either for research purposes or data in electronic medical records? Harmonizing research data is possible but not easy. A good example of the difficulty in such a task can be seen in the work by McCray and colleagues [30]. They worked with domain experts to construct an ontology that relates questions found in commonly used autism data structures. The work took a long time and involved many different sorts of experts. In principle, this work can be repeated in other scientific sub-domains. In practice, few researchers have thus far wanted to take on such a task or have been concerned about finding funding to support such work. Stronger inducements may be required to encourage post-hoc approaches to data harmonization.

There may be informatics approaches that can discover mappings between questions in data structures in a more automated fashion, but that is a difficult problem. Creating mappings between two structures where there is not some reference information that is known to be truly identical in those structures is an area where further research is needed. Until such tools exist, manual human curation seems to be the only path forward. That likely means that many legacy data sets will be lost.

Will the future of mental health informatics involve data from electronic health records (EHRs)? The answer is clearly yes, but there are still significant improvements that are needed in EHRs as they are used both to deliver care [31] and to provide data for clinical research [32] (see Chap. 16). Some recent results show how useful information can be derived from both structured and unstructured information in an EHR [33–35]. In terms of finding biomarkers to solve the subgroup problem, information from EHRs will likely end up being somewhere between helpful and essential. Use of EHR data to facilitate knowledge discovery is explored in detail in Chap. 1.

19.1.3   Training

The last major item to address is how to train the basic and clinical mental health research community to use the information that is becoming available and how to facilitate collaborations between informaticists and mental health researchers and care providers. These issues are not completely solved, but there has been a great deal of progress. The Sloan-Schwartz Program in Theoretical Neurobiology and other funding programs have provided the necessary initial funds to launch computational neuroscience and related fields such as computational psychiatry [36–40]. Informaticists interested in mental health certainly exist, including many of the contributors to (and readers of) this book. Their areas of research demonstrate a diverse range of interesting informatics approaches in mental health. We also need larger numbers of mental health informaticians. We hope that this book, and new courses that might use it—perhaps co-taught by experts in mental health and in informatics respectively—will help address this need.

The mental health research community will need training, both on how to deal effectively with large data sets and how to use modern informatics approaches as they collect data. For example, what is the best way to get researchers to use tools like the NDA validation tool on a daily basis? More broadly, where in their training can mental health researchers gain an understanding of data standards- what they are, what they do, and how MH research can benefit from their use? What approaches are best for building ongoing collaborations between informaticists and mental health researchers to understand the large data sets that exist and will continue to grow? Those collaborations will need to provide appropriate credit to both groups. Are there ways to create a virtuous feedback cycle where mental health researchers collaborate with informaticists on a regular basis to provide feedback to improve existing tools and data infrastructure?

Training for the mental health research community is one clear need, but there are infrastructure issues that also need to be addressed. One additional question is how to apportion credit for using data collected by someone else. Persistent identifiers assigned to a data set provide some of the needed infrastructure to give credit to those who initially measured the data. The concept of a "Data Descriptor" has been introduced along with journals to publish those descriptors, for example Nature Scientific Data [41]. But this type of formal data citation is not yet broadly used, by researchers *or* by APT (Appointments, Promotions, and Tenure) committees. An infrastructure similar to what PubMed and the Web of Science provide for publications is needed for data. Two initiatives to this end are the Google Dataset Search (https://datasetsearch.research.google.com/) and DataMed, developed by the NIH-funded biomedical and healthCAre Data Discovery Index Ecosystem (bio-CADDIE) consortium [42]. Once these tools and resources become more broadly used, training of APT committees, of peer reviewers, and of many others involved in the research enterprise will be needed to ensure that both those who collect or generate data and those who use it get appropriate credit.

19.2   Making a Difference Now: Informatics and a Learning Health System for Psychosis

Twenty years ago, the Institute of Medicine (IOM, now the National Academy of Medicine or NAM) envisioned "learning health care" for the United States, where evidence-based treatment, measurement-based practice, and informatics come together to promote high quality services and to further scientific discovery [43, 44]. As was discussed in Chap. 1, a learning healthcare system (LHS) is bidirectional. Information generated by the research community informs clinical care, and observations made during clinical care suggest areas where additional research is needed. Recent advances in treatments for first episode schizophrenia [45, 46], coupled with innovations in clinical assessment, data mining, and performance feedback [47], create new opportunities for building a learning health care system for persons in the early stages of serious mental illness (SMI). The case study below shows how we can create a mental health informatics framework to provide the sort of virtuous feedback cycle needed to optimize health care delivery.

In 2015, the NIMH announced the Early Psychosis Intervention Network (EPINET) as a platform for delivering, studying, and refining evidence-based care for those at greatest risk for early SMI. Several foundational activities ensued, including an expert consensus process to identify standard data collection protocols for early psychosis clinical services and translational research [48, 49], a multi-site evaluation of early psychosis programs using common measures and centralized data aggregation and analysis [50]; and a stakeholder meeting [51] to explore opportunities and barriers to adopting harmonized assessment methods in "real-world" treatment settings. Based on these endeavors, NIMH invited proposals in 2018 for learning health care projects that apply informatics to improve intervention effectiveness, service delivery, and health outcomes in clinics offering evidence-based care to persons experiencing an initial episode of psychotic illness.

NIMH currently supports five regional networks and a national data coordinating center under the EPINET initiative. Each regional network links six or more participating clinics through standard clinical measures, uniform data collection methods, data sharing agreements, and integration of participant-level data across service users and settings. Working closely with the regional networks, the national data coordinating center will harmonize clinical assessments across programs and combine regional datasets into a national repository of early psychosis common data elements, clinical measures, and de-identified person-level data. Together, the national EPINET initiative includes 58 early psychosis programs in nine states. NIMH estimates that approximately 5000 persons will be enrolled and followed in these programs over the course of the five-year award, generating up to 10,000 clinical assessments each year. Data collected by regional networks will be submitted to the data coordinating center every 6 months and then deposited in the NIMH Data Archive.

EPINET regional networks will employ analytic platforms and data visualization tools that can rapidly translate large amounts of clinical service data into usable information for network stakeholders, including patients, family members, clinicians, program administrators, and scientists. Data reporting tools will promote a variety of learning health care functions within the networks, including treatment fidelity monitoring, measurement-based practice, and quality improvement analyses. Likewise, the national data coordinating center will employ "big data" tools to explore variation across early psychosis programs in treatment fidelity/quality, service delivery, and treatment response and plot individual clinics' performance against outcomes observed across all regional networks. Combined, these informatics resources will allow individual programs to monitor learning health care metrics in real time, and to compare local performance to results obtained across the national early psychosis ecosystem.

Through the national data coordinating center, EPINET will possess many of the computational building blocks mentioned earlier in this chapter: large samples of similarly ascertained subjects; informed consent for data use and sharing; common measures administered in consistent manner; data scientists to assist with analysis workflow; and long-term data storage in the NIMH Data Archive. Eventually, the coordinating center will offer a secure, web-based portal to allow extramural scientists to query de-identified EPINET data for research purposes. Through this mechanism, NIMH hopes to promote large-scale, practice-based research on the EPINET platform to improve diagnosis, intervention effectiveness, and clinical and functional outcomes in early psychosis. Future translational research efforts are also envisioned. These second-wave studies will link early psychosis clinical programs to research centers exploring early psychosis risk factors, mechanisms of illness progression, and novel treatment targets and interventions.

Mental health informatics will help facilitate these studies, in part by disaggregating early psychosis clusters into more homogeneous subpopulations. Should the EPINET study achieve its goals, it is easy to imagine that this framework can be used to create a learning healthcare system for other diagnostic groups.

19.3   Conclusion

There is a pressing need to use the tools of mental health informatics to improve our understanding of mental illness and other complex diseases. Defining the subgroups in complex diseases is probably the most important question that needs to be solved by informaticians collaborating with mental health researchers and clinicians. There are still significant challenges with findability and interoperability for data that come from mental health researchers and clinicians. Some solutions to these challenges were discussed above, but there is work to be done both on in infrastructure and in training. The EPINET case study shows what can be done today. Creating a similar virtuous feedback cycle in areas other than early psychosis should be possible using the lessons learned as EPINET progresses. Undoubtedly there will be challenges, but there is reason for optimism that the EPINET approach will be replicable in other areas of mental illness. The stage is set to allow mental health informatics to transform the practice of treating mental illness.

References

1. Zhou T, Zhu H, Fan Z, Wang F, Chen Y, Liang H, Yang Z. History of winning remodels Thalamo-PFC circuit to reinforce social dominance. Science. 2017;357(6347):162–8. https://doi.org/10.1126/science.aak9726.
2. Horstmann A. It wasn't me; It was my Brain – obesity associated characteristics of brain circuits governing decision-making. Physiol Behav. 2017 Jul 1;176:125–33. https://doi.org/10.1016/j.physbeh.2017.04.001.
3. Bedrosian TA, Nelson RJ. Timing of light exposure affects mood and brain circuits. Transl Psychiatry. 2017;7(1):e1017. https://doi.org/10.1038/tp.2016.262.
4. VanBuecken DE, Greenbaum CJ. Residual C-peptide in type 1 diabetes: what do we really know? Pediatr Diabetes. 2014;15(2):84–90. https://doi.org/10.1111/pedi.12135.
5. Cuthbert BN. Research domain criteria: toward future psychiatric Nosologies. Dialogues Clin Neurosci. 2015 Mar;17(1):89–97. https://doi.org/10.1016/j.ajp.2013.12.007.
6. Insel TR, Gogtay N. National Institute of Mental Health clinical trials: new opportunities, new expectations. JAMA Psychiatry. 2014;71:745–6. https://doi.org/10.1001/jamapsychiatry.2014.426.
7. Zhang C, Kolodkin AL, Wong RO, James RE. Establishing wiring specificity in visual system circuits: from the retina to the brain. Annu Rev of Neurosci. 2017;40:395–424. https://doi.org/10.1146/annurev-neuro-072116-031607.
8. Hurko O, Ryan JL. Translational research in central nervous system drug discovery. NeuroRx. 2005;2(4):671–82.

9. Litvina E, Adams A, Barth A, Bruchez M, Carson J, Chung JE, et al. BRAIN initiative: cutting-edge tools and resources for the community. J Neurosci. 2019;39(42):8275–84. https://doi.org/10.1523/JNEUROSCI.1169-19.2019.
10. Reininghaus U, Bohnke JR, Chavez-Baldini U, Gibbons R, Ivleva E, Clementz BA, et al. Transdiagnostic dimensions of psychosis in the bipolar-schizophrenia network on intermediate phenotypes (B-SNIP). World Psychiatry. 2019;18(1):67–76. https://doi.org/10.1002/wps.20607.
11. Drysdale AT, Grosenick L, Downar J, Dunlop K, Mansouri F, Meng Y, et al. Resting-state connectivity biomarkers define neurological subtypes of depression. Nat Med. 2017;23(1):28–38. https://doi.org/10.1038/nm.4246.
12. McCarroll SA, Feng G, Hyman SE. Genome-scale Neurogenetics: methodology and meaning. Nat Neurosci. 2014;17(6):756–63. https://doi.org/10.1038/nn.3716.
13. Bonney R, Shirk JL, Phillips TB, Wiggins A, Ballard HL, Miller-Rushing AJ, Parrish JK. Next steps for Citizen science. Science. 2014;343(6178):1436–7. https://doi.org/10.1126/science.1251554.
14. Ramos KM, Grady C, Greely HT, Chiong W, Eberwine J, Farahany NA, et al. The NIH BRAIN initiative: integrating Neuroethics and neuroscience. Neuron. 2019;101(3):394–8.
15. Wilkinson MD, Dumontier M, Aalbersberg IJ, Appleton G, Axton M, Baak A, et al. The FAIR guiding principles for scientific data management and stewardship. Sci Data. 2016;3:160018. https://doi.org/10.1038/sdata.2016.18.
16. Sayers EW, Agarwala R, Bolton EE, Brister JR, Canese K, Clark K, et al. Database resources of the National Center for biotechnology information. Nucleic Acids Res. 2019;47(D1):D23–8. https://doi.org/10.1093/nar/gky1069.
17. Tennenbaum JD, Bhuvaneshwar K, Gagliardi JP, Hollis KF, Jia P, Ma L, et al. Translational bioinformatics in mental health: open access data sources and computational biomarker discovery. Brief Bioinform. 2019 May;20(3):842–56. https://doi.org/10.1093/bib/bbx157.
18. Tobi H, Kampen JK. Research design: the methodology for interdisciplinary research framework. Qual Quant. 2018;52(3):1209–25. https://doi.org/10.1007/s11135-017-0513-8.
19. Busby B, Lesko M. August 2015 and January 2016 hackathon participants and Federer L. closing gaps between open software and public data in a hackathon setting: user-centered software prototyping [version 2; peer review: not peer reviewed]. F1000Research. 2016;5:672. https://doi.org/10.12688/f1000research.8382.2.
20. Hall D, Huerta MF, McAuliffe MJ, Farber GK. Sharing heterogeneous data: the National Database for autism research. Neuroinformatics. 2012;10(4):331–9. https://doi.org/10.1007/s12021-012-9151-4.
21. Barch DM, Gotlib IH, Bilder RM, Pine DS, Smoller JW, Brown CH, Huggins W, Hamilton C, Haim A, Farber GK. Common measures for National Institute of Mental Health funded research. Biol Psychiatry. 2016;79(12):e91–6.
22. Chow M, Beene M, O'Brien A, Greim P, Cromwell T, DuLong D, Bedecarre D. A nursing information model process for interoperability. J Am Med Inform Assoc. 2015;22(3):608–14. https://doi.org/10.1093/jamia/ocu026.
23. Van Essen DC, Smith SM, Barch DM, Beherns TE, Ugurbil K. WU-MINN HCP consortium. Neuroimage. 2013;80:62–79. https://doi.org/10.1016/j.neuroimage.2013.05.041.
24. Bookheimer SY, Salat DH, Terpstra M, Ances BM, Barch DM, Buckner RL, et al. The lifespan human connectome project in aging: an overview. NeuroImage. 2019;185:335–48. https://doi.org/10.1016/j.neuroimage.2018.10.009.
25. Sommerville LH, Bookheimer SY, Buckner RL, Burgess GC, Curtiss SW, Dapretto M, et al. The lifespan human connectome project in development: a large scale study of brain connectivity development in 5–21 year olds. NeuroImage. 2018;183:456–68. https://doi.org/10.1016/j.neuroimage.2018.08.050.
26. Howell BR, Styner MA, Gao W, Yap PT, Wang L, Baluyot K, et al. The UNC.UMN baby connectome project (BCP): an overview of the study design and protocol development. NeuroImage. 2019;185:891–905. https://doi.org/10.1016/j.neuroimage.2018.03.049.

27. Fan Q, Witzel T, Nummenmaa A, Van Dijk KRA, Van Horn JD, Drews MK, et al. MGH-USC human connectome project datasets with ultra-high B-value diffusion MRI. Neuroimage. 2016;124(Pt. B):1108–14. https://doi.org/10.1016/j.neuroimage.2015.08.075.
28. Glasser MF, Smith SM, Marcus DS, Andersson JL, Auerbach EJ, Beherns TE, et al. The human connectome Project's neuroimaging approach. Nat Neurosci. 2016;19(9):1175–87. https://doi.org/10.1038/nn.4361.
29. Casey BJ, Cannonier T, Conley MI, Cohen AO, Barch DM, Heitzeg MM, et al. The adolescent brain cognitive development (ABCD) study: image acquisition across 21 sites. Dev Cogn Neurosci. 2018;32:43–54. https://doi.org/10.1016/j.dcn.2018.03.001.
30. McCray AT, Trevvett P, Frost HR. Modeling the autism Spectrum disorder phenotype. Neuroinformatics. 2014;12(2):291–305. https://doi.org/10.1007/s12021-013-9211-4.
31. Evans RS. Electronic health records: then, now, and in the future. Yearb. Med. Inform. 2016;Suppl 1:S48–61. https://doi.org/10.15265/IYS-2016-s006.
32. Cowie CR, Blomster JI, Curtis LH, Duclaux S, Ford I, Fritz F, et al. Electronic health records to facilitate clinical research. Clin Res Cardiol. 2017;106(1):1–9. https://doi.org/10.1007/s00392-016-1025-6.
33. Lyalina S, Percha B, LePendu P, Iyer SV, Altman RB, Shah NH. Identifying phenotypic signatures of neuropsychiatric disorders from electronic medical records. J. Am. Med. Inform. Assoc. 2013;20:e297–305. https://doi.org/10.1136/amiajnl-2013-001933.
34. Liu Q, Woo M, Zou X, Champaneria A, Lau C, et al. Symptom-based patient stratification in mental illness using clinical notes. J Biomed Inform. 2019;98:103274. https://doi.org/10.1136/amiajnl-2013-001933.
35. McCoy TH Jr, Yu S, Hart KL, Castro VM, Brown HE, et al. High throughput phenotyping for dimensional psychopathology in electronic medical records. Biol Psychiatry. 2018;83(12):997–1004. https://doi.org/10.1016/j.biopsych.2018.01.011.
36. Catani M, de Schotten MT, Slater D, Dell'Acqua F. Connectomic approaches before the connectome. NeuroImage. 2013;80:2–13. https://doi.org/10.1016/j.neuroimage.2013.05.109.
37. Dauce E, Perrinet L. Computational neuroscience from multiple levels to multi-level. J Physiol Paris. 2010;104(1–2):1–4. https://doi.org/10.1016/j.jphysparis.2009.11.001.
38. Huys QJM, Maia TV, Frank MJ. Computational psychiatry as a bridge from neuroscience to clinical applications. Nat Neuro. 2016;19:404–13. https://doi.org/10.1038/nn.4238.
39. Nayak L, Dasgupta A, Das R, Ghosh K, De RK. Computational neuroscience and neuroinformatics: recent progress and resources. J Biosci. 2018;43(5):1037–54.
40. Sejnowski TJ, Koch C, Churchland PS. 1988. Computational Neuroscience. Science. 1988;241(4871):1299–306. https://doi.org/10.1126/science.3045969.
41. NPG (2014) About scientific data. https://www.nature.com/sdata/about. Retrieved 13 Sept 2020.
42. Chen X, et al. DataMed–an open source discovery index for finding biomedical datasets. J Am Med Inform Assoc. 2018;25(3):300–8.
43. Institute of Medicine. Crossing the quality chasm: a new health system for the 21st century. Washington, DC: National Academies Press; 2001. https://iom.nationalacademies.org/Reports/2001/Crossing-the-Quality-Chasm-A-New-Health-System-for-the-21st-Century.aspx
44. Institute of Medicine. Best care at lower cost: The path to continuously learning health care in America. Washington, DC: National Academies Press; 2013. http://iom.nationalacademies.org/Reports/2012/Best-Care-at-Lower-Cost-The-Path-to-Continuously-Learning-Health-Care-in-America.aspx
45. Kane JM, Robinson DG, Schooler NR, Mueser KT, Penn DL, Rosenheck RA, et al. Comprehensive versus usual community care for first episode psychosis: two-year outcomes from the NIMH RAISE early treatment program. Am J Psychiatr. 2016;173(4):362–72. https://doi.org/10.1176/appi.ajp.2015.15050632.
46. Correll CU, Galling B, Pawar A, Krivko A, Bonetto C, Ruggeri M, et al. Comparison of early intervention services vs treatment as usual for early-phase psychosis: a systematic review, meta-analysis, and meta-regression. JAMA Psychiat. 2018;75(6):555–65. https://doi.org/10.1001/jamapsychiatry.2018.0623.

47. Nossel I, Wall MM, Scodes J, Marino LA, Zikha S, Bello I, et al. Results of a coordinated specialty care program for early psychosis and predictors of outcomes. Psychiatr Serv. 2018;69:863–70. https://doi.org/10.1176/appi.ps.201700436.
48. Dixon L, Jones N, Loewy R, Perkins D, Sale T, Huggins W, et al. Tales from the clinical services panel of the PhenX early psychosis working group. Psychiatr Serv. 2019;70:514–7. https://doi.org/10.1176/appi.ps.201800585.
49. Ongur D, Carter CS, Gur RE, Perkins D, Sawa A, Seidman LJ, et al. Common data elements for national institute of mental health funded translational early psychosis research. Biol Psychiatry Cogn Neurosci Neuroimaging; Jun 29, 2019; 5(1):10–22. Pii: S2451–9022 (19)30174–0 https://doi.org/10.1016/j.bpsc.2019.06.009
50. Rosenblatt, A., Dixon, L., Goldman, H. et al. The mental health block Grant ten percent set aside study final report; 2019.
51. https://www.nimh.nih.gov/news/events/2017/fep/harmonizing-clinical-data-collection-in-community-based-treatment-programs-for-first-episode-psychosis.shtml.

Index

A

Accountable care organizations (ACOs), 431, 432
Actigraphy data, 456
Acute myeloid leukemia (AML), 3
Acute Residential Treatment (ART) programs, 87
Advanced practice practitioners, 92
Advanced practice providers (APPs), 85
Affective Norm for English Words (ANEW), 332
Affordable Care Act (ACA), 94
Affordable Healthcare Act (ACA), 431
Affymetrix, 273
Agile model, 43
AllOfUs biobank, 412
All of Us Program, 267
Alzheimer's Disease Neuroimaging Initiative (ADNI), 208
Alzheimer's disease (AD), 276, 278, 282, 288, 289
American Academy of Neurology (AAN), 417
American National Standards Institute (ANSI), 429
American Psychological Association (APA), 417
Amyloid-β, 289
Analysis Data Model (AdaM), 398
Analytic methods, 236–238
Annotation and Image Markup (AIM), 200
Anthropomorphism, 488
Antisocial personality disorder (APD), 173
Anxiety and Depression Association of America (ADAA), 418
Anxiety disorders, 74
Apache Software Foundation, 398

Apparent Diffusion Coefficient (ADC), 195, 196
Application programming interface (API), 324, 433
Area under the ROC curve (AUC), 254
Assessment of illness
    diagnostic clinical interview, 106–109
    family history, 107
    HPI, 107
    medical history, 107
    mental status exam, 107, 108
    past psychiatric history, 107
    social history, 107
ATLAS dashboard, 381
Attention mechanisms, 335
Audio/Visual Emotion Challenge (AVEC), 406
The Autism and Developmental Disabilities Monitoring network database, 326
Autism Biomarker Consortium for Clinical Trials (ABC-CT), 418
Autism Diagnostic Observation Schedule 2nd Edition (ADOS-2), 226
Axiom, 174

B

Backward elimination, 246
Bag of words (BoW) vectors, 331
Behavioral Risk Factor Surveillance System (BRFSS), 375
The Belmont Report, 496
Between-person (inter-individual) mechanistic reasoning, 308, 309
Bidirectional long-short term memory (BiLSTM), 335

© Springer Nature Switzerland AG 2021
J. D. Tenenbaum, P. A. Ranallo (eds.), *Mental Health Informatics*, Health Informatics, https://doi.org/10.1007/978-3-030-70558-9

Big data, 267, 268
  behavioral data repositories, 405, 406
  biological data repositories, 403–405
  challenges, 419
  clinical administrative data
      repositories, 406–408
  constructing large data repository, 416
  developing data repositories in mental
      health, 417, 418
  electronic health records, 409, 410
  FAIR guiding principles, 400
  governance, 397
  machine learning algorithms, 396
  metadata, 399
  multi-modal data repositories, 410–414
  opportunities, 418
  practical challenges of using data
      repositories, 413
    missingness, 413, 414
    psychiatric diagnosis, 414
  refined scientific knowledge repositories,
      402, 403
  requirements analysis, 415, 416
  secondary usage, 400, 401
  submitting data to a large data
      repository, 417
  supervised machine learning, 396
  technical infrastructure, 397–399
  using large data repository, 416
  volume, velocity, and variety, 394, 395
Binary Alignment Mapping, 270
Binary vector, 331
Biobanks, 401
Bioinformatics
  biomarker discovery (*see* Biomarker
      discovery)
  knowledge discovery and application,
      288, 289
  mental health vs. medical conditions, 288
Biological theory, 62, 64
Biomarker discovery
  big data, 267
  bioinformatics, 267, 268
  cellular attributes, 285, 286
  DNA copy number, 282
  epigenetics, 279
  genomics (*see* Genomics)
  imaging, 283
  metabolomics, 277
  microbiome, 284
  miRNA (*see* MicroRNA (miRNA))
  physiological function, 268
  proteomics (*see* Proteomics)

  transcriptomics (*see* Transcriptomics)
  translational bioinformatics, 266, 267
Biomedical Informatics, *see* Informatics
Biomedical Informatics Research Network
      (BIRN), 207
Biophysical models, 256, 257
Biopsychosocial model, 68, 109
Bipolar-Schizophrenia Network on
      Intermediate Phenotypes (B-
      SNIP), 508
Block grant funding, 95
Borderline personality disorder (BPD), 279
Brushing, 373

C
Calibration curve, 254
California Consumer Privacy Act (CCPA), 498
Cancer Imaging Phenomics Toolkit
      (CaPTk), 283
Causal networks, 240, 241
CDS Hooks, 442
Cellular attributes, 285, 286
Center for Epidemiologic Studies Depression
      Scale Revised (CESD-R), 457
Center for Information Technology Leadership
      (CITL), 435
Center for Reproducible Neuroimaging
      Computation (CRNC), 209
Centers for Medicare and Medicaid Services
      (CMS), 433
Centers of Excellence in Genomic Science
      (CEGS), 324
Cerner Corporation (Cerner), 435, 437
ChIP-chip, 279
ChIP-sequencing (ChIP-seq), 278, 279
Chromatin immunoprecipitation (ChIP), 278
Chromosomal aberrations, 270
Classification models, 257
Classification system, 172, 173
Clinical Data Acquisition Standards
      Harmonization (CDASH), 398
Clinical Data Interchange Standards
      Consortium (CDISC), 398
Clinical decision support (CDS), 43
Clinical element model (CEM), 511
Clinical global impressions (CGI) scale, 383
Cloud computing, 267
CLPsych shared task, 342
Clustering, 250, 336
Cluster models, 258, 259
CMS Interoperability and Patient Access Act
      final rule, 433

Coding regions, 275
Coding systems, 41
Co-expressed genes, 275
COGITO study, 308
Cognitive-behavioral model, 66
Cognitive behavioral therapy (CBT), 113
Cognitive model, 66
Common Agreement, 496
Common data elements (CDEs), 156, 175, 176, 511
Common data models (CDMs), 398
Community/county mental health care center, 90
Computable phenotyping, 38
Computational Health Informatics Program, 442
Computational model
    biophysical models, 256, 257
    classification models, 257
    cluster models, 258, 259
    connectionist models, 257
    data-driven approaches, 241–244
    machine learning
        deep learning, 252
        semi-supervised learning, 251
        supervised learning, 249, 253–255
        unsupervised learning, 250, 251, 255, 256
    policy, ethical, and safety issues, 260, 261
    predictive models, 257, 258
    preprocessing
        dimensionality reduction, 245
        feature extraction methods, 247
        feature selection methods, 245–247
        range of activities, 244
    process, 236
    regression models, 257
    reinforcement-learning models, 257
    reporting models, 259, 260
    theory-based approaches, 238
        causal networks, 240, 241
        dynamical systems, 238–240
Computational psychiatry, 306, 307
Computerized physician order entry (CPOE), 440
Computerized psychometric assessments, 459
Concept mapping, 329
Conditional random fields (CRFs), 335
Connectionist models, 257
Consolidated Clinical Document Architecture (C-CDA), 180, 181
Consolidated Framework for Implementation Research (CFIR), 46

Construct validity, 220
Contemporary psychiatric diagnostics, 464, 465
Content standard, 163, 165
Content validity, 220
Continuum model, 60–62
Convergent validity, 220
Convolutional neural networks (CNN), 335
Copy number variation (CNV), 282
Coronavirus (COVID-19), 459
Corpus, 318
Count-based features, 332
COVID-19 pandemic, 90, 91
Credible, 437
Criterion validity, 220
Cures Act, 433
Cytoscape network visualization tool, 384

D
Data acquisition
    challenges, limitations and future directions, 230, 231
    computerized metrics, 229
    definition, 228
    smartphones and wearable devices, 229, 230
    social media usage, 229
Data analysis workflows, 510, 511
Data archives, 510, 511
Database management systems (DBMS), 38
Data-driven approaches, 241–244
Data harmonization, 509, 511, 513, 514
Data, Information, Knowledge, and Wisdom (DIKW), 36
DataMed, 342, 515
Data mining, 40, 41
Data relevant
    behavioral data, 226, 227
    environmental data, 228
    psychological data
        approaches, 225
        definition, 223–225
        history, 222
    social and interpersonal data, 227, 228
    types, 222
Data repository, 38
Data to knowledge (D2K)
    data and databases, 37, 38
    data mining and machine learning, 40, 41
    knowledge discovery, 36, 37
    NLP and text mining, 39, 40
    standards and interoperability, 41, 42

Data Use Agreements (DUAs), 397
"Death by 1,000 Clicks", 440
Deep learning, 41, 252, 335
Department of Health & Human Services
　　(DHHS), 429
Dependency parsing, 329
Depression screener Patient Health
　　Questionnaire (PHQ-9), 457
Descriptive metadata, 38
Diagnostic and Statistical Manual of Mental
　　Disorders (DSM), 69–72,
　　74, 75, 297
Diagnostic Interview for Anxiety, Mood, OCD
　　and Related Neuropsychiatric
　　Disorders (DIAMOND), 226
Dialectic behavior therapy (DBT), 113
Differentially expressed genes (DEGs),
　　274, 275
Digital Imaging and Communications in
　　Medicine (DICOM), 197
Dimensionality reduction, 245, 251, 360
Directed acyclic graph (DAG), 240
Discriminant validity, 220
DNA copy number
　　copy number changes, 281
　　data processing, 282
　　examples in mental health, 282
　　risk factors, 281
　　strengths and limitations, 282
DNA methylation, 278
Downstream analysis, 274
DrugBank, 403
Duration of illness (DOI), 106

E
Early onset Alzheimer's disease (EOAD), 289
The Early Psychosis Intervention Network
　　(EPINET), 515–517
Electroconvulsive therapy (ECT), 115, 460
Electronic health records (EHRs)
　　behavioral health components, 438
　　big data, 409, 410
　　current market share in United States
　　　hospitals, 436
　　definition, 434
　　disadvantages, 443, 444
　　improved efficiency, 441–443
　　information visualization, 376
　　landscape across medical and mental
　　　health care, 435, 436
　　neuroimaging, 192
　　patient safety and quality of care, 439, 440

PHRs (see Personal health records (PHRs))
　　proposed value of, 439
　　purpose of, 435
　　secondary uses for
　　　LHS, 445
　　　quality improvement, 445
　　　research uses, 444, 445
　　standards, 183
　　vendors in mental health field, 436, 437
Elsevier Pathway Studio software, 286
Embedded methods, 247
Emotional processing, 458
Encoding attribute values, 368
English sentiment analysis tools, 332
Environmental data, 228, 379
Epic systems corporation (Epic), 435
Epigenetics/epigenomics
　　data processing, 278
　　epigenome study, 278
　　examples in mental health, 279
　　strengths and limitations, 279
Epistemic cultures, 296
Epistemic injustice, 489
ESRI's ArcGIS geographic information
　　systems, 384
Ethical AI in mental healthcare
　　at data-level, 482
　　in deploying AI-based systems in
　　　practice, 483
　　designing AI-based systems, 483
Ethical, legal, and social issues (ELSI)
　　advocacy (see Patient advocacy)
　　AI, 482, 483
　　California Consumer Privacy Act, 498
　　confidentiality of substance use disorder
　　　records, 495, 496
　　General Data Protection Regulation,
　　　497, 498
　　genomics and mental health informatics,
　　　491, 492
　　HIPAA, 493
　　HIPAA Privacy Rule, 493, 494
　　HIPAA Security Rule, 494, 495
　　mHealth, 487 (see also Mobile health
　　　(mHealth) apps)
　　research regulations, 496, 497
　　stigma and data sharing, 481, 482
　　21st Century Cures Act, 496
Evidence-based medicine, 7
Evidence Generating Medicine (EGM), 7
Evoked potentials (EPs), 206
"Exhibition of American Negroes", 357
Explanatory models, 237

Extensible markup language (XML), 37, 166
Extraversion, Agreeableness,
        Conscientiousness, Neuroticism,
        and Openness to Experience, 223

F
Face validity, 220
Factor analysis, 302–304
FAIRSharing, 171, 172
Fast health interoperability resources (FHIR),
        181, 182, 441, 442
FASTQ file, 270, 274
Feature engineering, 329
Feature extraction methods, 245, 247
Feature selection methods, 245–247
Featurization, 329
Fee-for-service (FFS) payment model, 428
Fields, HL7 message, 179
Filter methods, 246
Findable, Accessible, Interoperable, and
        Reusable (FAIR), 38, 400, 511
Forward selection, 246
Functional magnetic resonance imaging
        (fMRI), 203
Future of mental health informatics
    brain function, 505, 506
    complex disorders, 507
    datasets, data storage, and
            workflows, 509–511
    data structures, 512, 513
    harmonizing and integrating across
            datasets, 511, 513, 514
    learning health system for
            psychosis, 515–517
    NIMH vision, 509
    top-down approach to clustering, 508
    training, 514, 515

G
Gene expression, 272
Gene ontology enrichment analysis, 286
General Data Protection Regulation (GDPR),
        497, 498
Generalized Anxiety Disorder 7-item scale
        (GAD-7), 457
Gene regulation, 273
Genetic data, 376, 377, 379
Genetic Information Nondiscrimination Act of
        2008 (GINA), 492
Genetic Links to Anxiety and Depression
        (GLAD), 412–413

Genome sequencing, 269
Genome-wide association study (GWAS), 133,
        271, 377, 405
Genomics, 266, 267, 269
    data processing, 270, 271
    DNA study, 269
    examples in mental health, 271, 272
    strengths and limitations, 271
GitHub, 326
GLoVe, 330
Google Dataset Search, 515
Gut-Brain-Axis (GBA), 284, 285

H
Haploview, 377
Healthcare Information Technology Standards
        Panel (HITSP), 429
Health information exchange (HIE), 428,
        431–435, 441, 444, 448, 449
Health Information Organization (HIO), 428
Health information technology (HIT),
        5, 16, 17
    ACOs, 431
    federal initiatives, 431
    FFS payment model, 428
    future directions, 449
    historical perspective, 429
    HITECH Act, 429, 431
    NAHIT definition, 428
    PCMHs, 432
    State Innovation Models, 433, 434
    timeline of important dates, 429, 430
Health Information Technology for Economic
        and Clinical Health (HITECH) Act,
        429, 431, 496
Health Insurance Portability and
        Accountability Act (HIPAA), 322,
        431, 484, 493
Health Level 7 International (HL7), 41, 179,
        180, 442
Health maintenance organizations (HMOs), 93
Health Resource and Services Administration
        (HRSA), 92
HEALthy Brain and Child Development
        (HBCD) study, 208
Hearing Voices Movement, 490
Hierarchical taxonomy of psychopathology
        (HiTOP), 301, 302
HIPAA Privacy Rule, 493, 494
HIPAA Security Rule, 494, 495
Histone modification, 278
History of present illness (HPI), 107

HITECH Act, 441
Hospital inpatient setting, 88, 89
Human Connectome Program, 513
Human Connectome Projects (HCP), 208
Human factors engineering (HFE), 44, 45
Human Genome Project, 269, 272
Hypertext markup language (HTML), 166

I

Icarus Project, 490
IL6 genes, 275
Illumina, 273
Imaging informatics, 283
Index Medicus, 402
Inference engine, 44
Informatics
    axes and translational spectrum, 33, 34
    comprehensive review, 35
    data to knowledge
        data and databases, 37, 38
        data mining and machine
            learning, 40, 41
        knowledge discovery, 36, 37
        NLP and text mining, 39, 40
        standards and interoperability, 41, 42
    definition, 32, 33
    history, 31
    knowledge to performance
        CDS, 43
        HFE, 44, 45
        software and knowledge
            engineering, 43, 44
    LHS, 22, 23
        overview, 5, 6
        role of, 17–19 (*see also* Mental health
            informatics (MHI))
    performance to data
        dissemination, 45
        evaluation models, 45, 46
        quantitative and qualitative
            methods, 46
    precision medicine, 20–23
    subdisciplines, 34
Informatics Consult approach, 17
Informatics for Integrating Biology & the
    Bedside (i2b2) consortium, 410
Informatics technologies
    consumer facing technologies
        smartphone based assessment, 457
        wearable devices, 456
    issues and challenges, 464–467
    technologies

computerized psychometric
    assessment, 459
coordination and continuity of
    care, 463
implications for mental health
    conditions, 458
mobile medical devices, 460
online support groups, 462
smartphone based assessment, 457
social media, 457, 458
specialized clinical information
    systems, 460, 461
telemedicine, 459, 460
web based and mobile applications,
    462, 463
Information extraction (IE), 39
Information model (IM), 174, 511
Information retrieval (IR), 39
Information visualization
    advances in, 384
    building visualizations, 363
    definition, 356
    displaying data, 365, 368–370
    electronic health records, 376
    environmental data, 379
    evaluation, 386, 387
    genetic data, 376, 377, 379
    information visualization, 358, 360
    interacting with data, 370, 371, 373
    interactive visualizations, 358, 360
    mobile health data, 379
    multiple displays of synthetic data relating
        social media use to the age of
        user, 366
    preparing data, 364
    successful techniques, 356
    survey and psychometric instrument
        data, 374–376
    tasks, 363
    two-dimensional embedding, 360
    two-dimensional representations of patient
        profiles, 360, 361
    uncertainty, 384, 385
    understanding user needs and goals, 364
    using data and predictive models, 380–384
    visual analytics, 358
    Visual Information Seeking Mantra, 363
    visualization tasks, 361, 362
    web-based tool, 380
    W.E.B Dubois' depiction of income and
        expenses of African Americans, 357
Inpatient settings, 88–90
Insertions and deletions, 270

Institutional Review Boards (IRBs), 397
Integrative paradigms, knowledge discovery
  disciplinary specialization, 296
  discipline-specific phenomena, 297
  DSM-5 classification, 297–299
  epistemic cultures, 296
  epistemology and limitations, 309–311
  integrative computational methods
    computational psychiatry, 306, 307
    factor analysis, 302–304
    network analysis, 304–306
    within- and between-person reasoning,
      308, 309
  RDoC, 299–302
Intelligence quotient (IQ), 223, 224
Intensive outpatient programs (IOP),
  87, 90, 112
Interactive data visualization, 356, 358, 359
Internal consistency, 219
International Classification of Disease
  (ICD), 69–72
International Classification of Disorders and
  Related Health Problems, 297
International Health Terminology Standards
  Development Organization
  (SNOMED), 449
International Neuroinformatics Coordinating
  Facility (ICNF), 209
Interoperability standards, 168
  C-CDA, 180, 181
  FHIR, 181, 182
  HL7 message, 179, 180
  technical, and semantic, 177
Interoperability Standards Advisory, 41
Interpersonal data, 227, 228
Inter-rater reliability, 220
Intuitive medicine, 20

J
Javascript library, 384
JavaScript Object Notation (JSON), 167
Jupyter scientific notebooks, 384

K
K-6 instrument, 375
Kaiser Permanente (KP), 448
Knowledge acquisition cycle
  data to information and knowledge, 131
  signal to data, 130, 131
Knowledge base, 44
Knowledge-based selection, 245

Knowledge crystallization, 361
Knowledge discovery, 8, 10–12, 14, 36, 37,
  218, 342
Knowledge Discovery in Databases (KDD), 37
Knowledge to performance (K2P)
  CDS, 43
  HFE, 44, 45
  software and knowledge
    engineering, 43, 44

L
Labeling/social reaction theory, 63
Late onset Alzheimer's disease (LOAD), 289
Latent Dirichlet Allocation (LDA), 336
Learning/behavioral model, 65
Learning health care system, 515
Learning health system (LHS), 343, 400,
  445, 509
  actionable knowledge, 4
  AML, 3
  conceptual shift, 5
  definition, 6, 7
  depressive disorders, 3
  diagnostic classification systems, 2
  factors, 4
  features of, 8, 9
  foundational requirements, 17
  informatics
    overview, 5, 6
    role of, 17, 18
  knowledge discovery, 8, 10–12, 14
  limitations of, 16
  paradigm, 14, 16
  translational science
    definition, 11–13
    limitations of, 12, 14
Lemmatization, 327
Leo natural language processing platform, 327
Lexical processing tasks, 327
Lexicons and ontology, 340–342
Linear discriminant analysis (LDA), 247
Linguistic Inquiry and Word Count Lexicon
  (LIWC), 332
Linked multi-modal data repositories,
  410–414
Liquid chromatography and mass
  spectrometry (LCMS)
  technique, 277
LocusTrack, 377
Logical Observation Identifiers Names and
  Codes (LOINC), 133, 136,
  176–177, 185–187

M
Machine learning (ML), 40, 41
  deep learning, 252
  descriptions, 241
  semi-supervised learning, 251
  supervised learning
    algorithms, 249
    evaluation, 253–255
  unsupervised learning
    algorithms, 250, 251
    evaluation, 255, 256
  workflow in, 243, 244
Magnetic resonance imaging (MRI), 202–204
Magnetic resonance spectroscopy (MRS), 204
Major depressive disorders (MDD), 281
Manhattan plots, 377
Mapping/alignment, 270
Mechanistic biomarkers, 267
Medicaid, 95
Medical Imaging Interaction Toolkit
    (MITK), 283
Medical Information Mart for Intensive Care
    (MIMIC) project, 206, 207
Medical Logic Modules (MLMs), 44
Medical providers, 83–85
Medical Subject Headings (MeSH), 183, 402
Medicare, 95
MEDITECH, 437
Mental distress, 60–62, 71
Mental healthcare professionals
  medical providers, 83–85
  psychiatric aides, technicians, and mental
      health workers, 87
  psychologists, 85, 86
  social workers, 86, 87
  tools, 83
Mental healthcare system
  mental health workforce disparity, 91–93
  payment models
    privately-funded insurances, 93, 94
    publicly-funded insurances, 89, 94, 95
  primary care and dental care shortage, 82
  professionals
    medical providers, 83–85
    psychiatric aides, technicians, and
        mental health workers, 87
    psychologists, 85, 86
    social workers, 86, 87
    tools, 83
  settings
    ART, 87
    inpatient, 88–90
    outpatient, 90, 91

  types of, 87, 88
  social and economic factors, 82
Mental health informatics (MHI)
  vs. behavioral health, 132
  biological, behavioral, and social sciences
    acquiring actionable knowledge, 135
    challenging, 135
    EHRs, 137
    epistemological differences, 137–142
    knowledge dissemination, 136
    LOINC and SNOMED-CT, 136
    points of intersection, 142, 143
    signal detection and data capture, 136
    training and licensure options, 137
  biopsychosocial model, 122
  definition, 121
  entities and phenomena of interest,
      122–125, 127
  ethical, legal, and social issues, 144
  mHealth, 143
  natural language processing, 143
  traditional health informatics
    behavioral, and social phenomena,
        133, 134
    data to information and knowledge, 131
    signal to data, 130, 131
    terminology and operational
        definitions, 126–129
Mental Health Information Systems, 461
Mental Health Professional Shortage Areas
    (MHPSA), 82
Mental health system
  access
    children and young adults, 104
    delays in care, 105, 106
    negative pathways, 104, 105
    primary care, 100–103
    problem identification, 99
    voluntary and involuntary care, 105
  assessment of illness
    diagnostic clinical interview, 106–109
    family history, 107
    HPI, 107
    medical history, 107
    mental status exam, 107, 108
    past psychiatric history, 107
    social history, 107
  definition, 56–59
  diagnosis and case conceptualization,
      109, 110
  DSM and ICD, 69–73
  genetic programming, 69
  identification, 72, 74–76

impact of, 55
limitations, 69
mental health care cycle, 98
mental illness, 60–62
pathogenic approach, 57
psychopathology, 62, 63
    biological theories, 62, 64
    biopsychosocial model, 68
    psychological theories, 65–67
    social theory, 67–68
salutogenic approach, 57, 58
somatic health, 59, 60
treatment
    components, 110
    monitoring, 115–117
    neuromodulation and surgical
        interventions, 113, 115
    pharmacotherapy, 113, 114
    psychotherapy, 113, 114
    setting, 111, 112
    social interventions, 113, 114
Mental health treatment
    components, 110
    monitoring, 115
        PROs, 116
        side effect, 116, 117
    neuromodulation and surgical
        interventions, 113, 115
    pharmacotherapy, 113, 114
    psychotherapy, 113, 114
    setting, 111, 112
    social interventions, 113, 114
Mental health vs. medical conditions, 288–289
Mental health workforce disparity, 91–93
Mental illness, 60–62, 337
Mental status exam, 107, 108
Messenger RNA (mRNA), 272
Metabolomics
    data processing, 277
    examples in mental health, 278
    strengths and limitations, 277, 278
    study of metabolites, 276, 277
Metadata, 399
Metagenomic sequencing, 284
Microarray chip, 273
Microbiome
    data processing, 284
    examples in mental health, 284, 285
    gut-brain-axis, 284
    strengths and limitations, 284
MicroRNA (miRNA)
    data processing, 280
    examples in mental health, 281

function, 280
    network of interactions, 280
    strengths and limitations, 281
MicroRNA-sequencing (or miRNA-seq), 280
Minders, 487
Minimum clinical data set (MCDS), 156,
        175–177, 184
Minimum Information about a high-
        throughput nucleotide SEQuencing
        Experiment (MINSEQE), 164
Minimum Information for Biological and
        Biomedical Investigations (MIBBI
        Project), 171
Missingness, 413, 414
Mobile app-based programs, 462
Mobile health (mHealth) apps, 143
    passive data collection, 485
    technical issue or limitations, 484
    telepsychiatry and telemental health,
        485, 486
    virtual helpers and providers
        caregivers, 487
        minders, 487
        personhood and AI, 488
        prostheses and implants, 487
        providers, 488
Mobile health data, 379
Mobile medical devices, 460
Mood 24/7, 457
Moon-shot type initiatives, 12
Multi-omics analysis, 279
Multivariate filter methods, 246
Multi-word term identification, 327
Mutation, 270

N
N-acetylaspartate (NAA), 204
Naive Bayes model, 255
Named entity recognition (NER), 39, 319
National Advisory Mental Health Council
        (NAMHC) Workgroup, 491
National Alliance for Health Information
        Technology (NAHIT), 429
National Brain Tumor Society (NBTS), 288
National Council for Prescription Drug
        Programs (NCPDP), 429, 449
National Health and Nutrition Examination
        Survey (NHANES), 375
National Health Interview Survey (NHIS), 375
National Health Service (NHS), 417
National Institute of Mental Health
        (NIMH), 417

National Organization for Rare Disorders
        (NORD), 418
Natural language processing (NLP), 39, 40,
        143, 199
    applications in mental health
        CLPsych shared task, 342
        knowledge discovery, 342
        lexicons and ontology, 340–342
        mental health detection, 337
        symptom and severity
            extraction, 340
    challenges, 344, 345
    corpus generation
        annotation of medical records, 323
        collecting and annotating social media
            data, 324, 325
        collecting medical records, 322
        de-identification of medical records,
            322, 323
        EHRs, 325
        generating a corpus from social media
            data, 324
        novel data sources, 326
        privacy with social media data, 325
        publicly available medical record
            datasets, 324
        tasks, 321
        using medical records as corpus, 321
    data processing
        analyzing natural language data, 333
        classification pipeline, 326
        count-based features, 332
        deep learning systems, 335
        featurization, 329
        preprocessing, 327–329
        rule-based features, 332
        rule-based systems, 334
        sentence and document vectors, 331
        sentiment and psycholinguistic
            features, 332
        sociability features, 333
        supervised machine learning systems,
            334, 335
        temporal features, 333
        term vectors, 330, 331
        unsupervised machine learning,
            336, 337
    data representations, 320
    ethical considerations, 345, 346
    goals, 318
    in mental health practice, 343, 344
    tasks, 318, 319
    workflow, 318, 319

Natural language understanding (NLU), 39
Nature Scientific Data, 515
Negation detection, 329
Network analysis, 304–306
Neuroimaging
    ADC, 195, 196
    anatomic and physiologic data, 196, 197
    behavioral health
        ADNI, 208
        BIRN, 207
        clinical images, 201
        CRNC, 209
        HCP, 208
        ICNF, 209
        MRI, 202–204
        neurophysiology workflows,
            206, 207
        nuclear medicine imaging, 204, 205
        rapid progress, 200, 201
        SMART, 201
    challenges and opportunities, 210
    data and standards, 199, 200
    data processing, 283
    examples in mental health, 283
    folate exposure and age-associated
        thinning, 194
    folic acid exposure and schizophrenia
        outcomes, 193
    neuroprotective effects, 192, 193
    PNC cohort, 192, 193
    quantitative imaging metrics, 192
    radiology workflow, 197–199
    strengths and limitations, 283
Neuroinformatics, 133
Neuromodulation, 113, 115
Neuron, 173
Neuroscience information Framework
        (NIF), 405
Next-generation sequencing (NGS)
        technology, 269
NIH-funded biomedical and healthCAre
        Data Discovery Index
        Ecosystem (bioCADDIE)
        consortium, 515
Nomological network, 220
Non-coding regions, 279
Normalization, 329
Normalized data matrix format, 274
Normative atlases, 195
Nuclear magnetic resonance (NMR)
        spectroscopy, 277
Nucleotides, 269
Nurse practitioners, 85

O

Obamacare, 94
Observational health data science and
    informatics (OHDSI), 381
Observational Medical Outcomes Partnership
    (OMOP), 398
One-hot (binary) vectors, 330
Online support groups, 462
"Open science" paradigm, 400
Outpatient settings, 90, 91

P

Partial hospitalization programs
    (PHP), 90, 112
Pathway enrichment analysis, 286
Patient advocacy
    barriers, 490
    Icarus Project, 490
    role, 489
    self-advocacy, 490
Patient-Centered Clinical Research Network
    (PCORnet), 398
Patient health questionnaire (PHQ-9),
    375–376
Patient Reported Outcome measures
    (PROs), 116
Payment models
    privately-funded insurances, 93, 94
    publicly-funded insurances, 89, 94, 95
Performance to data (P2D)
    dissemination, 45
    evaluation models, 45, 46
    quantitative and qualitative
        methods, 46
Personal health records (PHRs)
    definition, 446
    drawbacks, 448
    types, 446, 447
Pharmacotherapy, 113, 114
PharmGKB, 403
Phenome-wide association study
    (PheWAS), 377
Philadelphia Neurodevelopmental Cohort
    (PNC), 192
Physician assistants (PAs), 85
PhysioNet project, 206
Picture Archiving and Communication
    Systems (PACS), 198
PopMedNet, 410
POS tagging, 328
Postings, 324
Post-transcriptional regulation events, 274

Practical, Robust Implementation and
    Sustainability Model (PRISM)
    model, 46
Precision medicine, 267
    concept of, 19
    definition, 19
    genetic and genomic biomarkers, 22
    vs. intuitive medicine, 22
    learning heath system, 24, 25
    personalized treatment, 22
    role of informatics, 23–24
Predictive models, 257, 258
Preferred Provider Organizations (PPOs), 94
Preprocessing
    dimensionality reduction, 245
    feature extraction methods, 247
    feature selection methods, 245–247
    range of activities, 244
Pre-trained word embeddings, 331
Primary care provider (PCP), 102, 103
Principal component analysis (PCA), 247
Private insurance, 93, 94
Protected Health Information (PHI), 493
Protein structure, 276
Proteomics, 266, 268, 275–277
    data processing, 275, 276
    examples in mental health, 276
    protein study, 275
    strengths and limitations, 276
Psychiatric diagnosis, 414
Psychiatric formulation, 109
Psychoanalytic model, 65
Psychobiotics, 284
Psycho-educational interventions, 344
Psychological data
    approaches, 225
    definition, 223–225
    history, 222
Psychological theories, 65
    cognitive model, 66, 67
    cognitive-behavioral model, 66
    humanistic/existential perspective, 66, 67
    learning/behavioral model, 65
    psychoanalytic model, 65
Psychomerics
    definition, 219
    factor analyses, 221
    instruments, 375
    latent trait, 219
    nomological network, 220, 221
    reliability, 219
    statistical packages, 221
    validity, 220

Psychopathology, 62, 63
  biological theories, 62, 64
  biopsychosocial model, 68
  psychological theories, 65
    cognitive-behavioral model, 66
    cognitive model, 65
    humanistic/existential
      perspective, 66, 67
    learning/behavioral model, 65
    psychoanalytic model, 65
  social theory, 67, 68
Psychotherapy, 113, 114
PsycINFO®, 183, 402
Public insurance, 89, 94, 95
Putative small molecules, 277

Q
Qualifacts, 437
Quantification algorithm, 274

R
Random forest classifiers, 335
Raw gene expression data, 274
Reads, 270
Receiver Operating Characteristic (ROC), 253
Recurrent neural networks (RNN), 335
Reference genome, 270, 274
Regional Health Information Organization
      (RHIO), 428
Regression models, 257
Reinforcement learning, 41, 257
Relation extraction or ontology
      construction, 319
Reliability, psychometrics, 219
Reproducibility crisis, 400
Research Domain Criteria (RDoC), 299–302,
      324, 492
Residential settings, 89
Response Evaluation Criteria in Solid Tumors
      (RECIST), 200
Retinal variables, 369
Reverse-phased protein microarrays
      (RPPA), 276
Ribonucleic acid (RNA), 272
RNA sequencing (RNA-seq), 272
Rule-based features, 332
RxNorm, 449

S
Sanger sequencing, 269
Scalable vector graphics (SVG), 384

Scientific visualization, 356
Segments, 282
  HL7 message, 179
Semantic interoperability, 41, 178
Semantic processing tasks, 327
Semantic standard, 163, 168
SemEval, 332
Semi-structured data, 37
Semi-supervised learning, 41, 251
Sentence and document vectors, 331
Sentiment and psycholinguistic features, 332
Sentiwordnet, 332
Sequence learning algorithms, 335
Sequencing machine, 270, 274
Serotonin transporter gene (SLC6A4), 279
SERPINA3 genes, 275
Service Guidance Package, 461
Services Substance Abuse and Mental Health
      Services Administration
      (SAMHSA), 495
Severe and persistent mental illness
      (SPMI), 76
Shared Health Research Information Network
      (SHRINE), 410
Side effect monitoring, 116, 117
Skeel's taxonomy of uncertainty, 385
Sloan-Schwartz Program, 514
Smartphone based assessment, 457
SNOMED CT, 341, 342
Sociability features, 333
Social data, 227, 228
Social determinants of health, 357
Social interventions, 113, 114
Social media, 144, 457, 458
Social theory, 67–68
Social workers, 86, 87
Software as a Medical Device (SaMD), 260
Software or systems development life cycle
      (SDLC), 43
Somatic health, 59, 60
Specialized Clinical Information Systems,
      460, 461
Split-half correlation analysis, 220
SpotFile, 384
Standard Nomenclature for Medicine—
      Clinical Terms (SNOMED CT),
      136, 184, 186
Standards
  concept and knowledge representation
    CDEs and MCDS, 175–177
    definition, 172
    information model, 174, 175
    LOINC, 176–177, 185, 186
    MEDLINE, 183

MeSH, 183
minimum clinical data sets, 183
ontology, 173, 174
PsycINFO®, 183
semiotic triangle, 172
SNOMED CT, 184, 186
terminologies, 164–166, 172, 173
content standard, 161, 163, 164
data and information, 157, 159
definition, 160, 161
interoperability standards, 177
C-CDA, 180, 181
FHIR, 181, 182
HL7 message, 179, 180
technical, and semantic, 177
MINSEQE, 164
precision mental healthcare, 156
reporting models, 259, 260
repositories, 170–172
semantic standard, 168, 169
syntax standard, 166, 167
Standards development organizations
(SDO), 41
State Innovation Models (SIM) initiative,
433, 434
Stemming, 327
Stress theory, 60
Structured Clinical Interview for DSM-5
(SCID-5), 226, 454
Structured data, 37
Structured Query Language (SQL), 38
Substance use disorder (SUD), 495, 496
Substance Use–Disorder Prevention that
Promotes Opioid Recovery and
Treatment (SUPPORT) for
Patients and Communities
Act, 434
Substitutable Medical Applications and
Reusable Technologies (SMART),
44, 201, 443
Subsumption, 173
Supervised learning
algorithms, 249
evaluation, 253–255
techniques, 40
Supervised machine learning systems,
334, 335
Support vector machines, 335
Symptom and severity extraction, 340
Syntactic interoperability, 41
Syntactic processing tasks, 320, 327–329
Syntax standard, 163, 165, 167
Systematized Nomenclature of Medicine
(SNOMED-CT), 408

Systems biology, 287
Systems Engineering Initiative for Patient
Safety (SEIPS), 44

T
Tableau, 384
Targeted metabolomics, 277
Task, User, Presentation, and Function
(TURF), 44
Technical interoperability, 177, 178
Telehealth services, 90, 91
Telemedicine, 459, 460
Telepsychiatry, 90, 91, 111
Temporal features, 333
Term-Frequency Inverse Document Frequency
(TF-IDF), 331
Test-retest reliability, 219
Text mining, 39, 40
Threads, 324
Topic modeling, 336
Training data set, 244
Training set, 334
Transcranial magnetic stimulation (TMS),
115, 460
Transcriptomics
data processing, 273, 274
DNA microarray technology, 273
examples in mental health, 275
process of transcription, 272
RNA study, 272, 273
strengths and limitations, 274
Translational bioinformatics, 266–268, 290
Translational science
definition, 11–13
limitations of, 12, 14
Translocator protein (TSPO), 205
Transparent Reporting of a
multivariable predictive
model for Individual
Prognosis Or Diagnosis
(TRIPOD), 259, 260
Trusted Exchange Framework, 496
2008 Mental Health Parity and Addiction
Equity Act, 94

U
UK BioBank data, 203
UK Biobank process, 404
Uncoordinated conceptual pluralism, 309
Unified Medical Language System
(UMLS), 341
Univariate filter methods, 246

University of California, San Francisco
        (USCF) Health, 435
Unstructured data, 37
Unstructured Information Management
        Architecture (UIMA), 327
Unsupervised learning, 336, 337
    algorithms, 250, 251
    evaluation, 255, 256
    techniques, 40, 41
Untargeted metabolomics, 277
Unusual thought content, 305
US Department of Health and Human Services
        (HHS), 493
U.S. National Institutes of Health BRAIN
        Initiative, 507
US National Library of Medicine (NLM), 402
User interface, 44

V
Vagal nerve stimulation (VNS), 115
Validation data set, 244
Validity, psychometrics, 220
Variant Call File (VCF) format, 271

visJS2jupyter tool, 384
Visual analytics, 358, 359
VisualDecisionLinc (VDL), 383
Visual Information Seeking Mantra, 362, 363
Visualization abstraction, 365
Visual mapping, 365

W
Waiver of consent, 397
Waterfall model, 43
Wearable devices, 456
Web based and mobile applications, 462, 463
WebGestalt, 405
Whole exome sequencing (WES), 269
Whole genome sequencing (WGS), 269
Within-person (intraindividual) mechanistic
        reasoning, 308, 309
Word embeddings, 330, 331
Word sense disambiguation (WSD), 329
word2vec, 330
Workforce disparity, 91–93
World Health Organization (WHO), 3
Wrapper methods, 247